SECOND EDITION

# CANCER
## AND THE SEARCH FOR
# SELECTIVE
# BIOCHEMICAL
# INHIBITORS

SECOND EDITION

# CANCER
## AND THE SEARCH FOR
# SELECTIVE
# BIOCHEMICAL
# INHIBITORS

### E. J. HOFFMAN

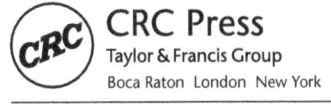

CRC Press
Taylor & Francis Group
Boca Raton  London  New York

CRC Press is an imprint of the
Taylor & Francis Group, an **informa** business

CRC Press
Taylor & Francis Group
6000 Broken Sound Parkway NW, Suite 300
Boca Raton, FL 33487-2742

First issued in paperback 2019

© 2007 by Taylor & Francis Group, LLC
CRC Press is an imprint of Taylor & Francis Group, an Informa business

No claim to original U.S. Government works

ISBN-13: 978-1-4200-4593-2 (hbk)
ISBN-13: 978-0-367-38893-5 (pbk)

### Library of Congress Cataloging-in-Publication Data

Hoffman, Edward J.
  Cancer and the search for selective biochemical inhibitors / Edward J. Hoffman.
-- 2nd ed.
     p. ; cm.
  Includes bibliographical references and index.
  ISBN-13: 978-1-4200-4593-2 (alk. paper)
  ISBN-10: 1-4200-4593-8 (alk. paper)
  1. Carcinogenesis. 2. Enzyme inhibitors--Therapeutic use. 3. Antineoplastic agents.
4. Materia medica, Vegetable. I. Title.
  [DNLM: 1. Neoplasms--drug therapy. 2. Antineoplastic Agents,
Phytogenic--therapeutic use. 3. Complementary Therapies. 4. Enzyme
Inhibitors--therapeutic use. QZ 267 H699c 2007]

  RC268.5.H63 2007
  616.99'4--dc22                                                    2006052548

**Visit the Taylor & Francis Web site at**
**http://www.taylorandfrancis.com**

**and the CRC Press Web site at**
**http://www.crcpress.com**

# Table of Contents

Preface ........................................................................................................ xi

**Chapter 1**  Crossroads ................................................................................ 1

Introduction ................................................................................................ 1
The Nutritional Brouhaha ........................................................................... 4
The Ponderables of Biochemistry ............................................................ 11
Troubles of Mind ...................................................................................... 17
What Seems to Work ................................................................................ 21
Scourges in the Making ........................................................................... 22
Remedies in Nature .................................................................................. 28
Poisons in Nature ..................................................................................... 33
From the Ordinary to the Bizarre ............................................................ 39
The Environment, Naturally and Not So Naturally ................................. 40
      Biomass ............................................................................................ 46
Where to Go from Here? ........................................................................... 46

**Chapter 2**  Cancer Origins and Characteristics ....................................... 59

Introduction .............................................................................................. 59
Cancer Formation and Oncogenes ........................................................... 62
Types of Cancers ...................................................................................... 63
Pleomorphism ........................................................................................... 65
Viral or Microbial Origins and Treatments ............................................. 67
Viruses and Lysogeny .............................................................................. 73
Viruses and Subviruses ............................................................................ 75
Antiviral Agents ....................................................................................... 77
Immune Reactions .................................................................................... 78
Vaccines .................................................................................................... 82

**Chapter 3**  Biochemical Insights ............................................................. 83

The Warburg Cancer Theory .................................................................... 84
Cell Metabolism ....................................................................................... 88
Enzyme-Catalyzed Metabolic Pathways ................................................. 92
      Glycolysis ......................................................................................... 95
      Production of Lactic Acid or Lactate ............................................... 97

Glutaminolysis ........................................................................................98
Tricarboxylic Acid Cycle......................................................................99
Overall Glycolytic Conversions ...................................................................100
Aerobic Glycolysis................................................................................101
Anaerobic Glycolysis............................................................................101
Cancer Cell Metabolism vs. Normal Cell Metabolism .....................................102
Selective Biochemical Inhibitors....................................................................104
Glycolysis Inhibitors.............................................................................104
Inhibitors of Lactic Acid or Lactate Formation from
Pyruvic Acid or Pyruvate........................................................105
An Update on Inhibitors for Cancer Cell Metabolism:
Glucose to Lactic Acid ............................................................106
Glutaminolysis Inhibitors....................................................................106
The Tricarboxylic Cycle and Respiration ........................................................107
Vitamins and Hormones as Inhibitors or Promoters .........................................109
Chemotherapy Drugs as Enzyme Inhibitors ...................................................118
More on Folic Acid ....................................................................................121
Enzyme Transformations.............................................................................123

**Chapter 4**   Starting at the Genetic Level ...........................................................125

DNA, RNA, and Protein Synthesis.................................................................125
The Functions of DNA ........................................................................126
The Functions of RNA.........................................................................127
The Ubiquitous Roles of Proteins .................................................................128
Genetics as Science ...................................................................................130
Digestive Processes....................................................................................134
Proteins.............................................................................................134
Carbohydrates.....................................................................................135
Fats .................................................................................................135
Proteases and Their Inhibitors......................................................................136
Protein Degradation Rates............................................................................138
The Influence of Antibiotics.........................................................................139
DNA Replication and Alteration ...................................................................143
DNA Repair ......................................................................................144
Carcinogens and the SOS Response.........................................................144
DNA Recombination............................................................................145
DNA Methylation................................................................................145
Chemoprevention ......................................................................................146
Commentary.............................................................................................148

**Chapter 5**   Enzymatic Biochemical Treatment Protocols...................................151

Enzymes..................................................................................................151
Enzyme Inhibitors.....................................................................................158
Enzyme Inhibition in Modern Medicine..........................................................159

Enzyme Inhibitors for Melanoma ......................................................... 164
Diet............................................................................................................. 164
Dietary Extremes ....................................................................................... 166
Iron in the Diet .......................................................................................... 168
Garlic and Allicin and Other Sulfur-Containing Compounds as
    Anticancer Agents ................................................................................ 172
Aberrations................................................................................................. 179
Immunity..................................................................................................... 180
Cancer Markers........................................................................................... 181
High-Tech vs. Low-Tech ........................................................................... 185
Footdragging on Using Enzyme Inhibitors............................................... 186

**Chapter 6** The Alternative Scene ........................................................ 189

An Introduction to Alternatives................................................................. 189
Some Alternatives, Information Sources, and Assessments ..................... 190
      Vitamin C ........................................................................................ 193
      Essiac Tea........................................................................................ 197
      Shark Cartilage................................................................................ 198
      Compound-X.................................................................................... 199
      Bloodroot......................................................................................... 200
      Condurango ..................................................................................... 201
      Cat's Claw ....................................................................................... 201
      Parasites.......................................................................................... 202
      Rabies ............................................................................................. 202
More About the Plant World ..................................................................... 204
Poisonous and Medicinal Plants................................................................ 213
Plants and Herbs as Agents Against Other Diseases ............................... 217
Selectivity .................................................................................................. 221
The Nitrogen Connection and Immunotherapy ........................................ 222
Alkaloids and Bioactivity.......................................................................... 227
Microorganisms and Immunity ................................................................. 228
In Short Summary ...................................................................................... 229

**Chapter 7** Surveying Anticancer Plant Substances............................. 233

Status of Plants Against Cancer ............................................................... 233
Laetrile Quandaries.................................................................................... 234
Plants of the American West and Southwest ............................................ 237
Chaparral..................................................................................................... 241
Other Plants and Herbs.............................................................................. 245
      South Africa .................................................................................... 246
      China ................................................................................................ 246
      Soviet Union ................................................................................... 248
      Mexico............................................................................................. 248
      Australia .......................................................................................... 249

Egypt and Israel ....................................................................................249
United States .........................................................................................250
Great Britain.........................................................................................255
Still Other Options......................................................................................267
Mystique Surrounding Cancer Cures ..........................................................275
Miscellaneous .............................................................................................276
Neo Tropica...........................................................................................276
Some Further Alternatives...........................................................................277
Successes vs. Failures...................................................................................278
Biological Response ....................................................................................279

**Chapter 8**   On Overcoming the Intractability of Cancer..................................283

Cell Resistance and Some Consequences .....................................................283
Alternative Treatment: The Status Quo.........................................................283
Controversies ..............................................................................................299
Heroic Efforts .............................................................................................304
More About Compound-X and the Like........................................................305
An Update on News and Views ...................................................................311
Cancer Directives........................................................................................316
The Continuing Legacy of Wayne Martin and Compatriots ..........................321
More of the Latest on Alternatives ..............................................................336
Magnesium..................................................................................................339
Peripherals..................................................................................................341
Subviral Agents: Prions ...............................................................................344
More on DNA..............................................................................................347
More on Diet ..............................................................................................349
The Navajo and Cancer ...............................................................................351

**Chapter 9**   Cancer Esoterica ....................................................................355

The Morphism of Cancer Cells.....................................................................355
Electromagnetic Phenomena and Cancer......................................................359
Some Inexplicables......................................................................................362
Metastasis, Resistance, and Aberrations ......................................................363
More on Immunity.......................................................................................368
Bioterrorism ...............................................................................................369
The Halogens and Cause and Cure...............................................................371
The Effect of Toxins in the Environment ......................................................373
More on Chemotherapy, Alkaloids, and Other Plant Biochemicals....................378
Recourses....................................................................................................380
Circling the Wagons ....................................................................................386
More on Genetic Modification or Engineering...............................................392
Vaccination and Cancer ...............................................................................395
Telomerase Inhibitors ..................................................................................399
Histone Diacetylase Inhibitors .....................................................................399

Markers for Monitoring Cancer Growth and Remission.........................................400
Moral and Ethical Quandaries.............................................................................400


**Chapter 10** The Inhibition of Cancerous Stem Cells.........................................403

The Subject of Stem Cells and Cancer................................................................403
Cancerous Stem Cells and Immunity..................................................................406
Inhibition of Cancerous Stem Cells....................................................................408
Tyrosine Kinase ...............................................................................................409
Plant Sources for Tyrosine Kinase Inhibitors .....................................................414


**Chapter 11** A Summing Up ..........................................................................417


**Bibliography** ................................................................................................425


**Index**...........................................................................................................449

# Preface

It goes almost without saying that one should view cancer personally and should anticipate its eventuality, whether in oneself, family members, or friends. The cancer victim, unfortunately, is too often a pawn in a vast money-making machine. The available information is conflicting, calling for discernment or "buyer beware caution" — with the poor and noninsured mostly forsaken. The seeking out of preferred modes of treatment reduces to an impasse between medical orthodoxy and alternative medicine. Inasmuch as medical orthodoxy is as close as one's family physician — and the success rates for conventional cancer treatments are too often dismal — the emphasis here will be otherwise: on alternative therapies.

We are therefore to a considerable degree also talking about manageable home therapies and keeping the costs down — way down — but at the same time these alternative anticancer therapies of choice are to be viable and, ultimately, death-defying, although, we can, of course, consider going to any of the numerous orthodox cancer clinics, which are of ever-increasing numbers, or to any of the few alternative cancer clinics available — if we are well endowed in the money department. One can even go outside the country, say, to alternative medical clinics in Mexico or Germany, etc. However, their charges are not "on the cheap," as is often the expectation.

A problem with alternative medicine is, of course, that it attracts much in the way of anecdote and hearsay; some people will claim almost anything. So what to believe? A resolution involves seeking the disclosure, in an understandable and unassailable fashion, of the underlying biochemical principles, whenever known, for alternative cancer therapies — a purpose of this exercise. Of particular concern are selectivity and the avoidance of conventional cell-toxic chemotherapy, with its adverse side effects, notably against the immune system — versus sometimes more vague and slower-acting alternative therapies.

Additionally, many or most of the alternative treatments may not work on a given patient, but trying to determine ahead of time the best route to pursue is like comparing political parties and campaigns, given the contentious standoff between medical orthodoxy and alternative medicine. One route to pursue is to try them all (or at least those few perceived as most promising), the everything-but-the-kitchen-sink approach as was advocated by the well-known physician Robert Atkins (now deceased). However, there is a matter of time and the potentially debilitating effects from treatment, whatever the treatment. The two go together, hence there is the need for a close and rapid monitoring system to see if the patient is responding in the right direction. Not only this, there is the need to counter any adverse side effects, like hyperallergenic anaphylactic shock. Enter, of course, the advisability or even necessity of working with a medical professional — and, needless to say, the more objective the professional, the better.

Causes and biochemical mechanisms for cancer formation are, to a degree, known — and to some extent can be avoided, environmentally and nutritionally, say, by the practices of what is called *chemoprevention*. However, when cancer does, in fact, strike, there is then the question of a preferred treatment or treatments — hopefully leading to immolation or at least to long-term remission. Surgical excision for solid tumors is at times successful, radiation less so, and conventional (cytotoxic, or cell-toxic) chemotherapy much less so, depending. So, if or when these orthodox therapies prove unsuccessful — which is too often the case — then what is to be the alternative? It is called *complementary and alternative medicine* (CAM) or by other names now, the latest perhaps being complementary, alternative, and integrative medicine (CAIM). The warfare then begins between medical orthodoxy, or establishment medicine, and the contrary. Never mind that in the case of cancer, especially, the choices are life-determining. And, obviously, anything that kills the patient will kill the cancer.

It is interesting to note that the central focus of study of conventional (cytotoxic) chemotherapy — indeed, all medicinal regimens — is the same as that of alternative and complementary medicine. The subject in both cases is, in general, that of biochemistry, or call it the "biochemical revolution." That is, both are ultimately concerned with cell metabolism and its various biochemical pathways and/or cycles for growth, maintenance, and modulation or immolation — which are embedded with, or controlled by, the proteinaceous biocatalysts called *enzymes*. In turn, the action of these enzymes — each specific to a particular biochemical reaction — is modulated or blocked (and rarely promoted) by a class of organic and inorganic substances broadly known as enzyme inhibitors.

In fact, much of modern medicine is based on enzyme inhibition, with the most famous instance being that of the antibiotics, which block one or another of the critical metabolic processes occurring in bacteria. Unfortunately, any given inhibitor is usually nonspecific to a particular enzyme, and may act against still other enzymes — even in the case of antibiotics, some of which become toxic to humans (although acting against cancer). This nonselectivity is the source of side effects, which may be either adverse or adverse in the extreme. (At the extreme end are poisons, being enzyme inhibitors that can, notably, shut down respiration and/or produce cardiac arrest.) So it is with conventional chemotherapy, where the side effects can be debilitating, sometimes even more so than the consequences of the cancer itself.

A key, therefore, is to find enzyme inhibitors that will selectively shut down cancer cell metabolism or growth without too adversely affecting normal cells. A notable example is that of antibiotics, previously mentioned, which will destroy bacterial (prokaryotic) cells in one way or another, but mostly do not affect human or mammalian (eukaryotic) cells. (There are exceptions, of course, for some antibiotics — including those acting as anticancer agents — are overtly toxic to humans.) This brings up the possibility that a large number of natural substances — as distinguished from synthetic substances — can act as readily available anticancer agents. Moreover, some are nontoxic, notably those used as foodstuffs. This distinction, between the synthetic and the natural, largely separates medical orthodoxy —

and the drug or pharmaceutical industry — from alternative (and folkloric) medicine. (And becomes an economic and political standoff, maybe more so than a scientific one.)

Nevertheless, although there are presumably many natural substances or extracts that can be — and have been — declared anticancer, there is the matter of effectiveness, which brings us to methods of administration, dosage levels, and frequency. Moreover, many of the anticancer substances can be toxic and extremely so, there sometimes being a fine line between life and death (as in the well-known case of digitalis for heart disease). This, in turn, may call for a close monitoring of vital signs by a medical professional, and the modification or abandonment of the treatment. (Hence, the oft-used caveat that the dosage *is* the poison.) Beyond this, the various means for assaying effectiveness — test-tube or *in vitro*, animal or *in vivo*, and human or clinical — do not necessarily give the same results. What works in one sort of test does not necessarily work in another or others. There is also the problem of biochemical individuality among humans. Moreover, there is a tendency for cancer cells to develop a resistance, say, to chemotherapeutic treatment, whereby the cells utilize other metabolic pathways.

An overriding complication is emerging, namely that of cancerous stem cells — stem cells being those that keep on proliferating no matter what. This aspect is explored in Chapter 10. A distinction can be made between "normal" cancer cells and a relatively few but significant super-active cancerous stem cells. Thus, the "normal" cancerous cells can be killed off by a standard treatment or therapy, whereas the initially few cancerous stem cells are immune to treatment and remain free to proliferate and spread or metastasize — and do so. (An analogy can be made to bacteria, where part of a bacterial population may develop a resistance to an antibiotic or may be inherently resistant. The usual course of treatment with an antibiotic is simply to overwhelm the bacterial population by the treatment or else to utilize a different — and stronger — antibiotic.) However, at the least, there seems to be a particular enzyme (or enzymes), or growth factor, that favors cancerous stem cell metabolism and proliferation, and the search is on to determine or develop inhibitors for this particular enzyme or growth factor. The problem may be that these countering substances — natural or synthetic — may also inhibit other, absolutely vital stem cell proliferations, such those generating new blood cells within the bone marrow. Thus, these further developments must walk a fine line.

Lastly, the ultimate word is always that of clinical successes, and for this reason it is advocated that a network of cancer clinical research centers (CCRCs) be instituted — or the equivalent — to serve initially as a court of last resort for advanced or terminal cancer cases, and later on for any case. These would be primarily staffed by M.D.s and D.O.s, and backed by a system of supportive pharmacologists, biochemists, botanists and ethnobotanists, biologists and zoologists, plus assorted naturopaths and the like — even if considered unconventional, but which are possibly a vital link in the therapeutic chain.

So ... instead of heading for the hospital emergency room, where the indigent are likely to be refused entrance, anyway, an advanced or terminal cancer patient could be taken to the nearest local CCRC. There, the patient would be treated (researched) using one or another, or several, alternative therapies, under the auspices of eminently qualified and objective M.D.s and/or D.O.s. This would circumvent the more usual scenario: an advanced cancer patient eventually goes to a non-M.D. or non-D.O., or whomever and whatever, as a "last resort" and "ray of hope," after medical orthodoxy has given up. In turn, if and when the patient dies, the non-M.D. or non-D.O., say, will reap the whirlwind from medical orthodoxy and the media, although never a word would be said if the patient had died under, or immediately after, orthodox treatment and care.

In the meantime, the choices are few. Either go with conventional medicine — surgery, radiation, or chemotherapy — or engage in alternatives, now more commonly called complementary and alternative medicine, or CAM. Here, as well, there are dilemmas: who are we to believe? Whereas chemo is most successful against blood-related cancers, such as leukemia, the prognosis is not at all clear with solid tumors or cancers, which are different. And the myriad anticancer substances — both natural and synthetic — do not necessarily translate into cures. Nevertheless, in some instances a positive track record exists. Consider, for example, the following: Massive dosages of vitamin C, preferably intravenous, as they are administered at the Riordan Clinic in Wichita (Center for the Improvement of Human Functioning International, 3100 North Hillside Avenue, Wichita KS 67219 [316-682-3100]) or by A. Hoffer, M.D., Ph.D., in Vancouver BC (2717 Quadra Street, Suite 3, Victoria BC Canada V8T 4E5 [250-386-8755]). There is also the antineoplaston therapy of Stanislaw Burzynski, M.D. (Burzynski Clinic, 9432 Old Katy Road, Suite 200, Houston TX 77055 [713-335-5697]), or Julian Whitaker, M.D., (4321 Birch St., Suite 100, Newport Beach CA 92660 [714- 851-1550]), and Coley's Toxins (Cancer Research Institute, 681 Fifth Avenue, New York 10022 [212-688-7515]). For the patient without the financial means, vitamin C may be the route of choice. Nevertheless, the intent herein is to pursue an array of possibilities.

It will be noted time and again that there is a difference between the metabolism of cancer cells and normal cells, and the determination of selective and nontoxic enzyme inhibitors for cancer cell metabolic pathways may provide the elusive "magic bullet." Lastly, it can be said that the exciting developments about selectively inhibiting or blocking cancerous stem cells, as described above, give an extra hope to cancer victims.

# 1 Crossroads

## INTRODUCTION

What should a person who has just been told that he or she has cancer do? This chapter has been written so that the patient does not have to start at ground zero, hunting for information and sources.

In fact, the time for a person to start reading up about cancer treatments and alternatives, specialized sources for help, and open-minded doctors is now, today, preferably before the disease strikes. It takes some sifting to settle on a strategy for dealing with cancer. The following pages are intended to provide this information in a compact, readily available fashion.

Of first importance are cures and causes. There is a notion that nothing is perfect; only, some cancer treatments are less perfect than others, and conventional treatments may be the least perfect of all. It is time, therefore, to consider alternative medicine, sometimes called *complementary medicine*, or *holistic medicine*, or *preventive medicine*.

(If time is of the essence, the concerned reader may wish to skip directly to the last chapter, Chapter 11, and at the same time consider that there is a dark side to conventional treatments. For biochemical insights of a more technical nature, Chapter 3 is more specific.)

The causes of cancer are inextricably linked with cures or containment; the one goes hand in hand with the other, from the claims for alternative remedies such as laetrile to the "refutations" of medical orthodoxy. As for the well-publicized laetrile controversy, it has been commented that if laetrile or some other alternative therapy, for instance, should indeed prove a deterrent or cure for cancer, the whole structure of the medical establishment would come tumbling down. This may be an overstatement, but cancer mythology and facts have been previously explored, for example, in *The Cancer Blackout*, by Nat Morris. Continuing our examination of some of the extant literature, there is a book called *The Politics of Cancer*, by S. S. Epstein and another by Robert N. Proctor titled *Cancer Wars: How Politics Shapes What We Know and Don't Know About Cancer.* Proctor, who teaches the history of science at Pennsylvania State University, takes on the political establishment more so than the scientific one, with television programs and documentaries sometimes coming under attack. Among other things, the efforts of medical research are challenged. In the introduction to Proctor's book, not only is the conclusion reached that the war against cancer is being lost, but also that the cancer research establishment itself is suspect (Proctor, 1994, pp. 4, 14, 15). The title of Proctor's first chapter is "A Disease of Civilization?" which provides grist for further speculation. A book by an academic press is James T. Patterson's history, *The Dread Disease: Cancer and American Culture*, which among other things traced the American Cancer Society (ACS) from its origins as the American Society for the Control of Cancer (ASCC).

There are a number of other books about the machinations that have been going on in the name of "cancer therapy correctness." Thus, Robert G. Houston has written *Repression and Reform in the Evaluation of Alternative Cancer Therapies*. John Heinerman leads off with a dynamic first chapter titled "Medical Science — A House Divided Against Itself" in his book on *The Treatment of Cancer with Herbs*, introduced by Robert Mendelsohn, M.D. Dr. Mendelsohn is the controversial but respected physician-author whose pyrotechnics light up *Confessions of a Medical Heretic* and other books, and some of his more pungent comments are highlighted by Heinerman.

Also, there is another book by Ralph W. Moss, first titled *The Cancer Syndrome* and published in a revised edition as *The Cancer Industry: Unraveling the Politics*. It is almost too infuriating to read, and once again illustrates the old French saying that the more things change, the more they stay the same. Moss, formerly with the Memorial Sloan-Kettering Cancer Center, sees the state of affairs not as a conspiracy but as the end result of the human failings of an all-powerful "cancer establishment," paralyzed by internal politics and egos. Cures outside the hallowed mainstream are not considered, and more unorthodox remedies such as vitamin C and even laetrile are not pursued, presumably because they are not patentable. Richard Walters, in the initial and concluding chapters of his book *Options: The Alternative Cancer Therapy Book*, is particularly damning about the orthodox cancer treatment establishment. He says that several fund-raising cancer agencies would be put out of business if cures were found.

A later book by Moss, *Questioning Chemotherapy*, takes a hard look at chemotherapy and its success rates, and lists the major chemotherapy drugs, their properties, and side effects. Largely ineffective against most cancers, the only surefire successes seem to be with blood-related cancers. In addition to a newsletter now called *The Moss Reports*, Moss is also involved in producing other publications (as per his phone number, 1-800-937-WELL). The lack of effectiveness of chemotherapy has been noted by others, for instance, by Georgia oncologist Guy Faguet, M.D., in *The War on Cancer: An Anatomy of Failure, A Blueprint for the Future*, published in 2005. A review is furnished by Ralph Moss in the August/September 2006 issue of the *Townsend Letter for Doctors & Patients*. Faguet's book has been endorsed by John Bailer III, M.D., and former editor of the *Journal of the National Cancer Institute*, and by Gerald E. Marti, M.D., Ph.D., who is Chief, Flow and Image Cytometry Section, Laboratory of Stem Biology, National Institutes of Health. Faguet speaks out against cytotoxic, or cell-toxic, chemotherapy and instead favors gene therapy, which requires much more research.

Ralph Moss has also written *Free Radical: Albert Szent-Györgyi and the Battle over Vitamin C*. Although Szent-Györgyi was awarded a Nobel Prize in 1937 for the discovery of vitamin C, there was considerable controversy at the time about who had discovered what. In Moss's biography of Szent-Györgyi, there is very little about cancer, and nothing about vitamin C and cancer although Szent-Györgyi claimed that he had a cure for cancer. Linus Pauling's notable work about vitamin C and cancer came along later. Along these lines, there is a substance called *Avemar* that is derived from fermented wheat germ, traceable back to Szent-Györgyi, as presented in an article by Dan Kenner in the August/September 2006 *Townsend*

*Letter for Doctors & Patients*. The theory is that there are two chemicals called *quinones* occurring in wheat germ that are liberated by the action of the yeast enzyme glucosidase and which chaperone cellular metabolism, thereby countering the hyper-metabolism of cancer cells, in the process serving as anticancer agents or at least modulating the adverse side effects of chemotherapy.

Also bridging the gap between the alternatives and the conventional is Michael Lerner's *Choices in Cancer Therapy: A Complete Guide to Conventional and Alternative Cancer Treatments, Including Nutrition — Mind-Body — Newest Drugs — Surgery — and Much More*. Lerner has also written another titled *Choices in Healing: Integrating the Best of Conventional and Complementary Approaches to Cancer*. Lerner confesses at the outset that though he has gathered much information in the 10 years or so spent on the project, he is not in a position to make specific recommendations for cancer therapy.

For the record, conventional treatments are described for the layman in *Choices* by Marion Morra and Eve Potts, into its third edition. A more technical exposition of conventional treatments is found in the massive *Cancer: Principles and Practice of Oncology*, edited by M.D.s Vincent T. DeVita, Samuel Hellman, and Steven A. Rosenberg, with 157 contributors.

More perspectives about the present state of affairs are found in the preliminaries of James H. Johnson's *How To Buy Almost Any Drug Legally Without a Prescription*. As a result of the thalidomide tragedies, the Food and Drug Administration (FDA) became supercautious about testing, recognizing that some drugs may have unsuspected long-term consequences. Unfortunately, the knife cuts both ways, and there is no doubt that many safe drugs have been needlessly excluded. An out has been provided, however, by permitting drugs to be purchased from foreign or overseas sources. This relaxation in policy was brought about by pressure from AIDS victims. In effect, the burden of proof is placed upon the patient. It is *caveat emptor*, or let the buyer beware.

Others continue to warm to the subject in a growing array of books and articles, with the Internet furnishing still more information. Along the way, there was *Death by Injection: The Story of the Medical Conspiracy Against America* by Clarence Eustace Mullins, considered sort of an "underground" exposé, not to mention Robert S. Mendelsohn's controversial *Confessions of a Medical Heretic*. There is also Paul Starr's Pulitzer-winning *Social Transformation of American Medicine*, published in 1982.

A Canadian physician, Dr. Guylaine Lanctôt, wrote an exposé titled *The Medical Mafia: How to Get Out of it Alive and Take Back Our Health & Wealth* about the medical situation in both Canada and the United States and has been harassed for his pains. Like Clarence E. Mullins, Robert S. Mendelsohn, and some others, she is skeptical about the widespread use of vaccinations. Earlier, in England, Donald Gould contributed a book with the similar title, *The Medical Mafia: How Doctors Serve and Fail Their Customers*. There seems to be enough dissent to go around, and more remains to be said about this resistance to medical orthodoxy.

Even milk has come under fire, with the assertion that the dairy industry has spent billions to influence the FDA and Congress, as well as the medical and scientific establishments (and price supports have become a fact of life). The exposé is Robert Cohen's *Milk: The Deadly Poison*, which emphasizes the contaminants that appear in milk: human-engineered growth hormones and pesticides, microorganisms such as those that cause bovine leukemia and bovine tuberculosis (not to mention the routine overuse of antibiotics, passed on to milk as well as meat products). The powerful growth hormone IGF-1 has in fact been implicated in the growth and proliferation of human cancer.

For more purely technical considerations about cancer and alternative therapies, there is John Boik's *Cancer and Natural Medicine: A Textbook of Basic Science and Clinical Research*, first published in 1995. With some 1200 or so references cited, it is a comprehensive and informative examination of the factors involved. This book takes up the initiation and growth of cancer cells, the processes of angiogenesis or vascularization by which a blood vessel network is formed in solid tumors, invasion and metastasis, and the effects of other factors, including the immune system. Beyond this, using conventional treatments as the baseline, Boik goes on to discuss Chinese therapies, the use of botanical agents, the effects of dietary macronutrients and micronutrients, the efficacy of still other agents, natural or synthetic, physical methods and psychological factors, and concludes with a discussion of research under way. The appendices list various substances noted to have antitumor or anticancer effects, provides an overview of many of the more common cancers, along with vital statistics, and furnishes other information of potential interest.

None of these references zero in on cures as such, but rather focus on treatments.

Lastly, for a couple of readable semitechnical accounts about cancer, both listed in the References, consider the following: Francis X. Hasselberger's *Uses of Enzymes and Immobilized Enzymes* (1978), and Matthew Suffness and John Pezzuto's chapter titled "Assays Related to Cancer Drug Discovery," in Vol. 6 of *Methods in Plant Biochemistry* (1991). Even if somewhat dated, much of the information nevertheless remains relevant.

## THE NUTRITIONAL BROUHAHA

The medical establishment has mostly gone out on a limb to the effect that supplemental nutritional factors play no significant role in our ills, for example, vitamins, minerals, and herbs (and such therapies as laetrile, etc.), as cures, remedies, or preventions. On the whole, osteopathic medicine — and, we may add, chiropractic — appears more receptive to the role of nutrition than does its M.D. counterpart.

Fortunately for all of us there are, and have been, some distinguished mavericks, both in and at the periphery of the medical profession, who have grabbed the initiative in nutritional medicine. Their findings have appeared, for instance, in the nutritional health magazine *Prevention* (founded by J. I. Rodale) and in other conventional and unconventional publications.

Nutritionist Adelle Davis was perhaps the progenitor, with her well-known series of books. (Her influence continues by virtue of The Adelle Davis Foundation, 116 Middle Road, Suite K, Montecito, CA 93108, 805-969-9076.) Among many other things, Adelle Davis was a strong proponent of including brewers' yeast or nutritional yeast in the diet. (Anecdotal evidence suggests that it will smooth out the heartbeat and a person's disposition as well. It also helps to keep off ticks, from both humans and dogs, and maybe keeps mosquitoes at bay. Another of Adelle Davis's therapies, unexpectedly, is common table salt against glaucoma.)

The ubiquitous Dr. Atkins and his organization came out swinging on the side of nutrition, with books, a newsletter, a line of supplements, and the Atkins Diet. Pediatrician Dr. Lendon Smith is another who promotes the nutritional approach in his books. Dr. Jonathan Wright has served the cause well through the years. Dr. Andrew Weil is a comparative newcomer. So is Dr. Julian Whitaker, a former associate of the famous chemist Linus Pauling. There is also Dr. Abram Hoffer, also a former associate of Linus Pauling. Both Dr. Whitaker and the Linus Pauling Institute have utilized the newsletter approach to disseminate information. The foregoing doctors are all M.D.s, sometimes with a Ph.D. attached, and are a part of a welcome and overdue trend within the medical profession. Some of the more prestigious medical schools now even offer courses in nutrition, reportedly, as many as half of them.

(An announcement by Elaine Zablocki in the January 2005 issue of the *Townsend Letter for Doctors & Patients* indicates that the University of Minnesota now offers holistic complementary and alternative medicine (CAM) education. Cited is Mary Jo Kreitzer, Ph.D., RN, who is an associate professor of nursing, and director of Nursing Practice and Research at the University of Minnesota Hospital and Clinic. Professor Kreitzer notes that the nursing profession has been oriented holistically from the very beginning. "It was Florence Nightingale, the founder of modern nursing, who wrote that the role of the nurse was to help patients attain the best possible condition so that Nature could act and self-healing could occur." It is added that Professor Kreitzer is the principal investigator for a $1.6 million National Center for Complementary and Alternative Medicine (NCCAM) curriculum grant and a $2.1 million clinical study funded by the National Institute for Nursing Research to assess "mindfulness mediation" for solid organ transplant victims.

There is the heritage of Linus Pauling, twice winner of the Nobel Prize, who faced off the opposition with his orthomolecular approach to the body's dysfunctions. In particular, he has long been known for his advocacy of megadoses of vitamin C. Then there are the two Drs. Shute, of Canada, who pioneered the intake of vitamin E for the heart, a regimen that is finally coming into vogue.

The subject is merging, along with the art of healing and conventional medical practice, into what is called *holistic* and sometimes *wholistic* medicine or maybe *Gestalt* medicine. (Holism: the whole is more than the mere sum of its parts; also called *synergism*. *Gestalt*: indicating that physical, psychological, and biological phenomena integrate, therefore, it is another applicable word.) Hans Holzer wrote a book titled *Beyond Medicine* about the evidence for unorthodox and psychic healing. The findings can be investigated anew.

In his bouts with illness, Norman Cousins, former publisher of the *Saturday Review* and author of *Anatomy of an Illness*, discovered that "happy people are healthy people," a finding endorsed by J. I. Rodale and others in *Prevention* magazine. (Cousins' successful battle against an incurable illness was supplemented with megadosages of vitamin C. He also mentioned a father who bootlegged vitamin-C-laden ice cream into the hospital for his seriously ill young daughter, who responded by getting well, much to the physicians' consternation.) An update has been provided from time to time, for example, in the September 1990 issue of the *Saturday Evening Post*.

A physician and surgeon, Bernie Siegel, has written *Love, Medicine and Miracles*, which further documents the powers of self-healing. In *Learned Optimism*, psychologist Martin Seligman compares the health of optimists vs. pessimists, with the former group emerging a clear winner. Not to mention Proverbs 17:22: "A merry heart doeth good like a medicine, but a broken spirit drieth the bones." "Humor rooms" are being placed in hospitals, which show old movies and videotapes and play recordings of the great comedians and comics of past times. There is the emerging field of gelotology, the science of laughter.

Another physician of consequence is Patch Adams, M.D., about whom a movie, *Patch Adams*, was made. His mission is carried out via the *Gesundheit!* Institute, dedicated to revolutionizing health care delivery by replacing greed and competition with generosity, compassion, etc. The particular Web site is www.patchadams.org/home.htm, although there are multiple listings of information on the Internet. The accompanying hospital project, ongoing, is located in Pocahontas County, West Virginia, but with an international impact.

We have, along the way, learned the importance of child–parent bonding, especially, maternal bonding, simple friendship or fellowship, and also the companionship of pets. Omar Khayyam ventured that each day spent fishing adds another day to one's life.

We learn that there is no such thing as completely objective testing. Everything sooner or later, in one way or another, becomes biased. The polygraph (lie detector), which scientifically monitors our nervous impulses, is found to be unreliable. It turns out there is also no such thing as a 100% placebo, although there is a placebo effect, which causes apparently neutral agents or methods to have a biased or beneficial effect, whether sugar pills or merely the fact of being tested (e.g., as observed in biorhythm studies). There is also talk of iatrogenic maladies or symptoms that are inadvertently introduced by the physician or researcher. (Hence the need for "double-blind" studies, in which the subject or patient does not know how he or she is being tested or what he or she is taking, and the doctor or researcher (the "tester") does not know what is being used, or maybe even does not know what the test is about.) Catchall descriptors, such as psychosomatic, and the power of suggestion have long been used to explain the unexplainable. But even if unexplainable, what difference does it make as long as it works? The subject is summarized, with examples, in *Your Emotions and Your Health* by Emrika Padrus and the editors of *Prevention*.

To mention more about the unexplainable, on or about February 22, 1993, on PBS, Bill Moyers reported on the mind–body connection in medicine. The two hour program was titled "The Mystery of Chi/The Mind–Body Connection," and was a segment of the PBS-series *Healing and the Mind*. (Additionally, the series has been made into a book by Bill Moyers, also titled *Healing and the Mind*.) A considerable portion of the program dealt with mysterious or unexplainable medical practices employed in China. Among them is the phenomenon called *Chi*, whereby a person may influence his own self or others, sometimes by the mere manipulation of the hands above the patient, in some respects similar to the laying on of hands. Healing may occur or the external forces may even be counteracted, the force working against itself. The traditional modes or models used for explanation in the West and the mechanistic interpretations based on cause and effect do not suffice in the mystical East.

This calls to mind the work of Dr. William H. Philpott, coauthor of *Brain Allergies: The Psychonutrient Connection*, who more recently coauthored *Biomagnetic Handbook: A Guide to Medical Magnetics, the Energy Medicine of Tomorrow*. There is, after all, something to magnetic fields and their effect on the body, or, in other words, to "auras," natural or induced. The inference is to extrapolate to such phenomena as hands-on or hands-off healing, maybe to water witching, and the ability of some persons to stop a clock or watch, etc.

Among other things, a disproportionate number of Chinese inexplicably live to a ripe old age, as do others in different cultures. This brings to mind Deepak Chopra's *Ageless Body, Timeless Mind*, published in 1993, which hit the best-seller lists.

Yet another report about unconventional medicine was CBS's *48 Hours*, aired on July 7, 1993. From October 26 to 28, 1993, WTBS-Atlanta contributed a program "The Art of Healing: Remarkable Stories of How We Heal Ourselves." The subject can be expected to be of ever-increasing interest, in spite of the resistance of the FDA to the use of vitamins, unorthodox medicine, and all that this implies, though the passage of the Dietary Health and Education Act in 1994 serves to counter much of this resistance.

An article in the *American Spectator*, January 1995, had considerably more to say about the FDA and its then commissioner, David Kessler. Written by James Bovard and titled "Double-Crossing to Safety," the reign of Kessler was characterized in the heading for the article in terms of a "hunger for regulations and addiction to power," which was just a warm-up. Bovard also mentioned that the wording in the Dietary and Health Education Act is so vague that it may actually give the FDA more power than it already has. The foregoing is only a part of what Bovard takes on in his book *Lost Rights: The Destruction of American Liberty*, published in 1994. Nor does Herbert Burkholz have too many good things to say in *The FDA Follies: An Alarming Look at Our Food and Drug Administration*.

A recurring critic of the FDA is William Faloon of the journal *Life Extension*; for example, he takes the FDA to task in the May 2004 issue for approving deadly drugs while delaying life-saving therapies. There have been several legal judgments made against the FDA, for example, as initiated by Durk Pearson and Sandy Shaw, authors of a prominent book also called *Life Extension* (most of which, interestingly, the FDA ignores.)

Even weather gets into the act. We are once again becoming more conscious of the mood swings that accompany changes in the barometric pressure, in terms of the elements, the emerging wind, rain, and snow. And there is the effect of the seasons, of warmth and cold, of sunlight and cloud, of daylight and darkness, and of moonlight and shadow, the life rhythms of the ancients.

There are such imponderables as why, during wartime, does the general level of health go up? (And why are more boy babies born?) A partial explanation for this in World War I is the use of unbleached flour, as the chlorine gas ordinarily used for bleach was utilized for the war effort. For World War II, perhaps it was "Lucky Strike green goes to war!" (That is, the green chemical compounds —

chromium oxide? — used to color the cigarette packs were needed in the war effort.) Or maybe not. Anyway, the Lucky Strike packs thenceforth stayed white.

Concerns with food additives have surfaced; the preservatives and flavor enhancers such as nitrites and nitrates, sulfites and sulfates, sodium benzoate, monosodium glutamate (MSG), etc., not to mention the synthetic dyes and flavorings. A compilation sometimes includes headache-producing or indigestion-inducing substances, with occasionally worse side effects that are of questionable benefit. (See for instance the January/February 1990 issue of the *Saturday Evening Post.* Also see George Schwartz's book about the effects of MSG, variously disguised as hydrolyzed protein and, presumably, calcium or sodium caseinate. Interestingly, MSG promotes the sense of taste rather than acting upon the food itself; similar to the room deodorizers that numb the sense of smell instead of removing the odor.) To read the list of ingredients on the label is, too often, enough to scare a party back to the drawing board. One wonders what possible purpose there could be for this seemingly senseless and random array of additives? Surely profit is a limp excuse, as more healthful foods are now a selling point.

In addition to additives, there are toxic substances that occur naturally and also during food processing or cooking. An example is the chemical acrylamide that is formed during the heating process for both French fries and potato chips. At higher temperatures, the naturally occurring amino acid asparagine reacts with the sugars and starches present to form acrylamide, which is thought to be a carcinogen. The State of California, for instance, is presumably taking steps to require warning labeling of fries and chips.

On occasion, the inference has been made that Alzheimer's disease, associated with advancing age, may be correlated with the presence of aluminum or its compounds in the body. (Or may not be, but prudence is said to be the soul of discretion .... For a more general treatment of the subject, there is, for instance, *Aluminum and Health: A Critical Review*, edited by Hillel J. Gitelman and published in 1989.) If this connection is indeed so, the American diet has some unpublicized opportunities for further modification. The aluminum compounds are a constituent of ordinary table salt (to make it pour more freely), of most baking powders, and of pickles (as alum), to name a few. (Unadulterated sea salt, with its trace elements, seems a better bet for the salt shaker. There is also a trend to use salt substitutes, including potassium chloride, instead of the ubiquitous sodium chloride, or common salt.)

The mania for food is another of the ponderables, somehow related to the drive for power, money, wealth, and success. Apparently, food addiction is one of the primary social satisfactions. In this country, it outstripped the needs of hunger, save for the underprivileged, by definition, long ago. The desire to pig up and pork out otherwise defies explanation. At the gatherings of the well fed, for instance, already bulging at the seams but still ritualistically stuffing it down amid the conversation, all are evidently fulfilling some sort of social need and filling in some sort of blank space in their lives, though there may be very little space to fill. Perhaps we are then speaking of an addiction, specifically a food addiction, or call it an eating disorder or a conditioned reflex (from our primitive ancestors, who gorged when the going was good, and the rest of the time did without). The result, whatever, is "weight."

(We seem to have outlived the desire and need for such backups as "steatopygia," which means the deposition of body fat in the buttocks.)

Obesity, or excess body weight, is therefore a subject of intense fascination. Whereas in earlier times a degree of avoirdupois was necessary for survival and was held in esteem, the opposite view is in vogue now, and we eternally try to shed the pounds. Sugar and fat are seen as the culprits.

Refined sugar, or sucrose, is viewed by some as addictive since its discontinuation produces withdrawal symptoms. In physical appearance, refined sugar looks like heroin, which has caused some talk. Otherwise, the descriptor "empty calories" is employed, apropos of a lack of nutritional value. For reasons not publicized, sugar seems to be part of most cookbook recipes, and it is a surefire way to ruin good cornbread.

William Dufty, in *Sugar Blues*, has dissected the subject exhaustively. Sugar is viewed as more of a "substance" than a food. Dufty also traces the role of sugar and the sugarcane industry in promoting slavery in the New World, with the encouragement of the Old world and its new-found craving for sugar. The African slave trade provided the workers for the sugarcane plantations, and the British and the Americans provided the ships for transport. Sugar has proved diabolical in unsuspected ways, from the very start. Cotton and American slavery came along later.

All of us favor sugar substitutes, now mostly in the form of the chemical aspartame, marketed under the trademarks NutraSweet® and Equal®. But this substitute has come under fire as having some adverse side effects. It is a chemical that in one way or another involves other chemical forms variously as reactants, in chemical bondings, or as decomposition products, notably phenylalanine and methanol, both regarded with suspicion for toxicity, especially the latter. Methanol, commonly referred to as methyl alcohol or wood alcohol, has long been known for its poisonous properties. Methanol has, at the same time, numerous industrial uses, including that of motor fuel. By comparison, ethanol (drinking alcohol or ethyl alcohol or grain alcohol) is reputed to be even more toxic than methanol, ounce for ounce absorbed. Fortunately, ethanol is absorbed into the bloodstream relatively slowly. (Whereas phenylalanine is a protein or amino acid, concentrated proteins are being reconsidered after the trouble with tryptophan.) As the temperature rises, thermal decomposition proceeds; hence the reason for not using aspartame in cooking. Similar effects that might occur in a person's stomach is further food for thought. A book by H. J. Roberts explores the subject and a citizens' network was founded, the Aspartame Safety Network, P.O. Box 780634, Dallas TX 75378. Still another book is *Bittersweet Aspartame, a Diet Delusion* by Barbara A. Mullarkey. The Christian Broadcasting Network, or CBN, once kept viewers up to date on its program, the *700 Club*.

Speculations are that there might still be a natural or synthetic sweetener awaiting discovery. Thus, the famous South American explorer Colonel P. H. Fawcett, in traversing the Brazil–Paraguay border, noted a small plant known locally as *Caahe-eh*, whose leaves were several times sweeter than ordinary sugar. (Could this be the South American herb now called *Stevia*, which is said to be 30 times sweeter than sugar?) Another, called *Ibira-gjukych*, had leaves with a salty taste. Common salt, or sodium chloride, is generally overconsumed, the idea being that maybe we need less sodium and more potassium in our diet, that is, a little more balance.

A recent article about Colonel Fawcett and his explorations, by David Grann, appears in the September 19, 2005, issue of the *New Yorker*. Grann retraced Fawcett's steps after his disappearance back in 1925. Fawcett was looking for a lost civilization in the headwaters of the Xingu River, a south/southwestern tributary of the Amazon, as had been reported by early-day Portuguese explorers. Most authorities thought this far-fetched, but the last few pages of Grann's article are breathtaking. He ran across an archeologist from the University of Florida who had been in the region for some ten years and had discovered the remains of a lost civilization, some twenty and more large sites. A particular site, for instance, might be a mile across, surrounded by a moat and was presumably backed up by a timbered palisade. The wooden buildings had long since decayed, but the sites contained much broken pottery or shards. The archeologist, Michael Heckenberger, and his team had reported on these findings in a few publications, for example, in *Science*, but his findings were not widely disseminated. Those who knew his findings have indicated that there might have been as many as a million inhabitants, though Heckenberger thought this figure was high. He agreed that the inhabitants had largely died off from the diseases introduced by the early white explorers, with only a few survivors remaining. Nevertheless, the layouts and interconnecting roads indicated to Heckenberger that this had been an advanced civilization for its time. Another book of related interest is *The River of Doubt*, by Candice Millard, which recounts former U.S. President Theodore Roosevelt's travails in exploring an unknown region of Amazonia.

In addition to common sugar, or sucrose, derived from sugarcane or sugar beets, already in hand are other naturally occurring sugars, such as glucose and dextrose (corn sugar), fructose and levulose (fruit sugar), lactose (milk sugar), and maltose (malt sugar), of varying sweetness. (The suffix "-ose" denotes a sugar or other carbohydrate.) There is, for example, sorbitol, derived from berries, cherries, and other fruits. The names sorbose, hexose, etc., are encountered. Of interest is xylitol, derived from tree bark, and similar in chemical structure to xylose, or wood sugar. (The prefix "xylo-" means wood.) It is being promoted for use in chewing gum, for instance, as an agent that fights tooth decay.

With regard to corn as the raw material, modern technology yields the product high fructose corn syrup, which is used in soft drinks and foods. The by-product is called *corn gluten meal*, which serves as livestock feed. Significantly, the meal also makes a great organic fertilizer, notably for lawns, where it acts against weeds, requires less watering, and the gluten content is a source for nitrogen-induced greenery.

The subject of intense sweeteners is briefly described in a section in the Hoffman cancer reference, which were noted to be either organic acids or peptides, with high intakes causing disturbances in the gut microflora. But the effect on tumor development was unclear (Hoffman, 1999, pp. 226, 227). Bringing matters up to date is an article by Burkhard Bilger in the May 22, 2006, issue of the *New Yorker* titled "The Search for Sweet." Noting the enormous sugar consumption, especially in the United States and dismissing saccharin, cyclamates, aspartame, and the like, considerable space is given to what became Splenda®, which was first encountered as 1,4,6.6-tetrachloro-1,4,6,6-tetradeoxygalactosucrose. It was discovered after adding highly toxic sulfuryl chloride liquid to a sugar solution, and has been subsequently improved upon. (The chlorine content discourages some parties from using it, despite the claim that it is made from sugar.) Another entry is called inosine monophosphate (IMP), which is synergistic with MSG. Many more possibilities have been uncovered, with sweetening effects thousands of times that of sugar, but none are as versatile or satisfying as ordinary sugar. The search continues, however.

(There are natural agents that can affect the craving for sugar or the metabolism of sugar intake. The licorice root is commonly mentioned. Another more exotic agent is said to be *Gymnema sylvestre*, or "Gurmar," herb marketed under the trade name *Sweet Away*.)

With regard to fats, we are developing fat substitutes, using which food will taste as good, but without the calories. And after the criminal prosecution of the authors of a book titled *Calories Don't Count*, it is found that, sometimes, maybe they do not. (More successful at fighting off the establishment was Dr. Andrew Ivy, at the time dean of the Northwestern University School of Medicine, whose endorsement of Krebiozen cancer therapy came under attack in the courts. But Dr. Ivy was acquitted.) Meantime, at Louisiana State University, it is reported that zoologist Albert Meier has made an intriguing discovery: Migrating birds and hibernating animals will build up fat in preparation for flight or hibernation, without any extra food intake. This is a rhythmic process, which in reverse could lead to a spontaneous weight loss in humans, for example, via the drug bromocryptine.

Cows' milk and its cream, or butterfat, and all those gourmet products such as butter and the many cheeses are presumably tough on the body plumbing because of the high fat content. About milk, however, the uniform practice of homogenizing the milk and cream together may lengthen the shelf life but does not do much for digestibility, although pasteurization has a lot going for it, namely, the elimination of milk-transmitted diseases such as tuberculosis. Speaking of indigestion, whereas most vegetable oils are derived from edible seeds or nuts, it is left to wonder about cottonseed oil as it hardly seems edible, though cattle apparently thrive on the leftover cottonseed cake. But we are not cattle. This also brings up the subject of hydrogenated vegetable oils, the semisolids used everywhere as butter substitutes or margarine for cooking and baking, but which are synthetics, that is, not found in nature. These also cause indigestion. The body sure needs a good alimentary canal to withstand this onslaught.

## THE PONDERABLES OF BIOCHEMISTRY

Basic to any discussion of life and life processes is the subject of cells, designated as *eukaryotes* and *prokaryotes* (e.g., in Voet and Voet, 1995, p. 2ff). The eukaryotes are distinguished by a membrane-enclosed nucleus containing their DNA and may be unicellular or multicellular, whereas prokaryotes lack this feature. Prokaryotes, by far the most numerous, are the cells of bacteria, whereas eukaryotes are the cells presumably of everything else — notably mammals, including humans, but also the cells of plants, which are distinguished by a rigid cell wall. Eukaryotes contain intracellular entities called *organelles* that perform various functions, including protein synthesis in mammalian cells. On the other hand, in plant cells, there are organelles called *chloroplasts*, the site of photosynthesis.

Viruses are excluded from this classification, being considered nonliving things, basically containing a strand or strands of DNA or RNA and lacking the metabolic apparatus to reproduce outside of host cells. Technically speaking, "Viruses are infectious particles consisting of a nucleic acid molecule enclosed by a protective capsid (coat) that consists largely or entirely of protein" (Voet and Voet, 1995, p. 841). In turn, there are what are known as *subviruses*, sometimes called *slow viruses*, and which merge into the *prions*, considered the possible cause of such diseases as *Alzheimer's* and *bovine spongiform encephalitis* (BSE, or mad cow disease) and the latter's human variant called *Creutzfeldt-Jakob disease* (CJD). The term *prion*, incidentally, stands for "proteinaceous infectious particle." (The word is that misdiagnosis may occur, in that what is called Alzheimer's disease may in some instances be Creutzfeldt-Jakob disease. In other words, CJD may be more common than it is thought to be.)

There is another microorganism called a *mycoplasma*, being the smallest microorganism capable of independent replication and growth, and it is sometimes viewed as a cross between a bacterium and a virus. It calls to mind that macro/micro/molecular entities may exist, ranging from fungi and bacteria down through viruses to subviruses and prions, even to various molecular-sized particles, pieces, or segments (say the fundamental particles of matter?). There is also the phenomenon called *polymorphism* or *pleomorphism*, in which an organism or entity can change from one form to another (say, a bacterium to a virus, or vice versa). This is a touchy subject in micro- or molecular biology, although apparently common enough in the macro world — take butterflies and their larvae, for example, or marine flagellates (red tide).

The prefix "myco-" signifies fungus, and appears in such categories as mycoplasma and mycobacteria, with the qualifier that these organisms may be plantlike, animallike, maybe even viruslike, etc., although the fungi or Mycota have their own separate kingdom (Hoffman, 1999, pp. 280–283). A specific example of a mycobacterium is the organism *Mycobacterium leprae*, the cause of leprosy, or Hansen's disease, in humans. These forms can also occur in certain animals, for example, in the nude mouse, the nine-banded armadillo, and the mangabey monkey: animals that have been utilized in trying to develop a vaccine. Moreover, there are two basic kinds of leprosy called *tuberculoid* and *lepromatous*. The former eventually yields to sulfone drugs, the latter is more intractable to treatment and may return unexpectedly at any time (Hoffman, 1999, p. 305). The traditional treatment of leprosy with chaulmoogra oil has long been proved ineffective, although several modern drugs have been tried, namely, rifampin, dapsone, and clofazimine, although with hepatoxic side effects. The BCG vaccine has also been tried, with widely disparate results.

An intriguing aspect was supplied by the once-famous roving correspondent Ernie Pyle in his book *Home Country*. A visit to Hawaii's Molokai leper colony is described in his chapter "The Leper Colony." There were a few patients who had a "reaction," in which a high fever occurs and the patient comes out of it "clean" (Pyle, *Home Country*, p. 242). Evidently, the patient's immune system rose to the occasion and destroyed the organism, in the same way it attacks other diseases. There was talk at the time of developing a machine to artificially induce fever in leprosy patients, but it was reported that nothing came of it. The subject is, therefore, that of hypothermia, which reportedly works on cancer patients at times.

In humans, there are different cells in each part of the body, which have been given various technical names. Of particular note here are the neurons, the cells of the nervous system, including the brain. They are the basis of the subject of biochemical communication, hormones as biochemical regulators of body processes, and of neurotransmitters for carrying instructions between neurons and from neurons to muscles or glands (Voet and Voet, 1995, p. 1261ff, 1291ff). With regard to neurotransmission, neurons are separated by interfaces or junctions known as *synapses* through which nerve impulses are carried (an electrochemical phenomenon) and have extensions called *axons* that carry impulses. (An impulse can be described as a burst or as a "go or no-go" phenomenon.) Among the more common neurotransmitters are positively charged potassium and sodium ions, and the negatively charged chlorine ion, described as acting through channels. Various neurotoxins block these channels with deadly results, e.g., manifested as a shutdown of respiration. Among these neurotoxins are tetrodotoxin, from the puffer fish (or fugu); saxitoxin, from the plankton known as the *red tide*; batrochotoxin, a steroidal alkaloid from the South American arrow-poison frog, *Phyllobates aurotaenia*; and venom from American scorpions.

Among the most important neurotransmitters are acetylcholine (ACh), amino acids and their derivatives, and certain polypeptides known as *neuropeptides*. In fact, the mammalian nervous system is said to employ over 30 different substances as neurotransmitters. For the record, among the amino acids and their derivatives (called *biogenic amines*) are many that are also hormonally active in the bloodstream, and include the catecholamines dopamine, norepinephrine, and epinephrine, as derived sequentially from tyrosine, whereas $\gamma$-aminobutyric acid (GABA), histamine, and serotonin are derived from glutamate, histidine, and tryptophan, respectively. The subject interfaces with the biochemical aspects of psychology, which may also be referred to as the *mind–body connection*, or *psychosomatics*.

Interestingly, the class of biochemically active substances called *alkaloids*, which are often toxic (sometimes extremely so) can act as neurotransmitters. Also relevant is the subject of enzymes and enzyme inhibitors, for alkaloids are also known enzyme inhibitors and may act against cancer cell metabolism. Enzymes are the catalytic agents for the various body processes, and along with catalysis, there are electrochemical phenomena involved — a manifestation somewhat similar to neurotransmission.

In inorganic catalysis, notably involving substances called the *Group VIII transition metals* of the periodic table, such as, nickel, iron, cobalt and their oxides, two states or degrees of oxidation are involved: a lower and a higher state. Thus, a catalyst is activated by a partial reduction with hydrogen or by a partial oxidation with oxygen or its equivalent to produce a heterogeneity throughout the catalyst composition. And a condition of compositional heterogeneity sets up minute or micro electrochemical forces, or emfs, which relates to catalytic activity (on a macro scale, for example, we would be speaking of a battery). Even platinum catalysts, perhaps the most active of metal catalysts, are found to have a coat of the oxide, indicating a condition of compositional and electrochemical heterogeneity.

It is interesting to note that certain platinum compounds or complexes have been found to act as anticancer agents, but also may act as carcinogens or mutagens, and/or toxicants (Chabner et al., in *Goodman and Gilman's Pharmacological Basis of Therapeutics*, 2001, pp. 1269–1271; Goyer, in Amdur et al., 1991, pp. 666, 667; *The Toxicity of Anticancer Drugs*, Powis and Hacker, 1991, p. 82ff.; various entries in Perry and Yarborough, 1994). The forms most studied are called *cisplatin* (or platinol, or DDP), *carboplatin* (CBDCA), and *iproplatin* (CHIP), as acronyms for their lengthy chemical names. Adverse side effects include kidney damage, hearing loss, and bone marrow suppression. In common with other anticancer agents, the dosage level is the poison.

Colloidal silver, available in health stores and of historical use, is occasionally touted as an anticancer, antifungal, and antibiotic agent. The arguments seesaw back and forth (on the Internet), with the admonition that much of the silver present may be ionic silver which can cause argyria, a graying of the skin. The antibiotic action is sometimes thought of in terms of a disablement of oxygen metabolic enzymes. (Bacterial or prokaryotic metabolism is extremely varied, however.) On the other hand, it could be a catalytic effect, even a consequence of oxidation-reduction reactions between metallic silver and its ions.

An update is furnished in the May 2006 issue of the *Townsend Letter for Doctors & Patients* in an article by Apsley, Holtert, Gordon, Anderson, and Buttar titled "Nanotechnology's Latest Oncolytic Agent: Silver, Cancer, and Infection Associations." The agents used were positive silver ion hydrosols composed of nanoclusters and even picoclusters, of the lowest size imaginable. *In vivo* (clinical) tests conducted in Central America produced striking results against female breast cancers. A treatment protocol against pancreatic cancer is also described, which has so far proved successful, with medical orthodoxy concluding that maybe the patient did not have pancreatic cancer after all.

To continue, an electrochemical- or polarity-induced condition of dissociation for the reactants can be inferred, followed by a reassociation into the products. With organic catalysts, such as enzymes, a condition of polarity is indicated in that one part of an organic molecule will appear positive relative to another, with the latter part having a negative connotation. This in turn may be inferred to confer a dissociation of the reactant or reactants, followed by a reassociation into the product or products.

It may also be noted that electrophilic behavior can contribute to mutagenesis and carcinogenesis (Klaasen and Eaton, in Amdur et al., 1991, p. 29). By "electrophilic" is meant a propensity to attract or share electrons to counteract an electron deficiency in the substance. Thus, it is noted that there are many electrophilic sites within the DNA that can readily react with electrophilic chemicals. (That is, the electrophilic sites share electrons with the electrophilic chemicals, a phenomenon also known as *covalent bonding*.) As another example, the amino acid guanine may undergo alkylation, which appears important in the mutagenicity and carcinogenicity of nitrosamines.

The inference is that organic enzymatic catalytic activity and carcinogenicity may share a common electrophilic ancestry. If this indeed has a bearing on anticancer agents, the resolution can be phrased in terms of finding natural or synthetic chemicals that will selectively counter or block this electrophilic behavior. Perhaps "electrophobic" behavior or an *antioxidant* is involved.

(In materials science, the word *antioxidant* pertains to an additive or agent that lessens the effects of oxidation, thus reducing degradation. Electrochemically, the word *oxidation* signifies the removal of electrons from a chemical entity and their capture by another oxidizing entity. In terms of hydrogen content, it can mean the removal of a hydrogen atom or atoms by, say, oxygen, in this case, to form water. Thus, in this context, antioxidant would denote something that prevents oxidation or, conversely, provides the inverse, called *reduction*. Reduction would, electrochemically, connote the addition of electrons; chemically, it would connote the addition of hydrogen. In any event, the net objective is to selectively inhibit or block a critical enzyme like lactate dehydrogenase, which is involved in cancer cell metabolism. This inhibiting or blocking action, generally could be either by oxidation or reduction, resulting in an electrochemical or chemical change.)

With this brief introduction, it may be inferred that there is a connection between the electrochemistry of the nervous system and the biochemical processes of the body. It is not yet fully understood but has the potential to negate cancer cell formation and metabolism.

Beyond this, however, we are adrift, as the mysteries that are the "spark of life" remain untouched. In other words, what distinguishes a "live" cell from a "dead" one, or a "live" virus from a "killed" virus? Or, more completely, what in the ultimate analysis distinguishes a live human being from a dead one? Can there be, or cannot there be, an inherent bio-physico-magneto-electro-chemical explanation at the most fundamental level? Or are we speaking of another domain, entirely, for example, metaphysics, literally beyond or apart from science?

Medicine continues to take many unexpected turns. There are theories and findings about the role of the body chemicals interferon and the endorphins, and their relation to well-being, both physical and mental. The term *phytochemicals*, which refers to plant, or plant-derived, chemicals, is among the newer buzzwords. There is talk of the interrelation between and among physicochemical and neuropsychological functions in terms of neurotransmitters, with neurologist Antonio R. Damasio's *Descartes' Error: Emotion, Reason, and the Human Brain* furnishing insights into this never-never land. (As an aside, there are apparently a few people whose chemical and electromagnetic aura is strong enough to disrupt a watch.) Bacterial strains resistant to the known antibiotics have developed, and are developing, calling for ever-new antibiotics, a situation like having a tiger by the tail. Another example regarding our increased consumption of carbonated soft drinks; there is concern about the phosphate content of these drinks depleting the calcium from our very bones.

(The preceding statement is part of a growing calcium deficiency problem, evidenced as osteoporosis, especially among the elderly, and is apparently reason enough to take calcium supplements along with vitamin D, which is supposed to aid in the body's calcium fixation. Not only do the elderly have a problem with calcium requirements, but also with the absorption of other nutrients, even if sufficiently abundant in the total diet; this is one of the many reasons geriatrics is such an inexact science. And magnesium may have as much or more potential than calcium in the future.)

There is also much talk about glucose, serotonin levels, and other chemical imbalances that may occur within the body. In many instances, specific food allergies are the prime suspect, including the use of food additives. There are problems with hormones and steroids (natural and injected or ingested) and with diethylstilbestrol (DES). And there are the environmental factors, weighed by Theron G. Randolph and Ralph W. Moss in *An Alternative Approach to Allergies: The New Field of Clinical Ecology Unravels the Environmental Causes of Mental and Physical Ills.*

Also, there is concern about trace, or "ultratrace," elements and their compounds, and how they may regulate bodily functions. Consider the fact, for example, that magnesium is vital to the functions of the heart, its rhythm, and its beat, and that inborn deficiencies may be responsible for crib deaths and other infant deaths, causes otherwise unknown. Magnesium is thought to quicken memory, whereas a deficiency may trigger Alzheimer's disease. Zinc, as another important example, is crucial for the proper growth of children and the proper healing of wounds. Lithium counteracts manic or depressive behavior and may be a factor in regulating ordinary mood swings, the ups and downs of daily life, to smooth out our coexistence on this earth. (About mood swings, one may consult Ronald R. Fieve's book of the same name.) However, too much of a lithium salt would be counterproductive; for example, lithium can adversely affect the liver and kidneys.

Some of the more recent publications about trace elements, trace minerals, or ultratrace elements or minerals, also described as micronutrients, include *Micronutrients in Health and Disease Prevention*, edited by Adrianne Bendich and C.E. Butterworth; *Trace Elements in Nutrition of Children*, edited by Ranjit Kumar Chandra; and *Trace Elements, Micronutrients and Free Radicals*, edited by Ivor E. Dreosti. The latter reference raises the important question of the undesirable health effects of the chemical agents called *free radicals*, and their control or eradication by such vitamins as E, C, and beta-carotene. There is a history of the health effects of trace elements going back to Henry A. Schroeder, who in the early 1970s wrote *Trace Elements and Man: Some Positive and Negative Aspects* and also *The Poisons Around Us: Toxic Metals in Food, Air, and Water*. Even further back there was Karl H. Schutte's *The Biology of Trace Elements: Their Role in Nutrition*, published in 1964.

The discussion about trace elements or minerals, their role, their optimal concentrations, and of how these may be vital to health and well-being continues. The water fluoridation controversy, of fluoride vs. tooth decay, is related. How much is not enough, and how much is too much? Not only with regard to fluoride addition to public water supplies, but with regard to the intervention of the state. Should the state doctor all municipal water supplies to maintain a uniform and apparently optimal mineral content? When is it and when is it not the state's business?

(Fluoride, in the form of stannous fluoride or tin fluoride, is said to be an enzyme inhibitor that blocks certain critical enzymes in oral bacteria. It is, however, also an inhibitor for other body enzymes, and the organic catalysts that support the myriad biochemical reactions occurring in the body, that is, the bodily functions. The more conventional explanation for fluoride's anticavity action is that it replaces calcium in the tooth surfaces or enamel with a hard calcaneus layer on the teeth, thereby making these surfaces more resistant to bacteria. But whichever way introduced, whether by the municipal water supplies or other sources, fluoride also has toxic effects or adverse side effects; the severity of the effect depends on the concentration level or dosage and on biochemical individuality. A recent critique is contained in *Our Stolen Future: Are We Threatening Our Fertility, Intelligence, and Survival? — A Scientific Detective Story* by Theo. Colborn, Dianne Dumanoski and John P. Myers. The reminder is of the Romans' use of malleable lead cooking vessels, affordable to the elites, and resulting in insidious lead poisoning among the ruling class, and this was thought to play a major role in the decline and fall of the Roman Empire. More is contained in Christopher Bryson's *The Fluoride Deception*, published in 2004, with a foreword by Dr. Theo. Colborn. The push for fluorides in dentistry is traceable back to the Manhattan Project, where fluorine was used in uranium enrichment, and any kind of adverse criticism was obstructed. Its purported dental benefits can be viewed as another case of "making a silk purse out of a sow's ear." An insert on p. 23 of the November 2005 *Townsend Letter* is titled "Fluoride Linked to Bone Cancer, Again." This specifically refers to osteosarcoma, a rare form of bone cancer.

In broader terms, our concerns are about side effects: the physical, chemical, and biological changes in body and mind that accompany diet and medication. Some of the side effects are benign: others are adverse. And each individual will react differently, in accordance with a part of our distinctive biochemical makeup, a fact emphasized by the noted University of Texas biochemist Roger Williams in *Free and Unequal*.

Aside from more routine methods and sources, hair analyses have been used to diagnose our bodily chemical deficiencies and excesses, and extended even to chart a record of drug intake. We are not only analyzed *post factum*, but we may also be programmed *ante factum*, that is, not only after but before the fact. A transcript of brain wave patterns can indicate personality and mood, and the changes in these patterns that are analyzed by a computer may be used as a lie detector.

## TROUBLES OF MIND

Psychiatric medication involves a dichotomy between free will and the use of mind-altering substances, natural or otherwise. Where is the line to be drawn? There is an old saying that everybody is a little crazy; some are just more so than others. When does "more so" become "too much"? The notation is that we are all affected to a degree by obsessive compulsive disorders (OCDs), with some of us severely so, or clearly so. Where, therefore, should the medication start and where should it end?

Or are we all to become zombies, having no personality, no disorders, no genius, no eccentricities, with any and all chemical dysfunctions of the body adjusted by drugs? This, in turn, will produce many other dysfunctions. The "happiness" pills and elixirs are the buzzwords of the moment.

There are those of us, nevertheless, who will for good enough reason settle for being average. On the other hand, there are those who perceive reality as so abhorrent that any sort of change or relief is welcome. What then? What has happened to a society or civilization where this feeling, this malaise, becomes pervasive? Can in fact the spiritual dimension, where truth is reality, rescue and revivify?

One may judge, therefore, that all is not exactly well with conventional psychotherapy. If there was criticism before, there is more now. Among the earlier critics was Karl Kraus, whose translated writings appear in Thomas Szasz's *Anti-Freud: Karl Kraus's Criticism of Psychoanalysis and Psychiatry* (1990), which is a new edition of Szasz's *Karl Kraus and the Soul Doctors*. For example, Kraus jested that "the psychiatrist unfailingly recognizes the madman by his excited behavior on being incarcerated." Thomas Szasz himself has written extensively on the subject, in *The Myth of Psychiatry: Mental Healing as Religion, Rhetoric, and Repression* (1988a). (It may be noted that the word *mythology* could be substituted for *myth*, the latter being perceived as a truth that can be expressed in no other way.) This volume of Szasz's polemics, along with a few others, is cited in the bibliography. Whether or not Szasz is 100% correct is open to debate, but his outlook certainly provides some alternatives to the way mental illness is viewed. There is, of course, the matter of degree, or as the saying goes, everyone is a bit crazy, and some more than others.

The most common and perhaps least talked about mental problems are depression and anxiety. The panic attack, or anxiety attack, is recognized as a fellow-traveler with depression. It has been called the "common cold" of psychological complaints. A state of misery is apparently the near-normal human condition. Not for nothing did Thoreau write about us leading lives of quiet desperation. This pervasive life crippler is slowly yielding to a nutritional and biochemical approach, which cannot be too soon.

A prominent name in nutritional therapy for mental disorders is that of Carl C. Pfeiffer of the Carl Pfeiffer Treatment Center, Naperville, IL, and of the Princeton Bio Center, Skillman, NJ. In addition to his clinical work, he has written, coauthored, or edited a number of books dating back through the years. His later books include the following: *Nutrition and Mental Illness: An Orthomolecular Approach to Balancing Body Chemistry* (1988b); *The Schizophrenias: Ours to Conquer* (1988a); and *The Healing Nutrients Within: Facts, Findings and New Research on Amino Acids* (1987). He had earlier written his *Updated Fact Book on Zinc and Other Micro-Nutrients* (1978) and *Mental and Elemental Nutrients: A Physician's Guide to Nutrition and Health Care* (1975). These books are mainly related to attention deficit disorder (ADD), as occurs in school-age children, and which may yield to a nutritional approach.

About the routine use of Ritalin for hyperactive children, especially in schools, there are some who maintain that this is due to boredom in class. An alternative approach getting good marks is individual schooling, as practiced by the Desiderata School at Longmont, CO. Named after the now-famous poem by Max Ehrman, originally published in 1927, there is a one-to-one correspondence similar to that of the famous educator Johns Hopkins and a student, sitting on opposite ends of a log. The key is individual instruction that reflects and challenges the student's very own interests, flexible scheduling, and informal meeting places. The dropout rate is said to be less than 1%.

Another prominent name in the field of mental problems is Priscilla Slagle, a psychiatrist M.D. who also prescribes the amino acids. Her book *The Way Up from*

*Down: A Safe New Program That Relieves Low Moods and Depression with Amino Acids and Vitamin Supplements* was first published in 1987. The first chapter is titled "The Horror of Depression." In the subsequent chapters, we find that such amino acids as L-tyrosine, tryptophan, L-phenylalinine, and GABA which are taken along with the B-complex and other essential vitamins and minerals, help relieve depression. There may be some side effects; for example, L-tyrosine and L-phenylalinine can also act as stimulants, something the patient may not necessarily want or need.

(Tryptophan was removed from the U.S. market after a contaminated batch that was manufactured overseas was responsible for disastrous consequences. Tryptophan is also said to have some undesirable side effects, as can about every other medication under the sun, especially at higher dosages. It can still be ordered from foreign sources, however. It is said to be as effective as the drug Prozac. What behind-the-scenes maneuvering may have been involved in the marketing, we do not venture to suggest here.)

Another possibility is the herb St. John's wort, which is increasingly cited as acting against depression, though it also has its detractors. Jean Carper, who writes an "Eat Smart" column for *USA Weekend*, lists and describes the effect of this herb against depression in both her column (i.e., July 11, 1997) and in her book *Miracle Cures: Dramatic New Scientific Discoveries Revealing the Healing Power of Herbs and Vitamins*, also published in 1997. Also prominently mentioned is celery seed extract against gout, feverfew for migraines, and glucosamine for arthritis, to name a few.

A highly regarded series is about *Smart Drugs*, written variously by Ward Dean, John Morgenthaler, and Steven Wm. Fowkes. The subtitle of Volume 2 in the series is partially self-explanatory: *New Drugs and Nutrients to Improve Your Memory and Increase Your Intelligence*. The series, however, covers a great deal more.

In the extreme, on a day-to-day basis in the trenches, there is Stephen B. Seager's *Psychward*, about how life goes on at County General in Los Angeles. It is the hidden world of the mentally ill. We recall here the old saying mentioned earlier that everybody is a little bit crazy, and some are just more crazy than others. There is, in turn, the corollary provided in Seager's book that everybody is a little sane, but some of us, maybe, are just more sane than others.

Depression and anxiety are found to be major biochemical problems, as most likely are other emotional or mental disturbances, even schizophrenia. It is a newly unfolding and exciting field. These disturbances are being found to be related to sleep disorders, which in turn are related to biochemical imbalances. Compounding the difficulty is not getting enough sleep in the first place. So writes Martin C. Moore-Ede of the Harvard Medical School in *The Twenty-Four Hour Society: Understanding Human Limits in a World That Never Stops*.

If biochemical imbalances do in fact occur, there is in turn the problem of first causes: what triggered the imbalance in the first place? (The same problem, of course, as with the occurrence of cancer.) The catchall term *stress*, frequently mentioned, is intertwined with the culture, medicines, allergies, other biochemical abnormalities, the simplicities and complexities of food and drugs, exposure to toxic or even not-so-toxic chemicals, and hereditary factors, that is, the genetic component, etc. As for narcotic drugs, it is being noticed that drugs used for pain control *per se* may not prove addictive — and that, for some mysterious reason, withdrawal symptoms do not usually occur if the drug is absolutely and unequivocally not available. There is, accordingly, a move to make opiates more routinely available for cancer patients. Not only can illness be made more painfree, but life itself can be extended.

There is, in the preceding text, the notion that biochemical imbalances or abnormalities are caused by many factors and may be counteracted or relieved by factors other than drugs or medicines. This is the premise of traditional psychiatry. It is a gray area, whether or not to use the drugs of biochemical psychiatry, which may be regarded as only an expediency and do not address root causes. There are, of course, the variables of dosage levels and length of medication, coupled with the fact that each individual case is probably unique. There is the question of will, of whether to confront life or run from life, a yes-or-no choice that may appear simple but is not simple at all.

Psychiatrist Peter D. Kramer takes a contemplative view of these issues and phenomena in *Listening to Prozac*. Whereas what Kramer calls "cosmetic psychopharmacology" can cause miraculous changes in personality, there is always the nagging question about the psyche itself, of just who a person is really supposed to be? In short, there is the ethics of the matter, and it may be said that once again science collides with metaphysics, religion, and theology, though this is not an area into which Kramer chooses to carry his explorations. As Kramer states in his introduction, the patient is not so much cured of illness as transformed. Also supplied is the memorable quote: "If the human brain were simple enough for us to understand, we would be too simple to understand it" (Kramer, 1993, p. 134).

Among those who take an even dimmer view of the wonder drug route is Peter R. Breggin, M.D., who has written, among other books on the subject, *Toxic Psychiatry: Why Therapy, Empathy, and Love Must Replace the Drugs, Electroshock, and Biochemical Theories of the "New Psychiatry"*. Breggin sees the medicines themselves as the cause of still other mental dysfunctions, especially over the long term.

There is also the indication that our mental outlook and our nervous system performance can be regulated by diet, and preferably by diet alone, especially by the B-complex vitamins, as found in natural sources such as as brewer's yeast. Brewer's or nutritional yeasts have high protein content of good quality and also desirable trace elements and other benefits. There are also the old standbys like onions and garlic to steady the nerves, and there has even been some talk about flower essences for alleviating depression (e.g., in *Natural Health*, May/June 1995, p. 80ff).

There is now the acknowledgment that nutritional factors are indeed being studied for their role in combating mental problems. Thus, for example, a review article in the scientific literature by Kathleen M. Kantak titled "Nutritional Aspects of Drug Action on Behavior," cited in the Bibliography, is representative. In this instance, the effects of (pure) tryptophan, magnesium/vitamin $B_6$, and vitamin C were examined, alone or in combination with drugs. There was an interaction even for such mental illnesses as schizophrenia, depression, autism, and hyperactivity.

There are still other factors at work. Thus, we may inquire variously about full-spectrum light for health and its relation to seasonal affective disorder (SAD), the effects of positive and negative ions in the atmospheric air, and the use of native herbs and plant medicines. Taking all these things a step further is Michael J. Norden, in *Beyond Prozac: Brain-Toxic Lifestyles, Natural Antidotes & New Generation Antidepressants*. Among other things, Dr. Norden stresses the importance of melatonin, a neurohormone related to serotonin, which is the principal hormone secreted from the pineal gland. It not only acts against anxiety and depression, and serves as an antiaging agent, but is also being studied in the treatment of cancer.

(Rose-colored glasses may indeed make the world look "rosier," whereas battery-powered wrist watches may have some unexpected and adverse effects, for example, on the wearer's memory, not to mention fluorescent lighting and its cyclic intensity; that is, its fluttering with 60-cycle alternating current. For more on this offbeat subject, there is the work of John Ott about the physiological effects of light and radiation.)

Not only does the vitality of the soil affect crop growth but in turn also human health. Even mental illness, which may be caused by nutritional deficiencies, can have apparently miraculous cures produced by diet. Such commonalities as garlic are seen as valuable additions to the mental health spectrum. The list can go onwards and upwards from there, as can be found in most health food stores.

## WHAT SEEMS TO WORK

Such ordinary matters as roughage in the diet are afforded a new importance, as is physical exercise. Acupuncture and reflexology have entered the scene, as have cycles, biorhythms, and the (adverse) effects of electromagnetic fields. The problems with electromagnetic fields are highlighted in Paul Brodeur's argumentative *The Great Power-Line Cover-Up*. Electric blankets have become suspect and are maybe better used only for taking the chill off before bedtime. (About the effect of the phases of the moon, it is better to leave the subject alone, or confine it to home gardening.) Chelation chemistry has been used to remove the fatty cholesterol deposits within our very arteries and veins and may be replaced by or assisted by certain vitamins, though the verdict is still out. The citations seem never-ending.

(The mention of, for example, the role of vitamin C [ascorbic acid] or vitamin E in the body functions and in various therapies is enough to start a discussion. Thus, to say that vitamin C can be used instead of sodium nitrate as a preservative for cured meats or sliced fresh fruit is not to cause alarm, but to admit that vitamin C could act as a chelating agent for removing heavy metals or arterial fatty deposits from the body is inadmissible. Much less acceptable is the suggestion that vitamin C possesses an antibiotic or antiviral action, especially against the common cold, as per Linus Pauling's work, and also that the body may need large amounts, as humans do not produce vitamin C internally as do most other animals. To state that vitamin E oil can act as an external healing agent for skin scars or burns is not so far out, but to admit that vitamin E taken internally might act against heart problems is a no-no.)

The dust is starting to settle on what does and does not work. The innovations are of a breadth and pace that can only be upsetting to organized medicine, which must necessarily remain cautious if not conservative, and play the devil's advocate to this "underground unorthodoxy." Particularly vexing to the professional establishment is anecdotal evidence, which by definition has not been subjected to scientific scrutiny, and therefore must be discounted. However, scientific evidence in turn needs verification by anecdotal case-by-case scrutiny.

Overriding all this is the profit motive, the force that drives a capitalistic economy. The yardstick of success for physicians, hospitals, and pharmaceutical companies is a return on investment, the higher the better. The conventional wisdom is that this will all prove beneficial for the patient. There is a gray area, however, which does not necessarily work for the well-being of the patient. In other words, if there are alternatives such as folk remedies, therapies, or cures for which the same physicians, hospitals, and pharmaceutical companies cannot show a profit or even a large enough profit, what then? Will these alternatives be then promoted, discounted, or even ruled against or made against the law? Laws and regulations, incidentally, are in large part written with the active support and acquiescence of the medical establishment.

Thus, in a legal sense, orthodox medicine must protect itself by establishing practices that are recognized by the medical body as the conventional wisdom. The peers protect their peers.

There is also the fact that medical insurance and Medicare will only pay for or pay on orthodox procedures and treatments, as established by the medical establishment. Logically speaking, it is another case of the vicious circle.

All this is especially vexing if medical orthodoxy cannot even come up with successful therapies or cures, for example, in the treatment of cancer. Hence, the emergence of unorthodox or alternative therapies — the *raison d'être* of the medical underground. It is obviously a catch-22 situation, and a time for investigation and reckoning.

## SCOURGES IN THE MAKING

Offsetting any reasons for optimism are indications of new scourges. Thus, the increased use of antibiotics is resulting in new strains of microbes or microorganisms that are tolerant or resistant to the same antibiotics which had formerly proved so effective. This situation is examined, for instance, in Jeffrey A. Fisher's *The Plague Makers* and in Stuart B. Levy's *The Antibiotic Paradox: How Miracle Drugs are Destroying the Miracle*. For these and other reasons, new or old diseases may become pandemic infections, affecting entire populations.

There have, for an unusual example, emerged especially deadly strains of "flesh-eating" bacteria causing the tissue-destroying disease *Group A streptococcal infection* (GAS), or *necrotizing fasciitis*. Though rare so far, there is the question of whether this is an old disease, or whether new species or strains have come about.

Influenza-type viruses, notably, have been found to have crossed the species barrier, for example, from ducks and swine to humans (recall the Spanish influenza epidemic of 1918 when 20 million lives were lost). There is, on the evidence, a genetic synthesis of an animal strain of virus with a human strain, producing deadly results sometimes. There are rumors that the rabies vaccine, derived from horses as the culture medium, will at times result in a delayed reaction, even after a period of years. This in itself can be fatal, but it is thought to be corrected by more modern vaccines. The facts about the production of antibodies and their side effects are not fully known. Reports are surfacing that the "hippie" generation was caused by the adverse bodily reactions of a certain percentage of individuals to a virus found in the rhesus monkeys used in the production of live polio vaccine Bookchin and Schumacher, *The Virus and the Vaccine*, 2004. This again may have resulted from a genetic synthesis between the monkey virus and a human virus. Where most persons overcome the viral infection, others are affected in different ways, to produce lethargy and other recurring or continuing flu-like symptoms. Newer findings indicate that these simian viruses may induce cancer. In fact, this is in line with findings that still other viruses are once again suspect in causing cancer, and the genetic mechanisms have been worked out.

Currently on the scene is the specter of AIDS, the ultimate social disease, which is said also to be derived from monkeys. (On the other hand, it has been advanced that the AIDS virus is the result of combining the bovine leukemia virus with the sheep visna virus, both of which are *retroviruses* capable of changing the genetic makeup of the cells they enter. The resulting virus was presumably introduced overseas in smallpox vaccine, and in the United States. with hepatitis B vaccine.) It therefore seems that the interface between humans and the animal world is fraught with unexpected hazards, some of the consequences of experimenting with viruses. So certain biblical codes may have emerged to keep these or other pestilences at bay. What may be occurring is a recycling of past experiences; it is called by the philosopher and historian Will Durant as the systolic and diastolic cycles of civilization.

For an early, comprehensive, and authoritative look at the AIDS situation, there was Randy Shilt's *And the Band Played On*. In quick order, there is discussed the discovery, the cover-up, the epidemic, and presumably everything else to know about this disease at the time of writing.

A political look is supplied by Michael Fumento in *The Myth of Heterosexual AIDS*. It has been said that AIDS is the first disease with "civil rights." Stephen Joseph, in *Dragon Within the Gates: The Once and Future AIDS Epidemic*, observes that an epidemic requires not only a microbe but also a social context. And in the case of AIDS, there has been an attempt to "democratize" the disease and to assume that everyone is liable, whereas the outbreaks are only within certain pockets of the population. These are those persons whose social habits put them at risk. At the same time, there is the distinct possibility that the disease can be controlled and eliminated within these population brackets. Their homogeneity, which puts them at risk, also makes it easier to contain the outbreak of the disease. (A counter to this argument is the widespread AIDS epidemic in Africa.)

On the other hand, a reassessment of the role of the AIDS virus (HIV) has been supplied by Peter H. Duesberg and Bryan J. Ellison of the Department of Cell Biology, the University of California, Berkeley. There are apparently reasons to suspect that the virus does not produce the AIDS disease. Instead, malnutrition, alcohol, drugs, and the routine use of antibiotics may cause the collapse of the immune system. (A partial counterargument is that AIDS also occurs among the affluent.) These conclusions were presented in an article by Duesburg and Ellison that appeared in the Summer 1990 issue of *Policy Review*. It caused a near riot, judging from the letters to the editor. It contained both the pros and cons, parts of which were published in the Fall 1990 issue. To say that a nerve was touched is an understatement. Another source of controversy has been a book by Paul Cameron titled *Exposing the AIDS Scandal*, published in 1988 and 1992.

Adding to the conflagration are statements by Duesberg that the drug zidovudine (AZT), used in the treatment of AIDS, may itself be a contributor to the disease. In other words, the research on AIDS has been misdirected.

Ellison and Duesberg followed up their earlier article with a book called *Why We Will Never Win the War on AIDS*, published in 1995, in which it is pronounced that the HIV virus is not the cause of AIDS, but there are instead simpler reasons. Going further, they describe a simple defense against AIDS. As a result of their unorthodox work and claims, however, they have been more or less banished from the orthodox scientific community and have lost research funding sources.

Within the ranks of medical orthodoxy, perhaps the most authoritative tome on the subject, to date, is *AIDS: What the Government Isn't Telling You: Censored* by Lorraine Day, M.D., author and surgeon, who has come under fire since. First published more or less privately, it is not what the establishment wants to hear. Nevertheless, Dr. Day has great credibility and the academic credentials to match, being from the University of California, San Francisco. Dr. Day brings up the unpleasant subject that the AIDS virus is a retrovirus and may have been introduced by the government as an agent for germ warfare. Furthermore, it is not a fragile virus, as commonly believed; it may be found even in saliva, and can be transmitted in ways yet unsuspected. For reasons of cost and practicability, blood supplies were not routinely screened for the virus, with the result that hemophiliacs, among others, have become innocent victims. Its virulence in the homosexual community can be traced in part to the incidence of other (social) diseases, which act to suppress the immune system, as was also pointed out by Duesberg and Ellison, of the University of California, Berkeley. Just where does all this leave the average citizen remains to be seen, but there is a sense of impending calamity in the air.

(For instance, the virus has been reported to remain on dental equipment, in and on the drills and other instruments, unless all the parts, inside and out, are systematically and sufficiently sterilized by heat, say, in the form of steam. It may be ventured that a trip to the dentist, if not to the doctor, should then seem more like Russian roulette.)

The AIDS disease has been studied from the standpoint of its etiology or origins, its demography or distribution by populations, and its epidemiology or spread and control. As for the disease itself, it seems the more that is found out, the less that is known. There are, and will continue to be, such books as *Rethinking AIDS Prevention: Cultural Approaches*, edited by Ralph Bolton and Merrill Singer, and *Rethinking AIDS: The Tragic Cost of Premature Consensus*, by Robert S. Root-Bernstein. (Root-Bernstein notes that the overuse of antibiotics will suppress the immune system, and there is an entire underground culture that routinely uses antibiotics excessively. For example, tetracycline is the antibiotic of choice for intravenous drug users. It is sold by the drug dealer along with the drug, as an antidote for using dirty needles.) The National Research Council and the Atlanta-based Centers for Disease Control and Prevention provide counsel and input and monitor the progression of the disease, though there has been no overt attempt at isolation and containment, as is routinely practiced for other epidemics of highly communicable diseases.

Marcus A. Cohen (2005a), in an article in the *Townsend Letter for Doctors & Patients*, furnishes some more inside information, namely, that not all AIDS cases are fatal, citing the work of Duesburg and others and an interview with Michael Ellner, president of HEAL (Health Education AIDS Liaison). The push for AIDS funding is presented as a reason for calling this disease fatal. (Nevertheless, the reported massive inroads of the disease in African populations should not be forgotten.) This was followed by an article in the October 2005 issue of the *Townsend Letter for Doctors & Patients*, which featured an interview with Roberto Giraldo, M.D., a physician in Colombia (Cohen, 2005b). The findings are much the same, stressing natural recoveries from AIDS and noting that the controversy has become increasingly political. In the November 2005 issue, it was noted that in Africa there are many other deadly, chronic diseases that are prevalent, such as tuberculosis, diabetes, malnutrition, malaria, etc., which are lumped into the category of AIDS because of similar symptoms (Cohen, 2005c). Thus, there are several definitions or criteria used for AIDS, the strictest being in the United States. If these criteria were applied to the host of miserable death-inducing conditions and diseases in poverty-stricken areas of Africa, AIDS would not be nearly as prevalent. The quote, "The AIDS figures out of Africa are pure lies, pure estimates" is eloquent. An article by Cohen (2005d) in the December 2005 issue of the *Townsend Letter for Doctors & Patients* pertains to an interview with Celia Farber, who has written extensively about AIDS in Africa, first-hand. The gist is that there is an epidemic of other sicknesses occurring apart from AIDS. However, AIDS is the buzzword as far as most of the media and public are concerned.

Celia Farber has an article on AIDS in the March 2006 issue of *Harper's Magazine*, where she mentions that a book is under way titled *Serious Adverse Events*, to be published by Melville House. The article, titled "Out of Control: AIDS and the Corruption of Medical Science," starts out reviewing the case of a pregnant lady who tested positive for HIV via a single test, but who was apparently healthy (with the comment supplied that pregnant women sometimes test positive). Although it turned out that she had not signed a consent form, the patient was given a regimen of two drugs for comparison, nelfinavir (trade name Viracept®) and nevirapine (trade name Viramune®), to which two other drugs were added, zidovudine (AZT) and lamivudine (Epivar®). There were increasingly adverse reactions, and the patient eventually died, though the baby was saved. The cause of death was attributed to liver failure due to nevirapine toxicity. The article later mentions Peter Duesberg, who had claimed that AIDS is a chemical syndrome caused by an accumulation of toxins from heavy drug use (and may be related to many other diseases), and is not caused by the HIV retrovirus. Moreover, Duesberg claims that cancer is not caused by retroviruses, but is caused by "aneuploidy," which is a chromosomal malfunction and is different from the "mutant gene" theory (Farber, 2006a, p. 52). For his troubles, Duesberg has long been cut off from government funding sources for his research.

(On p. 48 of the article, there is a footnote that states AZT brings DNA synthesis to a halt. AZT was shelved as a chemotherapy agent on account of this extreme toxicity.) It may be added that Farber's article produced an outpouring of counter-attacks in the letters to the editor. Farber's follow-up book *Serious Adverse Events: An Uncensored History of AIDS*, published in 2006, met with a similar response.

An episode of PBS's *Secrets of the Dead*, on or about August 30, 2005, about Black Death survivors also deserves mention. Backtracking case records into the medieval past of a particular village that was to a degree immune, geneticists found that a mutant gene going by the name *delta 32* (a mutant of the CCR5 gene, referred to as CCR5-delta 32) prevented some victims from dying of the plague, and with a person's double dose of the gene, exposure would not even cause sickness. When AIDS was investigated, it was found that the same delta 32 gene is involved, and exposure would not cause death, or even cause sickness, in the few persons who had inherited the gene.

(Interestingly, this mutant gene is found in the populations of Europe where the bubonic plague had occurred. The gene, however, was found not to occur in African populations, yet some individual Africans have proved resistant to AIDS. Additional information along these lines is furnished in Cohen [2005d]. This and similar articles by Cohen are described elsewhere.)

The controversy continued in a special issue of the *Townsend Letter for Doctors & Patients* for June 2006. In an article by Rebecca V. Culshaw, it was mentioned that AIDS cases increased rapidly starting in the early 1980s, peaked in 1993, and then declined rapidly, with the number of HIV-positive individuals now remaining constant at approximately 1 million. Strangely, HIV now occurs everywhere in the United States in all populations. In the same issue, Marcus A. Cohen recounts the unsettling case of Christine Maggiore, author of *What If Everything You Thought You Knew About AIDS Was Wrong?* whose dissenting views were rebuked by medical orthodoxy, including recriminations about the death of her daughter (Cohen, 2006).

As a final word, there is the premise in some quarters that AIDS and cancer are somehow connected, both being immunologically deficient diseases. There may be even more to consider. The AIDS virus is considered to mutate, to be ever-changing, so that no treatment can pin it down. This, however, is a characteristic known as *pleomorphism*, a phenomenon that has been connected with cancer-causing viruses or microbes, and one about which there is much disagreement (Walters, 1993, p. 16; Moss, 1992, pp. 490–492).

Legionnaires' disease, a form of pneumonia caused by the bacillus *Legionella pneumophilia*, was not known until 1976. The microorganisms, or germs, are found in such unsuspected places as air-conditioning ducts and cooling water towers. They have unique properties, different from those of any other bacterium previously encountered. A perplexing question follows: could this be a cross or a mutant? Cannot bacteria display the same sort of interactions as viruses? And other life-forms?

Perhaps the latest on the scene is the Four Corners virus, the cause of a pulmonary disease officially labeled as the adult respiratory distress syndrome (ARDS). The source has been found to be the feces from rodents such as deer mice that exist in the Four Corners area of the United States, where New Mexico, Arizona, Utah, and

Colorado conjoin. (Deer mice, or field mice, not coincidentally, are regarded as an ill omen in the traditions of the Southwestern Indians.) And, moreover, the same rodent species also exist elsewhere, as, apparently, does the disease, because there have been some newly emerging cases. There is a similarity to the hantavirus of Asia, though the Four Corners virus appears to be new. Inasmuch as the federal government was at one time involved in experiments on the hantavirus, there is the inference of some kind of connection between these experiments and all the other government experiments, and cover-ups, as regards nuclear testing and fallout and nerve gas testing and leakages, which occurred in the Four Corners area. Thus, some believe that there may be a connection, even so that viral mutations may have been caused inadvertently. Unexpected side effects are, in fact, a fact of life; the question of credibility, despite government denials and disassociations, therefore persists.

To the everlasting credit of modern medicine and public health measures, the scourge of the ancient world, leprosy, has largely been eliminated or controlled. Its infected hosts are no longer regarded as the unclean and to be cast out from society. (But there remains the question of the armadillo, which is prevalent around the southern United States and toward Argentina. It is implicated to be a carrier of a type of leprosy.)

There are, moreover, other unsuspected scourges on the horizon. Thus, there are emerging viruses from the destruction of the tropical rain forests or from other sources. This subject has been explored, for instance, by Richard Preston in the October 26, 1992, issue of the *New Yorker*, and also by John Langone in the December 1990 issue of *Discover*. The findings are that some of these viruses are lethal, as the human immune system does not respond to them. The subject is covered in *Emerging Viruses*, the title of a monograph contributed to by a number of specialists and edited by Stephen S. Morse of Rockefeller University, and published in 1993 by the Oxford University Press. Moreover, there is talk that the Gulf War, that is, Operation Desert Storm, may have unleashed its own brands of lethal viruses from the sands of the desert.

Preston has followed up his *New Yorker* article with a book titled *The Hot Zone: A Terrifying True Story*. It is mainly about the Ebola virus, which has a 90% fatality rate, and along with the Marburg virus, is another lethal African virus whose sources remain unknown, echoing the problems in tracking down the sources of the AIDS virus.

A book by Laurie Garrett with the title *The Coming Plague: Newly Emerging Diseases in a World Out of Balance* reminds us not only of these newer scourges, but details how the older, known diseases may unwittingly turn into epidemics.

Garrett contributed a section on the Ebola virus in an article by Bernard Le Guenno, published in *Scientific American*, October 1995. As the subtitle of the article proclaimed, the Ebola virus is a hemorrhagic fever virus, considered among the most dangerous biological agents so far known. With new ones discovered yearly, natural and artificial environmental changes further their spread.

Le Guenno explains that hemorrhagic fever viruses mutate rapidly owing to their genetic makeup. Whereas the genes of most living things are composed of DNA, the genes of these viruses consist of RNA, and must be converted by an enzyme called *RNA polymerase* (RNA-directed DNA polymerase, or reverse transcriptase).

Frequent errors occur in the conversion process, resulting in an accumulation of mutations. The commonly used name *retrovirus* denotes this conversion or reversion. These changes or mutations negate the development of a vaccine.

The connection, of course, is with cancer. And it seems that humankind only solves one riddle to be confronted by another.

## REMEDIES IN NATURE

We first consider the commonly encountered herb known as *rue* (*Ruta graveolens* of the family Rutaceae). It is a plant loaded with alkaloids and considered excessively toxic. Nevertheless, it surfaces as a herbal remedy for various ailments. Listed in Hartwell's *Plants Used Against Cancer*, it has also been used against rabies, at least according to European folklore, as set forth by John Heinerman in *Healing Animals with Herbs*.

The explorer Carl Lumholtz traveled among the Papago Indians of southwestern Arizona and northwestern Sonora, Mexico during 1909–1910, and furnished a report titled *New Trails in Mexico: An Account of One Year's Exploration in North-Western Sonora, Mexico, and South-Western Arizona 1909-1910* (1912), of which a reproduction is available from the Rio Grande Press, Glorieta, New Mexico. He noted, for instance, that these Indians had a secret cure for rabies (Lumholtz, 1912, pp. 184, 185). Previously, an earlier record of his travels in Mexico was published as *Unknown Mexico: A Record of Five Years' Exploration among the Tribes of the Western Sierra Madre; in the Tierra Caliente of Tepic and Jalisco; and among the Tarascos of Michoacan*, in two volumes (1902), of which a reproduction is also available. Here, he had been specific, writing of a cure using the juice of rue, as well as olive oil, deer rennet, grape vinegar, and lemon juice (Lumholtz, 1902, II, p. 347). It can be presumed that the last four ingredients are superfluous.

Although not of primary interest at this point, John Heinerman devotes considerable space later in his animal book to the cure of rabies using the herb elecampane (Heinerman, 1977, pp. 61–65). Elecampane (*Inula helenium* of the plant family Compositae) is also listed in Hartwell's compendium as an anticancer agent. Still other plant cures such as yarrow are set forth in Heinerman's book, dating back to Gervase Markham's *Cheape and Good Husbandry*, published in London in 1614. (This date is approximately the Elizabethan Age, which produced the great English herbalists John Gerard, John Parkinson, and Nicholas Culpeper.)

Bringing matters somewhat more up to date, it may be mentioned that the Papago Indians of the American Southwest and northwestern Mexico were reported by Joseph G. Lee, M.D., to have a rabies cure. The cure, interestingly, also involved rue. Thus, Dr. Lee, in an article titled "Navajo Medicine Man" in the August 1961 issue of *Arizona Highways*, describes rue as a Navajo remedy for rabies. Another is said to be dog lichen, *Peltigear canina*, which received its name as a folkloric cure for rabies. Nevertheless, most of us would no doubt prefer a modern version of the Pasteur treatment.

Interestingly, in the same August 1961 issue of *Arizona Highways* it is acknowledged by Dr. Lee that the Navajos had long been vaccinating themselves for smallpox, though they refused to say just how long. There was the hint that the vaccination procedure may have been passed up from Mexico, as the Spaniards carried smallpox into the Americas in the sixteenth century and may have also introduced vaccination.

Primitive remedies for hydrophobia and other illnesses have been set down by Claude Lévi-Strauss in his study *The Savage Mind*, and according to Lévi-Strauss may be examples of totem transference (Lévi-Strauss, 1966, pp. 8, 9). Thus, animals and plants are not first known as the result of their usefulness, but instead are assumed useful because they are first known.

Lumholtz observed as well that a tea made by steeping the twigs and leaves of greasewood, also called the *creosote bush*, serves admirably as an antiseptic for wounds and, taken internally, as an antidote for gastric disturbances (Lumholtz, 1912, p. 222). Caution is in order, however, for the leaves of the Wyoming species of greasewood, *Sarcobatus vermiculatus*, are known to contain oxalates (or oxalic acid, which are poisonous in quantity), as do spinach and rhubarb. At the least, body calcium may be tied up as the oxalate, to be lost from the body system. (Both violet- and yellow-blooming oxalis or wood sorrel, known colloquially as *sheepshowers*, contain oxalic acid, which provides the distinctive taste, even to the wine that can be made from these more-easterly plants.) Furthermore, this species of Wyoming greasewood is also known as a *selenium concentrator*, from the selenium occurring in the soil.

In short, the other species of greasewood are to be distinguished from the Wyoming species. For example, the common evergreen greasewood or creosote bush or chaparral of the American Southwest is an entirely different species, which has been called *Larrea mexicana,* but more usually is called *Larrea tridentata* or *Larrea divaricata*. Yet, other species are also called greasewood.

It has both been rumored and reported that a tea made from greasewood roots (as per the above, also called creosote bush or chaparral, and of the genus *Larrea*) presumably can be taken internally as a cure for arthritis — see, for example, Virginia Madison, in *The Big Bend Country of Texas*, and Charles Francis Saunders, in *Western Wild Flowers and Their Stories* (Madison, 1955, p. 221; Saunders, 1933, p. 287). In fact, it is said that an ointment made from the same greasewood or creosote bush roots can be rubbed on the afflicted joints and serves to remove aches and pains. The South American explorer Colonel P. H. Fawcett cited bloodroot (*Sanguinaria canadensis*) as being a surefire cure for advanced arthritis or rheumatism. (It has also been used in a toothpaste manufactured by the pharmaceutical company Vipont as a means of tarter control.) Colonel Fawcett further commented that there were a hundred remedies for everything he knew of, though the medical profession does not encourage their use (Fawcett, 1953, p. 182). He stated that the cures are often remarkable, and he speaks as one who has successfully used them, mainly as teas.

(Bloodroot is also used sometimes as a cure for cancer, e.g., in a substance called *Compound-X*, and likewise used is chaparral or creosote bush or greasewood, as it is variously called, and which will be detailed subsequently. At the least, a couple of other reported cancer cures hail from South America, namely, pau d'arco and cundurango or condurango, the condor vine, to be further discussed. Still another is called *cat's claw, or uña de gato*, also to be discussed.)

The greasewood or creosote bush or chaparral is also called by still other names. Thus, the Mexican people sometimes call it *Yerba hedionda* or "stink bush," for the leaves have an acrid, disagreeable odor (Madison, 1955, pp. 226–228). Alternatively, it is called *hediondilla*, the "little bad smeller," or *gobernadora*, the "governess," for its beneficial medicinal properties (Saunders, 1933, pp. 287, 288).

In her book about the Big Bend region, which is in the Chihuahuan desert, Virginia Madison includes a chapter on the "Botany of the Big Bend" that describes some of the other more interesting plants found here. Presumably, some or all of these unique plants should be further studied for their medicinal properties.

Other common plants have been used variously for teas and liniments: dandelion roots for poison ivy rash, the plantain leaf for insect bites and stings, aloe vera for almost everything, sunflowers for malaria, and the roots also for poison ivy rash, even snakebite. A partial mention is contained in Laura C. Martin's *Wildflower Folklore*. The doctrine of signatures enters into the folklore, whereby similarities in appearance between parts of a plant and parts of the human anatomy are supposed to suggest a connection, and hence a cure.

Still other information on native plant sources is contained in Michael More's *Medicinal Plants of the Mountain West* and in Melvin R. Gilmore's *Uses of Plants by the Indians of the Missouri River Region*.

Virgil J. Vogel has compiled and written *American Indian Medicine*. Kelly Kindscher has in turn authored *Medicinal Wild Plants of the Prairie: An Ethnobotanical Guide*, as well as *Edible Wild Plants of the Prairie: An Ethnobotanical Guide*. Other books include those by Alma R. Hutchens, *Indian Herbalogy of North America* and *A Handbook of Native American Herbs*, Daniel E. Moerman's two-volume *Medicinal Plants of Native America*, and *The Swimmer Manuscript of Cherokee Sacred Formulas and Medicinal Prescriptions* by James Vogel, issued by the Smithsonian Institution back in 1932. Further back, there was a rare effort by Dr. O. Phelps Brown titled *The Complete Herbalist*, which was published in 1875.

It is well known that the juice of the grape, or wine, serves as an antiseptic. It has a chemical kinship with phenol, which is alternately known as *carbolic acid*. Honey, in different ways, also serves as an antibiotic or disinfectant. And there is blackberry juice for diarrhea, cherry juice for gout, and more in the long list of native herbal remedies and folk medicines.

(Regarding arthritis and greasewood, the latest wrinkle going around is to spray a little WD-40 on the affected joint. Could this in fact be a totem transference?)

Homesteader J. O. Langford, in *Big Bend*, noted the medicinal properties of the green desert shrub popotillo. It appears that the Indians of Mexico, particularly, possess greater awareness of the value of plant life. Some of the flora of the more desertlike regions even require salt and alkali (sodium chloride and sodium carbonate) to flourish (Berlandier, 1980, II, p. 411). This is of potential value in the usage and desalination of brackish waters via irrigation, as is the growing of kelp and saltwater-active algae in an aqueous medium.

Another unusual plant of the American Southwest and Mexico is the bushlike guayule, which produces a form of natural rubber or latex, as do many other plants, even the dandelion, but not in sufficient quantity. The guayule, however, was employed during WWII when the Malaysian sources of natural rubber were cut off.

The southwestern jojoba plant is a source of high-quality lubricating oil, such as required in the automatic transmissions of automobiles and is a suitable replacement for sperm oil, the oil once obtained from the now-endangered sperm whale. Then there is the candelilla plant, which is used for candle wax, as the name infers.

The mystical regions of Mexico and the great Southwest have not only furnished the dietary staple maize, or corn, but are home to the hot pepper, of the genus *Capsicum*, whose active ingredient is called *capsaicin*. It characterizes the great cuisine collectively known as Mexican food, or "Tex-Mex," and has health-giving properties as well. Richard Schweid has written a book about this interesting plant and its history and uses, featuring the adjunct Louisiana hot sauce. For more books on this plant, Jim Robbins expounds at length in the January 1992 issue of the *Smithsonian*, and provides a Who's Who both in pepper authorities and in authoritative peppers. In the November 1992 issue of *Texas Highways*, Randy Mallory expands on the Jalapeño and other burning issues, and rates peppers in "Scoville heat units." Another book is Jean Andrews' *Peppers: The Domesticated Capsicums*, published by the University of Texas Press. This has been followed up with a cookbook by Andrews titled *Good and Hot: Capsicum Cookery*. At the end of his article in *Texas Highways*, Mallory also provides a few recipes. Amal Naj is the author of *Peppers: Hot, Hotter, Hottest*, part of which was condensed in the July 1993 issue of *Reader's Digest*. Whether there is a definite link to anticancer action or cures remains to be seen.

Back to South America, in the appendix of his book *The Rivers Ran East*, about exploring the headwaters of the Amazon, Leonard Clark lists many native Indian pharmaceuticals known at the time, approximately about 1946. Other descriptions contained in the text, if not specific, are certainly intriguing. Earlier, as has been indicated, Colonel P. H. Fawcett had made a number of entries in his journals, published as *Lost Trails, Lost Cities*. It may be assumed that many more are known today, as studies of the Amazonian rain forest proliferate, before time runs out, in the face of its continued destruction.

A key modern-day figure is ethnobotanist Mark J. Plotkin, who for many years has maintained a frequent visiting residency in Amazonia. His book, *Tales of a Shaman's Apprentice*, details some of the mysterious cures of this twilight world. Plotkin helped found the California-based Shaman Pharmaceuticals in 1987, which has in turn founded The Healing Forest Conservancy, a nonprofit organization. Another prominent name in collecting the mystery substances of the jungle is Mark Chandler, whose company is Inland Laboratories, based at Austin, TX. Chandler was profiled in an article by Toni Mack, which appeared in the May 23, 1994, issue of *Forbes* magazine. Inland's specialty is toxins, viruses, and other proteins, some of which are deadly in the extreme but might lead to new therapies. The news items continue to multiply; see, for instance, the May 1994 issue of *Profiles*, the magazine of Continental Airlines. Here, in an article about Belize, author Ray Scippa mentioned the Belizean Association of Traditional Healers, who are cataloguing the plants in a 6000-acre preserve of old-growth forest and submitting samples to the New York Botanical Gardens, which is in turn working with the National Cancer Institute to determine medicinal properties. Still another name, is David G. Williams [Mountain Home Publishing, P.O. Box 829, Ingram TX 78025, (210)367-4492].

Dr. Williams is no stranger to the jungle and publishes his own newsletter and other in-house publications, including *The Doctor's Worldwide Encyclopedia of Natural Remedies*.

Other Texas sources that sponsor expeditions to Amazonia include the Texas Pharmacy Foundation and the Austin-based American Botanical Council, whose director is Mark Blumenthal. Workshops are also sponsored at the Amazon Center for Environmental Education and Research. It is located in the 250,000-acre Amazon Biosphere Reserve, some 50 miles from the Amazon River port city of Iquitos, Peru. Blumenthal notes that out of the 250,000-plus plant species around the world, only about 5,000 have been investigated in detail for their human health potential. He further comments that each year an area of the rain forest roughly equal to the size of Indiana is being destroyed. He also mentions that somewhere out there in this plant pharmacopoeia may be a cure for cancer and AIDS, if it has not been already destroyed.

But now, in the reaches of the Amazon and in other scarcely known fecundities of plant and animal life, as the new generations of natives who do not know the traditional ways succeed the old, the chain may be irretrievably broken and the knowledge forever lost, along with the forest itself. This is a special concern of Mark Blumenthal. There is the question of whether science and technology are staying one step ahead of nature or one step behind.

Lastly, speaking of medical folklore in general, worldwide, mention should be made of Napralert, the University of Chicago's enormous database of biochemical and ethnomedical references. ("Napra" pertains to a therapeutic system.) A particular application of this database is described by Steven Kotler on p. 46 of the January 2005 issue of *Wired*. A Mayo Clinic researcher named Eric Buenz has been searching old medical textbooks and references for potential pharmaceuticals and treatments. In particular, the *Ambronese Herbal* is cited, a guide to some 1300 plants used against diseases in seventeenth-century Indonesia, as compiled by employees of the Dutch Indonesia Company.

Buenz was interested in plants that were mentioned in the old references but did not have a modern counterpart, as listed in Napralert. His computer search uncovered a few that did not have a match, and the search continues for others via the Kirtas Technologies book scanner, at about 1000 pages per hour.

For the record, the following plant species did not have a match with modern listings: lontar tree (*Licula rumphi*), used against TB and colitis and which may have potential as an anti-infective agent; mealy palm sago tree (*Metroxylon sagu*), for healing wounds and sores, with potential as an antibacterial agent; wild cadju tree (*Semecarpus cassuvium*), used against shingles, with potential as an antiviral, analgesic, and anti-inflammatory agent; anona tree (*Anona reticulata*), used against diarrhea and dysentery, with potential as an opiate; Maldivian coconut (*Lodoicea maldivica*), used against inflammation and fever, with potential as an anti-inflammatory and antipyretic (antifever agent); wild dragon tree (*Dracontomelon sylvestre*), used against gonorrhea, with potential as an antibiotic, anti-infective, and antitreponema agent. (The *Treponema* are a genus of parasites, including those causing syphilis and yaws.) It may be added that the particular genus for each of the plant species cited in the preceding text may also contain other species with medicinal properties.

Other guides from around the same time period, notably the Elizabethan Age, can be listed as follows: John Gerard's *The Herbal, or General History of Plants* (first published in 1597), which came to be known as *Gerard's Herbal*, John Parkinson's *Theatrum Botanicum* (1640), and *Culpeper's Complete Herbal* (about 1649–1653) by Nicolas Culpeper. The latter guide was translated into modern English by Graeme Tobyn, and titled *Culpeper's Medicine: A Practice of Western Holistic Medicine*. Later on there was George Graves' *Hortus Medicus*, published in 1834 and republished as *Medicinal Plants* in 1990.

Given that plant names, both common and scientific, sometimes change, the potential is viewed as a "pharmacological goldmine." Further information about anticancer plants is awaited, though Hartwell's *Plants Used Against Cancer* is a good reference point. Additionally, further citations about anticancer plants or herbals are contained throughout of the book you are now reading.

The ultimate question, of course, is whether these plant remedies really work, and if so, what the side effects are. Are they serious? Dosage levels and frequency, methods of administration, and biochemical individuality have to be considered. The bottom line becomes the risk/benefit trade-off.

## POISONS IN NATURE

Not that all plants are beneficial, directly or indirectly. Some are poisonous, such as Jimsonweed and the assorted nightshades, not to mention the hemlocks and the delphiniums or larkspurs. Alkaloids are a presence in plants called *locoweeds* or *crazyweeds* and can ruin a good horse. Grazing on larkspurs is a good way to wipe out a dairy herd overnight, although the Texas longhorns are said not to be affected. This anomaly may be due to the longhorns' nonselective grazing habits, which dilute the effects of the poison, or maybe they have a unique digestive and body chemistry.

Poisonous plants, by and large, are the most medically active in controlled doses, that is, in small or minute amounts. Digitalis, used for heart trouble, is obtained from the foxglove. Also there is atropine, derived from belladonna, or deadly nightshade, and used for such purposes as pupil dilation in ophthalmology. This is not necessarily a blanket endorsement, however, for there are poisonous plants that remain poisonous whatever the use.

There has been a succession of books dealing with poisonous plants. To list a few: *Poisonous Plants of the United States* by Walter Conrad Muenscher (1939); *Deadly Harvest: A Guide to Common Poisonous Plants* by John M. Kingsbury (1965), and Kingsbury's more comprehensive *Poisonous Plants of the United States and Canada* (1964); *Human Poisoning from Native and Cultivated Plants* by James W. Hardin and Jay M. Arena (1969, 1974); and *Poisonous Plants: A Color Field Guide* by Lucia Woodward (1985). We find that such medicinal plants as bloodroot, used for arthritis and cancer, have poisonous or toxic properties. With bloodroot (*Sanguinaria canadensis*) for instance, the poisonous component is an alkaloid called *sanguinarine* that can be selectively extracted and also used as a medicinal drug. Yew trees of the family Taxaceae contain the poisonous alkaloid *taxine* (Hardin and

Arena, 1974, p. 42). Nevertheless, the newly touted cancer drug Taxol is derived from the yew of the Pacific coast *(Taxus brevifolia)*.

However, it has been commented that research on the toxicology of poisonous plants has been sorely neglected (Kingsbury, 1965, p. 8). This is regrettable in more ways than one, as the poisonous plants are more biologically active and their study may yield clues to cures for such diseases as cancer.

Toxic substances can be divided into alkaloids, glycosides or glucosides, goitrogens, oxalates, phytoxins, and resinoids (Woodward, 1985, pp. 21, 22; Muenscher, 1939, p. 4ff). Other divisions or subdivisions can also be made. The alkaloids are complex substances that contain chemically bound nitrogen. Alkaloids of some 5000 different types have been identified and are found in about 10% of the plant or vegetable kingdom, irrespective of genera or species (Woodward, 1985, p. 21; Kingsbury, 1964, p. 19). The glycosides or glucosides are sugar related, and may be divided principally into cyanogenetic glucosides and saponin glucosides, though there are other divisions. The former will yield hydrocyanic acid upon hydrolyis; the latter are characterized by their ability to lather and act like soap. Muenscher further states that there are plants that cause dermatitis and photosensitization, and another class of plants is characterized as cyanogenetic, as previously noted, because they may produce hydrocyanic acid, or prussic acid. He speaks of introduced poisonous ornamental plants and plants whose seeds are poisonous. There are seleniferous plants that act as soil selenium concentrators, plants that produce an undesirable flavor in milk or milk products, and even plants that can cause mechanical injury, especially those armored with thorns or stickers. He provides examples of each of these categories.

Excluding cyanide, the principal toxic source in plants is from the alkaloids (Kingsbury, 1964, p. 18ff). This is surprising, considering the large number of other nitrogen-bearing compounds in plants, for example, the protein content. The alkaloids are all nitrogen-containing compounds with certain basic or alkali-like properties, such as forming salts with acids, and hence their name. Kingsbury provides a few specific examples of these compounds and their chemical structures out of the many possibilities: tropane, pyrrolizidine, pyridine, isoquinoline, indole, quinolozidine, and certain steroid alkaloids, for example, solanidine, veratramine, and delphinine. Kingsbury also includes a small number of polypeptides and amines, both classes of which are also nitrogen-containing compounds. Amines are a compositional unit of the polymers that comprise proteins, and polypeptides are but relatively shorter-length proteins. (It may be noted that these nitrogen-containing compounds are sometimes associated with various treatments for cancer.)

Some plants such as the milk vetches, even Wyoming's greasewood *(Sarcobatus vermiculatus)*, are known to selectively absorb selenium, which is toxic. Also referred to as locoweed, these plants are an added hazard to ranching in the high-selenium belt of southern Wyoming. A horse that grazes on these plants ends up becoming "hooked" and preferring them as feed to all other plants. The active ingredient is the selenium content and/or the alkaloid content. Moreover, newborn livestock exhibit deformities. In high enough concentrations, death is the outcome.

Climbing west from Laramie, Wyoming, for a specific instance, the highway skirts and overlooks the Big Hollow, which is notorious as a high-selenium rangeland. Here the selenium indicator plants (e.g., the woody aster and the milk vetches) demark the soil and even give off a characteristic selenium odor. Other major occurrences are along the Sweetwater River in west/central Wyoming. The Navajo Indian Reservation in northwest Arizona is characterized as being rife with selenium-bearing rock formations.

A book has been written about the harmful effects of selenium, especially from the point of view of the livestock business. Written by Tom Harris and titled *Death in the Marsh*, it is the result of a 10-year effort. A condensation appeared in the *High Country News*, February 10, 1992. (The *HCN* is perhaps the premier environmental news source for much of the Rocky Mountain West. Founded by Tom Bell at Lander, Wyoming, it is now published at Paonia, Colorado, on Colorado's Western Slope.) Harris refers considerably to the investigations of geologist J. David Love, who was featured in John McPhee's *Rising from the Plains*, and to the pioneering work of University of Wyoming chemist Orville A. Beath. It is observed that selenium indicator plants have largely proliferated over many parts of the range, probably owing to the plant parts and seed being spread out in the hay used for cattle feeding, by the presence of selenium in phosphate fertilizers, and by the processes of mining. This means that these plants produce water-soluble selenium compounds, which are then picked up by other plants and grasses. These are then grazed by wildlife and livestock, even if the same animals naturally avoid the selenium indicator plants. (The buffalo is an exception and is thought not to be affected by selenium.) The problem is thereby compounded. Needless to say, all this is not a popular subject in the livestock industry. In addition to lowering land values, there is the suspicion that the product may be tainted, ending up in the food chain, that is, the human food chain.

(The role of selenium as a trace element in the human diet is, apparently, a different matter. It may have beneficial properties and may even be essential, a subject that is being researched. For instance, in minute amounts, it may be a preventative for heart attacks, and there have been attempts to statistically correlate the presence of selenium in the soil with the prevalence or nonprevalence of certain diseases, including the incidence of cancer.)

In Wyoming, it is said that a cow that eats skunk cabbage on the 21st day of pregnancy will bear a calf with a Cyclops eye.

Weeds are sometimes an unknown hazard, either containing such commonplace chemicals as hydrocyanic-acid-releasing compounds or poisonous alkaloids of unknown complexity. The Cooperative Extension Service of the College of Agriculture at the University of Wyoming has issued two informative and comprehensive publications, with outstanding color photos. One is titled *Weeds and Poisonous Plants of Wyoming and Utah*, and the other, even more extensive, is titled *Weeds of the West*. Most of the poisonous plants are listed and described. The Phillips Petroleum Company, Bartlesville, Oklahoma, which also produces agricultural chemicals, notably fertilizers, once published a series of tracts on pasture and range plants, with superb artwork. Now out of print, one volume was titled *Poisonous Grassland Plants* and another, *Undesirable Grasses and Forbs*. Ben Green, the old horse trader, in

*The Village Horse Doctor: West of the Pecos*, has described his encounters, problems, and adventures with such poisonous plants as "yellowweed" in, about, and around Fort Stockton, Texas.

According to a dictionary, the term *yellowweed* could apply to a species of goldenrod, genus *Solidago*, or else to a species of ragwort that is also called *groundsel*, genus *Senecio*. According to the volume *Weeds of the West*, a particular species known as Riddell groundsell (*Senecio riddellii*), is poisonous to cattle and sheep, the toxic agents being pyrrolizidine alkaloids (PAs), as also the related species called *threadleaf groundsel*, *S. longilobus*, and *broom groundsel*, *S. spartioides*. In fact, it is noted on pages 89 and 90 of this book that the genus *Senecio* has more than 100 species that contain hepatotoxic PAs, out of a total of more than 1000 species in the genus, some of which are described in Ruth Ashton Nelson's *Handbook of Rocky Mountain Plants*. Other toxic species include the more common *S. jacobaea* and *S. vulgaris*. The fact that Ben Green wrote that he had developed an antidote is of more than passing interest, whatever the antidote was.

Hydrogen cyanide or hydrocyanic acid, sometimes called *prussic acid*, is formed in numerous plant species during the growth cycle, especially in early growth. This is a problem for both livestock and humans, and the contaminant is to be avoided or else removed, for example, by heating during cooking. It may be tied up in complex chemical structures, as in the case of the cassava or manioc root, which calls for a complicated refining process to produce edible tapioca.

The harvester of newly emerged poke greens from the pokeweed can remove parts of the plant that are poisonous by repeated boiling and washing, which are relatively easy methods; parts of the mature plant can prove fatal. On the other hand, preparation of the old-time remedy with the terrible taste, castor oil, from the even more poisonous castor bean requires a good deal of care. (Fortunately the poisonous component in the beans is not soluble in the oil produced.) The roots of the growing plant are equally fatal to the underground encroachment of moles into the garden, and plantings are made for this purpose. In both these plants, the deadly component is a kind of protein toxin found in certain snake venoms.

Moreover, the parts of many common flowering plants that are raised in homes and gardens can be lethal. And at certain times of the growing cycle, as noted, even ordinary forage can be harmful to livestock. Common ordinary Johnson grass can be a problem, as can growing alfalfa, which can be toxic early on.

There are poisonous principles in other common foods (Kingsbury, 1965, p. 22ff). For instance, lima beans contain (bound) hydrogen cyanide and those grown in South America contain more of it, which can lead to poisoning when fed to livestock. Eating large quantities of onions can provoke anemia. Cabbage, turnips, rutabaga, and other members of the cabbage family contain a chemical called L-5-vinylthiooxazolidone (VTO), which can lead to goiter by preventing the thyroid gland from utilizing iodine. Spinach and rhubarb are also mentioned as sources of oxalic acid, which depletes the body of calcium.

The common Irish potato and the tomato belong to the plant family *Solanaceae*, also called the *nightshade family* or the *potato family*. It is the same family to which the various nightshades belong, including belladonna. In fact, the potato and the tomato are of the same genus *Solanum*, and the leaves of both the potato plant and the tomato plant contain the poisonous alkaloid solanine. For this reason, the discarded vines should not be fed to livestock, much less humans. Additionally, the potato or tuber itself contains small concentrations of solanine, more so in the "eyes" (a reason for the custom of cutting out the eyes before cooking, though cooking tends to destroy or decompose the solanine). Moreover, potatoes sometimes have green skin and green sprouts. These contain much higher concentrations of solanine and should be avoided altogether, though it is said that the rest of the potato is considered edible if the green parts are first removed.

As for livestock and livestock diseases per se, in his explorations of Tibetan frontiers, Leonard Clark, in his book *The Marching Wind*, reported hearing of cures and controls for both rinderpest and anthrax from the fierce Ngolok tribesmen he encountered. (As previously noted, in his earlier book *The Rivers Ran East*, about exploring the headwaters of the Amazon, Colonel Clark listed many of the native Indian pharmaceuticals then known.)

Additionally, there are the numerous poisonous or near-poisonous species of the insect world, not to mention snakes. In a class by itself in the United States is the brown recluse spider, whose bite causes a sloughing off of the tissue around the wound, producing a cavity. The processes are complex, and a recognized authority is biochemist Collis Geren of the University of Arkansas. Another authority is Gary W. Tamkin, M.D., of the Highland General Hospital, Alameda Medical Center, Oakland, CA; he also holds the position of clinical instructor at the University of California, San Francisco.

The brown recluse spider is also called the *violin spider* or *fiddleback*, after the small violin-shaped marking on its back. (There is an occasional alert, e.g., an article appeared in the May 1993 issue of *Good Housekeeping* that was picked up by the press. A condensed version appeared in the September 1993 issue of the *Reader's Digest*.) Immediate treatment may involve the localized injection of steroids or cortisone. Later, a skin graft may be necessary. Other strange insect bites are also possible, with the black widow spider being the most infamous, its red hourglass marking a distinguishing feature, and the centipede is also suspected in many cases. Australia and other parts of the world have their own poisonous indigenous critters.

(For an entertaining look at these kinds of varmints, one may consult Roger M. Knutson's *Furtive Fauna: A Field Guide to the Creatures Who Live on You*. Included in the dossier are ticks, chiggers, mosquitoes, flies, bedbugs, and fleas. Knutson also wrote *Flattened Fauna: A Field Guide to Common Animals of Roads, Streets, and Highways*.)

We now turn to treatments and antidotes, including serums. One of the more drastic measures is called *intubation with charcoal* (of which mycologists who deal with poisonous mushrooms are well aware), whereby the patient's blood is withdrawn and cycled through a charcoal filter. The toxins are adsorbed by the charcoal. Unfortunately, other life-giving constituents of the blood are also adsorbed, making the treatment a dubious procedure at best. In the case of poisonous mushrooms, for instance, vomiting or a stomach pump may suffice, or a massive injection of penicillin, etc.

In another odd case, it has been reported that the Incas used a softening agent (a liquid) to fit their stone structures together without mortar (Fawcett, 1953, pp.

272, 273). It softened the stone surfaces to the consistency of clay, permitting a joining.

(Digressing still further, the Papagoes had their own version of the flood story [Lumholtz, 1912, p. 100, 103], in common with other peoples, as found by Velikovsky and reported in *Worlds in Collision*. Similarly, the Tarahumare Indians [also spelled "Tarahumara"] of the western Sierra Madre of Mexico not only had a deluge legend but a creation myth as well [Lumholtz, 1902, I, p. 296, 298]. Other than the Tarahumare, the Huichol Indians also had a tradition of the deluge and also of an ark [Lumholtz, 1902, II, p. 191]. The Tarahumare range over and through some of the most spectacular country in North America, the Sierra Madre Occidental, in which occurs the Barranca de Cobre [Copper Canyon], which in places is said to be deeper than the Grand Canyon of Arizona. The scenic railroad that traverses the area is a display of modern, and not-so-modern, ingenuity. Deep in the gorge flows a stream, the river Urique, where a traveler once provided a footnote about a colony of otters that were dangerous and life-threatening, providing a completely different view of the otter clan. Between detective stories, the prolific writer Erle Stanley Gardner was a wanderer in this part of the world, and his enthusiasm comes across in *Neighborhood Frontiers*. An update on the region is furnished in John M. Fayhee's *Mexico's Copper Canyon Country: A Hiking and Backpacking Guide to Tarahumara-Land*. Their prowess as long-distance runners, especially the girls, is described on pages 128 to 130 of John Heinerman's *The Spiritual Wisdom of the Native Americans*.)

In Ivan Sanderson's *Book of Great Jungles*, it is told how the forest floor of the jungle is impregnated with all kinds of molds and fungi that have an action similar to penicillin. Hence, to walk barefoot through the jungle, as the natives do, is healthy. The ways of the world are often beneficial for unsuspected reasons. (Incidentally, Alain Gheerbrant, on page 262 of his book *The Impossible Adventure: Journey to the Far Amazon*, noted that salicylic acid [aspirin] prevents mold from forming.)

Listings of bioactive/toxic plants found in the United States are presented in Appendix I of the first edition of the Hoffman cancer book. Listings of common garden or ornamental plants that have caused poisonings are cause for reflection and have been abstracted as follows from various poison control centers (Lampe, in *Toxicology*, pp. 804, 805). For the record, the listings include the following common names, not necessarily in any particular order: philodendron, jade plant, wandering Jew, Swedish ivy, dieffenbachia or dumbcane, asparagus fern, aloe, string-of-pearls, pothos, poinsettia, schefflera (of the Ginseng family), holly, pyracantha, pokeweed, yew, azalea, ornamental pepper, mountain ash, honeysuckle, apricot and other pits, horse chestnut, sweet pea, creeping Charlie, Jimsonweed, Oregon grape, tulip, nightshade, coleus (of the mint family), Brazilian pepper, rosary pea, pencil tree cactus, oleander, ixora, allamanda, coral plant, balsam pear, angel's trumpet, bischofia, hibiscus, sea grape, crown-of-thorns, croton, and bottlebrush.

The subject is further presented in Chapter 2 through Chapter 4 of the aforementioned Hoffman cancer reference, with particular emphasis on alkaloids as found in common garden vegetables and fruits (Hoffman, 1999, p. 154ff), and such other expected and unexpected sources for alkaloids and other toxic constituents (Hoffman, 1999, p. 160ff).

## FROM THE ORDINARY TO THE BIZARRE

In *A Thousand Miles of Mustangin'*, about a horse-gathering expedition down into the parts of Old Mexico in times past, Ben Green reminds us of the very common origins of penicillin. Here, an Indian medicine woman used bread mold to cure an infected horse bite on Ben's arm. Another annotation is that the ancient Chinese would induce a mold on a sliced orange half and use this against infections.

In Francis L. and Roberta B. Fugate's *Roadside History of Oklahoma,* the story is recounted about the settlers' baby who became seriously ill but was saved by a group of Cheyenne and Arapaho women. They wrapped the baby in blankets and placed him on a paddle used to retrieve bread from the Indians' beehive oven. After alternately "baking" the baby and bathing him for 10 days and nights, the baby recovered. Growing up healthy but with a limp, he was later diagnosed as having had spinal meningitis, a usually fatal disease at that time. Interestingly, the Indians' treatment was similar to that developed nearly a half-century later by the famous Australian nurse Sister Elizabeth Kenny to treat poliomyelitis.

The unexpected may turn out to be the commonplace, and the commonplace may turn out to be the unexpected. It is part of the mystery and mystique that surrounds us, which can range from the ordinary to the explainable and finally to the unexplainable, with regard to our concerns about cancer.

The health consequences from the world we live in can take more bizarre twists. Ergot, a fungus or mold found in cereal grains, such as rye used for bread, is noted to produce traces of lysergic acid. This is a component of the diethyl amide of lysergic acid, called *LSD*. It is said that the persons persecuted in the Salem, Massachusetts, witchcraft trials were inadvertently under the influence of this potentially hallucinogenic material, which affected some but not others (Hoffman, 1999, pp. 165, 177). We rely on modern fumigation practices to eliminate this problem from stored grains.

The common aspergillus fungus has been traced as the "agent" of the curse of the Pharaohs, whereby people have died after opening ancient tombs. The mold, present everywhere, grows to elevated concentrations in graves, vaults, and crypts and causes respiratory failure.

(The fungi, or Mycota, which include molds, yeasts, smuts, rusts, mildews, and mushrooms, have no chlorophyll, do not require sunlight, and therefore are saprobic or saprogenic, that is, living on other organic matter or organisms, or parasitic. They require moisture, however, but may or may not require air, that is, they may be either aerobic or anaerobic. Thus, some kind of fungus can be found most anywhere.)

Unexpectedly, care must be exercised in the use of honey. For honey, and indeed the very soils beneath us, contain botulinuses, the bacteria that produce the toxins leading to botulism. In most cases, the acidity of the human digestive system renders these microorganisms harmless. The digestive systems of infants and toddlers, however, are more or less neutral, which is why, in their case, honey is on the forbidden list. It has been advanced that botulism may be responsible for crib deaths.

## THE ENVIRONMENT, NATURALLY AND NOT SO NATURALLY

Consider the routine practice of using herbicides and pesticides on fruit and vegetable crops before, during, and after the harvest. Anybody who is complacent about the condition of fruits and vegetables at the store should read *Pesticide Alert* by Laurie Mott and Karen Snyder. (As washing is so often ineffective, it goes without saying that the outer layer or peeling of both fruits and vegetables should not be eaten. And don't be like the initiate who described bananas as pretty good except for being mostly core.)

The role of toxic chemicals in the environment, particularly in inducing cancer but also causing other health effects, is obscured by conflicting interpretations. There is a fog of semantic confusion about what is meant by poisonous vs. merely toxic, of acute vs. chronic, and of immediate vs. long term. Succinctly stated, the argument is about the time interval between "cause" and "effect." If the time interval is short, then the effect presumably can be connected with cause. If the time interval is long, as in the development of cancer, it cannot be readily "proved" to develop from a cause unless there is an irrefutable consensus of physical, chemical, and biological evidence, as in the case of asbestosis and black lung disease. The mechanisms of cause and effect become replaced by the ambiguities of statistics, which to a lay person can be used to prove or disprove most anything.

The situation is further complicated by the insidious and inexact usage of "threshold" limits. Any time the concept of a threshold or cutoff limit is introduced, it will run afoul of the idea of continuity. That is, if the threshold is exceeded by only a minute (or imperceptible or infinitesimal) fraction, then for all practical purposes, what is the difference? The answer, of course, is none. And if this minute fraction be exceeded by a successive minute fraction, then again the practical difference is nil, and so on. If a finite or discrete interval is adapted as a go or no-go criterion, then what is to be the situation within the interval? Is it to be a gray no-man's-land and therefore not defined? This paradox is not admissible, however, if a go or no-go decision is required within the interval.

(The idea of discontinuity vs. continuity is at the heart of the abortion or aborticide issue. The abortion and prochoice advocates argue that there is a matter of degree in pregnancy, a point before which a babe in the womb is not a human being. The antiabortion and prolife advocates argue that there is no such thing as a "little bit" pregnant and that life is life, human is human, and the human life in the womb is without sin. They further state that there is no point in growth at which it is possible to make the distinction between human life and nonlife. In other words, for example, what is the difference between exactly three months and one second, and three months minus one second? Or reduce the difference to milliseconds, microseconds, or nanoseconds, etc.)

However, the concepts of statistics and threshold limits introduce a dehumanization by which individual case studies can be ignored and put out of mind. The controversy over the effects of low-level and not-so-low-level radiation is a well-documented example, which is still largely unresolved. (As an aside, petals of the spiderwort can be used to detect low-level radiation. They will change color in about

2 weeks.) Many of the issues have been dealt with in at least a couple of books, for example, as reviewed by Thomas Powers in an article in the May 1994 issue of the *Atlantic Monthly*. In one book, *American Ground Zero: The Secret Nuclear War* by Carole Gallagher, the effect of nuclear radiation on the people and livestock in Nevada and Utah is dramatically highlighted. In the other, *Atomic Harvest: Hanford and the Lethal Toll of America's Nuclear Arsenal* by Michael D'Antonio, the mistakes and consequences of nuclear processing have been detailed.

The dispute over the use and effects of Agent Orange is another dilemma (Agent Orange is a mixture of 2,4-dichlorophenoxyacetic acid (2,4-D) and 2,4,5-trichlorophenoxyacetic acid (2,4,5-T) contaminated with dioxins, all of which are toxic in varying degree, depending on what is meant by the word). Among the later scientific studies is the large and comprehensive volume *Veterans and Agent Orange: Health Effects of Herbicides Used in Vietnam*, issued by the Institute of Medicine, Washington, D.C., in 1994. Now it is rumored that herbicides, or something as noxious, may have been used in the Gulf War, that is, in Operation Desert Storm.

A comparison of Michael Gough's detached explanation *Dioxin, Agent Orange* and Elmo Zumwalt's intensely personal account *My Father, My Son* says it all. It is the issue of statistics vs. the individual, of depersonalized science vs. humanness.

In each case, the argument can be made that the circumstance should be judged and decided on its own merits, with the recognition that each individual is unique and will react differently to a toxic agent. It will affect some adversely, and in others it may appear to have no effect. In a catchall way of expressing it, some individuals may exhibit an "allergic" response, others may not, or may in a lesser degree. It may all be in the genes. To be able to predict this individual response in advance is a formidable undertaking. It may involve, as the end goal, immunization. The fact that some persons will contract a disease when exposed and others will not is an enigma. Even when two persons are bitten by the same rabid animal, one might succumb and the other may not. These arguments, of course, apply to cancer also.

Also, by hand-picking the "fact-finding" committee consisting of the judge and the jury, any desired conclusion can be reached. So if perspective is needed, go behind the scenes and determine the background and interests of the individual committee members: who pays the salaries, who supplies the grants and contracts, who does business with whom, etc. In other words, find out which side of the bread is buttered.

(If one wants to explore what the technical experts have to say about the array of chlorinated organic chemicals and, in particular, dioxins and their spectrum of health effects, an examination of monographs by invited participants is recommended: consider *Dioxin: Toxicological and Chemical Aspects* and *Dioxins in the Environment*. Despite a variety of interpretations and an occasional disclaimer, the experimental and observed results indicate that at least some of these materials have serious and fatal consequences. The same recommendations can be made for the effects of low-level radiation or any other hazard. Popular and scientific accounts sometimes disagree; obviously one or the other may have an axe to grind. Nevertheless, sensationalism will at least bring things out into the open. Involved are large sums in claims and settlements and to what degree society must pay, directly or indirectly, for advancing technologies. The topic is dissected from a number of standpoints in *The High Cost of High Tech* by Lenny Siegel and John Markoff. Genetic engineering may have disastrous consequences in the future, as portended by Jeremy Rifkin in *Algeny*, by Charles Piller and Keith R. Yamamoto in *Gene Wars*, and by many others. It seems that there are side effects to everything. To think otherwise is akin to whistling in the dark.)

Examples of chlorinated compounds in the environment abound. Dichlorodiphenyltrichloroethane (DDT) is the most common example cited. Whether the use of DDT to control malaria is offset by its other impacts on the environment, e.g., the reproductive cycle of birds and other animals, is moot. (The chemical pyrethrum, described as a toxic, nonvolatile kerosene-type hydrocarbon, is an insecticide that was first derived from the flowers of a species of chrysanthemum and has emerged as a possible substitute for DDT. DDT and similar chemicals have since been synthesized, obviating the need for native sources from mountainous central Africa.)

Air pollution *per se* is for the most part tied in with automobile-derived pollutants, namely, *smog*, which is ozone related (ozone having the chemical formula $O_3$ as distinguished from normal molecular oxygen, or $O_2$), and with the loss of Freon refrigerants to the atmosphere, though there are plenty of other sources. The supplementing of gasoline with oxygenated fuels such as ethanol (ethyl alcohol) or methanol (methyl alcohol) is thought to alleviate the problem, but may cause still other problems. (The resulting mixture, with up to 10% oxygenated compounds, is uniformly called *gasohol*.) In particular, the use of MTBA (methyl *tert*-butyl alcohol) is thought to cause respiratory problems, inasmuch as other chemical pollutants such as formaldehyde may result from its combustion or partial combustion. The perception is that the newer cars, with efficient catalytic converters and computer-controlled air/fuel combustion mixtures, work well enough even with the conventional hydrocarbon gasoline.

(This is apart from global warming, which is caused by carbon dioxide emissions from combusting carbonaceous fossil fuels, for example, coal in power plants and gasoline in automobiles. Hence the push for a hydrogen economy; the hydrogen is to be produced by the steam gasification of fossil fuels however, which, also produces carbon dioxide as a coproduct. The carbon dioxide so produced, however, can be readily captured and then sequestered in porous underground formations or better yet, converted to biomass, for example, algae, by controlled photosynthesis using glass tubing in solar farms. The biomass can in turn be reconverted to hydrogen and carbon dioxide, thereby indirectly utilizing solar energy.)

To further elaborate on chlorine, there is the matter of the ozone layer and its depletion. Used as refrigerants and aerosol propellants, the freons or chlorofluorocarbons, also called CFCs, are usually viewed as the main culprits causing ozone depletion, a fact that has been well publicized. Their physical properties make them the ideal working fluid for all types of mechanical refrigeration. Normally stable and unreactive, their pressure-volume-temperature (PVT) characteristics during compression and expansion are unique for the purposes of refrigeration. Unfortunately, leakage is a fact of life, hence they also escape into the atmosphere and react with the ozone layer. (To what degree is a matter of argument and there is evidence that natural sources may be the primary agents and that the waxing and waning of the ozone layer may be a natural phenomenon. Furthermore, the theories for ozone depletion do not necessarily hold up.) Less ozone-reactive forms of refrigerants are now in use, however, such as hydrochlorofluorocarbons or HCFCs, which contain an atom or two of hydrogen in the molecule and hence have proportionately less chlorine and fluorine. (But the HCFCs may display more toxicity, that is, they may affect humans more. Furthermore, these substitutes are less efficient or effective as refrigerants, which means they reject more waste heat from the refrigeration cycle and, consequently, require more fuel or energy input for a given degree of cooling. Hence, they should be more effective for heat pumps, that is, for heating with the waste heat. All this is besides the cost incurred for the retrofit of existing systems.) The refrigerant used in newer cars requires different operating conditions and cannot be used in older cars, whose refrigeration system uses, or used, the material designated *R-12*. As noted, substitutes that are more environment-friendly have been developed.

The lower-molecular-weight hydrocarbons, namely, the liquefiable hydrocarbon gases, can alternately serve as refrigerants, although less effectively because they also combust. Carbon dioxide has long been known as a refrigerant, but requires more elevated working pressures. Possibly, it can be mixed with another, more readily liquefiable component. Deserving equal time for causing ozone depletion, moreover, is the hydrocarbon gas methane, the principal component of natural gas. It enters the atmosphere naturally via outgassing from the hydrocarbon-bearing formations of the earth.

(As regards the aforementioned gas, there is a further concern about global warming. Deep oceanic sediments and permafrost contain absolutely immense deposits of icelike methane or natural gas hydrates, which overlay or trap enormous additional reserves of methane or natural gas in the gaseous state, the earth being warmer with depth. If continued global warming should cause these hydrate formations to decompose, the effect would be sharply calamitous. The escaped methane will have about 20 times the atmospheric-warming effect of carbon dioxide. Although the wisdom is that the escaped methane would soon oxidize in the air, the oxidation will give off heat and additional carbon dioxide.)

As an alternative application for stationary refrigeration systems, there is always absorption refrigeration, as distinguished from mechanical refrigeration. This is a tried-and tested process of long standing. Here, a gas such as ammonia is absorbed into water, producing a chilling effect by an *endothermic heat of solution*. Its subsequent evaporation and separation from the aqueous phase completes the cycle.

A succession of books and articles have dealt with the effects of toxic chemicals on people and the environment, a hazard that accompanies industrialization. If there is any doubt that these compounds can be lethal, the horror that descended upon Bhopal, India, during the early morning hours of December 3, 1984, should be recalled. (It confirms that a large quantity of any toxic material should never be stored as such. The presumably nontoxic or less toxic reactants should instead be stored apart, to be mixed and reacted only as needed. Or better yet, manufacture the stuff from scratch only as needed.) Regarding the hypertoxic nerve gases from which organo/phosphorus/sulfur pesticides are derived, there is the unpublicized fact that a person only has about one minute to wash a drop from his skin before death intervenes.

Noteworthy are the works of Michael Brown and Lewis Regenstein, who survey the industry and the consequences. It all makes us wonder how the world will survive rampant industrialism, which, in the long run, may only be another phase in the cycle of civilizations. There is the thought that the omnipresence of toxic substances throughout the environment may arrest the course of civilization. The historic case was the use of lead cooking utensils, which insidiously poisoned the Romans and led to the decline of that empire. Adding to the damage was the spread and fallout of lead-bearing atmospheric pollutants from the smelters. Now, lead residues are ubiquitous, leftovers from the past, even though white lead paint has been phased out, and tetraethyl lead additives in automotive gasoline are no longer used. Furthermore, newer cars require unleaded gasoline.

Though lead water pipes are mostly a thing of the past, the replacement by galvanized-steel water pipes coated with cadmium-containing zinc gives pause for thought, especially with regard to the cadmium content. Added to this is the fact that newer construction uses copper pipes for household water, which can lead to low-level, long-range copper poisoning, which in turn may be related to mental illness. The protective mineral deposits from hard water offsets the risk to some extent. For soft water supplies, the risk is considerable.

Furthermore, lead-soldered "sweat" joints have been used for the fittings connecting copper piping, though more modern practice utilizes low-melting alloys such as those of antimony and tin. There is an analogy with the past use of malleable mercury or silver amalgams or alloys for dental fillings, to which all sorts of illnesses have been attributed, even those mimicking multiple sclerosis. The recommendation is to replace these fillings with modern nontoxic substitutes, such as ceramic, porcelain, plastics, or for the well-heeled, gold. (However, gold also amalgamates with mercury.) The fantastic modern adhesives or glues available to dentists have added a favorable extra dimension to dental work.

(With regard to copper and its alloys, and according to pioneer Kansan James R. Mead, there is the notation that Jesse Chisholm, after whom the famous Chisholm Trail was named, died from eating bear grease that had been kept in a copper or brass pot. However, the new omnipresence of mind- and body-altering drugs may make some of these metallic excursions in fallibility seem relatively minor, a world apart.)

Copper mining, for another instance, has left residues of lead and arsenic in the tailings produced. Though localized, these tailings are a serious environmental problem. The mining and processing of uranium ores has left radioactive residues, a different kind of problem. In fact, all mining practices have consequences in one form or another, whether it is acid leachate from sulfur-bearing coals in the East or mineral contamination from hard rock mining in the West. (The inference, of course, is that there is a connection with cancer incidence.)

The effects may be subtle and cumulative and may be noticeable only after a long time. Even the synthetic fibers or plastic goods used in clothing and sleepwear, as well as mattresses, may have minute effects on body and brain functions. Additives used in plastic containers or bottles are suspected to leach into the contents. For example, *Disphenyl A*, used in clear polycarbonate plastics such as in the lining of beverage cans, may mimic hormones. Not to mention the many electromagnetic effects, although usually miniscule, to which we are subjected. (For instance, see John N. Ott's *Light, Radiation, and You.*) The question to ponder is whether there are subtle and unexpected contributing factors for the aberrations of society, including cancer.

On a positive note, in addition to organic gardening and organic crop practices disfavoring the use of toxic agricultural chemicals, there is a machine on the market that literally vacuums the insect pests off the lettuce plants in the field. Called the *Salad Vac*, it is adaptable to other vegetable and crop growth. Maybe there is something to science and technology after all. Now, it remains to be seen if we could only be rid of the sulfite or sulfate solutions sprayed to freshen up the vegetables ....

Speaking further of varmints, and of vacuuming, Gay Balfour of Cortez, Colorado, has developed "Dog-Gone": a suction hose placed into the burrow deposits the prairie dogs, unharmed and frisky, into a tank on the back of a truck for relocation.

More about ecology and technology: Cattle are being fed gelatin capsules containing the seeds of desirable grasses, to be deposited at random in fresh manure piles, which practically ensures germination, especially in hard-to-reach places. A different use for manure is as "anaphage," or recycled feed.

Another problem is the detoxification of the hazardous wastes that are already present in the environment. Efforts are thwarted by the problem of how less toxic are the detoxification products in themselves? Thus, in incineration, for instance, what are the toxicities of all the final combustion products? Called *products of incomplete combustion*, or *PICs*, these are the myriad by-products and coproducts of the competing reactions that occur during combustion, and for that matter, during any chemical conversion, more or less. Can they ever be fully detected and analyzed? Or if selectively scrubbed, what is to be the disposition of the absorbed materials? What is called detoxification may be merely a further dispersion throughout the ecosphere, and a process of trading one set of problems for another.

Toxic waste disposal is another case of divide and conquer, where as long as only a minority are affected, there will be no great push for cleanup. As long as a technological solution can be stonewalled, there can be no commitment to detoxification and its costs. But cleanup faces a hard sell when money is the measure of all things. The problems are becoming ubiquitous, however, in unsuspected ways. For instance, inorganic phosphate fertilizers that contain low-level radioactivity have entered the plant-life chain, in tobacco, for instance, with their cancer-causing prognoses there are the micro-contaminants. (The tobacco habit, therefore, is suspect in more ways than one, not only from low-level radioactive species that may have been inadvertently picked up by the tobacco plant, but from the chemical sprays used in the growth cycle and in processing. This is in addition to the natural ingredients.)

As for environmental cleanup, the remediation of the mistakes in and of the past, the present, and the future does not seem to satisfy the true-blue environmentalists. They neither like the environment as it is nor show any indication for further change. They are strictly "anti-". These concerns were addressed in Ron Bailey's book *Ecoscam: The False Prophets of Ecological Apocalypse*. Another look is taken by Charle E. Davis in *The Politics of Hazardous Waste*. All this means that there will not be and cannot be any kind of absolute resolution to environmental problems.

The present problems are here to stay; at best, they just change their form. To recall an earlier saying, the more things change, the more they stay the same.

## BIOMASS

The total annual fixation of carbonaceous material by photosynthesis is an estimated 150–200 billion tons worldwide. This includes both terrestrial and oceanic fixation. The ultimate fate of a part of the biomass so generated is to either enter the food chain or to decompose or degrade, thereby contributing to the continuation of the life cycle of the planet in one way or another. The rest is interred in or laid down as sediment, part of which may over eons undergo physical, chemical, or biological metamorphosis into oil and natural gas, or into coal or other solid or semisolid carbonaceous materials. These metamorphoses may be related more to cataclysmic changes in the earth's makeup rather than the gradual changes of uniformitarianism.

In an article appearing in the December 1993 issue of *Discover*, Carl Zimmer took a look at the closure of the Earth's carbon balance for carbon dioxide and biomass. Not all of the carbon dioxide produced could be accounted for, suggesting that the rates of generation and degeneration of biomass are not equal, thereby leading to the scenario where there was a net accumulation of biomass.

On the other hand, the carbon dioxide levels of the atmosphere are increasing, indicating that not all of the carbon dioxide produced is being converted back into biomass. In this context, there is no net accumulation of biomass. In other words, *the inferences can be truly sobering, inasmuch as the world may be utilizing carbonaceous material at a rate that is greater than the rate at which it is being generated or renewed by photosynthesis.*

## WHERE TO GO FROM HERE?

The emphasis here is on CAM, as it pertains to cancer and its treatment. On the other hand, in perspective, the alternative to CAM is the conventional routes, about which the previously mentioned learned and more technical book *Cancer: Principles and Practice of Oncology* is not exactly optimistic. (Incidentally, at the time of this writing *Books in Print* carries over 300 titles starting with the word *cancer*, with a total of about 2500 having the word in the title. The Internet gives hits in the millions.) Edited by Vincent T. DeVita, Samuel Hellman, and Steven A. Rosenberg, all M.D.s, this huge 2489-page volume does not necessarily inspire confidence in conventional treatments, that is, surgery, radiation, and chemotherapy, and some of the drawbacks are also spelled out. Thus, for example, in the treatment of liver cancer by regional chemotherapy using intrahepatic infusion, we find that when the drug is injected into the cancerous liver nodules, there are the possibilities of the inadvertent perfusion of the stomach and duodenum, gastrointestinal ulcerations, and hepatic toxicity (DeVita et al., 1989, pp. 2287–2290), not to mention the ever-present possibility of infection (DeVita et al., 1989, p. 2384).

Also, general modern medicine largely confines itself to the illnesses of the temperate zone, i.e., the "developed" countries. Largely ignored are tropical diseases, the plague of the Third World. In A. A. Gill's collection *AA Gill Is Away*, in a section about the southern part of Africa, there is a chapter titled "I Don't Know What Makes You Angry ... " Gill substantiates the indifference of the West to curing and controlling the tropical diseases of Africa: sleeping sickness, malaria, AIDS, etc. Even when a pharmaceutical company makes a drug available on a license-free basis, there is none willing to step in and manufacture the drug. "Of the 1223 new medicines developed between 1975 and 1997, just thirteen were for tropical medicine. Only four sprang from the pharmaceutical industry's efforts to cure humans. None was found on purpose."

The foregoing leads to the issue of food supplies, one of the twin scourges of the underdeveloped countries. (The hand of man continues to get into the act, even if inadvertently. For one notable example, there is the record of irrigation along the Nile. The construction of barrages and dams on the River Nile provided the means for irrigation. This was perennial irrigation, whereby the water-saturated soils play host to the hookworm or fluke-causing bilharziasis, or schistosomiasis [Ludwig, 1939, pp. 591–593]. The effects of the Aswan High Dam should be recalled, in this context.) Not to be omitted, in any listing, are the benefits of modern plumbing and of large-scale public health measures. There too is the consideration of the Chinese attitude, in contrast to the Western doctrine of allopathy that is rooted in medical cures, where the doctor is paid only as long as one stays well, with payment cut off if sickness occurs.

We move now to medical ethics. At Houston, the Texas Medical Center has been regularly involved with the Institute of Religion, an independent center devoted to ethics, particularly medical ethics. So, hopefully, medical ethics is being given due thought. The larger problem is, how much is a life worth? Does not saving lives, properly managed, beget economic activity, the same as saving the environment? But first, what is "life"? And what is the difference between "saving" life and merely "maintaining" life? These are the dilemmas in human reasoning and understanding, where there is no absolute truth outside of a biblical or metaphysical context.

Even the charitable foundations and organizations, seemingly so devoted to the cause of good health, have come under fire in *Unhealthy Charities* by James T. Bennett and Thomas J. DiLorenzo. It seems that most, or at least a significant part, of the monies raised, goes to "overhead."

A claim has been made that most of the patients in the mental wards are there because of dietary deficiencies, and that excess sugar intake is a cause of chronic misbehavior of the nation's youth. As for the ritual and esoterica of drinking, consider wines, where sulfites are added, and other liquors, to which coloring agents, maybe, less charitably called dyes, may be added. With all the by-products and coproducts of fermentation, the higher alcohols or fusel oils, along with the aldehydes and ketones and all the rest, with additives of one kind or another, the wonder is that the consumers do not get sicker than they do. The best news would be the disclaimer: "Guaranteed not to make anyone sick." Although the higher alcohols are sometimes called *congeners*, as they will sometimes mix readily with other substances, their cumulative effect is anything but congenial.

If these comments somehow seem overly coarse, it should be kept in mind that, after all, we are talking of barnyard feed in one form or another, fermentation being merely a kind of digestion to produce offal, an intermediate product known more euphemistically in the trade as *beer*. But then, similarly, bacterial fermentations apply also for buttermilk, yogurt, sauerkraut, etc. All are forms of predigested or partially digested food, where microorganisms do part of the work.

(In a news item about the carcinogenic effects of beer and alcohol, an article by Dr. Joseph C. Anderson, assistant professor of medicine at Stony Brook University Hospital, Long Island, was cited. The article appeared in the September 2005 issue of the *American Journal of Gastroenterology*. Beer and alcoholic drinks were found to cause intestinal polyps, thus being precursors of colorectal cancer. Alcohol damages DNA, is immune suppressive, and favors a protein called *P-450*, a procarcinogen. However, red wine is considered anticancer. Maybe this has to do with the particular classes of anticancer organic compounds that produce its color. In fact, there was once an anticancer book written by Johanna Brandt titled *The Grape Cure*. Most commercial wines contain added sulfites, although so-called organic wines will contain no added sulfites, only those that occur naturally.)

There was a two-hour TV program on PBS on or about April 5, 1993, titled "Medicine at the Crossroads," presumably one of the many dealing with this subject that have already been, and will continue to be, aired. Whatever else this program may have portrayed, in its grappling between "high-tech" and "low-tech" medicine and Japanese medical practices in particular, the simple conclusion is, "Don't ever get sick." A humorous look at medicine through the ages was taken by Richard Gordon in *The Alarming History of Medicine: Amusing Anecdotes from Hippocrates to Heart Transplants*. And if the subject is at times not humorous, it is at least costly.

In Canada, however, all medical costs are covered for everyone. In a study by economist Victor R. Fuchs of Stanford University, it was found that U.S. doctors charged nearly two and one-half times as much for their services as did their Canadian counterparts. It must be said that Canada's economy remains as healthy as its citizens, in spite of this limited incursion into socialism. Or is it? Thus, consider the long waiting periods for vital care, causing some Canadians to visit the United States when the chips are down. The state of Hawaii has a universal health plan that seems to be practical and favorably thought of, and it is said to be modeled after what was proposed back in the Nixon administration. Nevertheless, there is Forrester's law lurking about, which states that in complicated situations, efforts to improve things often tend to make them worse, sometimes much worse, and on occasion, calamitous. Thus, the new operational buzzword is HMOs, or health management organizations. But they are not proving to be a panacea.

In the case of cancer, that is, advanced or metastasized cancer, a recommendation is that cancer clinical research centers, or CCRCs, be set up in new or existing facilities, as previously indicated. These would comprise a nationwide network, even worldwide, and would be staffed by M.D.s and D.O.s commonly supported by a variety of pharmacologists, botanists, herbalists, etc., who are familiar with the world of plants and plant medicines, the main source for alternatives. In a way, the Cancer Treatment Centers of America tend to fill this function at least partially, although there are only three locations, in the Chicago area, in Tulsa, and in Seattle. Both conventional and CAM therapies are offered, at the patient's discretion. It may be mentioned in passing that the CTCA no longer speaks of cures but of treatments, after they ran into trouble with the Federal Trade Commission (FTC) back in 1996.

Continuing in these directions, the December 2005 issue of *The Atlantic* lists award-
ees in a special section on Service to America Medals. Under Science and Environment, Subhashree Madhavan of the National Institutes of Health received the award.
Mentioning that cancer now surpasses heart disease as the leading cause of death
in the United States for persons under age 85, the citation notes that Madhavan is
the leader of a team called *Rembrandt*, the Repository for Molecular Brain Neoplastic
Data. It is described as the fullest and most analytically powerful database on brain
tumors and how they behave. Expectedly, other databases will emerge for other
cancer types. Will this be expanded to treatments and cures (i.e., remissions) and
CAM some day.

The present health care fiasco, which is a mess, was exposed in Walt Bogdanovich's *The Great White Lie: How America's Hospitals Betray Our Trust and Endanger
Our Lives*. A case of suspicions finally confirmed. For good measure there is Dave
Lindorff's *Marketplace Medicine: The Rise of the For-Profit Hospital Chains*. These
corporate health care chains, with big money and political power, can be blamed in
significant part for soaring medical costs. The health care quandary and further
brouhaha was covered by W. Halamandaris in *The Care Gaps*, in 1992.

As for interconnections among the pharmaceutical industry, world finance, and
government, there is Clarence Mullins' aforementioned *Death by Injection*, published as a kind of underground exposé. (Mullins has written other exposés about
the powers that be, as mentioned in the references.) Another in the same vein is by
James P. Carter, M.D., Ph.D., titled *Racketeering in Medicine*.

Speaking of pharmaceuticals, Marcia Angell, M.D., of the Harvard Medical
Schools has contributed *The Truth About the Drug Companies: How They Deceive
Us and What to Do About It*, published in 2004. She notes that drug companies
started to get the upper hand after 1980, when it was ruled that their research results,
although conducted under government auspices and funding, could nevertheless be
patented, instead of entering the public domain. As for the much-publicized costs
of R&D, Angell asserts that there are many other costs hidden under this umbrella.
Whereas the pharmaceutical companies used to promote drugs to cure the disease,
now "they promote disease to fit their drugs."

Another critique of the pharmaceutical industry, published at about the same
time, is by Jerry Avorn, who describes himself as a "pharmacoepidemiologist." Titled
*Powerful Medicines: The Benefits, Risks, and Costs of Prescription Drugs*, Avorn's
analysis is more statistically oriented, but he reaches essentially the same conclusions
as Angell.

Other books that cover the field are John Abramson's *Overdosed America: The
Broken Promise of American Medicine*, also published in 2004, and Greg Critser's
*Generation RX: How Prescription Drugs Are Altering American Lives, Minds and
Bodies*, published in 2005. The momentum is, therefore, building up.

For a specific case, there is an article by Michael Bennett in the November 2005
issue of the *Townsend Letter for Doctors & Patients* titled "Hospital-Spread Infection." Bennett's father died from the effects of a flesh-destroying disease caused by
nosocomial (hospital-acquired) bacteria, in this instance, a genetic variant of the
staphylococci. The figures supplied state that nosocomial infections in America's

hospitals have caused more than one hundred thousand deaths and more than 2 million injuries each year.

The same issue of the *Townsend Letter* contains an article by Jacob Teitelbaum, M.D., on "Treating Infections Without Antibiotics." Of note is the use of thymic hormone as well as vitamin C, the homeopathic remedy Oscillococcinum, etc. The article may be consulted for more. Also reviewed in the same issue is Bryan Rosner's *When Antibiotics Fail: Lyme Disease and Rife Machines with Critical Evaluation of Alternative Therapies*, the radio frequency Rife Machine itself being a possibility.

In the fall of 2004, Dr. David Graham, an FDA employee concerned with drug safety, claimed that new pharmaceuticals on the market were not always sufficiently evaluated as to safety, that is, to side effects, or biochemical individuality. Add to this the adverse interactions that can occur when two or more drugs are taken. The same caution, of course, applies to natural as well as synthetic medicines.

(Nothing was said, however, about the cytotoxic, or cell-toxic, chemotherapy drugs routinely used against cancer, which most often may have damaging side effects albeit amply documented.)

Specifically cited was the arthritis drug Vioxx®, along with others. This caused an uproar among drug companies and within the FDA, with charges of "junk science" hurled about, but Dr. Graham was supported by a whistleblowers' organization. This also brings up the question of what the term *junk science* is supposed to mean, although it is apparently considered synonymous with *quackery* — and which parties get to decide, and on what basis, what junk science is.

(A news item in the Spring 2005 issue of *Good Medicine*, a publication of the Physicians Committee for Responsible Medicine, or PCRM, is that Vioxx® was initially given the green light because of positive results in animals studies. This once again shows that *in vivo* studies and clinical studies do not necessarily correlate, notably so for the case of cancer. The same issue of *Good Medicine* extols the power of a plant-based diet in an article by T. Colin Campbell, Jacob Gould Schurman, professor emeritus of nutritional biochemistry at Cornell University, and Thomas Campbell. They are authors of *The China Story*, BenBella Books, 2005, confirming these conclusions, as per T. Colin Campbell's findings as director of the China Health Study, which the *New York Times* called "the most comprehensive large study ever undertaken of the relationship between diet and the risk of developing disease." Nor does PCRM recommend milk in the diet, the founder and president Neal D. Barnard, M.D., advocating other and better sources for calcium. The Autumn 2005 issue of *Good Medicine* follows up on this breaking story, emphasizing that *in vivo* experiments on animals do not necessarily correlate with human or clinical studies, and this divergence can be extended to anticancer drugs. There are differences in effects even among different animal species; the article mentions that penicillin was first judged ineffective against infections in rabbits, and if it had been tested on guinea pigs or hamsters, it would have even been declared toxic. Incidentally, PCRM is against the routine and inhuman use of animals to test drug efficacy, as there are other better ways, owing to advancing technologies and techniques.)

A mention of David Graham was made in PBS's *FRONTLINE* on or about December 14, 2004, the program title being "Dangerous Prescription." Most of the program was devoted to problems within the FDA and mentioned the fact that drugs against such conditions as elevated cholesterol, weight reduction, and rheumatoid arthritis were found to have some serious side effects for some people. Dr. Graham was also featured in an article by Mark Scherer in the May/June 2005 issue of *Mother Jones*. Among the highlights is that drug companies fund the FDA for speedy approvals, in that almost half of the FDA's $400 million drug evaluation program is funded by the industry.

(An article by Frazer Merritt in the November 2005 issue of *Z Magazine* highlights the problems that can be encountered by the patient. Titled "Pharmaceutical Outsourcing," the article is concerned with Merritt's taking a well-known antidepressant that in his case triggered a bipolar disorder called *hypomania* in its most severe form. However, he had not been forewarned of these side effects, even in the pharmacy's Patient Insert leaflets. He subsequently found mention of the mania/hypomania side effect on the Internet while searching under the brand name of the drug, and also found that the particular drug company and the FDA had known about this side effect since 1996. However, it turned out that information about a drug is disseminated via electronic drug information companies, or EDI companies, and the information supplied is not necessarily complete. A prior push for mandatory medication guides never made it through the legislative process, and today, the FDA has no power to regulate the drug information provided — or not provided. Among the reasons for nonregulation was that such comprehensive information guides could interfere with the doctor–patient relationship. Clearly, to a degree, patients are on their own.)

Supposedly, there is a voluntary computer information database called MEDWATCH (as distinguished from MEDLINE) that keeps track of instances as reported by physicians, and which are then relayed to the drug companies, but these companies may or may not inform the FDA. It is a fact that half the FDA's drug safety program is said to be funded by the drug companies. Many of the problems started in 1988 with pressure to fast-track the anti-AIDS drug approval. Before that the word was extreme caution because thalidomide had caused severe birth defects in babies of pregnant women who took the drug.

(Always foremost for evaluation is that of risks vs. benefits, a trade-off that can be vague indeed. In other words, where to draw the fine line? Most patients at risk are pregnant women and their fetuses. Hence, it can be added that there are plants and plant medicines that are suspect as well, not only as extreme poisons or toxicants, but as abortifacients and teratogens, which cause monstrous birth defects.)

Perhaps giving equal time, a succeeding program on *FRONTLINE*, aired on or about December 28, 2004, was titled "The Alternative Fix." Both pros and cons were aired as usual, and a most interesting aspect was the increased use of alternative medicines, as noticed by the practicing members of the medical profession. Moreover, CAM has increased clout in Washington by virtue of the financial growth of the alternative scene. Among the champions of alternative medicine and nutritional supplements are Tom Harkin (Democrat, Iowa) and Orrin Hatch (Republican, Utah).

Another aspect is the emerging use of various alternative therapies in certain hospitals, at the patients' discretion, for example, at Beth Israel in New York City. As a physician declared, with regard to homeopathy, there are matters that go beyond science and its explanations. (The buzzword is that these alternatives give hope for the otherwise hopeless victim.) Among those prominently interviewed was Nicholas J. Gonzalez, M.D., and two of his cancer patients, with a brief description of his cancer therapy, which notably involved coffee enemas and the consumption of 150 assorted but unspecified pills each day. It would have been informative, if time had allowed, to interview such as A. Hoffer, M.D., Ph.D., and Stanislaw R. Burzynski, M.D.

(A few names and Web sites for keeping track of what is going on in CAM have been posted by *FRONTLINE* on its Web site, as follows:

*Cochrane Collaboration Consumer Nework*
  http://www.cochraneconsumer.com/
  Provides summaries of recent clinical studies of CAM treatments and their
    results
*Center for Integrative Medicine*, University of Maryland
  http://www.compmed.umm.edu/
  Provides information and resources on CAM treatments aimed at both
    consumers and health professionals, including extensive lists of addi-
    tional resources and tips for assessing resource credibility
*Rowenthal Center for Complementary and Alternative Medicine, Columbia
University*
  http://rosenthal.hs.columbia.edu/
  Offers information on CAM therapies and resources for consumers, in-
    cluding tips for assessing the credibility of CAM information found on
    the Internet and additional questions to consider before beginning alter-
    native medicine treatments

Noteworthy is the fact that certain hospitals, as indicated earlier, utilize various alternative therapies. This merges with the previously advanced idea of creating CCRCs, as advocated herein. Unfortunately, there is a matter of costs for the patient — and really high costs at that — especially as alternative treatments are mostly uninsurable. The affluent do not face this problem. For most others, the financial difficulties become insurmountable. And this is a prime reason for the designation OCRC, inferring that the government could pick up the tab as it does for other research activities, as sponsored through the National Institutes of Health (NIH) and the NCCAM. There is, in addition, the incentive for individuals to try to cure themselves, an argument for keeping dietary supplements and herbs away from government regulation and interference. It should also be remembered that side effects can occur, as they also can with conventional pharmaceuticals. (A reason, of course, for counsel by medical professionals, whether speaking of alternatives or orthodoxy, if one can afford it.)

An earlier exposé of the pharmaceutical culture in similar vein was *Over Dose: The Case Against the Drug Companies* by Jay S. Cohen, M.D., published in 2001. The subtitle is *Prescription Drugs, Side Effects, and Your Health.* Interestingly, it received a favorable review in the *Journal of the American Medical Association.* Dr. Cohen's message is that standard drug dosages are stronger than needed for millions of patients and become a paean to drug industry profits. The result is an epidemic of adverse side effects, with seniors particularly at risk. Additionally, there is a compilation of useful drug information with references furnished. A sample chapter contains the title "When New Drugs Are Approved, the Experiment Is Just Beginning."

And so continues the joust in the United States over universal, mandatory, and government-controlled health care, or "socialized medicine," fueled by the rising costs of health care and medical insurance. As for the proposal of putting a cap on medical and doctor costs, a few have pointed out that maybe the same thing should be done for legal and legislative costs. Whereas socialism is often identified only with the equal distribution of wealth, there is the other hidden baggage carried along, namely, the control of everybody and everything by the government, which in turn is controlled by those elites who manipulate the government.

The nursing home industry was once excoriated by U.S. Senator Frank E. Moss and Val J. Halamandaris in *Too Old, Too Sick, Too Bad*. This was in 1977. The situation remains dismal, or more so, as the American family continues its breakup. It is a policy of self for self, with the impoverished elderly kept out of sight and out of mind, a hindrance to the aspirations and lifestyles of the younger generation. In some cultures, the elderly are revered; in others, the elderly are left out to die, a primitive form of euthanasia. But it should not be forgotten that what goes around comes around.

Regarding health insurance, John Krizay has updated the high cost of insurance, where it is a fact that on average only 35% of what was paid in was paid out in claims. The rest goes for overheads and acquiring a piece of America. (Even at that, some companies go insolvent. It is a situation of too many cuts from the cheese.) Moreover, the McCarran–Ferguson Act, passed in 1945, excludes the insurance industry from federal regulation, thus providing it with the power of a legal monopoly. The industry is thereby exempted from antitrust action, which would otherwise prevent price fixing, the mutual raising of prices, and denying coverage.

The general state of health itself can take some unexpected twists and turns. As may be noted, during World War I, chlorine was reserved for wartime needs rather than for bleaching flour. And, apparently, on a diet of bread from unbleached flour, the overall public health improved. There was less sickness, if we discount the flu outbreak of 1918. Another odd item is that during a doctor's strike, the death rate fell off.

Also to be noted is the very practical side of religion (e.g., Judeo-Christianity). Its codes are a guide to living and a fusion with life's meaning. Although there are arguments about the effectiveness of prayer, religion also fulfills social needs through the aegis of the churches. This function and its healing role are pointed out by James Lynch in *The Broken Heart: The Medical Consequences of Loneliness*.

In this context it is interesting to consider the mass mailing of a colorful and controversial 22-page brochure in the early days of January 2005. The heading was *Discover why one MD says "I HAVEN'T HAD A GLASS OF WATER IN 20 YEARS...".* Comments were added to the effect that "drinking tons of water" will "raise a stroke risk, bring on kidney failure, and encourage early Alzheimer's." (There was also a warning against fluoridated water, a by-product of aluminum production.) Paraphrasing other points raised: vegetarians die younger; coffee prevents cancer; massive strokes soar when cholesterol levels are below 200; when men eat more red meat, heart attacks plummet by 300%; testosterone can help some women cut breast cancer risk by 90%; and cortisone can be safe and act against arthritis. Other polemics provided are that sunshine is actually associated with lower melanoma occurrences, the consumption of fats by women does not correlate with breast cancer, DDT does not cause cancer and may even prevent breast cancer, and there is a test that exists for detecting cancer early enough. It is called *AMAS* but it should not be confused with mammography or the PSA (prostate specific antigen) test for prostate cancer. Neither is there an advocacy for calcium supplements, nor for CPR (cardiopulmonary resuscitation) as commonly practiced, not to mention soy products, and "enriched with iron," which can be treated like poison.

The protagonist is William Campbell Douglass, M.D., and the medium is a subscription to *Dr. Douglass' Real Health Breakthroughs*. There are testimonials from persons such as Jonathan V. Wright, M.D., a respected name in alternative medicine.

To continue, Dr. Douglass takes a closer look at the statistics for taking tamoxifen against breast cancer as compared to a placebo and speaks of a beverage that cuts off the blood supply to developing cancer cells. He indicates that laser light therapy is selective against cancer cells, does not harm normal cells, and makes chemotherapy obsolete. (The analogy is to Royal Rife's radio frequency treatments, described in Chapter 2.)

Additionally, hydrogen peroxide is said to be an effective anti-infective agent, even acting against cancer, but who would even think of drinking it? (In fact, Dr. Douglass is the author of *Hydrogen Peroxide: Medical Miracle*, Second Opinion Publishing, Atlanta, GA, 1996. The subject is given several pages in Richard Walters' *Options* in a chapter titled "Oxygen Therapies," published in 1993. The intravenous injection of hydrogen peroxide was noted to have received mixed opinions, in part related to dosage levels. As for efficacy, Walters' opinion is that the cancer patient is "probably more bewildered than before.")

Also, cattle fed on fatty foods such as coconut oil lost weight. And do not give up rich, meaty foods such as steak, eggs, prime ribs, lobster, bacon, etc. Instead of a carbohydrate burner, turn your body into a fat burner. In a way, the proposed diet is similar to Dr. Atkins' low-carbohydrate diet, which in turn was similar to the thesis of the book titled *Calories Don't Count,* igniting a controversy that once ended up in court with a judgment against the book's authors. But it was a different world back then, in the 1960s.

(Another low-carbohydrate diet, apparently one of many, is advocated by Ron Rosedale, M.D., of the Rosedale Metabolic Center of Denver, Colorado, as per *The Rosedale Diet* by Ron Rosedale and Carol Colman, Harper Resources, New York, 2004. Among other things, a proper balance is sought for the hormone leptin. And, by following this diet, less exercise is said to be needed — as also said by Dr. Douglass. Increasing leptin levels takes off weight, and leptin-rich sources include the following: nuts; avocado and olives; fish rich in omega-3 fatty acids, such as halibut, orange roughy, sardines, etc.; eggs (omega-3 enriched); chicken and turkey; goat cheese; most vegetables; tea, etc. To these can be added the fact that fish oil capsules rich in omega-3 fatty acids can apparently counter joint problems, as in the knees.)

Suspending judgment, it can at least be said that the wordings in Dr. Douglass' brochure no doubt must be presented so as to pass the test of law and cannot be adjudged as patently erroneous and incriminating. As for an (impartial) assessment, such would require large-scale independent clinical testing, and even then the results would be open to interpretation and argument. It is further confirmation that the individual patient or victim (and his or her family, and physician, if any) must be the court of last resort, or it is a case of every man for himself. It seems to be a no-man's-land. It almost implies that it is much better to stay healthy and not get sick, and to live for about 115 years.

And so it goes, with most of the rest of the information out there. This is a reminder that the Quackwatch Home Page has put out a list of some nonrecommended periodicals, some 197 in number, which are described as "untrustworthy because they promote misinformation, espouse unscientific theories, contain unsubstantiated advice, and/or fail to distinguish between reliable and unreliable sources of advice." Among those cited are the following: *Dr. Campbell's Real Health Breakthroughs, Good Medicine, Life Extension, Noetic Sciences Review, Prevention, Psychology Today, Townsend Letter for Doctors & Patients, Journal of Orthomolecular Medicine, Blaylock Wellness Report, Dr. Atkins' Health Revelations, Health and Healing* (Julian Whitaker, M.D.), *The Perlmutter Report, Second Opinion* (William C. Douglass, M.D.), and *Self Healing* (Andrew Weil, M.D.).

The foregoing listing is like a *Who's Who* and *What's What* in alternative medicine. The gauntlet has been thrown and the joust continues, with medical orthodoxy (still) questioning nutritional supplements such as vitamin E, and their statistics are sure to be contested. It all seems more like a presidential race, the public relations machine of the Republicans vs. that of the Democrats, rather than objective science.

(It may be added that Quackwatch has had some reversals in the courts, as per an article on pp. 27 and 28 of the February/March 2006 issue of the *Townsend Letter for Doctors & Patients*. The force behind Quackwatch, Dr. Stephen Barrett, had sued Dr. Tedd Koren, a chiropractor who had allegedly made some uncomplimentary statements in a newsletter. The case was thrown out of a Lehigh Valley, Pennsylvania, court by Judge J. Brian Johnson. Dr. Koren was represented by the well-known health freedom advocate, attorney Carlos F. Negrete of San Juan Capistrano, California, by attorney James Turner of Swankin & Turner, Washington, D.C., and also local Pennsylvania attorney Christopher Reid of Laub, Seidel, Cohen, Hof & Reid. Turner's experience dates back to the 1960s when he joined consumer advocate Ralph Nader and his organization Nader's Raiders. During the course of events, it came out that Barrett had not been a licensed physician since the early 1990s nor was he a Medical Board Certified psychiatrist, and had had no formal legal training. Also, it was mentioned that Barrett had lost 40 other similar defamation lawsuits. Barrett's role as a medical expert to the FDA, FTC, and other government agencies was cited, as were his participations in many interviews, such as with *Time*, ABC's *20/20*, NBC's *Today Show*, and PBS programs.)

In late 2004 it was reported that more than 400 mg of vitamin E per day increased the death rate. This was, of course, contested, for instance, by Wayne Martin and by Alan R. Gaby, M.D., in the February/March 2005 issue of the *Townsend Letter for Doctors & Patients*, who challenged both the statistics used and the interpretation. Not only this, but there may be extraneous factors involved such as copper intake, which may have an effect. Dr. Gaby mentions the four kinds of naturally occurring vitamin E, namely, alpha-, beta-, gamma-, and delta-tocopherol. He writes that gamma-tocopherol may be more effective than the alpha-tocopherol generally consumed (with the possibility that the mixed tocopherols may be most effectual of all). There are two forms of alpha-tocopheral, being D-alpha-tocopherol and L-alpha-tocopherol. (The prefix pertains to the effect on the rotation of light passed through the substance, the D-form having a "right-handed" effect, and the L-form a "left-handed" effect.) The equal mixture of the two is called D,L-alpha-tocopherol and is cheaper to produce commercially. The mixture is sometimes called *synthetic vitamin E* (and it is generally assumed to be less active).

Dr. Gaby also went to bat in the November 2005 issue of the *Townsend Letter for Doctors & Patients* about an editorial appearing in the *New England Journal of Medicine* about "Studying Herbal Remedies." In part, the editorial said that herbal echinacea was found to be ineffective against common colds, at least in healthy persons. Gaby's critique was that the assessment in the *NEJM* was in effect neither comprehensive nor rigorous but biased.

Speaking further of statistics and their manipulation, as an aside, there is *200 Percent of Nothing: An Eye-Opening Tour Through the Twists and Turns of Math Abuse and Innumeracy* by A. K. Dewdney, a professor of mathematics, which was published in 1993 and 1996.

If cancer is thought of more as a statistic, the volume *Cancer Stories: Lessons in Love, Loss, and Hope* (Temple and Beeson, 2004) brings us back to reality. The School of Journalism at West Virginia University conducted a Cancer Project, with journalism students individually assigned to cancer patients, notably at the university's Mary Babb Randolph Cancer Center. The final result, edited by John Temple and Joel Beeson, with an Introduction by Jennifer Roush, contains photo essays that chronicle the experiences and ordeals of cancer patients. A DVD accompanies this award-winning documentary, recipient of a 2004 Midwestern Regional Emmy.

Why is not a surefire selective cure or cures for cancer in evidence? This query is made in light of a vast pharmacopoeia of bioactive plants and plant extracts that reportedly act against cancer. References include Jonathan Hartwell's compendium *Plants Used Against Cancer* and others, as in this book and elsewhere. Whereas most reported anticancer plant medicines are derived from medical folklore, anecdote, and hearsay, there are fewer screened *in vitro* (in the test tube or petri dish), and still fewer screened *in vivo* (in mice), with a dearth of (positive) clinical studies on humans. (The word is that *in vitro* and *in vivo* tests do not necessarily translate to humans, and vice versa.) In any event, these plants and plant substances can furnish a point of departure, but the cautionary note is to beware, calling for discernment, and professional medical counsel and care in the event of toxicity.

A reasonable question is whether there are not some cures already in existence, held in abeyance by the interminable wrangling between medical orthodoxy and alternative medicine? Such wrangling can of, course, be viewed as political and economic, as well as scientific. Given that many or most of the unorthodox treatments may not be substantiated with documented cures – the same holds true for orthodox medicine – it can still be asked if there are not a few that can pass the clinical test of objective scrutiny. This can be backed by impartial scientific explanations, for example, in terms of selective enzyme inhibitors. Again, we have come back to the subject of CCRCs or their equivalent.

# 2 Cancer Origins and Characteristics

## INTRODUCTION

Although much is known about the processes of cancer formation, or carcinogenesis, comparatively little is known about the processes of cancer regression. The former will be explored as an introduction to the latter, and both involve the biological and chemical functions of the body, stated in terms of normal cells vs. cancerous ones. Surgical excision and radiation treatment are excluded from the discussion, though they can be selective if, say, the solid tumor is localized and has not yet spread or metastasized — and if the operations or treatments in themselves do not cause metastasis.

It should be emphasized that there are all kinds of biochemically active, or bioactive, compounds or substances that will destroy cancer cells — and will destroy normal ones as well, and even kill the patient. For instance, some of the lesser-known antibiotics will kill cancer cells as well as bacterial cells, but are also lethal to the patient.

We will examine in detail enzymes and enzyme inhibitors, enzymes being the proteinaceous substances that catalyze the myriad biochemical reactions or processes that occur in the body. Almost without exception, there is one enzyme specific to each biochemical reaction. (What may be called supporting reactions, side reactions, or simultaneous reactions may also be involved and, in fact, may be a necessity.) In turn, there are other proteinaceous substances, or still other chemical substances, that will inhibit, block, modulate, or control the action of enzymes, and on rare occasion, even accelerate or promote the action. Known as enzyme inhibitors, such substances may affect more than one enzyme, or many different enzymes; that is, they may have side effects, or in other words, are nonselective. These inhibitors may be generated internally, or more likely may originate from external sources. That is, they may be designated as medicines. In fact, modern medicine is more and more viewed as encompassing enzymes and enzyme inhibitors. Broadly, this may be viewed as the utilization of biologically active or biochemically active substances, that is, bioactive substances, either natural or synthetic.

The examples are numerous, and include the routinely used antibiotics, which selectively act against certain vital enzymes in bacteria cells, or prokaryotes, but fortuitously do not affect human or mammalian cells, or eukaryotes, at least in the dosages used, although there may be side effects. Fluorides in drinking water or toothpaste act against critical enzymes in oral bacteria, but more generally, they also act as inhibitors for still other enzymes, which sounds a cautionary note for fluoride use. The conventional chemotherapy drugs act against enzymes involved in

DNA/RNA/protein synthesis, not only for cancerous cells, but for all cells, hence the designator *cytotoxic*.

The most famous of the antibiotics is penicillin, which is, more broadly speaking, a chemotherapy agent. Its predecessors were the synthetic dyes known as sulfona-mides, or the "sulfa" drugs, considered the first in line of the chemotherapy agents, but they were largely superseded by the more effective penicillin and subsequent antibiotics produced from fungal sources. Although penicillin, a chemical compound in its pure state that is derived from the pencil-shaped fungus or mold of the genus *Penicillium*, was first discovered by Alexander Fleming in 1928, its further devel-opment over the next 12 years was due to Howard Florey, an Australian transplanted to England, along with Florey's assistants, notably Ernst Boris Chain. In fact, Fleming, Florey, and Chain jointly shared a Nobel Prize in 1945 for their work. Details are furnished in Gwyn Macfarlane's *Alexander Fleming: The Man and the Myth* (1985). In a more recent volume (2004), *The Mold in Dr. Florey's Coat: The Story of the Penicillin Miracle*, author Eric Lax wonders why the other Oxford coworkers did not receive a greater degree of recognition.

The investigations were originally concerned with lysozymes, which are enzymes occurring in mucus secretions (for instance, the mucous membranes in the nose) and which act as antibacterial agents. Thus, a vitamin A deficiency will cause the mucus secretions to cease in the intestine, which is followed by a bacterial invasion of the intestinal tissue (Macfarlane, 1985, p. 161). There is an inference that this may be the way vitamin A works against cancer, inasmuch as the action of gut flora or bacteria can be anticancer but can also produce all sorts of carcinogens.

(However, there are the beneficial gut and other flora, which may be destroyed by antibiotics — an ongoing issue, along with the buildup of bacterial immunity to drugs. Thus, there is Jessica Snyder Sach's article in the September 2005 issue of *Discover*, titled "Are Antibiotics Killing Us?" The argument is furnished that drugs that target bad bacteria will destroy a lot of good bacteria, upsetting the ecological balance in our bodies. A further quotation says it all: "For every cell in your body, you support 10 bacterial cells that make vitamins, trigger hormones, and may even influence how fat you are. Guess what happens to them when you pop penicillin." This illustrates the eternal trade-off between beneficial effects and side effects.)

An interesting fact is that curare acts against tetanus (Macfarlane, 1985, p. 163). Unfortunately, curare is highly toxic, being an alkaloid-containing mixture (e.g., tubocurarine) derived from South American plants, notably of the genus *Chonendron* of the family Menispermaceae, and of the genus *Strychnos* of the family Logani-aceae. In minute, closely monitored doses curare or its purified alkaloids are of value as a muscle relaxant. In higher doses it is deadly, acting against respiration and causing death by suffocation, the fate of animals (or humans) shot by South American Indians. (And it indicates the horrible action of the alkaloid strychnine and other poisonous substances.)

It is interesting to note that *in vitro*, *in vivo*, and clinical tests can produce anomalies or exceptions, one of the perplexities in assaying drugs. Thus, it was later found that *in vivo* tests showed penicillin toxicity to guinea pigs (Macfarlane, 1985, p. 184). If these had been tested first, quite possibly the use of penicillin would have been delayed or abandoned. As it was, a penicillin mixture was clinically tested first on a human patient and found to be nontoxic (although it was to be subsequently found that certain individuals are allergic to penicillin).

It so turned out that penicillin does not affect mature bacteria cells, but only the progeny resulting from division (Macfarlane, 1985, p. 246). It prevented the cell walls from forming in the new cells, thereby acting as an inhibitor for the biochemical processes involved. The specific enzymes blocked have since been determined, and are routinely cited in most biochemical and microbiological textbooks or references.

The conventional chemotherapeutic drugs used against cancer are in the main cytotoxic, or cell toxic, therefore acting against normal cells as well as cancerous ones, too often with debilitating results. Although, in talking about enzymes and enzyme inhibitors, or medicines, the subject in general is that of chemotherapy or biochemotherapy, it must be emphasized that the drugs or substances used are to be *selective*, affecting normal cells only minimally or not at all; that is, are safe. In other words, the objective is *selective* chemotherapy or biochemotherapy.

In fact, what are called poisons are the most bioactive of substances, and in minute dosages are sometimes employed for medicinal purposes; hence, the some-times-used term *poisonous and medicinal* as applied, say, to plants or plant-derived substances. The most overt toxic effects are generally against the heart or against respiration, causing cardiac arrest or suffocation. In other cases, somewhat less deadly, the substance may act against the immune system or against the liver and kidneys, or still other body processes or organs. These toxic actions of varying degree are commonly referred to as side effects, although adverse effects may be more appropriate.

In essence, therefore, we are speaking about biochemical cellular processes, stressing the selective inhibition of cancer cell metabolism, by indigenous or exog-enous agents, from within or without, and which, if and when and to the degree it works, may be referred to as a selective biochemical cure, or at least a therapy.

By metabolism or primary metabolism is meant the biochemical processes, sequences, or pathways by which cells grow and proliferate, and are sustained. The various steps involved are each selectively catalyzed by a particular enzyme, which may in turn be inhibited, blocked, controlled, or modulated by other substances called enzyme inhibitors. As had been noted the latter may be internally generated or may be administered from external sources. The action can therefore be described as biochemical, both of the enzymes and of the inhibitors.

Particular emphasis will be placed on plants or plant-derived substances, whose myriad chemical constituents are commonly referred to as phytochemicals or plant chemicals, some of which are especially biologically active, or bioactive, and some of which may selectively act as inhibitors for the critical enzyme or enzymes involved in cancer cell metabolism.

For our purposes carcinogenicity means oncogenicity, where the latter pertains to the formation of oncogenes, the cancer-causing entity at the genetic level. Whereas these and other terms may provide elaborate ways to talk about the causes, initiation, and formation of cancer, for example, from viruses, they do not necessarily project to the cure or cures. For this, the subject of enzyme inhibitors is of paramount interest, as it pertains to cancer cell metabolism, which in the main proceeds by what may be called anaerobic glycolysis — a finding of the German biochemist Otto Warburg, to be elaborated upon subsequently.

Of prime consideration with regard to curative powers will be the specific mention of known plant or herbal substances and other chemicals that may act as enzyme inhibitors for the controlling step in cancer cell metabolism by anaerobic glycolysis. This controlling step involves the formation of lactic acid or lactate by the catalytic action of one or more forms of the enzyme lactate dehydrogenase. In this way, the opportunity is afforded for cancer cell growth to be modulated, controlled, or blocked, that is, inhibited. A more recent development concerns the enzyme telomerase, which is involved in regulating cellular growth and aging, and for which the identification of inhibitors or modulators will be most timely.

Of parallel concern is melanoma, involving the enzyme tyrosinase, for which there are known enzyme inhibitors. Blood-related cancers such as leukemia, whose origin is different from that of solid tumors, apparently respond more favorably to certain cytotoxic chemotherapy agents, but here again a selective anticancer agent with no side effects would be most welcome. (There is a parallel action, that antileukemic drugs in fact destroy the overproliferating white blood cells.)

## CANCER FORMATION AND ONCOGENES

Aside from an inherited propensity, the more usual causes of cancer are considered to be viruses, chemicals, and radiation. These may be said to be carcinogenic or cancer-causing, and may be called carcinogens, albeit this label is generally reserved for chemicals. The intermediate result is the formation of oncogenes, the tumor-forming genetic entity in the chromosomes of the body cells, which may also be inherited. (The prefix "onco-" signifies tumor or cancer.)

Oversimplifying the ever-evolving complexities, it may be said that a chromosome is the structural unit proper in the cell nucleus that carries the genetic information, whereas the genes are the functional or operational units represented in the chromosome. Furthermore, a gene can be described as a segment on a length of DNA. The chromosome is the physical entity, and the genes figuratively represent the information and instructions, with each gene carrying its own set of information and instructions. The entire array of information and instructions may be called the genome, and can connote either an individual cell or the total organism. The genome therefore stands for the entire complement of DNA and RNA information or coding for protein synthesis, and cellular growth and death.

It has been found, moreover, that cancer-causing chemicals may be formed by the bacterial flora in the intestinal tract or gut, an important factor being diet. (As an example, the consumption of hydrogenated vegetable oils or *trans*-fatty acids is coming under increasing suspicion.) This intestinal reservoir can also be a source of myriad viruses, labeled *enteroviruses*, in humans and in animals. Both chemicals and viruses may be transferred to body fluids and subsequently enter cells. This latter phenomenon may be related to, and abetted by, what are called stress proteins or heat shock proteins and molecular chaperones, which enhance the transfer of substances across cell walls, including carcinogens, or cancer-causing chemicals.

It is for instance well known, or at least well inferred, that radiation and many chemicals are a more or less direct cause of genetic aberrations, and the aberrant entity may in turn be called an oncogene, as previously noted. Industrial chemicals in particular are routinely tested and screened for carcinogenicity, notably for their ability to produce bacterial mutations (mutagenicity) by what is usually called the Ames test.

Less well known are the ways in which a virus acts, and which may be more indirect or insidious, causing other strange or poorly understood diseases as well. That is, a virus may invade a cell and combine with the chromosomal genes to become what is called a provirus or protovirus, the parent entity for forming oncogenes. Beyond this, even venoms, toxins, or drug chemicals are potentially suspect as carcinogenic or oncogenic agents, although the cancer formation may be noticeable only over the long term, and the effect cannot be traced to first cause.

The sequence is similar to that of what is referred to as *lysogeny*, in which two different modes may occur. In one mode, the usual course for viral infections, the virus invades the host cell and follows the familiar lytic mode. That is, the virus is replicated in the cell such that the cell lyses or self-destructs, releasing the replicated progeny viruses to infect other cells. (In this context, the virus — or viral or virus particle, or virion — is sometimes referred to as a *prophage*, the suffix "-phage" indicating something that "eats" or destroys cells.) In the other mode, called the *lysogenic life cycle*, the virus transmits its DNA to the host-cell chromosome and is accordingly designated a provirus, whose genes continue to be so expressed, initiating and maintaining a transformed or malignant, or oncogenic state. (A provirus or protovirus signifies the parent form that results in the formation of oncogenes.) These viruses may exist in a latent form, to be induced by various factors or agents to multiply and infect other cells, producing tumors.

## TYPES OF CANCERS

It may also be noted, as per an *Encyclopedia Britannica* article, subsequently to be cited, that retroviruses are often defective and require the assistance of other, nondefective helper retroviruses. (In retroviruses, which are commonly associated with cancer, the RNA provides the cellular instructions rather than the DNA.) Usually, these helper viruses are involved in transforming fibroblastic cells, as in connective tissue, and the result is malignant sarcomas. Otherwise, without assistance, the defective retroviruses will act to transform blood cell precursors, and the end result is leukemia.

The preceding paragraph shows that there is indeed a difference between blood-related cancers and solid malignancies, related to the origins. Solid tumors or malignancies may in turn be distinguished as sarcomas or carcinomas. Sarcomas are defined as malignancies in the nonepithelial tissues or cells such as of connective tissue, lymphoid tissue, cartilage, bone, etc., whereas carcinomas are malignancies occurring in epithelial tissue, the tissue that lines free surfaces or body cavities, and which consists of one or more layers of cells with little intercellular substance.

It may be added that melanomas, which may or may not become malignant, constitute still another category, with the differences in chemotherapeutical treatment, for one thing, constituting prima facie evidence. More definitively, pigment cell biology is relevant to melanoma. Thus, melanoma originates in cells called melanocytes, the source for the manufacture of the pigment melanin. The conversion of the well-known amino acid tyrosine to levadopa via an enzyme named tyrosinase is involved. The levadopa is subsequently oxidized to melanin. Melanoma cells, however, contain much more tyrosinase than normal melanocytes. Thus, the biochemistry or metabolism for malignant melanoma is uniquely different from that for other cancer cells.

Because cancerous cells mimic the normal cells from which they originate, cancers may be classified on the basis of their origin. Thus, there may be more than 100 different kinds of cancer, or perhaps 300, or even as many as 600, depending on — or, in the limit, equal to — the number of different kinds of cells in the body. (Moreover, as will be subsequently discussed, this mimicry prevents the body's own immune system from distinguishing cancerous cells from its own normal cells, although it can immediately recognize foreign cells and react accordingly.)

However, there is what is known as cancer of unknown primary (CUP). In other words, the cancer has metastasized, and in some cases it is found not to be possible to trace the cancer back to its primary origins (although cellular identity may be a clue, because cancer cells are known to mimic the body cells where they originate). This complicates the treatment, because a given chemotherapeutic cancer drug will presumably be more effective against a particular kind of cancer. This underlines the fact that a universal therapeutic drug would be most welcome — a drug effective against all kinds of cancer. In turn, will (or must) such a drug be synthetic or derived from natural sources? And, of course, can or does such a drug already exist, natural or synthetic?

Regarding the number of different cancers that may exist, Ralph W. Moss furnishes "A New View of Cancer's Origins" in his column "The War on Cancer" in the May 2005 issue of the *Townsend Letter for Doctors & Patients*. Thus, Moss mentions that in work at the University of Massachusetts Medical School, scientists led by Professor Jean Marie Houghton, M.D., Ph.D., found that stomach cancer may be linked to a type of undifferentiated stem cell that originates in the bone marrow. An infection of the bacterium *Helicobacter felis* (related to *Helicobacter pylori* in humans) would cause an influx of bone-marrow-derived stem cells, called BMDCs. These stem cells would attempt to repair the injury produced by the infection. The team found that it was these stem cells and not the stomach cells that produced the cancer. The implication is that there may be a similar occurrence with other forms of cancer, giving rise to a unified theory for cancer. This notion is not new, however, and is tied in with the idea that inflammation causes cancer. The quote is supplied that "the link between infection, chronic inflammation, and cancer has long been recognized." More than this, there is a link between cancer and bacteria, as per the past work of Coley, Livingston, and Eleanor-Jackson, some of which is cited elsewhere. (And to this may be added the phenomenon known as pleomorphism, whereby bacteria themselves may transform or be transformed, as described in the following section.)

## PLEOMORPHISM

In the work of researcher Virginia Livingston on a cancer vaccine, there is mention of an ever-changing or form-changing, or pleomorphic, microbe designated *Progenitor cryptocides* or PC, which presumably may be the source, or a source, of cancer. Always present, it is noted to occur in especially high concentrations in cancer patients, and apparently can vary in size and shape down to that of a miniscule virus and back again. Injected into animals, it has been observed to cause cancer. The subject is examined in separate chapters in Walters' *Options: The Alternative Cancer Therapy Book* (1993), Moss's *Cancer Therapy: The Independent Consumer's Guide to Non-Toxic Treatment and Prevention* (1992), and Pelton and Overholser's *Alternatives in Cancer Therapy: The Complete Guide to Non-Traditional Treatments* (1994).

Other researchers identified the microbes as different species of the genera *Staphylococcus* and *Streptococcus* (Pelton and Overholser, 1994, p. 179). Dr. Livingston, however, did not claim her discovery to be unique, and commented that the same microorganism had long been observed by other researchers (Walters, 1993, p. 78).

Speaking further of infectious germs, Dr. Livingston advised against eating chicken and eggs (calling to mind the poultry abstinence of the Navajos, to be more fully described elsewhere — for example, in Chapter 8 — and their low natural cancer incidence). She similarly advised against beef (the mostly cancer–free Navajos eat mutton, boiled for a long time). Milk products are also better avoided (Walters, 1993, pp. 76, 77). In fact, Walters comments that the cancer microbe exists in chicken, meat, and dairy products. Commenting that many dressed chicken carcasses have tumors, Walters states that "Dr. Livingston believed that nearly 100 percent of chickens on American dinner tables have the active, pathological form of the cancer microbe, which she believed transmittable to humans." In another expert opinion, it was said that about 40% of all human cancers are derived from chicken and eggs. In one investigation, 90% of the chickens sold in New York City were found to have cancers attributed to a microbe much smaller than a bacterium — indicating a virus. Not only this, 80 to 90% of domestic cattle carry a leukemia virus. Both Switzerland and Sweden, incidentally, keep milk from leukemic cows off the market. (Not to mention that commercial feedlots have been called a breeding ground for disease and death, as per Jeff and Jessica Pearson's *No Time but Place: A Prairie Pastoral*, 1980, pp. 146–149.)

About pork, there is the comment that the blood of a person who eats pork will be indistinguishable from that of a cancer patient for 8 or 9 hours after eating (Lynes, *Cancer Cure*, 1992, p. 123).

The preceding statement was included in a chapter about AIDS in Lynes' book *The Cancer Cure That Worked!* which also remarked about the pleomorphism that is said to exist between viruses and bacteria. The book states further "that AIDS is cancer, and that cancer is AIDS." To these can be added, the mutations found to occur in the AIDS retrovirus or other retroviruses can be alternately regarded as merely a case of pleomorphism — or vice versa. We are here maybe talking about semantics, therefore. Because most conventional authorities see only the dead viruses after successive increments of time, any such phenomenon is regarded as stepwise or discontinuous, and is therefore described as a series of mutations. Those who speak of pleomorphism see the phenomenon as a continuum in terms of live viruses.

Ralph Moss concludes his book *Cancer Therapy* with a chapter about the work of microbiologist Gaston Naessens. (The Livingston Method was discussed by Moss in a prior chapter.) An elementary living particle is described that Naessens calls a "somatid," but which can be seen only through a special, proprietary microscope which Naessens called a "somatoscope." The somatoscope is said to observe the behavior of a minute living organism beyond the reach of ordinary microscopes — as distinguished from electron microscopy, where the organisms first have to be killed. Naessens is reported to have observed somatids existing in all biological liquids, notably blood, and he notes that under stress their life cycle changes, possibly leading to cancer.

As a treatment, Naessens used a mixture of nitrogen-containing camphor, called 714X (and said to be trimethylbicyclonitraminoheptane chloride). It is injected directly into the lymph system, and the nitrogen content is stated to be the active ingredient. Not only has Naessens' treatment been discounted by medical orthodoxy, but his work on somatids has been coolly received by conventional microbiology. Richard Walters (1993) *Options* and Pelton and Overholser (1994) furnish more information.

Other characteristics ascribed to somatids include a strong resistance to temperature extremes, radiation, and death of the host. Called elementary particles of life, they conceivably correspond to the "microzymes" of the French scientist Béchamp, a rival and contemporary of Pasteur. (Whereby, a "microzyme" or microenzyme can be construed as a minute biological form of one kind or another that displays enzymatic or biocatalytic action, accelerating a biochemical reaction or reactions.)

The Naessens treatment had a positive encounter on the TV program *Good Morning America* on April 7, 1995. A patient named Billy Best, of Norwell, MA, was interviewed, and he also made an appearance on *Dateline* and other programs. The Naessen theory received favorable notices in a book published in 1991 by Christopher Bird titled *The Persecution of Gaston Naessens: The True Story of the Efforts to Suppress an Alternative Treatment for Cancer, AIDS, and Other Immunologically Based Diseases.*

If the recoveries using 714X are for the most part true, then it is indeed amazing, even unto a temporary remission from deadly pancreatic cancer (e.g., Walters, 1993, p. 34). It was reported to have prolonged the patient's life beyond expectations, with the patient remaining painfree — although the attending physician called 714X no panacea. Others such as Ralph Moss are not yet convinced about the treatment.

If all this seems farfetched, there is a reminder that subviral particles exist, for example, prions, as implicated in mad cow disease, or bovine spongiform encephalitis (BSE), or similar diseases of the nervous system in both animals and humans. Furthermore, the term *pleomorphism* is not unknown in treatises on microbiology or biochemistry.

## VIRAL OR MICROBIAL ORIGINS AND TREATMENTS

Early on and along the way, the concept emerged that cancer may be linked to viruses or other microorganisms or microbes. (A wart is an example of a benign tumorous mass caused by a virus.) There is even the idea that such other effects as chemicals and radiation may trigger a cancer-causing virus. Seeing how viruses may mutate, or maybe undergo pleomorphic changes, it appears there are lots of possibilities. It is a subject area with its own appellation, namely "viral oncology."

Viruses are elementary microorganisms or molecular organisms structured at the DNA and RNA level, and so in one way or another, we may at the same time be speaking also of changes in the genetic code that involve what we call viruses. An opinion increasingly held is that only a small proportion of cancers are in fact direc tly virus related; they are instead caused by "oncogenes," inherited or induced, and counteracted by "suppressor genes." (The word root "onco-" is derived from the Greek transliteration *onko*, meaning mass or bulk.) Obviously, however, something causes cancer, and what is needed is a cure, not a reason.

Industrial chemicals such as benzene are notorious for causing chromosome damage, which implies genetic damage. The same for the effects of radiation and radioactivity. Whether or not "viruses" act as the intermediary may be only academic, because the whole business is at the DNA and RNA level, or molecular level, anyway, as are viruses. It may be more a game of semantics.

Nevertheless, we would settle for an inoculation to immunize against cancer, all cancers, and get it over with once and for all. That is, presumably if we could just determine which and what viruses cause the different cancers. So in one way or another there is a continuing search for universally effective cancer vaccines, in a class with polio vaccines, an ideal yet to be realized, though Virginia Livingston, M.D., is credited with an earlier attempt; see Chapter 7 of Walters (1993). The problem may, however, be much more complicated than merely developing antibodies for a specific virus, as we are here talking about genetic codes.

And right away, the question must be asked, if cancers are in part virus caused, then why are not some cancers at least contagious, as are other viral diseases? Or is this a distinguishing factor between cancer-causing viruses and other kinds of viruses? In other words, are we here speaking of special kinds of viruses, maybe of pleomorphic viruses vs. monomorphic viruses? It is a subject for future discussion.

Inasmuch as a virus can be described as some sort of elementary combination of DNA or RNA, there is the school of thought that the answer to cancer may lie in the fundamental chemistries of DNA and RNA and their modification, be it by genetic engineering or whatever you call it (presumably a long-term line of research). All this, of course, presupposes that what we think of as viruses are somehow connected with cancer; that is, that cells can be, and are, invaded by viruses, sometimes causing cancer.

Speaking further of viruses and microbes, there remains the continuing question of just which specific microorganisms may cause cancer. We turn next to the efforts of Royal R. Rife and radiotherapy.

A treatment that did not survive — at least in its original embodiment — has been referred to as radiotherapy, or by various other names. It is included in a chapter titled "Bioelectric Therapies" in Walters (1993). An entire book has been written about it: *The Cancer Cure That Worked!: Fifty Years of Suppression* by Barry Lynes (1992). The method was developed by Royal Raymond Rife, and involved a specially built electromagnetic frequency generator, called the Rife generator. Royal Rife was a scientist and inventor located in San Diego, but who originally hailed from Nebraska. Walters comments that there have since been numerous other generators built supposedly on the same principles, but which do not reproduce the same phenomena, and may be hazardous. Additionally, Rife is said to have constructed a very powerful light microscope with which he could view live bacteria and even live viruses.

(It may be noted in passing that electromagnetic radiation is also regarded as a cause of cancer or other adverse effects, depending on the wavelength, intensity, and exposure. Examples include x-rays, cosmic rays, microwaves, radiation from high-voltage electrical power transmission lines, even sunlight. Not to mention radioactivity and its associated gamma rays, as well as alpha and beta particles, and other radioactive products or by-products from nuclear reactions.)

Four forms of the cancer microbe were discovered, varying from a fungus to a bacillus to a virus. (Bacteria are considered by some microbiologists to be a special, elementary, and ambiguous form of fungi or Mycota.) One of the forms, called a monococcoid, occurred in the blood of some 90% of cancer patients. Furthermore, Rife concluded from his observations that these minute life-forms are pleomorphic, that is, they can metamorphose from one form to another (as per the subsequent work of Livingston and of Naessens). Apparently harmless bacteria can become disease-producing viruses.

By 1932, Walters notes, Rife had used his electromagnetic generator, called a *frequency instrument*, to destroy the cancer microbe as well as the typhus virus, the herpes virus, and other viruses in cultures and in experimental animals. Starting in 1934, the Rife generator was used successfully to treat human cancer patients in a simple 3-minute burst every third day. Complete remissions were attained. But Rife ran afoul of the usual machinations, and by 1939 had been virtually forced out of business. A partner of Rife, John Crane, was subsequently tried in 1961 and spent 3 years in jail. The FDA still bans the Rife-like treatments for human medical use, though some apparently are still around, skirting the ban, but Walters advises caution in considering their use.

(The duplication and improvement of Rife's equipment and results is certainly a subject for further research. And there are stirrings in these directions, as presented under the heading of Magnetic Field Therapy in the *Alternative Medicine Yellow Pages*. More specifically, the following names and addresses are included: Enviro-Tech Products,17171 SE 29th St., Choctaw, OK 73020; Bio-Electro-Magnetics Institute, 2490 West Moana Lane, Reno, NV 89509-3936, (702)827-9099; Dr. Wolfgang Ludwid, Silcherstrasse 21, Horb A.N.1, Germany, FAX: 011-49-7451-8648. Also, there is a flyer issued by Natural Energies, Inc., 1825 Tamiami Trail A6#108T, Port Charlotte, FL 33948, 702-579-4027, which describes what is named the ProWave© Model 101, a system that sells for $2495.00. It is said to utilize solid-state electronics, and to apply the radio frequency energy via electrodes rather than beaming it through the air. A disclaimer is proffered, to be signed prior to purchase.)

In Chapter 2 and Chapter 3 of Lynes' book about Rife's work in the 1930s, some of the intrigues that went on behind the scenes are described. For one thing, the idea of pleomorphic viral and bacterial changes was greeted with hostility, in particular by a Dr. Rivers of the Rockefeller Institute, who was strongly opposed to the notion. The Rockefeller Institute was not only a source of funding for medical research, but wielded great power in the halls of professional recognition. For another, after the demonstrated efficacy of Rife's methods, others had the notion of grabbing a share of his success. One person named was none other than Dr. Morris Fishbein, who virtually ran the American Medical Association, and who wanted "in," and when rebuffed, threw the entire weight of the AMA against Rife and his associates. Another opponent was Dr. Cornelius P. Rhoads, afterwards a strong advocate of chemotherapy, who at the time was first at the Rockefeller Institute and then director of the Memorial Sloan-Kettering Cancer Center. In turn, there were the ties to the American Cancer Society, the National Cancer Institute, the FDA, and the doctors, pharmaceutical companies, and private research institutes. This armada of organized opposition was more than could be overcome.

The effect of electromagnetic radiation on the body is little understood. In small dosages it may activate the immune system, or else it might act as an inhibitor to the enzyme-catalyzed anaerobic metabolism of cancer cells, which involves the glucose–lactic acid cycle. In larger doses the effects can apparently be damaging to the body, though the degree may vary with the individual. There is a similar effect for radioactive substances, namely, radon gas. The latest word is that small or minute levels of radon exposure may be beneficial in that it stimulates the body's immune system, whereas higher exposures have a disastrous track record. These trace exposures are another facet of homeopathy, a premise being that traces of an agent that causes a disease are said to act instead against the disease.

In the work of Virginia Livingston on a cancer vaccine, described earlier, the subject of viral pleopmorphism was introduced. However, the notion that a cancer-causing viral entity exists brings up the matter of contagion. Yet, the distinction is generally made that cancer is not contagious — whereas AIDS, say, is. The classic experiment is to introduce cancer cells into a healthy animal or person, and nothing happens; whereas if the victim already has cancer, it is another story. This may not be the end of the matter, however, for there is the question of introducing the blood from a cancer victim into a healthy victim or animal, as happens with the transmission of AIDS. If the viral-microbial theory for cancer holds, one should beware.

The trouble with pleomorphism is when it is assumed that viruses can change or assemble into bacteria, and bacteria can change or decompose into viruses. (We adopt the convention that a virus is composed of a core of nucleic acid with a coat of protein plus maybe a lipid or fatty material and carbohydrate material. Bacteria are unicellular microorganisms, with a nuclear substance surrounded by a membrane and cell wall.) Ordinarily, a virus may invade a bacterial cell, but this presupposes the existence of both. And it may be not so much whether transmutations can occur, however, but how do they occur? In the latter regard, there is the fact that some bacterial cells contain genetic elements or pieces of DNA called *plasmids*, which can function as viruses. Thus, viruses possibly may originate as a fragment of cellular nucleic acid that has become independent of the host cell. (See, for instance, the topic "Virus" in the *Encyclopedia Britannica.*) And, conversely, we may reason that these viruses or plasmids may recombine to form a bacterial cell.

In any event, the idea of pleomorphic microbes is not generally accepted, and the controversy dates back to the previously indicated argument between the famous French chemist Louis Pasteur (1822–1895) and his chief rival, French microbiologist Antoine Béchamp (Walters, 1993, pp. 78, 79). Pasteur believed in nonchangeable microbes (reportedly, later renounced), whereas Béchamp spoke in terms of more fundamental "microzymes" that can grow or evolve into bacteria, given the right circumstances. That is, the size, form, or identity of any strain of bacteria depends on the circumstances or conditions, and accordingly it can change into a disease-producing strain.

The German bacteriologist Guenther Enderlein (1872–1968) also came to believe in pleomorphism, and that harmless bacteria in the body can change into disease-causing bacteria or fungi (Walters, 1993, p. 16). He is said to have developed medicines to cause a reversion back to the harmless form. A medical doctor and homeopath, Dr. Abram Ber, who practices in Phoenix, AZ, is reported to use the Enderlein remedies with success. Two others also cited who use the Enderlein medicines are Harvey Bigelson, M.D., of Scottsdale, AZ, and Erik Enby, M.D., of Gothenberg, Sweden.

The matter of growth in size in a liquid medium is particularly vexing, apparently in that some sort of virus-like submicroscopic particles or life-forms — if that is the word, and whatever a virus is supposed to be — will somehow grow or coalesce and end up as larger bacteria-like life-forms. This may not be too radical an idea, because we accept the fact that cells divide, and we also accept the fact that cells grow or multiply as multicellular organisms.

An autogenous vaccine (from a culture of the patient's own bacteria) was developed by Dr. Livingston and is said to have had a success rate of 82% or higher, though Walters calls for caution in these figures (Walters, 1993, p. 80). The Livingston Foundation Medical Center, located in San Diego, CA, was in 1990 forbidden to continue the use of autogenous vaccines by California health officials, though nonautogenous vaccines were still used.

Dr. Livingston first viewed *Progenitor cryptocides* as attacking the "genetic" memory of the nucleus of healthy cells, causing them to proliferate. A later viewpoint was that *P. cryptocides* causes infection, lowering the immune response, which enables the cancer cells to multiply. In other words, cancer is an immune-deficiency disease (Walters, 1993, pp. 74, 75).

In further comment, AIDS is also an immune-deficiency disease, and therefore there is an implied connection with cancer. Moreover, the AIDS virus is also described as ever-changing, which complicates finding a cure. Thus, there is a similarity with Dr. Livingston's findings.

(This brings up the point that it would be desirable to have a simple test to measure and rate the activity of the immune system, and more and better ways to activate or stimulate the immune system.)

Another mechanism that surfaced was Dr. Livingston's discovery that *P. cryptocides* could produce a hormone nearly identical to the human hormone named *human chorionic gonadotrophin* (HCG), called "the hormone of life and death." It is also present as *choriogonadotropin* (CG) in various cells, including cancer cells. Her findings were confirmed at several orthodox laboratories, and it was shown that all cancer cells, animal or human, contain CG. Furthermore, Dr. Livingston found that abscisic acid neutralizes CG, and as such is "nature's most potent anti-cancer weapon." Abscisic acid is a plant hormone and vitamin A analog commonly present in such foods as carrots, mangoes, avocados, tomatoes, lima beans, and green leafy vegetables. Because cancer patients lose their ability to break down vitamin A in the liver to make abscisic acid, she recommended drinking carrot juice containing dried liver powder, in that the liver enzymes break down the vitamin A to form abscisic acid. Newer research confirms that vitamin A is a significant factor in protecting the body from cancer. Thus, a group of vitamin A analogs called *retinoids* have been used to cause cancer cells to develop into normal cells, a process called *differential therapy*. Human abscisic acid is believed to serve the same function, breaking down vitamin A into retinoids (Walters, 1993, pp. 75, 76).

Accordingly, and on account of the foregoing, and to further paraphrase from Walters (1993), the Livingston anticancer diet emphasizes nonprocessed fresh vegetables and fruits and whole grains, raw or slightly cooked, and abetted by vitamins, minerals, and enzymes to help the body build immunity (Walters, 1993, p. 76). Refined flour and white sugar are not to be used, and salt and high-sodium foods are discouraged, though potassium-rich fruits and vegetables are encouraged. Most animal products are also forbidden because, in addition to the virus-microbe problem, they may be charged with toxins, synthetic hormones, antibiotics, and pesticides that subvert the immune system (Walters, 1993, p. 76). This kind of diet has become virtually a standard.

If all this seems out of the ordinary, read on.

The concluding chapter of Moss (1992) is about the pioneering work of microbiologist Gaston Naessens, as has been described earlier, and which involved an elementary living particle which he called a "somatid," against which a mixture of nitrogen-containing camphor, called 714X, is injected into the lymph system, the nitrogen being the active ingredient. Speaking further of nitrogen-bearing compounds, in Moss 1(992) for instance, both hydrazine sulfate and urea are provided separate chapters as anticancer agents. Whereas urea is apparently a common-enough chemical, a source for hydrazine sulfate is the Syracuse Cancer Research Institute, Presidential Plaza, 600 East Genesee St., Syracuse, NY 13202, (315)472-6616. It may be observed that both hydrazine sulfate, $N_2H_4H_2SO_4$, and urea, $H_2NCONH_2$, contain bound nitrogen, designated by the symbol "N." A confirmation is furnished in a letter from Wayne Martin that appeared in the November 2005 *Townsend Letter for Doctors and Patients*. He cited the previously reported work of Professor Evangelos Danopoulos of Athens, Greece, that had appeared in *Clinical Oncology* in 1983, where oral urea was used to treat liver cancer and colorectal cancer. That this treatment worked was evidenced by a patient in Singapore, and another in Australia for breast cancer. Dosage levels quoted were 15 g of urea per day. Needless to say, there was opposition within medical orthodoxy.

More details are provided by Walters (1993) and Pelton and Overholser (1994). Returning to Naessens' work, he found that somatids — whatever they are — tend to be indestructible, not being affected by strong acids or by nuclear radiation, or by temperatures as high as 200°C (392°F) or higher, and surviving the death of their host (Walters, 1993, p. 35). He thus concluded that somatids were, in fact, elementary particles in the chain of life. They presumably correspond to the "microzymes" of Béchamp, previously mentioned.

As for the specifics of the Naessens therapy, as has been noted, the mixture called 714X is injected into the lymph system at the groin area. For the record, recommended daily dosages of the serum are presented at the end of the chapter in Pelton and Overholser (1994). There is a cautionary note that vitamin E and vitamin B12 should not be taken at the same time as 714X, a caution also mentioned in other references: *Alternative Medicine: The Definitive Guide*, p. 574; *An Alternative Medicine Definitive Guide to Cancer*, pp. 32, 504.

(In *Alternative Medicine: The Definitive Guide*, a practitioner cited who used 714X and other alternative therapies is Harvey Bigelson, M.D., of Scottsdale, AZ. Additional resources are found in *An Alternative Medicine Definitive Guide to Cancer*, e.g., p. 781ff.)

A most interesting side feature is that Naessens claims that the condition of somatids in the blood can be used to detect the initiation of cancer up to 18 months before clinical symptoms appear (Walters, 1993, p. 31). It may also be mentioned in passing that there is the Ames bacterial test, which serves as an indicator of possible cancer activity in the body (Heinerman, 1984, p. 152).

(For additional information about the Naessens 714X therapy, there is, or was, an address and phone number in Canada: C.O.S.E., Inc., 5270, Fontaine, Rock Forest, Quebec, JIN 3B6, (819)564-7883 — if the phone is answered. A list of U.S. doctors who administer 714X is presumably available. Other information — some conflicting — is available from the British Columbia Cancer Agency, or BCCA, at Vancouver, which can be accessed on the Internet. With instructions provided, 714X is or was also available by mail for home injection. An interested party could also consult Genesis West-Provida, P.O. Box 3460, Chula Vista, CA 91902-0004, (619)424-9552, which is a referral point for a clinic in Tijuana, Mexico. In particular, there is, or was, Writers and Research, Inc., 4810 St. Paul Blvd., Rochester, NY 14167, (800)488-4332. Writers and Research has published a book about 714X and its use, titled *Do No Harm*, and has been involved with supplying the serum. The latest word is that cooperation is maintained with the FDA, and that administration of 714X must be by a physician. For an update, consult the Internet.)

As has already been mentioned, the Naessens treatment received an electrifying boost on the TV program *Good Morning America* on April 7, 1995, with some apparently amazing recoveries reported (e.g., Walters, 1993, p. 34). It may be added, however, that Ralph Moss in his monthly column in the *Townsend Letter* was not overly enthusiastic about the Naessens therapy, although Naessens' theories about pleomorphism were of much interest.

In sum, the viral or microbial theories or mechanisms of cancer formation and its cure seem for the most part plausible. If these theories can be tied in with the cancer-forming consequences, say, of radiation and chemicals — and they seemingly can — and with the anticancer effects of other agents, in particular plants and herbs, this would round out the picture. As such, it will furnish a way to unify cancer theory at the most elementary level.

The concept of pleomorphism may very well tie in with the fact that nearly 600 different kinds of cancer cells reportedly have been identified. And that one kind of cancer may lead to another, or secondary, cancer. That is, cancer may not only metastasize or spread as the same kind of cancer, but a new kind may occur (that is, in different kinds of cells). If, say, viruses are involved in cancer formation, and can change from one kind to another, then the different kinds of cancer-causing viruses could be legion. And this, of course, may be an obstruction to the development of a general vaccine, as is in the case of AIDS. (It may be reemphasized that the work of Dr. Livingston was aimed at autogenous vaccines, specific to the particular patient.)

Whether or not the foregoing will meet with the approval of the medical establishment is ultimately immaterial, for at this level it is a microbiological and biochemical issue in basic science. All this aside, what really counts is how well the treatment works.

## VIRUSES AND LYSOGENY

The 15th edition of the *Encyclopedia Britannica*, published in 1974, under the category Viruses has a section titled "Viral DNA Integration," with subsections on Lysogeny and on Malignant Transformation. The discussions are of a technical nature, with the latter subsection of particular interest. Virus families or viruses occurring in animals and known to produce malignant transformations are cited, and are divided into DNA viruses and RNA viruses, the latter also involving retroviruses. The DNA viruses include the papova viruses or Papovaviridae, the most common of which are the papilloma viruses, the cause of polyps (e.g., warts). Another family is the adenoviruses or Adenoviridae, first noticed in human tonsils and adenoids, but not suspected as cancer causing. The herpes viruses or Herpesviridae are suspect, however; for example, the Epstein-Barr virus is known to produce Burkitt's lymphoma, often fatal in children.

Significantly, the RNA viruses or retroviruses, or Retroviridae, are the most widespread of the transforming viruses, affecting nonbacterial species from yeasts to humans. The characteristic enzyme called RNA-dependent DNA polymerase, or reverse transcriptase, is vitally involved. As a matter of record, the end result is what is known as double-stranded DNA, or dsDNA, which in turn can have some far-reaching results that were further spelled out in the *Encyclopedia Britannica* article. Also noted is that the retroviruses are most usually animal specific; that is, they do not ordinarily cross species barriers.

There are animal viruses, plant viruses, and bacterial viruses called *bacteriophages*. Animal viruses include mammalian viruses, both human and otherwise, avian viruses, and no doubt reptilian viruses. Additionally, there are insect viruses, from which, oddly enough, plant viruses may have evolved. (Some insects may carry an enormous load of viruses, but remain unaffected, although this is not necessarily the case for humans. Bee stings, for instance, have been correlated with melanoma occurrences, but whether these are attributable to viruses or to the toxins is apparently not known.) There are also fungal viruses and protozoan viruses (affording a potential mode of treatment or cure for malaria). The virus families are referred to as the

Viridae, and in some the nucleic acid is DNA and in others RNA, with both types occurring in animals. Large viruses, such as the poxviruses or Poxviridae, may contain enzymes such as RNA polymerase, involved in RNA synthesis.

(Viruses and bacteria are potential agents for treating cancer if they can be made to act selectively against cancer cells, that is, if they can work as pathogens for cancer cells only. Thus, the bacteria known as BCG, for Bacillus Calmette-Guerin, is a weakened strain of the microbe *Mycobacterium bovis*, which is used worldwide as a vaccine for tuberculosis. BCG is said to stimulate the immune system and thereby act against cancer. The treatment is described, for instance, in Ralph Moss (1992), but its effectiveness against cancer, so far, seems to be against bladder cancer, where BCG is injected directly into the bladder. As such, it has entered mainstream medical practice. Of further note are Coley's toxins, of bacterial origin, to be further described subsequently.)

Crossovers in fact do occasionally occur between viruses, as in the case of the human influenza virus, where past epidemics and outbreaks have been traced to crossovers or mutations with duck and swine viruses. The notion may, of course, be extended to the AIDS virus and to the Marburg and Ebola viruses. There is the remote prospect, even, that these may be of plant or insect origin. And there are concerns that decimating tropical rain forests may unleash unsuspected and unknown viruses, with adverse consequences.

In a brief book by former well-known herbalist and author Hanna Kroeger of Boulder, Colorado, titled *Free Your Body of Tumors and Cysts*, it was stated that tumors are caused by fungi as well as viruses. Among those caused by fungi she lists hard tumors, a tumor formed by the fungus maduromycates as found in India, and prostate cancer. As for the kinds caused by viruses, she lists the following four virus classifications: papilloma and papilloma combined with Epstein-Barr, Epstein-Barr with herpes, herpes with another virus, and retroviruses.

With regard to retroviruses, it is indicated that these were originally found in animals such as mice and apes, and are involved in the diseases hepatitis C, adult T-cell leukemia, hairy cell leukemia, lymph cell leukemia, peripheral T-cell lymphoma, non-Hodgkins lymphoma, breast cancer, lupus, multiple sclerosis, and brain tumors. Noting that retroviruses can change their genetic makeup — that is, mutate — and may lie dormant for years, it is further stated that HIV and AIDS may be induced by the presence of hookworm, giardia, and amoeba. Multiple sclerosis and lupus will occur if nickel and lead (possibly acting as catalysts) are present in the body.

The assertion is repeated that polio vaccine derived from Rhesus monkeys was contaminated with the monkey or ape virus named Simian 40. It is a retrovirus, harmless to apes and other animals, but in humans may affect the nervous system, and may be responsible for mental disorders, in turn manifested in crime, even in suicides. Not to mention cancer.

Astounding numbers of viruses of different kinds may occur in meat products. Although there are concerns, and rightly so, about bacterial contamination — for example, the species *Escherichia coli* or *E. coli*, and the genus *Salmonella* — little or nothing is said about viruses. These viruses may occur naturally or by contamination, a prime repository being the intestinal tract or gut, as previously noted. Sometimes described as disease ridden, feedlots are getting a bad name.

The word also is that isolated societies or cultures that follow a vegetarian diet — such as in parts of Mongolia — also have a low cancer incidence. The Hunzas of the Himalayas, who are noted for their long life spans, are lactovegetarians.

(Among other hazards, as per the Navajos, is that of radiation-induced cancers of workers in the uranium mines, and of children playing around radioactive mine tailings. Newer on the scene is the use of depleted uranium, or DU, in munitions, which ends up as dust, spreading over the land and into the atmosphere. For instance, according to an article by Paul Likoudis in the November 8, 2004, issue of the *American Free Press*, this has resulted in radioactive poisoning, occurring in and after both the Gulf War and the Iraq War, with much higher cancer rates and birth defects. There is apparently a reluctance even to talk about this sort of thing, as will be subsequently reported in discussing Duff Wilson's *Fateful Harvest*, about toxic chemicals being included in the fertilizer that was spread on crop soils in Washington State.)

Dairy products contain both microbes and viruses, for instance, polio and hepatitis viruses, which is a good and sufficient reason for pasteurization as a partial remediation. Also occurring is the bovine leukemia virus, or BLV, said to be related to HIV. A high proportion of U.S. milk cows are said to be infected, and milk from the United States cannot be exported to certain European countries. For more on the subject there is Jeremy Rifkin's *Beyond Beef: The Rise and Fall of the Cattle Culture* (1992).

## VIRUSES AND SUBVIRUSES

Whereas DNA is the main source of genetic information, other information can also be carried in RNA (Gray, in Devlin, 1986, p. 873). This occurs in the sequence of bases that constitute RNA, and which serves as the genome in several viruses. (In genetic parlance, a genome can be viewed as the abstraction that represents all the genetic information, whether at the molecular level or for the organism as a whole.) Normally, however, RNA does not serve as the genome in eukaryotic or in prokaryotic cells, but rather is found in the tumor viruses and other small RNA viruses such as poliovirus and reovirus.

Viruses can be defined as infectious particles that consist of a nucleic acid molecule surrounded by a protective coat made up of protein (Voet and Voet, 1995, pp. 841, 1074). The virus particle is known as a *virion*; the protein coating is called a *capsid*. In more complex viruses, the capsid may be encased by an envelope derived from a host cell membrane.

When adsorbed by a cell, the virus insinuates its nucleic acid, whereby the viral chromosome redirects the cell's metabolism to produce new viruses, which in turn initiate further infection. The virus has no metabolism of its own, and can be described as the ultimate parasite. Viruses are not considered living organisms, and in the absence of the host cell, are biologically inert, the same as any other large molecule. Viruses called bacteriophages, which infect bacteria, have been used to study bacterial genetics as well as viral genetics. And because viruses have no metabolism, their presence is indicated by the death of the host cell.

It is noted that mutant or wild-type phages or viruses may occur (Voet and Voet, 1995, p. 842). Thus, we may be speaking of genetic crossovers, such as for influenza viruses that invade humans as well as animals, and even of such incidences as of the Marburg and Ebola viruses.

Furthermore, as viruses in a sense "eat" the host cell, and hence may be called "phages," for example, bacteriophages, there may be a connection with what is called pleomorphism, in which viruses or microbes are thought to change their form or makeup. That is, if a virus eats or destroys bacteria, then there is nothing left but a virus, or virus particle, called a virion.

Infecting plants and bacteria as well as animals, viruses are divided into helical and spherical viruses, and their great simplicity as compared to cells assists in the study of gene structure and function, though viral modes of gene replication are more varied (Voet and Voet, 1995, p. 1076). No particular mention is made of cancer-causing viruses in the reference.

However, in a section on subviral pathogens, it is commented that our ideas about infectious agents are still evolving (Voet and Voet, 1995, p. 1113ff). Thus, two types of subviral agents have been discovered that cause infectious diseases. One is the viroid, composed of a small single-stranded RNA molecule. The other is the prion, which is apparently only a protein molecule.

It is thought that viroids are similar to what are called introns. In the language of genetic codes, an intron is the noncoding sequence in what are designated mRNA molecules, as compared to the exon, which is the coding sequence (Gray, in Devlin, 1986, p. 906).

Prions are now thought to be what were formerly called "slow viruses," because the resulting diseases took months or years or decades to develop (Voet and Voet, 1995, p. 1116). These particular diseases pertain to the mammalian nervous system. None of the diseases exhibit inflammation or fever, indicating that the immune system is neither activated nor impaired by the disease. As has been indicated, the word prion stands for "proteinaceous infectious particle," and the protein itself is called PrP, for prion protein.

(A mycoplasma is the smallest microorganism capable of independent replication and growth. These mycoplasmas may be regarded as a cross between a bacterium and a virus. The inference is that there may be an extended spectrum of micromolecular entities ranging from fungi and bacteria down through viruses to subviruses — even to various molecular-sized particles, pieces, or segments — and back up again.)

The foregoing brief discussions about viroids and prions serve to illustrate that there are many unknowns left to be uncovered. Cancer causes and cures may very well lie in this domain, and may tie in with some of the unconventional cancer therapies — e.g., the work of Naessens, Livingston, Rife, and others, whose findings about pleomorphism seem to have upset the conventional wisdom about microorganisms.

As an interesting adjunct, 1974 Nobel Prize cowinner Christian de Duve, in an article in the April 1996 issue of the *Scientific American*, advanced the idea that human or mammalian eukaryotic cells evolved from bacterial prokaryotic cells. That is to say, tiny, primitive bacteria were transformed into the large, intricately organized cells of humans and other mammals. One can wonder if the processes are ongoing, and reversible.

## ANTIVIRAL AGENTS

The most pervasive and well-known antiviral agent is, of course, the immune system, in terms of the immune response. Certain types of white blood cells, collectively called lymphocytes, leave the blood vessels and patrol the intercellular regions looking for foreign invaders (Voet and Voet, 1995, p. 1207). The lymphocytes arise from precursor cells in the bone marrow, as do all blood cells. The lymphocytes eventually return to the blood by way of the lymphatic vessels after interacting with such lymphoid tissues as the thymus, lymph nodes, and the spleen.

(Lymphatic cancer, or cancer of the lymph glands, can occur, and a treatment is described by Rudoph Ballentine, M.D., on page 328 of *Radical Healing*. The treatment involved what was called *Silica* 1M, described as a "daring and deep-acting prescription." The patient's swollen lymph nodes soon opened and started draining, and continued for months. When the discharges finally stopped, the openings healed, and the patient's good health returned, and continued.)

The two types of immunity recognized are cellular immunity and humoral immunity. The former protects against virally infected cells, fungi, parasites, and foreign tissue. Its functions are carried out by T lymphocytes, or T-cells, which develop in the thymus. Humoral immunity ("humor" meaning fluid) is most active against bacterial infections and viral infections outside the cell. Its functions are carried out by proteins called antibodies or immunoglobulins. The antibodies are generated by B lymphocytes or B-cells in the bone marrow.

Another action of the immune system is to raise the body temperature, another way of killing off the invader's body.

Vitamin C (ascorbic acid), besides its other purposes — for example, in preventing scurvy — is a suspected antiviral agent, though the point is controversial and not settled. In other words, the effectiveness of vitamin C as a cure or preventive for the common cold is still argued (see the work of Linus Pauling), though recognition has come about that vitamin C at least alleviates its symptoms (Chaney, in Devlin, 1986, p. 1227). To which may be added, that the common cold is caused by a virus, and if vitamin C is not always effective, neither is the immune system, or we would never get sick in the first place.

Vitamin C "enhances the utilization of folic acid, either by aiding the conversion of folate to tetrahydrofolate or the formation of polyglutamate derivatives of tetrahydrofolate" (Chaney, in Devlin, 1986, p. 1226). Inasmuch as folic acid has a number of roles in body chemistry, including that of an anticancer agent, there may be further connections with the benefits of vitamin C that are yet to be spelled out.

Another characteristic of ascorbic acid, $C_6H_8O_6$, is that it is closely related chemically to glucose, $C_6H_{12}O_6$ (Chaney, in Devlin, 1986, p. 1225). Whether or not this chemical resemblance has a desirable effect on some of its properties is fuel for speculation. For the record, its main biochemical role is said to be that of a reducing agent in certain important hydroxylation reactions, for example, of lysine and proline in protocollagen. It is therefore important in maintaining normal connective tissue.

It may be commented also that ascorbic acid or ascorbate or vitamin C serves as an enzyme inhibitor. Jain's handbook (1982) lists a number of enzymes or phenomena that may be affected: adenylate cyclase; ATPase, Na, K; catalase; catechol *o*-methyl transferase; ferredoxin-NADP reductase; glucose-6-*p*-dehydrogenase; lipase; oxygenase, fatty acid; peroxidase; phosphodiesterase, cAMP; tyrosinase; and urea levels. Zollner's handbook (1993) lists the following affected enzymes: *o*-aminophenol oxidase; catalase; β-glucuronidase; GTP cyclohydrolase I; hydroxymethylglutaryl-CoA reductase; and lactoylglutathione lyase. Whether these inhibiting actions by vitamin C in some way involve the immune system and cancer repression evidently is not known. The enzyme catalase, incidentally, catalyzes the decomposition of hydrogen peroxides to water and oxygen (Voet and Voet, 1995, p. 9). Whether or not its inhibition would be beneficial under the special circumstances remains to be determined.

As a final note, there is the observation that antiviral agents act to inhibit the replication of nucleic acids. There is a connection with anticancer agents, which are enzyme inhibitors for DNA processes. In a way, the connection is obvious, in view of the fact that viruses are but pieces of DNA. A search of Medline indicates that antiviral agents being clinically tested include inhibitors for the enzymes called nucleoside phosphorylases and M-deoxyribosyltransferases.

These are but a few of the possibilities for antiviral agents. Many more lie in the myriad plant substances called phytochemicals or plant chemicals, a subject that is part of medical folklore. It does not take long to see why there is dissension about the complete role of nutrients and foreign substances in body biochemistry, in that it has not all been figured out yet, at least not in commonly accepted terms and theories. In other words, the completed rationale hasn't made its way into the treatises and textbooks.

## IMMUNE REACTIONS

The bodily reactions to the ingestion of plants or herbs, or their extracts, decoctions, or teas, may be a mild fever and the sweats from time to time, which are the symptoms produced when the immune system acts against such invaders as viruses. And the white cell blood count may be expected to rise at the same time, again a manifestation that the body is trying to fight off something or the other — the ingested or injected quasi poison and the tumor, at the same time.

Thus, microorganisms have been used in cancer treatment. For example, Moss has a chapter about Coley's Toxins, a mixed bacterial vaccine, in the treatment of cancer (Moss, 1992, pp. 407–412). Moss calls the discovery of these toxins one of the most remarkable happenings in the history of cancer therapy. Discovered in the late nineteenth century by William B. Coley, M.D., chief surgeon at Memorial Hospital (now the Memorial Sloan-Kettering Cancer Center or MSKCC), who undertook a 40-year experiment in treating and even curing cancer. Coley's Toxins may be regarded as the basis for modern immunotherapy.

Coley's Toxins are the by-products from two common bacteria, *Streptococcus pyrogenes* and *Serratia marcescens*. The toxins can cause a fever anywhere from slightly above normal to 105°F, and a pulse rate of 100 or more, and accompanying chills. In other words, flu-like symptoms. To quote directly from Moss's book:

Unlike conventional chemotherapy, such side effects, while unpleasant for the patient, are not emblematic of an immunity-destroying process. Quite the opposite, they are the result of pushing the immune function to the limit of excitability. The increase in bodily temperature, for example, seems to function as a biological form of *heat therapy*.

Impressive cure figures were reported, 45–50% and higher. Moss reports that the effects of Coley's Toxins have been studied extensively for over 30 years by Dr. Frances Havas, professor (emeritus) in the Department of Microbiology and Immunology, Temple University School of Medicine, at Philadelphia. Dr. Havas has stated that Coley's methods would be less dramatic and effective today than 100 years ago, for two main reasons. People have received so many antibiotics by now that their immune systems are less responsive than back in the prepenicillin days. Furthermore, many or most patients have already been treated by conventional methods such as chemotherapy, which decimates the immune system. Sporadic investigations have continued, particularly in Germany and China, sometimes with complete success and at other times with partial success.

Inasmuch as other species of bacteria produce toxins of varying lethality, there is apparently a potential for other such bacteria-derived vaccines to activate the immune system, although it would no doubt be a very risky, even deadly approach. A safety factor would consist of antibiotic action against the bacteria itself. A comprehensive listing of bacilli and their associated diseases, with first, second, and third choices for antibiotics, is presented in Chapter 43 of *The Pharmacological Basis of Therapeutics*, as authored by Chambers and Sande.

(Of interest is the fact that Section IX of the aforesaid reference, titled "Chemotherapy of Microbial Diseases," has eight chapters dealing with antimicrobial agents. Thus "chemotherapy" can be used in a general sense to signify a broad spectrum of treatments against various diseases. An examination of the chapters shows the intimate role of enzymes and inhibitors in diseases and their treatment. Moreover, the effectiveness of antibiotics, is not necessarily a foregone conclusion, for there are exceptions and there are side effects. It is a tribute to modern medicine that the subject has been studied in such great depth. We await, therefore, the successful and immediate resolution of the war against cancer.)

As for bacterial toxins per se, the reference is *The Pharmacology of Bacterial Toxins* by Dorner and Drews (1986). Without going into detail, by and large the toxins are composed of peptides or polypeptides, a very few of which are cited below, with their sources, as obtained from various references:

Cholera — *Vibrio cholerae* toxin (CT).

Gastroenteritis — *Escherichia coli* heat-labile enterotoxin (LT), where "entero" signifies intestinal.

Staph infections — *Staphylococcus aureus* enterotoxins are composed of single polypeptide chains (of 239 to 296 amino acid residues).

Botulism — *Clostridium botulinum* toxin is composed of polypeptides or proteins designated A through G with molecular weights of 200,000 to 400,000. The species *Clostridium perfingens* has heat-labile protein enterotoxin and a molecular weight of about 36,000. Botulism toxin is in fact among the most deadly known. There is a similarity with the deadly vegetable proteins ricin (from the castor bean plant, *Ricinus communis*) and abrin (from the rosary pea or jequirity, *Abrus precatorius*).

Of perhaps special interest are *Micobacterium tuberculosis* toxins, for which a vaccine has been developed known by the name Bacillus Calmette-Guérin (BCG), derived from *Microbacterium bovis*.

Many bacteria of course have their origins in food (Miller, in Amdur et al., 1991, p. 845; *Role of the Gut Flora in Toxicity and Cancer.*)

A recent development is the possibility that bacterial toxins may act against colon cancer. That is, the microbes that produce diarrhea do so by generating a toxin that is apparently an anticancer agent. The subject was discussed in *Science News Online* for the week of February 15, 2003 (Volume 163, No. 7, p. 100). The bacterium under consideration was the ubiquitous *Escherichia coli*, and the observation correlates with the fact that colon cancer occurs less frequently in regions of the world where *E. coli* is more common. The work of clinical pharmacologists Giovanni M. Pauli and Scott A. Waldman was cited, both of Thomas Jefferson University in Philadelphia. They prepared a synthetic version of the *E. coli* enterotoxin (intestinal toxin), and *in vitro* experiments showed that these enterotoxins halved the proliferation of human colon cancer cells. A side effect noted was an influx of calcium ions into the cells, which relates to reports that dietary calcium can act against colon cancer. These findings have caused considerable interest among other specialists, with the results to be reported in the *Proceedings of the National Academy of Sciences*.

Interestingly, snake venoms variously contain both peptides and enzymes, even lactate dehydrogenase, as well as various inorganics such as of sodium, potassium, calcium, magnesium, and such metals as zinc, iron, cobalt, manganese, and nickel (Russell and Dart, in Amdur et al., 1991, p. 756ff). Therefore, various amino acids comprising proteins or polypeptides can contain elements other than carbon, hydrogen, oxygen, and nitrogen — and, assuredly, sulfur. Of parallel or maybe opposing interest is the use of various peptides as anticancer agents — as per Stephen Hall's *A Commotion in the Blood* (1997a), and Burzynski therapy. (Hall also had an article in *Atlantic Monthly*.)

The subject in general is that of toxicants or toxic agents, which produce the toxins or else are in fact the toxins — such as alkaloids occurring in plants. The subject of toxic agents is presented at great length in Unit III of *Casarett and Doull's Toxicology: The Basic Science of Poisons* (Amdur et al., 1991). The agents encompass pesticides, metals, solvents and vapors, radiation, animal (reptiles, amphibia, marine animals of various sorts, and arthropods — spiders and the like), and plants.

Another pioneer in immunotherapy was Josef Issels, an M.D. from Germany, retired, whose methods have been called *Issels' Whole Body Therapy* (Walters, 1993, p. 82ff). His work was continued at the Panama City Clinic in Panama City, Florida. Issel's therapy induces a fever, a practice used in Europe for centuries. Modern medicine views fever with alarm, and as something to be counteracted with antibiotics. By giving a "fever shot" once a month to raise body temperature to as high as 105°F for a couple of hours, the level of disease-destroying leukocytes in the blood is increased. At the same time, the lymphocytes generate antibodies that destroy microbes and toxins. For an active fever, the drug Pyrifer is injected, which is made from coli bacteria. For a passive fever, hyperthermia is induced by ultra short waves or microwaves with the patient inside a chamber. The foregoing and other methods used have been catalogued with success rates of as high as 17% for terminal patients. It is noted that in patients with a fast-growing cancer, the previously long-term immunotherapy is combined with chemotherapy (Walters, 1993, p. 85).

There are other ways to describe the immune system and its functioning. In a chapter in Walters (1993) on the Revici therapy, after the work of Dr. Emanuel Revici, health is described as a balance between lipids and sterols, the former comprising fatty acids or esters, the other fatty alcohols such as cholesterol. Aside from this, the overall body defense system is said to consist of four phases. When a foreign substance or antigen such as a virus or microbe invades the body, the antigen is first broken down by enzymes, followed by the lipidic phase, then by the coagulant antibody phase, and concluded by globulinic antibodies. AIDS is regarded as a "quadruple pathological condition." In the course of treatment for cancer, selenium compounds are used, noted elsewhere as antitumor agents. (Gallium nitrate, for instance — also declared toxic — has been similarly proposed.) The theory and results so far have been subject to dispute. The theory is considered complex, but there are also some remarkable cancer remissions reported. An address in New York City can be supplied for Romanian-born Dr. Revici, now deceased, but Dr. Revici's niece Elena Avram carries on his work, described in William Kelly Eidem's book *The Doctor Who Cures Cancer*, published in 1997.

An update on Dr. Revici is furnished by Marcus A. Cohen's article "Emanuel Revici, MD: Efforts to Publish the Clinical Findings of a Pioneer in Lipid-Based Cancer Therapy — Part 1," published in the August/September 2004 issue of the *Townsend Letter*. (There were ultimately to be four parts.) Considerable data about Dr. Revici's background are presented, starting with his date of birth in Romania on September 6, 1896. Receiving his doctorate in medicine and surgery in 1920 from the University of Bucharest, he in turn took up the study of advances in chemistry related to lipids and cell metabolism. Opting to settle in Paris in 1936, he was forced to flee in 1941, finally ending up in Mexico City — but along the way having aided the Allies by surreptitiously carrying microfilm information from the French underground. After successfully establishing a clinic in Mexico City, he later decided to immigrate to the New York City area. There, New York's Office of Professional Medical Conduct (OPMC) chose to revoke his license in 1993, but the state education department was able to restore his license in 1997. Among his medical discoveries is the fact that adjacent carbon atoms in bioactive molecules will carry identical charges, a fact now widely recognized, and ostensibly an extra-energetic configuration.

Part 2 of the foregoing article was published in the October 2004 issue of the *Townsend Letter*. It is noted that Dr. Revici's sojourn in Mexico City was greeted by a letter in the August 18, 1945, issue of the *Journal of the American Medical Association* (*JAMA*). Signed by the journal, and not naming names, it was nevertheless titled "A Mexican Treatment for Cancer — A Warning." An associate of Dr. Revici named Gaston Merry was of the opinion that the powers that be wanted to "work along the ideas of Revici and to claim the paternity of some of his ideas." Revici, however, subsequently relocated to the United States and formed the Institute of Applied Biology (IAB) in Brooklyn, which specialized in clinical cancer research. Moreover, the research reports were made public, and sometimes published as articles during the 1950s and 1960s. In the meantime, Dr. Revici prepared a book manuscript titled *Research in Physiopathology as Basis of Guided Chemotherapy, With Special Applications to Cancer.* The prestigious technical book publisher D. Van Nostrand undertook publication, but Revici's work was blacklisted by the American Cancer Society, which markedly reduced book sales and ended circulation of Revici's findings.

Whatever the case and however described, the immune system, and its deficiencies and its stimuli, all seem irrevocably linked to the causes and cures of cancer.

## VACCINES

The idea has understandably emerged that cancer may be linked to viruses or other microorganisms or microbes. In consequence, therefore, we would like to have an inoculation and immunization against cancer, all cancers, and get it over with once and for all. So in one way or another there is a continuing search for both specific and universally effective cancer vaccines, in a class with polio vaccines, and an ideal yet to be realized. Giving due acknowledgement, Virginia Livingston, M.D., is credited with an earlier attempt, as has been mentioned, see Chapter 7 of Walters (1993). It will continue to be a subject of further interest.

# 3 Biochemical Insights

It is appropriate to reemphasize that the famous German biochemist Otto Warburg, who received a Nobel Prize in 1931 for later work, found that cancer cell metabolism, by and large, is anaerobic — that is, does not require oxygen — whereas normal cell metabolism is aerobic. Thus, cancer cell metabolism involves primarily the conversion of blood sugar or glucose (or its polymer, glycogen) ultimately to lactic acid or lactate by an enzyme-catalyzed anaerobic fermentation rather than the oxidation of glucose ultimately to carbon dioxide and water as occurs with normal cells. If a way can be found to nullify the specific enzyme catalysts required, then conceivably this could lead to a cure for cancer. (The pioneering work of Warburg is reviewed in a book by Hans Krebs titled *Otto Warburg: Cell Physiologist, Biochemist and Eccentric.* The original papers of Warburg and coworkers are produced in *The Metabolism of Tumors: Investigations from the Kaiser Wilhelm Institute for Biology, Berlin-Dablem,* edited by Otto Warburg. Warburg's results on tumor cell glycolysis and respiration were first published in 1923.) However, cancer cell metabolism is complex, and is partly aerobic, with many reaction intermediates, and has led to much controversy, as pointed out in Alan C. Aisenberg's *The Glycolysis and Respiration of Tumors,* published back in 1961. A later development is that glutaminolysis, the conversion of the nonessential amino acid glutamine mainly to lactic acid or lactate, also occurs in tumor cells (Eigenbrodt et al., 1985, II, p. 141ff; Hoffman, 1999, pp. 23, 24). Moreover, other amino acids can be so converted, by the processes of aminolysis. The metabolism of cancer cells is beginning to appear more and more complicated.

In this regard, the production of lactic acid from sugars by lactic-acid-forming bacteria is an industrial process of long standing. If the enzyme or enzymes produced by the bacteria were to be confronted and extrapolated to the human condition, and inhibitors in turn identified, perhaps this would lead to something important like a cure for cancer. This notation also applies to the production of lactic acid from another compound called glutamine. And it may provide a rationale for the action of anticancer agents, in that they may serve to destroy or inhibit the enzyme-catalyzed metabolism of cancer cells.

Speaking further of enzymes, in brief mention there are enzymatic treatments that have been used against cancer. These include such enzymes as trypsin, chymotrypsin, ficin, papain, bromelin, fungal proteases, deoxyribonuclease, lipase, and calf thymus extracts. The subject is reviewed in a chapter of biochemist Francis X. Hasselberger's *Uses of Enzymes and Immobilized Enzymes,* in which mention is also made of the Wobe-Mugos enzyme mixture, as used in Germany and Europe (Hasselberger, 1978, p. 145ff). The mixture can be given orally, rectally, or injected into the abdominal muscles, but is most effective when injected directly into the tumor, where it literally dissolves the tumorous tissue. The animal and plant enzymes used are obtained from beef pancreas, calf thymus gland, and the plants *Pisum sativum* (a variety of pea), *Lens esculenta* (a variety of lentil), and the papaya tree (Hasselberger, 1978, p. 142).

Here, however, the emphasis will be on enzyme inhibitors per se, as they pertain to cancer cell metabolism — that is, inhibitors or blockers for certain critical biochemical reactions occurring in the conversion of glucose to pyruvic acid or pyruvate, and then to lactic acid or lactate.

## THE WARBURG CANCER THEORY

The theory advanced by Nobel laureate Otto Warburg, outlined earlier, is that normal cells undergo the aerobic oxidation of glucose, whereas cancer cells undergo an anaerobic fermentation to lactic acid or lactate (the neutralized form), followed by the conversion of the lactic acid or lactate back to glucose. Warburg's results were first published in 1923, and have since produced a great deal of controversy, as the situation is much more complicated than appears at first glance, and is becoming more so. Some of the work along the way has been described in Alan C. Aisenberg's *The Glycolysis and Respiration of Tumors*, published in 1961. For one thing, both anaerobic and aerobic glycolysis occurs in cancers or tumors, although the first route is predominant. Later investigations indicate that the amino acid glutamine also plays a role.

Concomitantly, in the liver and muscle tissue the glucose is converted to and exists in a form called glycogen, by a process called *glycogenesis*. Glycogen is a high-molecular-weight branched-chain polymer or polysaccharide composed chiefly of glucose units or monomers. The conversions are catalyzed by various enzymes that are highly specific to each particular conversion. In the terminology used, the conversion of glycogen to lactic acid or lactate is called *glycogenolysis*, and the reconversion of lactic acid or lactate back to glycogen may also be called glycogenesis, confusingly, as is the conversion of glucose to glycogen. In general, we may speak of *glycolysis*, the enzymatic conversion or breakdown of sugars and other carbohydrates.

(Glucose, also called dextrose or corn sugar, may exist in several forms. It is what is called optically active, with the usual form exhibiting the dextrorotatory property, and is known as dextroglucose, written D-glucose or d-glucose. In turn there are the $\alpha$ and $\beta$ phases, depending on the particular range of conditions. For the purposes here, however, the word "glucose" suffices, with the chemical formula $HCO(CHOH)_4CH_2OH$ or the simple stoichiometric formula $C_6H_{12}O_6$ — although a more complicated ring structure is involved.)

Fermentation, in its restricted sense, is the anaerobic enzymatic conversion of carbohydrates to other useful products. The most well-known example is no doubt the production of ethyl alcohol or ethanol from the sugar resulting from the conversion of malted grains. Although yeast is listed as the agent causing or catalyzing the fermentation, the actual agent is an enzyme or enzymes produced by the yeast, which may be either unknown or unspecified. Another example occurs in putrefaction, for example, the anaerobic digestion of organic wastes, producing chiefly methane and carbon dioxide, or so-called sewer gas.

Enzymes are proteinaceous structures at the molecular level that specifically catalyze certain biochemical reactions, or that as coenzymes may take part in the reaction. Some vitamins, for instance, are related to coenzymes. The subject of enzymes or enzymology is an expanding field, with a corresponding proliferation of books and articles.

The anaerobic conversion of glucose (or molasses) to lactic acid is an industrial process of long standing, for which the microorganism used is named *Lactobacillus delbruckii*. This bacterium is the source of the enzyme, which is not routinely specified. (The enzyme is one form or another of lactate dehydrogenase, as will be further detailed in the sections titled "Glycolysis," and "Production of Lactic Acid or Lactate" below.) The conversion is called *homolactic fermentation* as compared to *heterolactic fermentation*, because the product is almost entirely lactic acid. The general subject area is that of bacterial metabolism (e.g., in the *McGraw-Hill Encyclopedia of Science and Technology*).

Other microorganisms that produce homolactic conversions are notably of the genus *Streptococcus*. This is most interesting in that *Streptococcus* is such a common source of infections. Thus it can be projected that possibly here is a mostly unsuspected cause of cancer, although maybe indirectly — or at least the genus could be supportive of cancer growth.

It may be added, moreover, as has been indicated, that a species of *Streptococcus* was identified as the elusive *Progenitor cryptocides*, the pleomorphic microbe found in the research by Dr. Virginia Livingston to be a source of cancer. Conversely, a species of *Streptococcus* is used in what are called Coley's toxins as an immunological treatment for cancer. This seems to be a common enough paradox, that cause and cure are somehow entwined. That is, the causes of cancer may at the same time cause the body to attempt to fight off the cancer. Or as the saying goes, for every action there is a reaction.

There is also an enigma buried here. Should or should not a cancer patient take antibiotics if an infection is indicated? Is the infectious microbe in fact causing cancer or reacting against cancer? Or doing more of the one than the other? It is a research area that requires a sensitive test to determine whether the cancer is on the upswing or on the downswing (the subject of monitors).

Although various microorganisms or bacteria are listed as the agents for fermentation, as noted earlier the actual agents are enzymes produced by the microorganisms. Thus it may be said that the sources for enzymes in general are bacteria, fungi, and yeasts. Whether the particular enzyme involved in the body reactions is the same enzyme involved in say, the industrial formation of lactic acid remains conjectural at this point, for it could as well, be another. (The conversion of sugars to lactic acid remains a long-standing industrial process as per H. Benninga's *A History of Lactic Acid Making: A Chapter in the History of Biotechnology*.) Suffice to say that biotechnology is an expanding field, and involves among other things the production of penicillin and the other antibiotics by fermentation processes. There is of course an equal or surpassing interest about enzymology in medicine proper.

Central to applying Warburg's theory is the suppression of cancer by the use of inhibitors that would break or inhibit the glucose–lactic acid cycle. The existing cancer cells would atrophy and not be replaced. Presumably the hydrazine sulfate therapy developed by a certain Joseph Gold (of the Syracuse Cancer Research Institute) would act in this manner. Moreover, and importantly, a believable theory, explanation, or mechanism is provided. That the medical establishment tends to concur can be illustrated by the fact that the hydrazine therapy was removed from the ACS unproven methods blacklist in 1982 (Walters, *Options*, 1993, p. 49). However, as Michael Lerner finds in *Choices in Healing*, after the positive reports the negative reports started to filter in.

(As a reminder although we may be talking of anticancer agents, in the strictest sense we are not necessarily talking of cures. In fact, the FDA does not permit claims to be made for cancer cures, although it is permissible to speak of cancer therapies or cancer treatments.)

The anticancer role of nitrogen-bearing compounds may be that of substances that inhibit or break, in one way or another, the enzyme-catalyzed reactions in the glucose–lactic acid cycle. The topic of enzyme inhibitors is in itself an expanding subspecialty within the field. Enzymatic reactions and enzyme-breaking actions are involved, for instance, in the efficacy of antibiotics and in other unexpected areas.

These enzyme-breaking or enzyme-inhibiting substances may be predominantly nitrogen-bearing compounds, as represented for instance by the poisonous alkaloids and cyanogens of plant origin. Or they may be still other kinds of substances, for example, the compound named nordihydroguaiaretic acid, or NDGA, the main active ingredient of chaparral or creosote bush (*Larrea tridentata*), which is commonly found in the American Southwest. For instance, in work by Dean Burk of the NCI it was shown that NDGA inhibits both aerobic and anaerobic glycolysis, particularly the latter (Walters, *Options*, 1993, p. 135). Antioxidants may also play this role. It could even explain the beneficial action of chemotherapy drugs in small amounts. And may take in the subject of homeopathy, not to mention enzyme therapy. In fact, this enzyme-breaking or enzyme-inhibiting property may account for the wide variety of anticancer substances found in nature, as compiled in Hartwell's *Plants Used Against Cancer*, and those cited in other listings of herbal remedies or treatments.

If the foregoing speculations are correct, at least in part, then there is the problem of making the enzyme-breaking or enzyme-inhibiting actions more effective. The goal should be not merely enzyme inhibiting, but enzyme breaking, and maybe enzyme destroying. In other words, the object is to find a *selective* "poison" for the enzyme catalysts involved. That is, a poison that will act only on the particular enzyme or enzymatic reaction, and not on other enzymes, and not on the rest of the body.

Furthermore, in order to nullify the enzyme-catalyzed conversion or conversions, it may be required that the enzyme-breaking substance or poison be "activated," or that various poison enhancers be added. The latter may be the role of creatine, for instance, in enhancing the effectiveness of urea as an anticancer agent. In one way or another, this may also be the role of electromagnetic radiation as an anticancer agent.

Although microorganisms per se are easily poisoned by metallic substances, whether this can be extrapolated to enzymes is moot — though it provides a point of departure. And it is worth noting that such metallic substances as germanium and selenium compounds are observed to be anticancer agents. Arsenic, for instance, is listed in J. Leyden Webb's *Enzyme and Metabolic Inhibitors*. In a general way, we may also be speaking of so-called heavy metals and their compounds, which in higher concentrations are toxic, but potentially may act as anticancer agents in very low or trace concentrations (homeopathy again!) As for some well-known industrial catalyst poisons, nickel compounds foul up the anaerobic digestion of organic wastes, and vanadium compounds adversely affect petroleum-refining catalysts. Sulfur compounds are notorious as metallic or inorganic catalyst poisons, although sulfided metals sometimes serve as catalysts for certain kinds of reactions, such as hydrogenation. Even electromagnetic fields or radiation may have a catalytic or anticatalytic effect. The subject of catalysis, in fact, often seems more of an art than a science, but presumably involves compositional heterogeneity and electrochemical phenomena.

(It is interesting to note that sulfur-containing vegetables such as garlic and onions, as well as the cruciferous members of the mustard family, such as cabbages and broccoli, are considered anticancer agents in their dietary effects. These effects conceivably may involve poisoning the enzyme or enzymes favoring the glucose–lactic acid cycle, the feature of anaerobic cancer cell metabolism.)

A further development (related to Warburg's work) concerns what is called *apoptosis*, whereby billions of body cells perish each day to be replaced by new cells. There is an enzyme called apopain that determines whether the cells live or die. This enzymatic effect on apoptosis may possibly be inhibited or favored by an additive, which potentially may be of interest in the treatment of cancer. This again brings up the point that some of the myriad biologically active plant substances may act in such a way or other ways.

As a concluding statement, the fact that a treatment works for some, at least some of the time, is an indication that it should be perfected rather than rejected. Nor is it always necessary to understand how a treatment works, for what we are most interested in are results. For example, we may never know exactly how antibiotics work, other than that they are enzyme inhibitors. This, in spite of all the biochemical formulas and equations, and the lengthy, technical, and encyclopedic treatises on the subject. For every answered question always leads to further questions. Ditto for the immunizations against various viral diseases, such as polio and smallpox — though we seem almost at a point that for some diseases the only new cases seem to be from the vaccination itself. Nevertheless, we are most grateful that antibiotics and immunizations most often do work, and we'll accept the same for any treatment of cancer.

It is commonly said that everyone has cancer cells, but they are kept in check presumably by the action of the body's immune system. In this respect, cancer is like other viral diseases, such as polio, which most times may be thrown off with the symptoms of a little fever and a runny nose, as with a common cold. The exceptions are, of course, where the trouble starts.

The fact that cancer gains a foothold may thus be a sign that the immune system did not work satisfactorily or was overwhelmed. Therefore, an argument can be advanced against compromising or depleting the immune system with, say, chemotherapy; the body needs all the help it can get. Rather, it is the signal to go on with something else, say, an anticancer agent that will negate further cancer growth by inhibiting or destroying the enzyme-catalyzed anaerobic metabolism of the cancer cells. If this thesis is correct, then the search is for the best anticancer agents to do this, and the correct dosage and frequency, which may have to be tailor-made for the individual patient.

Whether this regimen may be described as therapeutic, or after the fact, there is also an interest in prophylactic regimens before the fact, as in the development of inoculations against cancer, similar to smallpox or other serious diseases. At the moment, however, therapeutic regimens remain at the forefront of interest. Nevertheless, whereas Virginia Livingston's or similar cancer vaccination theories and practices were once ignored or blacklisted, now there is a revival of interest in this same kind of therapy. In particular, a vaccine therapy was studied for metastatic malignant melanoma at the John Wayne Cancer Institute of Saint John's Hospital and Heath Center at Santa Monica, California, as was described by Donald L. Morton and Andreas Barth in the July/August, 1996, issue of *CA — A Cancer Journal for Clinicians*, a review publication of the American Cancer Society.

The use of chemotherapy, on the other hand, notably of the drug dicarbazine, has been judged unsatisfactory for advanced or metastasized melanoma. Accordingly, cancer vaccines have been tried with a degree of success. These vaccines are made from attenuated whole cells, cell walls, specific antigens, or nonpathogenic strains of living organisms. (The last-mentioned source underscores the sometimes-observed correlation between resistance to bacterial infections and to cancer.) There are, in fact, a large number of known serum melanoma-associated antigens (MAAs) that induce an immune response. The initial response, however, is much slower than with cytotoxic chemotherapy agents, taking 4 to 6 weeks to manifest.

That cancer vaccines may conceivably work is not surprising, given the previously mentioned work of Dr. Virginia Livingston and others. In fact, there is a vaccine for feline leukemia. Some of the latest findings are reviewed in *Exploring the Biochemical Revolution* in a section on Arousing the Immune System Through Vaccines, and although aimed more at viruses per se, there may be a connection to cancer formation, since viruses are recognized as a primary cause of cancer. One version would involve injecting the DNA from a particular microbe, which would cause an immune response by the host. Another mode would be to inject a vaccine into an edible fruit or vegetable. Whether the extrapolation can be made to cancer remains to be seen.

## CELL METABOLISM

As has been indicated, the biochemistry of cancer and its treatment may be fundamentally expressed in terms of the differences in metabolism between cancerous cells and normal cells. By metabolism is meant the biochemical processes by which blood sugar or glucose (or its polymer, glycogen) is converted to energy and end products. The essential differences date back to the investigations of German biochemist Otto Warburg, first published in the 1920s, as previously noted. Thus, Warburg observed that cancer cells undergo anaerobic behavior, which does not require oxygen, whereas normal cells undergo aerobic behavior, which requires oxygen. The fuel or energy source is principally glucose or its equivalent, although such amino acids as glutamine may be involved to a limited degree. It may be added that such anaerobic processes are sometime referred to as *fermentation* (although there are aerobic as well as anaerobic "fermentations").

We may further distinguish cells as prokaryotic and eukaryotic. Prokaryotes are bacterial cells (and blue-green algae cells), whereas eukaryotes comprise all other cells. The eukaryotes have a membrane-enclosed nucleus or organelle, which contains their DNA, which encodes the genetic information. The remainder of the cell is, in fact, made up of membrane-enclosed organelles having different functions, bound together as the plasma, in turn enclosed by an outer membrane. Prokaryotes do not have a nucleus, having only a simple unicellular structure, though colonies of independent cells may exist. On the other hand, eukaryotes may be both unicellular and multicellular. Viruses, as distinguished from bacteria, are considered nonliving entities because they cannot reproduce outside the host cell. For the present purposes here, only eukaryotes or eukaryotic cells are of interest.

The foregoing brings up the matter of "genes," which in an abstract sense are hereditary units of action or function, about which there is apparently not a complete consensus. In any event, each such genetic unit can evidently be shown to occupy a specific locus or segment in a length of DNA, and in a chromosome, a gene may change into different forms called *alleles*, the fundamental basis of mutations.

The partial or overall cellular conversion process by which glucose is converted or utilized may be called glycolysis, whereas the utilization of some other reactant or nutrient, such as the nonessential amino acid called glutamine, is called glutaminolysis, and so forth. For cancerous cells, the main and final end product from glycolysis is lactic acid, also called lactate. For normal cells, the main and final end products are carbon dioxide and water, the same as for simple combustion. There are, of course, intermediate products, principally a compound called pyruvic acid, or called pyruvate in its neutralized form. Both anaerobic and aerobic glycolysis yield pyruvic acid or pyruvate as an intermediate. Its further conversion marks the overall difference between anaerobic and aerobic glycolysis, the former yielding lactic acid or lactate, the latter carbon dioxide and water.

More generally, the term *metabolism* can refer to any biochemical reaction or reaction sequence; the involved substances are known as metabolites, and may be reactants and reaction products (or intermediates). In its more usual usage, however, metabolism, or primary metabolism, pertains to biochemical reaction sequences or conversions that are the primary source of energy. These life-sustaining biochemical reactions are designated exothermic, meaning that heat energy is given off. The quantity of heat so furnished (or evolved) can be designated the heat of reaction. This energy may be converted to, or make an appearance as, still other forms of energy — kinetic energy, or energy of motion, being one form. What is called chemical or biochemical energy is stored as biomass, namely, as carbohydrates, fats, and/or proteins, for subsequent utilization. Carbohydrates and fats in foodstuffs are the main energy sources, being ultimately converted to glucose by digestive processes. Proteins or amino acids are also convertible for energy purposes.

In more restricted usage, the term *metabolite* is reserved only for reaction products, with the primary metabolites being those produced from energy-giving biochemical reactions; whereas the products from all other kinds of reactions can be called secondary metabolites.

Furthermore, there may be great differences in the quantity of energy furnished by different reactions. In the case of anaerobic cancer cell metabolism, the overall heat of reaction is minimal. In the aerobic metabolism of normal cells, the heat of reaction is much larger — equivalent to the heat of combustion. Glutaminolysis, by comparison, does not give off much energy.

The cancer problem and solution can be viewed as that of inhibiting, blocking, poisoning, controlling, regulating, or modulating cancer cell metabolism without adversely affecting normal cell metabolism. The focus thus shifts to enzymes and enzyme inhibitors, whereby cancer cells can be selectively "starved."

Each and every biochemical reaction in the body is catalyzed or favored by a unique proteinaceous substance called an enzyme, and a sequence of biochemical reactions will require a separate and distinct enzyme for each individual reaction or reaction step. (Moreover, there may be a supporting reaction or reactions involved as well.) Such reaction sequences are commonly called "pathways." Some of the reaction steps and corresponding enzymes may be more significant than others, in that they may control the overall conversion rate. In other words, a slower reaction or reactions in the sequence tends to control the overall conversion rate.

This subject is biochemical or organic catalysis, and for the technically inclined there is a fairly recent four-volume elaboration of various reaction mechanisms, titled *Comprehensive Biological Catalysis: A Mechanistic Reference*, edited by Michael Sinnott and published in 1998.

As indicated, any or all of these enzymes or enzyme catalysts may be modulated, regulated, poisoned, blocked, or inhibited by another substance or substances, organic or inorganic, and proteinaceous or otherwise. These latter substances may be said to *deactivate* the *active* catalytic sites, or receptor sites, as they may also be called — a terminology adopted from the explanations of inorganic catalysis. Modern drug therapy is based on enzyme inhibitors, antibiotics being the outstanding example, with the antibiotics blocking vital enzyme-catalyzed pathways in bacterial metabolism.

What are commonly regarded as poisons serve to act as enzyme inhibitors, severely interfering with a life-sustaining process such as respiration or the functioning of the heart. The drugs of conventional cytotoxic chemotherapy also act as enzyme inhibitors, interfering, for instance, with the DNA/RNA/protein synthesis pathway — processes that will be further described subsequently. All cells are affected to a degree in using chemotherapy, in particular the faster-growing cells such as in hair filaments, and notably those that comprise the immune system and gastrointestinal tract, with anemia a possible side effect.

Thus, it is of primary importance that enzyme inhibitors be selective toward a certain enzyme, and not adversely affect other enzymes; that is, it should not produce pronounced side effects or adverse effects. Fortuitously, this is mostly the case for the common antibiotics used, in the dosages prescribed, and which therefore in the main attack bacterial rather than human cells. (Some lesser-known antibiotics are toxic even to humans, that is, are toxic to normal human cells.) As previously indicated, conventional cytotoxic chemotherapy drugs unfortunately attack normal cells as well as cancer cells, and all too often more so.

In essence, therefore, the objective is to determine what substances could interfere with cancer cell processes, but not normal cell processes, the criterion being interference with cancer cell metabolism as distinguished from normal cell metabolism. A statement made by Donald Voet and Judith G. Voet in their treatise on biochemistry is still relevant (Voet and Voet, 1995, p. 595): "Attempts to understand the metabolic differences between cancer cells and normal cells may one day provide a clue to the treatment of certain forms of this deadly disease."

This difference is underlined by the observation of biochemist Robert A. Harris that glucose consumption under anaerobic conditions may be 20 times greater than under aerobic conditions (Harris, in Devlin, 1986, p. 353). That is, a much higher utilization of glucose is required to meet the energy demands of anaerobic glycolysis, as occurs for cancer cells — in that the glucose ends up as lactic acid or lactate instead of carbon dioxide and water, the normal products of aerobic glycolysis. This is reflected in the fact that anaerobic conversion has a much lower overall heat of reaction than normal aerobic conversion.

The foregoing considerations do not touch on the causes of cancer in the first place. The overall conventional thinking is that cancers are of genetic origin, whether inherited or induced, their basis ultimately residing in our chromosomes and genes. Speaking of induced cancers, attributed to external causes or sources, a general consensus is that cancers are viral-related, radiation-related, and chemical-related. This was reflected in the landmark three-volume treatise *Origins of Human Cancer*, published back in 1977, and edited by H. H. Hiatt, J. D. Watson, and J. A. Winsten, with the individual chapters by authorities in their respective fields.

(In Book B of the aforementioned *Origins of Human Cancer*, published in 1977, there is a chapter by Wattenburg et al. on the study of inhibitors for chemical carcinogenesis as caused by the application of such carcinogens as BP or benzo(a)pyrene to rats and mice. The antioxidants BHA (butylated hydroxyanisole) and BPT (butylated hydroxytoluene) acted as suppressants or anticancer agents, but, of course, not as cures. These findings were significant as these compounds are commercial food additives. Other compounds tested included disulfiram (Antabuse, tetraethylthiuram disulfide), benzyl isothiocyanate, and selenium compounds, as well as various compounds used as chemopreventives. The final verdict is still out.)

Viruses, once considered perhaps the foremost cause of cancer, were subsequently discounted, only to be later reconsidered. For a mechanism or theory has been provided by which a virus invades the chromosome to produce cancer-forming genes, or oncogenes. At the same time, radiation and chemicals certainly cause chromosomal/gene damage, presumably creating oncogenes. As for viral causes, it can be added that a virus itself is only a segment of protein of uncertain makeup and characteristics, and there are even subviruses called *prions*. We have to accept that these are virus-related phenomena that may never be fully understood.

Expanded, more technical versions of the foregoing subject areas were included in Part 1 of this author's *Cancer and the Search for Selective Biochemical Inhibitors*, published in 1999. A synopsis of Part 1 comprises the remainder of this chapter. The paradigm used is cell metabolism, which provides a systematic way to analyze cancer and its suppression in terms of enzymes and enzyme inhibitors. Although matters can be taken to increasingly micro levels — say to DNA and its encoded genetic information — enzymes and their inhibition relate more directly to the macro world about us, and are emphasized.

The remaining contents of this chapter serve to support subsequent findings about cancer, and illustrate the overall complexity of the subject. The challenge is to manage and apply this information toward immolating cancer cells. There is always the dilemma of overstatement vs. understatement. But when medical folklore opines that a (inexpensive) herbal or other substance acts against (or even cures) cancer, the skeptic wants to know if this could indeed be true. Understanding the reasons for possible anticancer action requires us to explore some underlying bio-chemistry.

## ENZYME-CATALYZED METABOLIC PATHWAYS

Metabolism — that is, primary metabolism — signifies the ways by which energy is supplied to cells; it is the means by which life and growth are sustained. Fundamentally, it is related to the exothermic aerobic processes of normal cell respiration, which involve the biochemical conversion of glucose or its equivalent sugars, or blood sugars, a process ultimately involving oxygen, and known as glycolysis, or aerobic glycolysis. These are the enzyme-catalyzed steps that ultimately yield carbon dioxide and water, and at the same time produce energy, signified by the term *exothermic*. The energy produced may be broadly designated as thermal energy, or heat; other manifestations also occur, particularly cellular growth or proliferation.

Cellular growth is manifested in the classes of substances known mainly as proteins, fats, and carbohydrates. Additionally, there is the metabolic support of the myriad body functions, of maintaining body temperature, and of permitting body motion. In other words, the subject is that of chemical or biochemical energy stored as biomass or body mass, of thermal energy manifested as body temperature, and of kinetic (and potential) energy changes manifested as body motion (in an external gravitational field).

Aerobic glycolysis first involves a ten-step conversion of glucose to pyruvic acid or pyruvate, called the Embden–Meyerhoff–Parnas pathway, followed by its further conversion to carbon dioxide and water via what is variously called the tricarboxylic acid cycle, or citric acid cycle, or Krebs cycle after its discoverer. The net products discharged from the cycle are carbon dioxide and water, with recycle of a further product called oxaloacetic acid or oxaloacetate. Successive organic acids that contain three carboxyl groups (-COOH), are initially involved in the cycle starting with citric acid or a neutral salt of citric acid (citrate). Hence the designator *tricarboxylic*.

What we call anaerobic glycolysis also involves the same ten-step conversion of glucose to pyruvic acid or pyruvate. However, the pyruvic acid is instead further converted to lactic acid or lactate in a single step catalyzed by an enzyme called lactate dehydrogenase (and sometimes called lactic acid dehydrogenase).

Although the carbohydrate glucose or its polymer glycogen is regarded as the fundamental fuel or nutrient, other carbohydrates may be involved, even nitrogen-containing amines, or amino acids. Thus, for example, there is the role of glutamine, a nonessential amino acid (that is, glutamine can be produced internally by body processes), in cancer cell metabolism. Referred to as glutaminolysis, the utilization of glutamine may be incorporated into the metabolic loop. It is illustrative of how both normal and cancerous cells may utilize still other fuel sources such as proteins, which are made up of chains of amino acids. Thus, other amines or amino acids also metabolize, though glutamine is the predominant amino acid.

Illustrative diagrams showing the principal biochemical reactions are portrayed in Figure 3.1 through Figure 3.4. To summarize, these biochemical reactions are divided into the following categories:

1. Glycolysis, the ten-step sequence producing pyruvic acid or pyruvate, which occurs in all cells, normal or cancerous.
2. Anaerobic conversion of pyruvate to lactate, as occurs in cancer cells.
3. Glutaminolysis, the conversion of glutamine, which may occur simultaneously.
4. Aerobic tricarboxylic acid cycle, which oxidizes pyruvate to carbon dioxide and water as end products and liberates energy, as occurs in normal cells.

The convention is to denote each forward reaction step by an arrow, for convenience represented downward ($\downarrow$). For reversible reactions, in both directions, a double arrow is used ($\uparrow\downarrow$). The particular enzyme catalysts are specified for each step, along with whatever supportive reactions occur, with both reactants and products shown. Further, a positive or negatively charged atomic or molecular entity is called an ion (or radical), and may be designated a positive ion by a (+) superscript, and a negative ion by a (−) superscript. An increase of positive charge (or lesser negative charge) is termed *oxidation*, and a decrease in positive charge (or greater negative charge) is termed *reduction*. Oxidation can also correspond to the addition of oxygen, which takes up an electron but in the process itself becomes "reduced." Reduction can correspond to the addition of hydrogen, which loses an electron but in the process itself becomes "oxidized." In other words, both oxidation and reduction occur simultaneously, the terminology depending on which way the electrons move. (Such oxidation-reduction reactions are sometimes abbreviated as *redox* reactions.)

It may be further observed that the appropriate reactants, intermediates, and products may be represented either in the acid form or the "-ate" form, the latter designating the negative ionic form (or anion), which exists in combination with a positively charged ion (cation), for instance, the hydrogen ion, denoted as $H^+$. (That is to say, in the conventions used for an electric potential difference between electrodes, an anion, which is negatively charged, will travel to the positively charged anode, and the cation, which is positively charged, will travel to the negatively charged cathode.)

Consider for example the pyruvic acid/pyruvate product of glycolysis, which may be written equivalently as

$$CH_3COCOOH \Leftrightarrow CH_3COCOO^- + H^+$$

where the first term on the right is the pyruvate form. For the further production of lactic acid/lactate, say, the equivalence is

$$CH_3CH(OH)COOH \Leftrightarrow CH_3CH(OH)COO^- + H^+$$

where the first term on the right is the lactate form. The hydrogen ion may be replaced by some other positively charged ion, such as the sodium ion, $Na^+$ or potassium ion, $K^+$. We will not be further concerned about this notation, but only mention it here for completeness.

Plants also undergo the same metabolic respiration processes, whereby the plant energy sources such as sugars undergo respiration to yield carbon dioxide and water. This is accompanied by transpiration, the elimination of water vapor to the atmosphere via the leaves, as derived from soil water and its nutrients, and also from respiration. (And which influences climate, notably via the tropical rain forests.) More details about plant biochemistry are furnished in the standard references and textbooks, e.g., in *Plant Physiology* by Frank B. Salisbury and Cleon W. Ross (1985).

In plant photosynthesis the opposite of respiration occurs, whereby carbon dioxide and water are converted to organic material, say, by what is called the Calvin cycle, yielding first either a three-carbon compound or else a four-carbon compound, and, in turn, the myriad other plant-generated compounds (Salisbury and Ross, 1985, p. 195ff). The initial three-carbon compound, called 3-PGA for 3-phosphoglyceric acid, results in what are called the C-3 plant species. By far the most numerous, the C-3 plant species include all gymnosperms, pteridophytes, bryophytes, and algae, as well as most trees and shrubs. Most C-4 plant species are monocotyfledons, especially grasses and sedges. (Monocotyledon seedlings having one emerging leaf, whereas dicotyledons have two emerging leaflets.) The C-4 plant species include the important agricultural crops sugarcane, maize (corn), and sorghum, as well as numerous range grasses.

Sunlight is the photochemical energy source for the photosynthetic conversion, which can be termed endothermic, indicating that energy has to be added. Photosynthetic processes are also enzyme-catalyzed, the green substance, the magnesium-containing chlorophyll, serving that purpose. Interestingly, the C-4 species are the fastest growing and most efficient, yielding the most biomass per unit of photosynthetic energy expended. Photosynthetic conversion rates range from 0.6 to 2.4 micromoles of $CO_2$ converted per second per square meter of leaf surface, for agave, to 20 to 40 for corn or maize (Salisbury and Ross, 1985, p. 218).

Ideally, the C-4 plant species would represent the best prospects for controlled or greenhouse photosynthesis from added carbon dioxide sources. Unfortunately, there is an upper limit to the carbon dioxide concentrations that can be utilized in greenhouse gases. Whereas normal atmospheric air may contain about 340 μl of carbon dioxide per liter (340 parts per million, or ppm), or 0.000340 mole fraction, or say 0.034 volume percent, the upper limit is around 1000 μl of carbon dioxide per liter (or 1000 parts per million, or ppm), or 0.001 mole fraction, or 0.1 volume percent, whereby toxicity occurs (Salisbury and Ross, 1985, p. 224).

Interestingly, algae can stand up to 50,000 ppm of carbon dioxide. Thus, it is a prime candidate for the regeneration of carbon dioxide via controlled photosynthesis in glass-tubed solar farms, to yield biomass (and water). The carbon dioxide source would be from the steam gasification of coal or other fossil fuels to yield hydrogen ($H_2$) and carbon dioxide ($CO_2$):

$$C + H_2O(g) \rightarrow H_2 + CO_2$$

where the separated hydrogen serves as a clean-burning fuel for power generation, or even for automobiles provided the hydrogen storage problem can be successfully resolved.

Of course, with a carbon dioxide buildup in the atmosphere from fossil fuel combustion (causing global warming), normal atmospheric concentrations continue to be exceeded. Thus, algae may provide a resolution.

## GLYCOLYSIS

The ten-step glycolysis pathway producing pyruvic acid or pyruvate is diagrammed in Figure 3.1. Also known as the Embden–Meyerhoff–Parnas pathway, after its discoverers, this sequence occurs in both aerobic and anaerobic glycolysis. The main biochemical reactions are catalyzed by enzymes, and at the same time require supportive or complementary reactions. The faster reactions approach a condition of chemical equilibrium. The slower reactions are controlling, and may be influenced by inhibitors or promoters. Other chemical compounds or substances entering into glycolysis via the supporting reactions are, for the record, designated as follows:

ATP — adenosine triphosphate
ADP — adenosine diphosphate
$P_i$ —orthophosphate ion, in any ionization state
$NAD^+$ — nicotinamide adenine dinucleotide, oxidized form
NADH — nicotinamide adenine dinucleotide, reduced form
$H^+$ — hydrogen, oxidized form, or hydrogen ion

Still other substances and minutiae may enter, but are not shown. Generally speaking, the various enzymes encountered are named according to their functions, using the suffix "-ase," and these organic catalysts may be regarded as proteinaceous.

The names of the enzymes involved in the ten successive glycolysis reaction steps, as per Figure 3.1, are: (1) hexokinase, (2) hexose phosphateisomerase, (3) phosphofructokinase, (4) aldolase, (5) triosphosphate isomerase, (6) glyceraldehyde-3-phosphate dehydrogenase, (7) phosphoglycerate kinase, (8) phosphoglyceromutase, (9) enolase, and (10) pyruvate kinase.

(Note: There is a systematic nomenclature for classifying the enzymes by function, as follows: oxidoreductases involve oxidation-reduction reactions; transferases involve the transfer of functional groups; hydrolases involve hydrolysis reactions with water; lyases involve the elimination of a group to form double bonds; isomerases involve isomerization to a different structure but with the same chemical composition; ligases involve the formation of a chemical bond simultaneously with ATP hydrolysis. There are in turn subclasses and sub-subclasses, and a subclass that

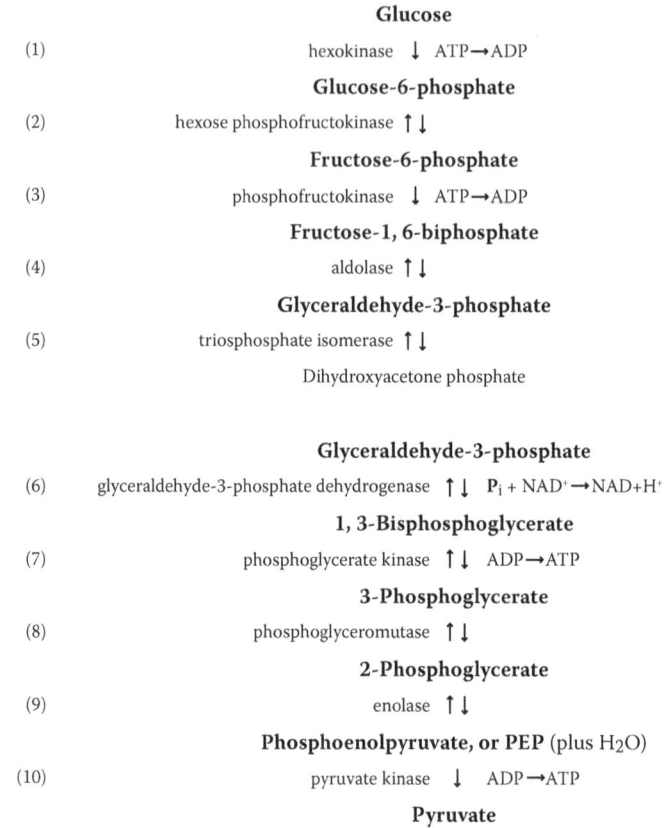

**FIGURE 3.1** Glycolysis conversion sequence yielding pyruvic acid or pyruvate, with enzymes and supportive reactions shown. (Based on information in Voet and Voet, *Biochemistry*, 1995, p. 446; Harris, in *Textbook of Biochemistry*, 1986, p. 334.)

will be of special interest is the kinases — as per tyrosine kinase in Chapter 10 — and which are phosphoryl-transfer enzymes involving ATP. In the glycolysis pathway steps 1, 3, 7, and 10 variously involve kinases. For the record, the phosphoryl group involved in the transfers may be written symbolically as $-(PO_3)^{2-}$, where the superscript signifies two negative charges.)

As has been previously indicated, one or another (or several, or even all) of the particular enzymes may each be inhibited, blocked, poisoned, controlled, regulated, or modulated by other substances. Thus, the glycolytic pathway is affected by such inhibitors or poisons as 2-deoxyglucose, sulfhydryl reagents, and fluoride (Harris, in Devlin, 1986, p. 346). Fluoride is a potent inhibitor of enolase, the enzyme for Reaction 9 in glycolysis, as shown in Figure 3.1 (which can give pause for the common use of fluorides for dental hygiene purposes.)

Furthermore, the activity of phosphofructokinase (PFK), the enzyme that controls glycolysis by regulating Reaction 3, for instance, has been found to decrease sharply when switching from anaerobic to aerobic metabolism. This is said to

Pyruvate

lactate dehydrogenase $\downarrow$ NADH + H + $\longrightarrow$ NAD$^+$ + 2[H]

Lactate

**FIGURE 3.2** Anaerobic conversion of pyruvic acid or pyruvate to lactic acid or lactate with enzyme and supportive reaction shown. (Based on information in Voet and Voet, *Biochemistry*, p. 464; Harris, in *Textbook of Biochemistry*, p. 334.)

account for a pronounced drop in the overall glycolysis rate for aerobic conditions as compared to anaerobic conditions. In other words, cancer cells, which undergo anaerobic glycolysis, will have a much greater glycolysis rate than normal cells.

Still other substances may accelerate or promote the glycolytic reactions, some of which may be related to genetic causes. For instance, there may be a genetic predisposition to promote the activity of the enzyme or enzymes involved in cancer cell metabolism.

## PRODUCTION OF LACTIC ACID OR LACTATE

The production of, say, lactic acid from pyruvic acid is sometimes called homolactic fermentation. The enzyme involved in the one-step conversion is lactate dehydrogenase in one form or another. A schematic diagram for the conversion is shown in Figure 3.2. We omit further details about the conversion.

Another bioconversion that can occur will instead yield an alcohol. Thus, with different enzymes (from yeast cultures), aldehyde can be produced from pyruvic acid or pyruvate (the enzyme is pyruvate decarboxylase), then ethyl alcohol or ethanol (the enzyme is alcohol dehydrogenase), the overall process being called anaerobic alcoholic fermentation (Voet and Voet, 1990, p. 464). This is the classic means of making alcoholic beverages from sugars (starches are first converted to sugars, e.g., in what is called mash, via the enzyme amylase, as produced from young barley sprouts by the process of malting).

In the formation of lactic acid or lactate, there may be a buildup of lactic acid in body tissues, an occurrence called *lactic acidosis* (Harris, in Devlin, 1986, pp. 357, 358). Normally, the lactic acid will be oxidized to the end products carbon dioxide (or $CO_2$) and water (or $H_2O$), or else will converted back to glucose in the liver, by gluconeogenesis. (The entire process, glycolysis to lactic acid or lactate followed by gluconeogenesis back to glycogen or glucose, is called the *Cori cycle*.) Decreased oxygen availability favors an increase in lactate production and a decrease in lactate utilization. Intense muscular exertion will also favor lactic acid or lactate in accumulations well beyond those used in the tricarboxylic cycle. Bicarbonate can be administered as a counter, however. Whether these phenomena could be related to cancer growth or remission has presumably not been investigated.

Glucose may also exist in the form of its polymer, glycogen. Regarding glycogen and its synthesis and degradation, the regulatory enzymes involved are variously activated by a chemical compound called adenosine monophosphate, or AMP (Harris, in Devlin, 1986, p. 391ff.). These enzymes are in turn further regulated by a substance with the acronym cAMP, or cyclic AMP. It is reported, furthermore, that in acting as a hormone regulator, cAMP also serves as a cancer inhibitor, and is assisted by the amino acid arginine (Boik, 1996, p. 48). These are some of the indirect means by which cancer can potentially be controlled.

Thus, natural agents said to raise cAMP levels to inhibit cancer include the species *Andrographis paniculata* (of the plant family Acanthaceae), *Polyporus umbellatus* (of the fungal family Polyporaceae), *Salvia multiorrhiza* (of the plant family Labiatae), *Ziziphus jujuba* (of the plant family Rhamnaceae), *Cnidium monnieri* (of the plant family Umbelliferae), *Actinidia chinensis* (of the plant family Actinidiaceae), *Aconitum carmichaeli* (of the plant family Ranunculaceae), *Cinnamomum cassia* (of the plant family Lauracae), and the alkaloid caffeine. All families, genera, or species are variously listed in Hartwell's *Plants Used Against Cancer* except for *Andrographis* and *Actinidia*.

The situation is complex, but illustrates the fact that there may be many as yet unsuspected anticancer agents, and which act by unsuspected means.

## GLUTAMINOLYSIS

For documentation purposes, a much-abbreviated reaction scenario for glutaminolysis is shown in Figure 3.3. Glutamine is an amino acid, and glutaminolysis is only part of the more general topic of the metabolism of amino acids, which is covered in the standard texts and references on biochemistry.

That cancer cell metabolism may alternately be supported by glutaminolysis or aminolysis is an additional complication in attempting to suppress cancer growth.

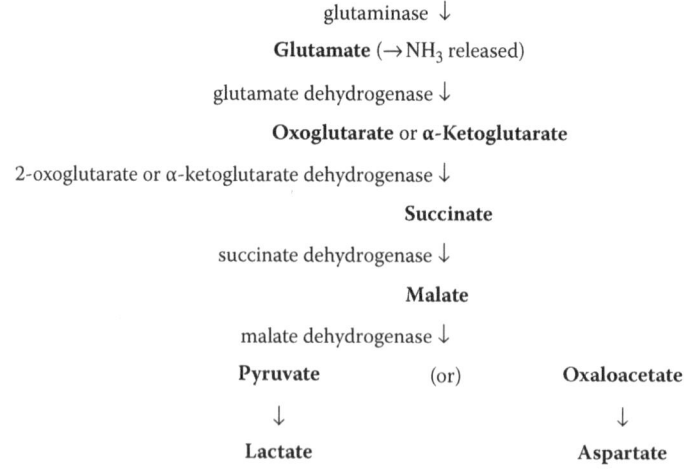

**Glutamine** ($\leftarrow H_2O$ added)

glutaminase $\downarrow$

**Glutamate** ($\rightarrow NH_3$ released)

glutamate dehydrogenase $\downarrow$

**Oxoglutarate** or **α-Ketoglutarate**

2-oxoglutarate or α-ketoglutarate dehydrogenase $\downarrow$

**Succinate**

succinate dehydrogenase $\downarrow$

**Malate**

malate dehydrogenase $\downarrow$

**Pyruvate**      (or)      **Oxaloacetate**

$\downarrow$          $\downarrow$

**Lactate**          **Aspartate**

**FIGURE 3.3** Glutaminolysis as it may interface with the tricarboxylic acid cycle, with enzymes shown. (Based on information in Eigenbrodt et al., 1985, pp. 145, 153; Voet and Voet, *Biochemistry*, 1995, p. 741; Diamondstone, in Devlin, 1986, p. 583). Under carbohydrate or glucose restrictions, all lactate will be produced from glutamine rather than from glucose via glycolysis.

## Tricarboxylic Acid Cycle

The tricarboxylic acid cycle can be thought as completing aerobic glycolysis to yield carbon dioxide and water, plus energy, by oxidizing the pyruvic acid or pyruvate obtained at the end of glycolysis proper. The organic acids involved in the cycle have three carboxylic groups per molecule, and hence the name. The carboxylic group can be denoted as -(C=O)-OH, or simply as -COOH, of which citric acid is an example, with its formula representable as $HOC(CH_2COOH)_2COOH$.

As documented in Figure 3.4, a substance called coenzyme A or CoA enters the tricarboxylic acid cycle. It is vital to the initiation of the cycle, and occurs in other body processes. Its complicated chemical structure is diagrammed in most biochemistry textbooks (e.g., by Olson, in Devlin, 1986, p. 270; and by Voet and Voet, 1995, p. 826). Conceptually, it can be viewed as a consortium of chemical compounds

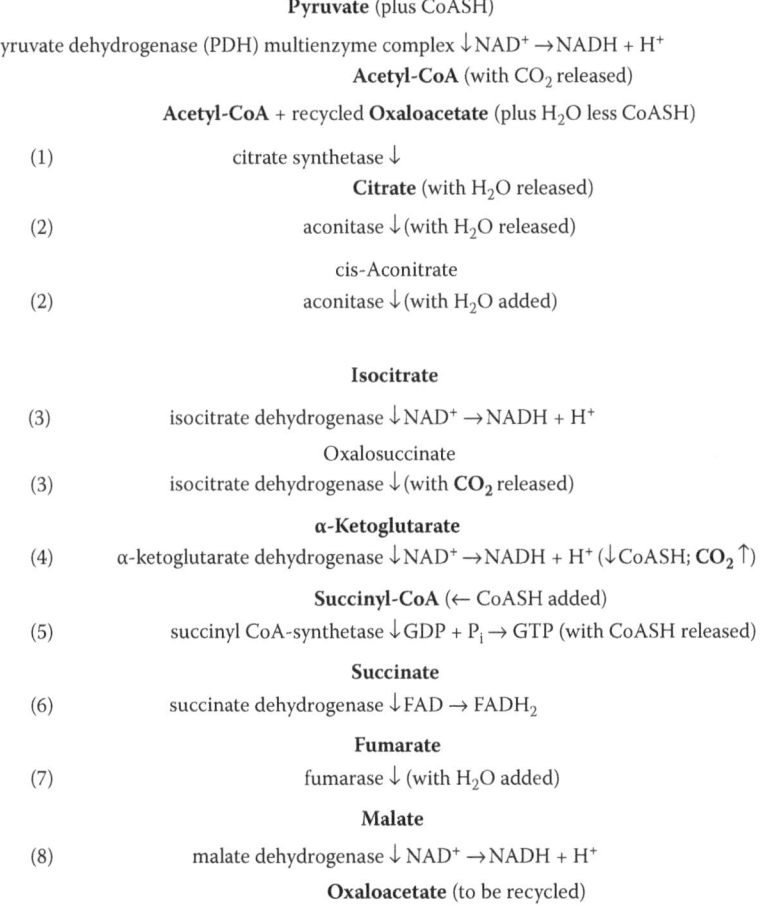

**Pyruvate** (plus CoASH)

pyruvate dehydrogenase (PDH) multienzyme complex $\downarrow NAD^+ \rightarrow NADH + H^+$

**Acetyl-CoA** (with $CO_2$ released)

**Acetyl-CoA** + recycled **Oxaloacetate** (plus $H_2O$ less CoASH)

(1)                          citrate synthetase $\downarrow$

**Citrate** (with $H_2O$ released)

(2)                          aconitase $\downarrow$ (with $H_2O$ released)

cis-Aconitrate

(2)                          aconitase $\downarrow$ (with $H_2O$ added)


**Isocitrate**

(3)            isocitrate dehydrogenase $\downarrow NAD^+ \rightarrow NADH + H^+$

Oxalosuccinate

(3)            isocitrate dehydrogenase $\downarrow$ (with $CO_2$ released)

**α-Ketoglutarate**

(4)      α-ketoglutarate dehydrogenase $\downarrow NAD^+ \rightarrow NADH + H^+$ ($\downarrow$ CoASH; $CO_2 \uparrow$)

**Succinyl-CoA** ($\leftarrow$ CoASH added)

(5)            succinyl CoA-synthetase $\downarrow GDP + P_i \rightarrow GTP$ (with CoASH released)

**Succinate**

(6)            succinate dehydrogenase $\downarrow FAD \rightarrow FADH_2$

**Fumarate**

(7)                          fumarase $\downarrow$ (with $H_2O$ added)

**Malate**

(8)            malate dehydrogenase $\downarrow NAD^+ \rightarrow NADH + H^+$

**Oxaloacetate** (to be recycled)

**FIGURE 3.4** Tricarboxylic acid cycle with enzymes and supportive reactions shown. (Based on information in Voet and Voet, 1995, *Biochemistry*, p. 539; Olson, in Devlin, 1986, p. 280.)

variously called β-mercaptoethylamine, pantothenic acid, adenine, and d-ribose. Biosynthesis occurs in the body, starting with pantothenic acid, and is completed in a succession of reactions, each catalyzed by a particular enzyme (Diamondstone, in Devlin, 1986, p. 671; Voet and Voet, 1995, p. 826). Alternately, it may be considered as existing also in what is called the thio (-SH) form and written as CoASH. Another form is obtained by replacement of the (-H) above with an acetyl group ($CH_3CO$-) to yield what is referred to as acetyl-CoA, which could as well be written as acetyl-CoAS or acetyl-SCoA. In other words, the sulfur content is always present.

(The foregoing illustrates the intrinsic and vital role of the B vitamin called pantothenic acid in normal aerobic metabolism. Furthermore, by favoring aerobic glycolysis, it may act as an anticancer agent by countering the anaerobic metabolism associated with cancer. Conversely, a deficiency could discourage aerobic glycolysis, thereby contributing to anaerobic glycolysis, that is, cancer cell metabolism. Thus, nutritional requirements can be related to cancer formation or its inhibition.)

Some other substances entering the tricarboxylic acid cycle are the following:

$NAD^+$ — nicotinamide adenine dinucleotide, oxidized form
NADH — nicotinamide adenine dinucleotide, reduced form
$H^+$ — hydrogen, oxidized form, or hydrogen ion

GTP — guanosine triphosphate
GDP — guanosine diphosphate
$P_i$ — orthophosphate ion

FAD — flavin adenine dinucleotide
$FADH_2$ — flavin adenine dinucleotide, hydrogen, reduced form

where nicotinamide, guanosine, and flavin are variously nitrogenous compounds, with flavin signifying the B vitamin called riboflavin, or $B_2$. Again, we see that B vitamins are essential to life processes.

A distinguishing feature of the substances listed previously is the presence or absence of a phosphate group or groups, again underscoring the prominent role of phosphates in life processes. As a point of departure, it may be noted that what are called nucleotides form the monomeric units of the polymers that comprise nucleic acids, and are thereby connected to the composition of DNA and RNA (Voet and Voet, 1995, pp. 795, 796). The loss of a phosphate group or groups yields what is called a nucleoside.

## OVERALL GLYCOLYTIC CONVERSIONS

In anaerobic glycolysis, by definition, no oxygen is present and the tricarboxylic acid cycle cannot proceed, and only lactic acid or lactate is the end product. In aerobic glycolysis, both the tricarboxylic acid cycle and lactic acid or lactate formation can occur. In the preferred limit, only the tricarboxylic acid cycle is assumed to occur.

Here, the two routes can be compared. In the one, in the limit, lactic acid or lactate formation can be assumed not to proceed during aerobic glycolysis, with carbon dioxide and $H_2O$ as the final products. In the other, only lactic acid or lactate will be the final product during anaerobic glycolysis.

## AEROBIC GLYCOLYSIS

This is the normal body process whereby glucose or blood sugar is converted ultimately to carbon dioxide and water. Following the ten-step conversion of glucose to pyruvic acid, the pyruvic acid is then converted to the end products of carbon dioxide and water via what is variously called the tricarboxylic acid, or citric acid, or Krebs cycle. The conversion is strongly exothermic, fueling the body's internal processes and its external activities.

Consider the phenomenon referred to as spontaneous human combustion (SHC), as publicized from time to time (e.g., as was reported in *Arthur C. Clarke's Mysterious Universe*, shown on the Discovery Channel, for instance, on October 22, 1996, and was mentioned in Charles Dickens' *Bleak House*). If this weird phenomenon does indeed occur, it could instead be referred to as spontaneous ignition, followed by combustion. And if it is at least conceivable for aberrations to occur among the enzyme-catalyzed reactions involved in the metabolism of glucose or other carbohydrates to yield $CO_2$ and $H_2O$, then conceivably there may be a case. Ordinarily, body metabolism reaction rates are miniscule as compared to the direct combustion or combustive oxidation of conventional fuels. If enzyme promoters exist, however, there is the possibility that runaway metabolic processes occur, similar to those in the ignition and further combustion of carbonaceous materials. If so, ample air or oxygen supply would also be required for this extremely unlikely scenario.

In further comment about spontaneous combustion, there is the example that rags soaked in linseed oil or hydrocarbon solvents will ignite if the heat of oxidation (or heat of combustion) is not dissipated or controlled. The practice is to store these materials in air-tight containers or else spread them out for heat dissipation. The storage of low-rank coals, particularly, has this problem, and coal storage piles require monitoring. Some dried low-rank coals are even pyrophoric, bursting into flame on exposure to air. Brazil nuts from the Brazil-nut tree, species *Bertholletica excelsa* of the family Lecythidaceae, must be raked and turned when stored to avoid spontaneous ignition and combustion. It may be said, therefore, that spontaneous ignition and combustion is a common enough phenomenon.

As for the human body system, a fever can be induced by reducing the heat normally dissipated to the surroundings. The phenomenon can be viewed in terms of the caloric intake, without heat dissipation. If this heat is not dissipated, the body temperature would continue to rise inordinately.

## ANAEROBIC GLYCOLYSIS

Adding all the chemical equations involved, the overall net conversion of glucose to lactic acid is slightly exothermic, which indicates that not much metabolic energy results. In consequence, the anaerobic glycolysis rate must increase manyfold to support the equivalent bodily energy requirements. Thus, in partial confirmation, anaerobic glycolysis rates have been observed that are 20 times aerobic glycolysis rates (Harris, in Devlin, 1986, p. 353). A noticeable consequence is that the body loses weight so as to meet its energy requirements.

## CANCER CELL METABOLISM VS. NORMAL CELL METABOLISM

The initial part of the glycolysis sequence or pathway producing pyruvic acid or pyruvate is the same for both anaerobic and aerobic glycolysis. It would seem that this part should not be inhibited or otherwise interfered with, and only the anaerobic fermentation to yield lactic acid or lactate should be blocked, this being the main distinguishing feature of cancer cell metabolism.

There are other factors to consider, however, such as cancer cells having an abnormally high glycolysis rate, causing a buildup of lactic acid product. This will in turn reduce the activity of PFK (phosphofructokinase enzyme), which falls off under acidic conditions. Thus Reaction 3 of Figure 3.1 should expectedly be inhibited, thereby reducing the glycolysis rate. In spite of this, however, the glycolytic enzymes are still in such high concentrations that glycolysis remains at high levels (Voet and Voet, 1995, p. 595). Even under aerobic conditions, cancer cells produce much more lactic acid than expected, and in fact the glycolytic pathway will form pyruvic acid or pyruvate much faster than can be utilized by the tricarboxylic cycle of normal cells (Voet and Voet, 1995, p. 595). The conversion to lactic acid or lactate is apparently favored whatever the conditions, indicating that cancer cell metabolism is sustained no matter what.

The inference from the foregoing, therefore, is that the enzyme-catalyzed conversion of pyruvic acid or pyruvate to lactic acid or lactate should somehow be blocked.

There is also another possibility. Looking at the other reactions, that are involved in glycolysis, consider the slower or controlling reactions, which are Reactions (1), (3), and (10) of Figure 3.1, which are catalyzed, respectively, by hexokinase, phosphofructokinase (PFK), and pyruvate kinase. Their inhibition in part or in totality could conceivably slow down the formation of pyruvic acid or pyruvate, and in turn slow down the production of lactic acid or lactate, thereby acting against cancer cell metabolism. This could also act against the tricarboxylic acid cycle, however; that is, against normal cell respiration or metabolism.

A few inhibitors of these several enzymes are provided in Voet and Voet (1990). These include glucose-6-phosphate as an inhibitor for hexokinase, as it is a reaction product. Also, ATP and citrate are listed as inhibitors of PFK, and ATP is an inhibitor for pyruvate kinase, as it is a conversion product. Other inhibitors are tabulated in Appendix A of Hoffman's *Cancer and the Search for Selective Biochemical Inhibitors* (1999). On the other hand, Voet and Voet (1990) list a few activators or promoters for PFK, including ADP, fructose 6-phosphate (which is a reactant), fructose 1,6-bisphosphate (which is a product), the ammonium ion, and the orthophosphate ion $P_i$. The situation can get complicated.

An inhibitor for lactate dehydrogenase would block the formation of lactic acid or lactate, the main distinguishing feature of cancer cell metabolism. This would alternately favor the normal oxidation of pyruvic acid or pyruvate via the tricarboxylic acid cycle. As a qualification, cancer cells also apparently undergo a degree of oxidative metabolism, though the conversion to lactate or lactic acid occurs to a much greater extent.

There are some other reactions that occur, additionally or alternatively, indicating that cancer cells as well as normal cells have some escape routes for survival. These other effects have been analyzed as follows in terms of high and low glucose concentrations, and glutaminolysis.

A comparison of the glycolysis route for cancer cells at high and low glucose concentrations vs. that of normal cells has been provided by Eigenbrodt et al. (1985, p. 144). The analysis is involved, to say the very least, and here only the rudiments will be presented as based on a previous synopsis (Hoffman, 1999, p. 21ff). The ultimate objective would be to determine if the enzyme inhibitors for the particular controlling enzyme reactions can be linked to anticancer agents, known or unknown. For the record, the features are as follows, as per the effect of glucose concentrations:

(1)  Regulation of glycolysis by oxygen in normal cells: Reaction 3 of Figure 3.1 is controlling under normal aerobic conditions, being slower than the other reactions. This is partially offset by a high capacity to convert the product of Reaction 3 on to pyruvate.

(2)  Regulation of glycolysis by oxygen in tumor cells at high glucose concentrations: In tumor cells, there is a heightened activity of the enzyme hexokinase in Reaction 1, of the enzyme phosphofructokinase in Reaction 3, and of the enzyme pyruvate kinase in Reaction 10, all of which produce a high glycolytic capacity. The formation of pyruvate by Reaction 10 will be decreased, however, by the presence of alanine, phenylalanine, and ATP, which inhibit the enzyme pyruvate kinase. This will be eventually offset by the buildup of reaction intermediates. Tumor cells, as compared to normal cells, use almost the total glycolytic capacity, independent of how much oxygen is present. That is, in tumor cells, it apparently makes no difference whether an aerobic or anaerobic condition exists for conversion to lactic acid or lactate to occur.

(3)  Regulation of glycolysis by oxygen in tumor cells at low glucose concentrations or with alternative reactant energy sources other than glucose (e.g., glutamine): At low glucose concentrations, the levels of fructose-1,6-bisphosphate produced by Reaction 3 are very much lower than at high glucose conditions (for instance, there is a much lower concentration of glucose initially). The result is a deactivation of the enzyme pyruvate kinase for Reaction 10. No conversion to pyruvate occurs, and no ATP is synthesized. (Thus, little or no pyruvate is available for oxidation via the tricarboxylic acid cycle, or for fermentation to lactic acid.) On the other hand, conversion of the ATP yields the orthophosphate ion $P_i$, which in turn activates glutaminase for the conversion of glutamine. Thus

glutaminolysis proceeds as per Figure 3.3. The end result is a proliferation of the tumor cells.

A conclusion reached by Eigenbrodt et al. (1985) is that the metabolic behavior of tumor (or cancer) cells differs from normal cells in that the former show increased anaerobic glycolysis and glucose uptake, enhanced glutaminolysis; enhanced nucleic acid (DNA) synthesis capacity, and enhanced lipid synthesis (p. 143).

(The molecules called lipids include the fatty acids, which are relatively small molecules compared to the macromolecules that are proteins, nucleic acids, and polysaccharides (Voet and Voet, 1995, p. 16). Proteins, of first importance, are polymers of amino acids; nucleic acids are polymers of what are called nucleotides; and polysaccharides are polymers of sugars.)

Tumor cells, however, also show a reduced pyruvate and acetyl-CoA oxidation rate as involved in the tricarboxylic cycle. There is a lower sensitivity to oxygen, and a lower growth hormone requirement. Thus, as a potential anticancer measure, there is the objective also of enhancing respiration or oxygen uptake, thereby favoring the tricarboxylic acid cycle over lactic acid or lactate formation.

Thus, it may be concluded that perhaps the simplest way to inhibit cancer cell metabolism is merely to block the enzyme lactate dehydrogenase for the conversion of pyruvic acid or pyruvate to lactic acid or lactate.

## SELECTIVE BIOCHEMICAL INHIBITORS

The cancer problem can be viewed as a search for ways to suppress cancer cell proliferation by means of the foregoing routes (Figures 2.2 and 2.3), which pertain to tumor cells. The agents of interest are enzyme inhibitors, which have been explained as acting in several different ways, for example, by chemically reacting with the enzyme, and by adsorption on the enzyme surface, either at so-called active sites, or at least adjacent to these active sites.

Inhibitors determined for the controlling enzymes involved in cell chemistry have been listed elsewhere (Hoffman, 1999, Table A-1 through Table A-3 of Appendix A), as obtained from Jain's *Handbook of Enzyme Inhibitors* (1982) and Zollner's *Handbook of Enzyme Inhibitors* (1993). The breakdown is for glycolysis, lactate formation, and glutaminolysis. Some of the more common and simpler chemicals or compounds serving as enzyme inhibitors for one or another of the various reaction steps are as follows, as derived from the Jain and Zollner references. Many more, natural or synthetic, no doubt remain to be discovered, as both the Jain and Zollner references are dated. The sequences presented here parallel those presented by Hoffman (1999).

### Glycolysis Inhibitors

Inhibitors may serve any of the several (ten) sequential steps involved in the glycolysis pathway. A partial listing includes certain metallic or mineral substances, notably calcium and magnesium (as the ions $Ca^{++}$ and $Mg^{++}$). These are among the essential minerals found in the diet. Lithium is another inhibitor, which is notably used in treating depression. The phosphate ion is reported to be an inhibitor, as is the sulfate ion. Chromium acts as an inhibitor in the form of an ATP complex, where adenosine is the principle component of ATP (and ADP).

It may be added that sulfides or disulfides, which are found to be glycolysis inhibitors, also act as poisons or inhibitors for such inorganic catalysts as nickel or nickel oxide catalysts.

Various sugars make the listings, denoted by the suffix "-ose." Various amino acids also make the listings, denoted by the suffix "-ine," notable examples being L-alanine and L-phenylalanine, commonly associated with nutritional supplements. Arginine, an essential amino acid (not manufactured in the body), is said to be an inhibitor. The suffix "pyridoxal" is listed as an inhibitor, whereby it may be noted that pyridoxine (or pyridoxin) is called vitamin B6.

Estrogen is represented by the synthetic hormone diethylstilbestrol or DES.

Citric acid, found in citrus fruits, is listed as an inhibitor, and also occurs as a reaction intermediate in the metabolic tricarboxylic acid or citric acid cycle. Ethanol or ethyl alcohol makes an unexpected appearance as an inhibitor, as does glycerol. The ubiquitous alkaloid ingredient of coffee, better known as caffeine, is listed as an inhibitor (in fact, coffee enemas are sometimes used in folkloric cancer treatments). Creatine, a nitrogenous compound found naturally in the body, is an inhibitor, and is a known anticancer agent, for example, as used with urea in a mixture called Carbatine.

Fatty acids make the list, especially lauric acid and unsaturated oleic acid. Flavianic acid is a precursor in the preparation of the essential amino acid arginine and the nonessential amino acid tyrosine. Moss (1992) has a chapter about using arginine in the treatment of cancer. Tyrosine interestingly enters the picture as a component of the enzyme tyrosine kinase, the latter in the role of an inhibitor for cancerous stem cells, to be described in Chapter 10.

The chemical compound quercetin, listed in the compilation of inhibitors, is considered an anticancer agent, at least in a folkloric sense. It occurs naturally in chaparral or the creosote bush (*Larrea tridentata*); in fact, chaparral itself is considered an anticancer agent.

(We remind the reader that the term "anticancer agent" is to be distinguished from "cure.")

Not resolved, however, is whether the inhibition of glycolysis per se can be an effective inhibitor of cancer cell metabolism, inasmuch as glycolysis is also involved in normal cell metabolism.

## INHIBITORS OF LACTIC ACID OR LACTATE FORMATION FROM PYRUVIC ACID OR PYRUVATE

By virtue of what is called the law of mass action, the buildup of product itself works against the conversion reaction. Thus, the very buildup of lactic acid or lactate product serves as an inhibitor. (Albeit pyruvic acid is also listed as an inhibitor in the compilations, but which is a reactant for the conversion to lactic acid.) Another inhibitor listed is oxalic acid, a naturally occurring component of such vegetables as spinach and rhubarb, and which becomes toxic in large amounts. The common chemicals salicylic acid (aspirin) and urea are both listed as inhibitors, and are both known as anticancer agents. Serotonin, the brain neurohormone or neurotransmitter, makes the listing. It is derived from the essential amino acid tryptophan, and is more often known as a vital mind relaxant.

## AN UPDATE ON INHIBITORS FOR CANCER CELL METABOLISM: GLUCOSE TO LACTIC ACID

Inasmuch as anaerobic glycolysis to produce lactic acid or lactate occurs in cancerous cells, a partial update on inhibitors is presented in Table 3.1, notably as presented in the second edition of Zollner's compendium (1993). Of special interest is allicin as an inhibitor for lactate dehydrogenase. Itself a sulfur compound, it is formed from a precursor sulfur compound called alliin by the action of the enzyme alliinase. Both alliin and alliinase occur naturally in garlic, and the conversion to allicin normally occurs with mastication of the garlic. Allicin is a transient sulfur-bearing compound, decomposing on standing, and must be utilized fresh or near fresh. Garlic contains still other organic sulfur compounds that are potential enzyme inhibitors.

## GLUTAMINOLYSIS INHIBITORS

According to the previously cited reference (Hoffman, (1991), Appendix A), some dyelike materials show up as inhibitors of glutaminolysis. Thus, the agents listed as bromcresol (or bromocresol) green and bromcresol purple are dyes derived from sulfonephthalein, starting with the compound called *meta*-cresol. Cresols in turn are related to phenol or carbolic acid, and to the coal–tar mixture called creosote. Phenolic-type compounds are also known to occur in chaparral or creosote bush (genus *Larrea*), hence its alternate common name.

(Phenolphthalein, another organic dye (red), is used as an acid-base titration indicator, and also in a laxative [e.g., in Ex-Lax®]. It is in itself sometimes considered to be an anticancer agent. Having the same chemical formula but different structures, the three cresol isomers — *ortho*-cresol, *meta*-cresol, and *para*-cresol — serve variously as the starting materials for such industrial chemicals as the herbicides DNOC and MCPA, are also used in plastics or resins, and can be converted even to the common food antioxidant known as BHT.)

Albizzin, considered an anticancer agent, comes from a tree of the genus *Albizzia*, family Leguminosae. It is found in India and Malaysia, and is listed in Hartwell's compendium *Plants Used Against Cancer* (1982b).

The metallic ions of copper ($Cu^{++}$), lead ($Pb^{++}$), and mercury ($Hg^{++}$) are listed variously as enzyme inhibitors for glutaminolysis. However, not only can they be poisonous to humans, but they can also be poisons or inhibitors for inorganic catalysts.

Ammonia ($NH_3$), listed as an enzyme inhibitor, has a kinship with urea and such other ammoniacal inorganic compounds as hydrazine sulfate. Not only may they be potential enzyme inhibitors for glutaminolysis, but also for other metabolic reactions. Both urea and hydrazine sulfate are known to have been tried against cancer, apparently with mixed results.

## TABLE 3.1
## Update on Enzymes and Inhibitors Involved in Anaerobic Glycolysis

### Hexokinase or Hexosekinase
*n-Acetylglucosamine; Allicin, *Allos 6-phosphate; *Chromioum-ATP complex; *Copper (Cu++);
*L-cystamine; Dihydrogiesenin; Disulfiram; *Disulfides; Gafrinin; Geigerinin; *Glucose 6-
phosphate; *Glutathione oxidized; Griesenin; 4′,5′,7-Hydroxy-3,6-methoxyflavonone; 4-
Hydroxypentenal, 2-(p-Hydroxyphenyl)-2-phenylpropane; Ivalin; *Glycerol; *Lauric acid; *Lyxose;
*Magnesium (Mg++); *Mannoheptulose; *Mannose; *Nucleotides; o-Phthalaldehyde; Quercetin;
Vanadate oligomer; Vermeerin; *Xylose, D-,

### *6-Phosphofructokinase or Phosphofructokinase
Argeninephosphate; Caffeine; Calcium (Ca++); Citric Acid; Creatine phosphate; Ethanol, Fructose
diphosphate; Glucose 6-phosphate; Glycerol; Lauric acid; NADH; Oleic acid; Phosphoenolpyruvate
(PEP); Pyridoxal-5-phosphate; Phyrophosphate ion; Pyruvic Acid.

### *Pyruvate Kinase
Alanine; Amino acids; AMP, Anions; Butyric acid; Calcium (Ca++); Creatine phosphate;
Diethylstilbestrol (DE); Fatty acids; Lithium (Li+); Phenylalanine; Phosphate; Pyhridoxal-5-
phosphate; Pyrophosphate; Pyruvic Acid, Quercetin; Sulphate; Tris.

### *Lactate Dehydrogenase
Allicin (in Zollner, 1989); Arsenite ion; ATP; Butyric acid, 2-3-epoxy; 3GA-destran; Estradiol, 17-
B; Fatty acids; Glycerate; Butynoic acids; Lactic acid; L-maleic acid; Mandelic acid;
Mononucleotides; NAD; NADH.

* Appears in Appendix A of Hoffman (1999).

*Source:* From Zollner, H., *Handbook of Enzyme Inhibitors*, in two volumes, VCH, Weinheim, FRG,
1993; (*) from Zollner, H., *Handbook of Enzyme Inhibitors*, VCH, Weinheim, FRG, 1989; Jain, M.K.,
*Handbook of Enzyme Inhibitors*, Wiley, New York, 1982.

The unusual material labeled Tris has the lengthy chemical name tris(2,3-dibro-
mopropanol)phosphate, where "tris" stands for a certain amine group. It was once
used as a fire retardant for clothing or nightwear, and although an enzyme inhibitor,
it is also suspected of being carcinogenic. (This is not an unknown contradiction,
for whether a substance is anticancer or procancer may depend on the dosage as
well as other factors.)

The listings of this chapter can be viewed as incomplete, here and elsewhere,
given the many naturally occurring substances from the plant world and mineral
world, yet to be tested (not to mention synthetic compounds). The bioactive alkaloids,
for example, are prime possibilities.

## THE TRICARBOXYLIC CYCLE AND RESPIRATION

Glycolysis and the tricarboxylic cycle are fundamental to respiration, that is, the
uptake and utilization of oxygen from the air. If respiration is shut down, suffocation
results. It is the way in which many poisons act, for instance, the deadly South

American poisonous mixture called curare. Curare is derived from certain members of the genus *Strychnos*, and contains a number of toxic alkaloids (strychnine being a familiar name for such an alkaloid). Thus, enzymes in glycolysis and the tricarboxylic cycle proper are of fundamental concern, for their blockage or inhibition could prove fatal. Inhibitors for enzymes involved in the carboxylic acid cycle are listed in Appendix B of Hoffman (1999).

Arsenic poisoning requires a special mention. The enzymes affected are notably pyruvate dehydrogenase and α-ketoglutarate dehydrogenase, as well as other enzymes (Voet and Voet, 1995, pp. 547–548; Harris, in Devlin, 1986, pp. 348, 349). The result, unfortunately, can be overinhibition, shutting down respiration. Chronic arsenic poisoning occurs with smaller, cumulative dosages. Microamounts possibly may act to stimulate the immune system, a thesis of homeopathy, for example.

(Interestingly, small amounts of arsenic have been used to put back the spring in the step, and the shine on the coat, of older and decrepit horses, as Ben Green writes in *Horse Tradin'*. Neither Jain (1982) nor Zollner (1993) include arsenic as an enzyme inhibitor per se, but list enzymes inhibited by arsenate and arsenite ions, that is, by compounds of arsenic.)

Both enzymes mentioned previously pertain to the tricarboxylic acid cycle proper, and are apparently vital to sustaining respiration. Accordingly, inhibitors can lead to undesirable and sometimes life-threatening consequences. Enzyme inhibitors for pyruvate dehydrogenase are more commonly known, those for α-ketoglutarate dehydrogenase less so. In the Jain reference respiration inhibitors are treated as a special category.

Among the other notations is that acetaldehyde is to be avoided, it being a respiration inhibitor. It is related to ethyl alcohol or ethanol and also to acetic acid, but not necessarily to citric acid as involved in the carboxylic acid or citric acid cycle. Alkaloids are expectedly respiration inhibitors, and anesthetics can have respiration inhibition as a side effect. Aromatic acids such as phenol are bad news, as are arsenate, cyanide, isothiocyanate, and thiocyanate. The heavy metals cadmium, cobalt, copper, ruthenium, vanadate, and zinc are regarded as health risks, if not for respiration, for other reasons.

(The cyanide and cyanate ions inhibit many enzymes, as cataloged in both Jain's and Zollner's handbooks, which have extensive listings for enzymes that are inhibited or poisoned. The copper ion in the cupric form $Cu^{++}$ has many entries. Frontiersman Jesse Chisholm, namesake for the famous Chisholm Trail, died after eating bear grease stored in a copper container.)

The inclusion of fatty acids is a surprise, but maybe not for that called "guaiaretic acid, nordihydro," better known as NDGA or nordihydroguaiaretic acid. It is an ingredient in chaparral or creosote bush, and was formerly used commercially as an oxidation inhibitor in various applications (note that oxidation inhibitors are viewed as beneficial for a number of purposes, including cancer suppression).

The hormone progesterone shows up as an inhibitor. Interestingly, so does sucrose, or common table sugar.

The alkaloids papaverine and theophylline are listed as inhibitors, but not strychnine. However, many or most alkaloids should be suspect, depending on the dosage level.

## VITAMINS AND HORMONES AS INHIBITORS OR PROMOTERS

If enzymes do not act or only act slowly, they can be stimulated or promoted by small ionic or molecular entities called *cofactors* (Voet and Voet, 1995, pp. 337, 338). Examples of cofactors include metallic ions such as the zinc ion $Zn^{++}$, and also organic molecules called coenzymes, such as $NAD^+$ (nicotinamide adenine dinucleotide, in the oxidized form).

If the necessary cofactors cannot be synthesized within the body, they must be ingested via the diet. The terminology then becomes that of vitamins, which can be regarded as precursors of coenzymes. Nutritional deficiencies in fact served as the impetus for discovering many vitamins, i.e., coenzymes. For instance, a component of $NAD^+$ is better known as nicotinamide (or niacinamide), and its carboxylic acid analog is called nicotinic acid (or niacin). The human vitamin deficiency known as pellagra yields to supplements of niacin or niacinamide.

The vitamins that are coenzyme precursors are all water soluble, whereas the fat-soluble vitamins such as vitamin A and vitamin D are not components of coenzymes, though vital to the diet (and, strictly speaking, vitamin D can be classified as a hormone rather than a vitamin).

Vitamins are not synthesized in the body, at least not in the amounts needed. On the other hand, hormones are produced within the body, to be secreted by specific glands. For example, vitamin D in the form called cholecalciferol ($D_3$) is technically a hormone, being synthesized in the skin from the ultraviolet irradiation of 7-dehydrocholesterol, a metabolite or metabolic product of cholesterol. On the other hand, an almost identical form called ergocalciferol ($D_2$) is synthetically prepared by the irradiation of ergesterol from yeast, and is the type used in nutritional supplements and fortified foods. It is therefore a vitamin (and large doses are considered toxic).

(Interestingly, vitamin C, or ascorbic acid, is a vitamin in human nutrition, since a necessary enzyme is missing to convert what is called gulonolactone to yield ascorbic acid (Ungar, in Devlin, 1986, p. 719), whereas in animals such as the rat or dog, this enzyme is naturally present, so that ascorbic acid could then be called a hormone.)

As a matter of record, Table 3.2 lists vitamins, chemical names, and stoichiometric chemical formulas. In many or most cases, however, the vitamin structure is too complicated for any kind of simplified representation.

Vitamins that may act as enzyme inhibitors are listed in Table 3.3, as found in Jain (1982) and Zollner (1993).

The effects of vitamins and various foodstuffs on cancer continue to be a subject of interest and controversy, as are of course the effects of using other plant and herbal substances. With regard to vitamins, Frank L. Meyskens authored the *Modulation and Mediation of Cancer by Vitamins*, published in 1983. This was followed by another volume titled *Vitamins and Cancer*, edited by Meyskens and Prasad, and published in 1986. A further update is furnished in *Vitamins and Minerals in the Prevention and Treatment of Cancer*, edited by Maryce M. Jacobs and published in 1991.

**TABLE 3.2**
**Vitamins**

| | | |
|---|---|---|
| Vitamin A | Retinol | $C_{19}H_{24}\text{-}CH_2OH$ |
| Vitamin B1 | Thiamine hydrochloride; thiamin chloride | $C_{12}H_{18}Cl_2N_4OS$ |
| Vitamin B2 | Riboflavin; lactoflavin; vitamin G | $C_{17}H_{22}N_4O_6$ |
| Vitamin B6 | Pyridoxin | $C_8H_{11}NO_3$ |
| Vitamin B12 | Cobalamine; cyanocobalamin | $C_{63}H_{90}N_{14}O_{14}PCo$ |
| Folic acid | Pteroylglutamic acid (PGA); folacin; vitamin Bc; vitamin M | $C_{14}H_{11}N_6O_2\text{-}(C_5H_7NO_3)_n\text{-}OH$ where n = 1–7; $C_{19}H_{19}N_7O_6$ for n = 1 |
| Niacin | Nicotinic acid; 3-pyridinecarboxylic acid | $(C_5H_4N)COOH$ |
| Pantothenic acid | | $HOCH_2C(CH_3)_2CH(OH)CO\text{-}NHCH_2CH_2COOH$ |
| or $N(\alpha,\gamma$-dihydroxy-$\beta,\beta$-dimethylbutyryl)$\beta$-alanine | | $C_9H_{17}NO_5$ |
| Vitamin C | Ascorbic acid; antiscorbutin | $CO\,(COH)_3CHOHCH_2OH$ $C_6H_8O_6$ |
| Vitamin D | Calciferol | $C_{28}H_{44}O$ |
| Vitamin E | $\alpha$-Tocopherol; 5,7,8-trimethyltocol | $C_{14}H_{17}O_2\,(C_5H_{10})_3\,H$ |
| Vitamin K | Phthiocol; 1,4-naphthoquinone, 2-hydroxy-3-methyl- | $C_{11}H_8O_3$ |

*Source:* Adapted from Table 1.1 in Hoffman, *Cancer and the Search for Selective Biochemical Inhibitors,* CRC Press, Boca Raton, FL, 1999.)

For a general look at the subject, there is the *Handbook of Vitamins,* second edition, edited by Lawrence J. Machlin and published in 1991. Another is by Sheldon Saul Hendler and a board of medical advisors, most or all M.D.s, titled *The Doctors' Vitamin and Mineral Encyclopedia,* published in 1990. This reference also covers herbs, amino acids, and other substances, and has numerous citations in the index about cancer, but no definite, sure-fire remedies.

Further information about herbal substances will be presented in subsequent chapters and sections, including particulars about garlic and its compounds.

The subject of hormones, along with neurotransmission, has been included under the category of biochemical communications in the Voet and Voet reference (Voet and Voet, 1995, p. 1261ff). These chemical messengers called hormones serve to communicate intercellular signals, as do nerve-transmitted electrochemical signals in higher animals. Hormones may be divided into polypeptides and amino acid derivatives, and the reference provides a tabulation (Voet and Voet, 1995, p. 1263). In a manner of speaking, therefore, and based on their composition, hormones may be regarded as proteins.

## TABLE 3.3
## Vitamins and Hormones as Enzyme Inhibitors

### Vitamins

| | | | |
|---|---|---|---|
| Vitamin A | Retinol | Retinol inhibits β-glucuronidase. Retinoic acid inhibits estrogen sulfotransferase, glutamate dehyrogenase, metaplasia; shows **antitumor activity**. (The suffix "-metaplasia" means development.) β-Retinoic acid inhibits hyperplasia. 13-*cis*-Retinoic acid inhibits **carcinogenesis**. Vitamin A topical application **increased incidence of rous sarcomas** in chickens Vitamin A acid (retinoic acid) inhibits alcohol dehydrogenase. | $C_{19}H_{24}$-$CH_2OH$ |
| Vitamin B1 | Thiamine hydrochloride; thiamin chloride | Thiamine derivatives inhibit **glucose synthesis**, transketolase (yeast), phosphodiesterase (snake venom), thiamine triphosphatase, thymidylate kinase. Thiamine antagonists inhibit acetylcholinesterase. | $C_{12}H_{18}Cl_2$$N_4OS$ |
| Vitamin B2 | Riboflavin; lactoflavin; vitamin G | Inhibits daminoacid oxidase, FAD pyrophosphylase, galactonolactone dehydrogenase, glutamate racemase, riboflavin synthetase. *Inhibits cytochrome-B5 reductase. | $C_{17}H_{22}N_4$$O_6$ |
| Vitamin B6 | Pyridoxin | Inhibits alanine racemase, **malate dehydrogenase**, pyridoxamine pyruvate transami. Vitamin B6 antagonists inhibit **adenocarcinoma** growth. *Inhibits alanine racemase, pyridoxamine-pyruvate aminotransferase. | $C_8H_{11}NO_3$ |
| Vitamin B12 | Cobalamine; cyanocobalamin | Cobalamin analogs inhibit ethanolamine deaminase. (Ethanolamine is an industrial solvent that selectively absorbs the acid gases $CO_2$ and $H_2S$.) Cobalamin derivatives inhibit ribonucleotide reductase. Hydroxy-cobalamin inhibits diol dehydratase. | $C_{63}H_{90}N_{14}$$O_{14}PCo$ |

**TABLE 3.3 (CONTINUED)**
**Vitamins and Hormones as Enzyme Inhibitors**

### Vitamins

| | | | |
|---|---|---|---|
| Folic acid | Pteroylglutamic acid (PGA); folacin; vitamin Bc; vitamin M | Inhibits **thymidylate synthetase**. Pteroylglutamate derivative inhibits **dihydrofolate reductase**. *Both pteroyl-$\alpha$-glutamic acid and pteroyl-$\gamma$-glutamic acid inhibit 5-methyltetrahydropteroyltriglutamate-homocysteine methyltransferase. | $C_{14}H_{11}N_6$ $O_2$- $(C_5H_7N$ $O_3)_n$-OH where n = 1–7: $C_{19}H_{19}N_7$ $O_6$ for n = 1 |
| Niacin | Nicotinic acid; 3-pyridinecarboxylic acid | Inhibits catecholase, D-aminoacid oxidase, fatty acid synthesis, lipolysis, nicotinamide deaminase, NMN aminhydrolase, phenol oxidase, tributyrinase. Nicotinic acid derivatives inhibit accumulation of nicotinic acid, lipolysis. **Nicotinamide** inhibits ADPR polymerase, cytochrome P-450 reductase, **diphtheria toxin**, IMP dehydrogenase, NAD glycohydrolase, NAD nucleosidase, NADase, nucleoside pyrophosphatase, mixed function oxidation, CAMP phosphodiesterase, poly ADPR synthesis, prostaglandin A1 metabolism, T-RNA methylase, xanthine oxidase, 6-phosphogluconate dehydrogenase. ***Nicotinamide** inhibits NAD ADP-ribosyltransferase, NAD(P)nucleosidase, unspecific mono-oxygenase. | $(C_5H_4N)C$ OOH |
| Pantothenic acid | $HOCH_2C(CH_3)_2CH(OH)C$ $O$-$NHCH_2CH_2COOH$ or $N(\alpha,\gamma$-dihydroxy-$\beta,\beta$-dimethylbutyryl)$\beta$-alanine | | $C_9H_{17}NO_5$ |

## TABLE 3.3 (CONTINUED)
## Vitamins and Hormones as Enzyme Inhibitors

### Vitamins

| Vitamin C | Ascorbic acid; antiscorbutin | Inhibits adenylate cyclase, Na,K-ATPase, catalase, catechol $o$-methyltransferase, ferredoxin-NADP reductase, glucose-6-P dehydrogenase, lipase, fatty acid oxygenase, peroxidase, cAMP phosphodiesterase, tyrosinase, **urea levels**. Ascorbic acid derivatives inhibit ascorbate-2-sulfate sulfohydro, dehydro-ascorbic acid. L-ascorbic acid inhibits β-acetylhexosaminidase. *Ascorbate inhibits $o$-aminophenol oxidase, catalase, β-glucuronidase, GTP cyclohydrolase I, hydroxymethylglutaryl-CoA reductase, lactoylglutathione lyase. | CO (COH)$_3$ CHOHC H$_2$OH C$_6$H$_8$O$_6$ |
|---|---|---|---|
| Vitamin D | Calciferol Vitamin D2 inhibits ATPase | | C$_{28}$H$_{44}$O |
| Vitamin E | α-Tocopherol; 5,7,8-trimethyltocol | Inhibits arachidonate peroxidation, Na,K-ATPase, **glutamate dehydrogenase**, fatty acid oxygenase. Tocopherol analogs inhibit phosphodiesterase. *Inhibits lipoxygenase. | C$_{14}$H$_{17}$O$_2$ (C$_5$H$_{10}$)$_3$ H |
| Vitamin K | Phthiocol | 1,4-Naphthoquinone, 2-hydroxy-3-methyl-vitamin K1 inhibits incorporation of glucosamine. 2-chloro-vitamin K1 inhibits prothrombin levels. Vitamin K3 inhibits aniline hydroxylase. | C$_{11}$H$_8$O$_3$ |

| Hormones | Origins | | |
|---|---|---|---|
| *Polypeptides* | | | |
| Corticotropin-releasing factor (CRF) | Hypothalamus | Corticotropin analogs inhibit adenylate cyclase. | |
| Gonadotropin-releasing factor (GnRF) | Hypothalamus | Human chorionic gonadotropin inhibits release of A-amylase. | |

## TABLE 3.3 (CONTINUED)
## Vitamins and Hormones as Enzyme Inhibitors

| Hormones | Origins | |
|---|---|---|
| Thyrotropin-releasing factor (TRF) | Hypothalamus | Inhibits growth hormone biosynthesis. |
| Growth hormone-releasing factor (GRF) | Hypothalamus | **Growth hormone inhibits glucose consumption.** **Growth hormone derivative inhibits pyruvate dehydrogenase.** |
| Somatostatin | Hypothalamus | Inhibits accumulation of cAMP, cAMP levels, parathyroid hormone action, release of CCK, release of **growth hormone**, release of **insulin**. |
| Adrenocorticotropic hormone (ACTH) | Adenohypophysis | Inhibits DNA synthesis in adrenal tumor cells; inhibits replication in adrenocortical cells. ACTH analogs inhibit adenylate cyclase, fatty acid synthesis. ACTH derivatives inhibit lipolytic action, cAMP synthesis, corticosterone synthesis, and ACTH activity. |
| Follicle-stimulating hormone (FSH) | Adenohypophysis | |
| Luteinizing hormone (LH) | Adenohypophysis | Leuteinizing hormone inhibits cholesterol synthesis. Luteinizing hormone inhibits sterol synthesis. |
| Chorionic gonadotropin (CG) | Placenta | |
| Thyrotropin (TSH) | Adenohypophysis | Inhibits interferon action. |
| Somatotropin (see **growth hormone**) | Adenohypophysis | |
| Met-enkephalin | Adenohypophysis | |
| Leu-enkephalin | Adenohypophysis | Enkephalin inhibits neuronal firing. |
| J-Endorphin | Adenohypophysis | Inhibits acetylcholine turnover. Has opiatelike activity in mice. Endorphin inhibits cAMP formation. |
| Vasopressin | Neurohypophysis | Forms conductance channels across planar by: layer. **Inhibits carbon dioxide synthesis.** |
| Oxytocin | Neurohypophysis | Oxytocin analog antagonizes oxytocin action on uterus and mammary gland. Oxytocin analogs inhibit binding to oxytocin recepter, uterus contraction. Oxytocin derivatives inhibit binding of oxytocin, oxytocin effects. |

## TABLE 3.3 (CONTINUED)
## Vitamins and Hormones as Enzyme Inhibitors

| Hormones | Origins | |
|---|---|---|
| Glucagon | Pancreas | Inhibits contraction of dog papillary muscle, **fatty acid synthesis**, **glycogen synthesis**, vasoconstriction in dog artery. |
| Insulin | Pancreas | Inhibits lipolysis, adenylate cyclase, binding of NSILA, cAMP levels, cathepsin D, incorporation of thymidine, lipase, PEP carboxykinase synthesis, phosphorylase, protein kinase, **protein synthesis**. |
| Gastrin | Stomach | |
| Secretin | Intestine | |
| Cholecystokinin (CCK) | Intestine | |
| Gastric inhibitory peptide (GIP) | Intestine | Gastric secretion inhibitor blocks secretion of acid. |
| Parathyroid hormone | Parathyroid | Inhibits ATP–P$_i$ exchange, **glycogen synthesis**, **respiration**. Analogs inhibit bovine enzyme; adenylate cyclase. |
| Calcitonin | Thyroid | Lowers calcium, **glucose**, phosphate, and potassium levels. |
| Somatomedins | Liver | Inhibits binding to insulin receptor, NSILA binding. |
| *Steroids* | | |
| Glucocorticoids | Adrenal cortex | Glucocorticoid receptor inhibitor inhibits binding to DNA. |
| Mineralocorticoids | Adrenal cortex | Corticosteroids inhibit binding of calcium, collagen synthesis, prostaglandin synthesis, release of prostaglandins. |
| Estrogens | Gonads and adrenal cortex | Estradiol, stilbesterol, and methyltestosteron, inhibit bile acid metabolism. Estrogens inhibit binding of estradiol, cortisone reduction, **glucose-6-P dehydrogenase**, steroid D4-5B-reductase, steroid NAG transferase. |
| Androgens | Gonads and adrenal cortex | Derivatives bind to specific proteins. The resulting complex migrates into the prostate cell nuclei, where they appear to regulate gene transcription. Derivatives inhibit aromatase in the human placenta. |

## TABLE 3.3 (CONTINUED)
## Vitamins and Hormones as Enzyme Inhibitors

| Hormones | Origins | |
|---|---|---|
| Progestins or progesterones | Ovaries and placenta | Inhibits aldehyde dehydrogenase, amylase, **induction of collagenase** (which is modulated by cAMP), DNA repair and replication, DNA synthesis. *Inhibits aldehyde oxidase, cholesterol acyltransferase, retinol fatty-acyltransferase. |
| Vitamin D or calciferol | Diet and sun | Vitamin D2 inhibits ATPase. |
| *Amino Acid Derivatives* | | |
| Epinephrine | Adrenal medulla | Inhibits adenylate cyclase, CA-ATPase, uterus contraction, drug metabolism, lipogenesis, PE *N*-methyl transferase, **phosphofructokinase**, release of β-glucuronidase, release of tyrosine A-KG transaminase. |
| Norepinephrine | | Inhibits binding of penoxybenzamine in aorta, permeability of water, pigmentation, serotonin levels, tryptophan levels, tryptophan 2,3-dioxygenase, tyrosine hydroxylase, tyrosine transaminase. |
| Triiodothyronine (T$_3$) | Thyroid | Inhibits protein synthesis, secretion of prolactin. |
| Thyroxine (T$_4$) | Thyroid | Inhibits alcohol dehydrogenase, glutamate dehydrogenase, glutamic dehydrogenase, lipid peroxidation, **malate dehydrogenase**, oxidative phosphorylation, thyroid transaminase. L-thyroxine inhibits nicotinamide deaminase, cAMP phophodiesterase, triglyceride levels. |

*Note:* Zollner (1993) in the main does not include hormones as enzyme inhibitors. Items that may be of particular interest are in boldface.

* The tabulation is adapted from Appendix Z in Hoffman, *Cancer and the Search for Selective Biochemical Inhibitors,* CRC Press, Boca Raton, FL, 1999.

*Source:* From M.K. Jain, *Handbook of Enzyme Inhibitors, 1965-1977,* Wiley, New York, 1982; (*) from H. Zollner, *Handbook of Enzyme Inhibitors*, VCH, Weinheim, FRG, 1989, 1993. The list of vitamins is according to Table 1.1 of Hoffman (1999). The list of hormones is from Voet and Voet, *Biochemistry,* New York, 1995, p. 1263.

Hormones as well as vitamins also serve as enzyme inhibitors, as also presented in Table 3.3, which lists the enzymes inhibited corresponding to the tabulation provided in the Voet and Voet reference (Voet and Voet, 1995, p. 1263).

Hormones are classified by the distance within which they act. Autocrine hormones act on the same cell that releases them. An example is interleukin-2. Paracrine hormones act on cells close to the cell that releases them. Examples are prostaglandins and polypeptide growth hormones. Endocrines act on cells at a distance. Examples are the endocrine hormones insulin and epinephrine, which are released into the bloodstream by endocrine glands. (The term *endocrine* signifies internal secretions directly into the bloodstream, whereas the term *exocrine* signifies secretions through a duct.) A table of various endocrine hormones is provided in the cited reference. Most hormones consist variously of polypeptides, amino acid derivatives, or steroids. Some examples of sources and functions are as follows.

Of note is the pancreas, which serves as an exocrine gland for producing various digestive enzymes. It also secretes insulin and glucagon, which regulate blood glucose levels, and somatostatin, which regulates the insulin and glucagon secretions.

The gastrointestinal hormones are secreted into the bloodstream by cells lining the gastrointestinal tract, and are no doubt affected by the ravages of chemotherapy, which in particular attacks the cells of the gastrointestinal tract.

Thyroid hormones regulate metabolism.

Parathyroid hormone along with vitamin D and calcitonin (a polypeptide hormone) regulate calcium metabolism.

The adrenal glands, which are divided into the medulla (core) and the cortex (outer layer), furnish catecholamines and steroids, respectively. The catecholamines are hormonally active, and consist of norepinephrine and epinephrine. Steroids variously affect carbohydrate, protein, and lipid metabolism, regulate the salt/water losses of the kidneys, and affect sexual development and function. Androgens and estrogens fall in the last-mentioned category. Another adrenal hormone of note is ACTH, or adrenocorticotropic hormone. Cortisol is an adrenal product, which can be converted to cortisone.

The hypothalamus and the pituitary gland act together to control much of the endocrine system. Included is regulation of the growth hormone GH, also called somatotropin.

No effects pertaining to cancer were noted in the foregoing Voet and Voet reference. Two chapters on the biochemistry of hormones are provided by Frank Ungar in *Textbook of Biochemistry* (Devlin, 1986). Again, no direct connection with cancer was mentioned. There are, however, some interesting inferences about thyroid hormone functions dealing with oxygen consumption and thermogenesis (Devlin, 1986, pp. 753, 754). Increased oxygen consumption and heat production go together, and correlate with increased thyroid activity.

In further comment about increased thyroid activity, there is the contention that higher body temperatures (hyperthermia) act against cancer. If so, this suggests increased capacities for the tricarboxylic acid cycle, manifested as an increased aerobic glycolysis rate. Noting that cancer cells in the main undergo anaerobic glycolysis, its inhibition should favor a significant increase in aerobic glycolysis. This in turn could presumably could raise body temperatures and act against cancer.

The effect corresponds to the immune system raising body temperatures to induce a fever and fight off an infection — in this case, cancer cells.

Observing that iodine is associated with increased thyroid activity, the foregoing reference states that obesity implies what is called "reduced ATPase enzyme activity." (ATPases are proteins that transport ATP, or adenosine triphosphate, across cellular membranes.) This may connect with obesity, and by a stretch of the imagination, with cancer.

## CHEMOTHERAPY DRUGS AS ENZYME INHIBITORS

Conventional chemotherapy drugs act as inhibitors for enzymes, notably for critical enzymes that pertain to DNA/RNA/protein synthesis. The idea is that by blocking one or another or all of these enzymes, cancer cell growth and proliferation will be stopped. Unfortunately, these drugs are nonselective, acting against normal cells as well, and are therefore categorized as cell toxic, or cytotoxic.

A basic consideration will involve the subject of what are called nucleotides, which are the fundamental chemical structures contributing to cellular functions. Divided into the two classes named purines and pyrimidines, they are precursors to both DNA and RNA. The purine and pyrimidine nucleotides are formed *de novo* (anew) in the cell from amino acids, ribose, formate, and carbon dioxide (e.g., Cory, in Devlin, 1986).

(Deficiencies in the synthesis of these nucleotides result in such diseases as gout, the Lesch–Nyhan syndrome, orotic aciduria, and immunodeficiency diseases, which may include cancer.)

Thus, a large number of substances have been tested as inhibitors for the steps in purine and pyrimidine metabolism (Cory, in Devlin, 1986, p. 674ff). Included are both synthetic compounds and compounds isolated from plants, bacteria, fungi, etc. The substances may be further classed as glutamine antagonists, antifolates, and antimetabolites. Whereas the first-mentioned substances are toxic in the extreme, the latter two classifications have been of main concern although they are toxic enough in their own right.

Enzyme inhibitors used as chemotherapy drugs take advantage of the fact that enzymes and enzyme inhibitors are sometimes chemically or structurally similar (Voet and Voet, 1995, p. 355). A notable example is the chemo drug methotrexate (or amethopterin), which is similar to the chemical compound called hydrofolate. In consequence, methotrexate binds to an enzyme called dihydrofolate reductase. This in turn blocks the enzyme from converting dihydrofolate to tetrahydrofolate, the latter being essential in the biosynthesis of the DNA precursor thymidylic acid. This action is nonselective, however, affecting both normal and cancerous cells, although there is the hope or supposition that cancer cells may be more affected.

The subject of enzyme inhibitors and their action is complex, but a few guidelines exist (York, in Devlin, 1986, p. 165ff). Thus, inhibitors can be classed as competitive, noncompetitive, and uncompetitive — even a buildup of reaction product can inhibit enzyme activity — and still other enzymes can inhibit (or promote) activity.

Competitive enzyme inhibitors are generally similar to the enzyme itself, binding to the active enzyme sites to block activity, whereas a noncompetitive inhibitor binds at different sites. An irreversible inhibitor chemically reacts with the enzyme, as distinguished from the more loose association denoted as bonding.

The foregoing gets around to the purposes and action of drugs or medicines. Generally speaking, this comes under the catchall heading of chemotherapy. The modern concept of a drug is that of inhibiting a specific enzyme in a specific metabolic pathway. The applications include antiviral and antibacterial action, and also antitumor action. The foremost problem is that of side effects or adverse effects, for inhibitors will usually affect more than one enzyme, and thus may affect other biochemical processes in different degrees. The attempt therefore is to limit toxic side reactions, for some degree of toxicity is apparently unavoidable. A known exception is cell-wall biosynthesis in bacteria, which is blocked by the fungal-derived antibiotics, which are mostly nontoxic to humans in the dosages used.

In different words, it has been said that "there are no critical metabolic pathways that are unique to tumors, viruses, or bacteria" (York, in Devlin, 1986, p. 167). The host cell is affected by the drug as well, but the anticipation is that the disease-causing organism will be more quickly affected, for example, bacteria, in the case of using antibiotics..

With respect to the previous statement that "there are no critical metabolic pathways unique to tumors," an exception can be made in the case of glycolysis, for glycolysis rates are many times greater for cancer cells than for normal cells. Not only this, but cancer cells are predisposed to produce lactic acid or lactate rather than undergo normal metabolism. Therefore, there is the incentive for not only slowing down glycolysis, but especially for blocking lactate or lactic acid formation and glutaminolysis. This approach has been spelled out previously, naming the controlling enzymes involved, and listing some known inhibitors for those enzymes. Inhibition of the particular enzymes involved may in fact be the role played by many unorthodox anticancer agents, both organic or herbal, and inorganic.

Modern chemotherapy can be viewed as beginning with the sulfur-containing sulfa drugs (York, in Devlin, 1986, p. 167). The general formula for these chemical compounds is $R-SO_2-NHR'$, where R and R' represent arbitrary molecular groups. The simplest and most well known is sulfanilamide, which inhibits the action of $p$-aminobenzoic acid (PABA), this being required for bacterial growth. That is, bacteria must synthesize folic acid from $p$-aminobenzoic acid, but as sulfanilimide is structurally similar to PABA, the necessary enzyme dihydropterate synthetase will substitute sulfanilamide for PABA. The bacterium is therefore deprived of folic acid or folate, which prevents it from growing or dividing. Fortuitously, humans obtain folic acid or folate from external sources, and the sulfanilamide is not otherwise harmful at the dosage levels used.

What are called antifolate drugs pertain in general to blocking the biosynthesis of purines and pyrimidines, the heterocyclic bases used in the further synthesis of DNA and RNA, where folic acid is required as a coenzyme (or vitamin) for the enzyme dihydrofolate reductase. The previously mentioned compound called methotrexate or amethopterin (4-amino-$N^{10}$-methyl folic acid), being a structural analog of folate or folic acid, locks up the enzyme dihydrofolate reductase, which in turn blocks the synthesis of a thymidine nucleotide necessary for cell division.

In this way, methotrexate has been successfully used in the treatment of childhood leukemia, as cell division depends on thymidine in addition to other nucleotides. Unfortunately, rapidly dividing cells are especially sensitive, as in bone marrow. Not to mention that prolonged usage will cause the tumor cells to produce ever-larger amounts of the reductase enzyme, thereby becoming resistant to the drug.

What are in general called antimetabolites show a similarity with a reactant; that is, they are analogous with, or are analogs to, a reactant. An example is the chemotherapy drug 5-fluorouracil (5-FU or 5Ura), which is an analog of the fundamental building block thymine, whereby a methyl group is replaced by fluorine. Thymine, along with adenine, guanine, or cytosine, is one of the four basic building blocks in the nucleotides that form the DNA molecule and its encoded genetic information. As such, 5-FU acts as an irreversible inhibitor for the action of the enzyme thymidylate synthase, also called thymidylate synthetase, which is necessary in DNA synthesis (Voet and Voet, 1995, pp. 812–816; Cory, in Devlin, 1986, p. 677).

The drug 6-mercaptopurine is another example. It is an analog of a compound involved with adenine and guanine, two of the basic four constituents of nucleotides and, in turn, of DNA synthesis. This drug therefore acts as an antimetabolite, competing in most reactions involving adenine and guanine and their derivatives. By acting against all cells, normal or otherwise, it also acts against cancerous cells.

The pertinent descriptor is cytotoxic, or cell toxic, meaning these drugs act inclusively against both normal and cancerous cells. In other words, these drugs are poisons. Further specific information about the array of drugs that have been used is furnished by Ralph Moss in *Questioning Chemotherapy* (1995). The degree of success is included, which in the main is depressing, the few positive exceptions being for blood-related cancers such as leukemia.

The connection has been made with nucleotides and their synthesis into DNA and RNA.

"Since nucleotides are obligatory for DNA and RNA synthesis in dividing cells, the metabolic pathways involving the synthesis of nucleotides have been the sites at which many antitumor agents have been directed" (Cory, in Devlin, 1986, p. 628). Some inhibitors have already been mentioned, with others in the offing. These inhibiting substances can be said to be not commonly known outside the specialized chemical world, with the exception of folic acid.

Apart from chemically synthesized bioactive substances and naturally occurring bioactive substances, the alternative is the production of bioactive substances from natural sources, and leads in turn to the much-studied and infamous bacterium *E. coli*, short for *Escherichia coli*.

Studied over the years from both a biochemical and a genetic standpoint, the prokaryote *E. coli* is found in the colon of higher mammals, and members of the genus *Escherichia* are collectively known as coliform bacteria (Voet and Voet, 1995, pp. 4, 5). Its DNA encodes some 3000 proteins, with a resulting cellular totality of perhaps 6000 different kinds of molecules comprising proteins, nucleic acids, polysaccharides, lipids, and other varieties. Glucose is predominantly metabolized, and lactose less so (Glassman, in Devlin, 1986, p. 952). If no glucose is available, lactose suffices, with the necessary enzyme ($\beta$-galactosidase) increasing a thousandfold.

(Still other bacteria or prokaryotes may require only simple compounds for their nutritional or metabolic requirements, e.g., those commonly designated by the chemical formulas $H_2O$, $CO_2$, $NH_3$, and $H_2S$ [Voet and Voet, 1995, pp. 4, 5]. Others may even utilize the ferrous ion $Fe^{2+}$, and for some, light energy becomes the energy source, via the processes of photosynthesis, in which $H_2O$ and $CO_2$ are converted to organic matter. The latter bacteria are known as *cyanobacteria* ("cyano," inferring the presence of the -CN, or cyanide, group), described as the green, chlorophyll-containing organisms found in or around water, formerly called blue-green algae. Species of cyanobacteria growing on the roots of legumes convert atmospheric nitrogen into organic nitrogen compounds. Another, less-known form of photosynthesis utilizes such sulfur compounds as hydrogen sulfide, or $H_2S$, and thiosulfates, even hydrogen or organic compounds.)

In gene cloning, the DNA of the desired gene is introduced into the *E. coli* cells (Glassman, in Devlin, 1986, pp. 986, 995). Called genetic engineering, the objectives are to produce useful proteins such as insulin, blood-clotting factors, growth factors, hormones, interferon, etc., and to use cloned normal human genes to replace the defective genes causing diabetes, sickle cell anemia, and hemophilia.

As for cancer treatment, the end objective is to replace the DNA or RNA of cancer cells with DNA or RNA from normal cells. But, of course, how this can be achieved and how effective it will be are unanswered questions.

## MORE ON FOLIC ACID

Folic acid, or folate, is frequently mentioned as a treatment against cancer. There are many natural folate-containing foods, including leafy green vegetables and fruits such as oranges (Moss, 1992, pp. 42–44). John Heinerman also gives special mention to folic acid in his book *The Treatment of Cancer with Herbs*.

In combination with vitamin B12, its more usual function is as a preventive and treatment for certain kinds of anemia, such as, pernicious anemia. More recently, it has been prominently cited for the prevention of birth defects. Its role as an enzyme inhibitor is much less publicized.

A couple of relevant books are *Folate in Health and Disease*, edited by Lynn B. Bailey (1994), and *Apricots and Oncogenes: On Vegetables and Cancer Prevention* by Eileen Jennings (1993). The latter emphasizes folic acid and beta-carotene, and it is mentioned that folic acid deficiency may be a major cause of colon cancer and breast cancer. It is relevant to mention here that carrots, a source of beta-carotene, are a folkloric anticancer agent, and also contain traces of bioactive alkaloids, for example, daucine, putrescine, and pyrrolidine, as well as other bioactive compounds. (Folate is commonly used as a carrier for the chemotherapy drug 5-FU, although the folate has anticancer action in itself.)

In a study by Kearney et al. (1995) of the Department of Nutrition, Harvard School of Public Health, low folic acid levels were found to correlate with an increase in cancerous intestinal polyps, as well as with cancer in general.

Folic acid may occur in several forms, the most common being polyglutamarate derivatives that ultimately get converted in the intestines into tetrahydrofolate by the action of the enzyme dihydrofolate reductase (Chaney, in Devlin, 1986, p. 1219ff.). Note, for instance, the chemical connection with the use of 5-FU.

Folate deficiency is said to inhibit DNA synthesis, a consequence of which is that the maturation of red blood cells is slowed, causing anemia. As for folate deficiency during pregnancy, this can be the side effect of drugs that interfere with folate metabolism.

In a reiteration of the action of chemotherapy agents, in describing the formation of tetrahydrofolate from folic acid, antifolates have been defined as compounds that inhibit this conversion by blocking dihydrofolate reductase, which in turn blocks the formation of thymidylate (e.g., Cory, in Devlin, 1986, p. 674ff). At the same time, antifolates also block the formation of thymidylate by acting as an inhibitor for thymidylate synthase, a fact that has been stressed, besides inhibiting or blocking dihydrofolate reductase. The action is twofold. Folic acid is listed as an inhibitor for both of these enzymes. Furthermore, the chemotherapy drug methotrexate, or MTX, is an antifolate that is very similar chemically to folic acid.

On the other hand, as previously indicated, the action of 5-fluorouracil (5-FU, or FUra) becomes that of an antimetabolite. Further described as a pyrimidine analog with no biological action in itself, it is converted in the body to other cytotoxic (cell-toxic) agents that act as the antimetabolites; that is, act against cellular metabolism.

The use of 5-FU, or FUra, in cancer therapy has therefore been noted to have some adverse consequences or side effects (Cory, in Devlin, 1986, p. 677): " ... the incorporation of 5-FUra into RNA has serious effects on normal RNA metabolism and is a factor in the cytotoxicity of this agent." That is, the RNA of normal cells, as well as that of tumor cells, is compromised. (Significantly, the reference further states that the nucleosides thymidine and uridine may act as antidotes, rescuing the FUra-treated cells from the action of the FUra.)

Also mentioned is that a high concentration of the compound hydroxyurea inhibits DNA synthesis, but with very little effect on RNA (Cory, in Devlin, 1986, p. 678). The inhibiting action is against the enzyme ribonucleotide reductase, blocking the formation of DNA. The similarity with urea as an anticancer agent may not be coincidental.

All things considered, then, folic acid (or one of its derivatives) should be further studied as an anticancer agent, especially as it has been listed as an inhibitor for the same enzymes inhibited by the usual cytotoxic chemo agents. It is a substance natural to the body, and not some mysterious chemical or questionable plant or animal extract. Effective dosage levels and the best method of administration would have to be determined and the side effects established. If most doctors are reluctant to give even B12 or B-complex shots, megadoses of folic acid may not be on the cards. As with other cancer treatment alternatives, the patient may have to look at avenues other than medical orthodoxy.

(Speaking of side effects, folic acid and its analogs and derivatives inhibit other enzymes. These other enzymes are listed in Jain's handbook (1982), and the listing includes thymidylate synthetase or synthase, as well as dihydrofolate reductase, the enzymes blocked by antifolates, as previously indicated.)

The foregoing speculations seem worthy of independent clinical trials, the measure for credibility, for folic acid and some of its derivatives may be key to the regulation and control of cancer cell growth and proliferation, although there may not be much money in folic acid for Big Pharma.

A search of Medline will yield a few items of information about the use of folic acid and its hazards, especially in supplemental megadoses. Thus, there have been clinical trials conducted at the University of Arizona as part of a Southwest Oncology Group Intergroup study (Childers et al., 1995). The comparison involved a predisposition to cervical cancer, but found no significant difference between those tested and the controls. Oral dosage levels of 5 mg (5000 mcg) per day were used, whereas a vitamin supplement will have a nominal 400 mcg. (As a further reference dosage, up to 1 g per day has been reported.) A qualifier is, of course, that the tests did not pertain to actual, developed cervical cancers, and that the control group may have had sufficient folic acid in their diet. Also, should the folic acid have been taken intravenously?

Another article brings up toxic side effects that may occur with folic acid and its analogs or derivatives, and in the context of thymidylate synthase antagonists or inhibitors (Jackman and Judson, 1994). In it, adverse effects against the kidneys were noted.

Another article, by S.R. Snodgrass, appeared in the Spring 1992 issue of *Molecular Neurobiology*, which deals with vitamin neurotoxicity. Tests on animals showed that high dosages of folate directly into the brain or cerebrospinal fluid produced seizures and excitation. However, folate toxicity in humans is rare, though fatal reactions to intravenous injections of the B vitamin thiamine have occurred. However, the conclusion was that megadose vitamin therapy is more hazardous to peripheral organs than to the nervous system. Moreover, a high vitamin intake could itself produce diseaselike symptoms, and vitamin administration directly into the brain should be avoided. The issues are clouded by biochemical individuality: different patients will react differently.

As for the chemoprevention program sponsored by the National Cancer Institute, it seems odd that investigations using these kinds of substances against cancer had to wait until the 1990s to commence, for it was known by about 1980 at the latest — and very possibly much sooner — that folic acid and some of its derivatives were inhibitors or blockers for the enzymes thymidylate synthase and dihydrofolate reductase. (The year 1982, for instance, was the publication date of *Textbook of Biochemistry*, edited by Thomas M. Devlin, and also of M.K. Jain's *Handbook of Enzyme Inhibitors*.) Comprehensive clinical tests on folic acid, particularly, as an anticancer agent should no doubt have been conducted years ago, based on the biochemical knowledge then already available, not only on folic acid, but on many of the myriad other possibilities mentioned in Jonathan L. Hartwell's *Plants Used Against Cancer* (1982).

## ENZYME TRANSFORMATIONS

An additional problem with the proliferation of cancerous cells is that there may not only be quantitative changes in the levels of the enzymes responsible, but qualitative changes also (Cory, in Devlin, 1986, p. 665). Thus, the chemical structure of the enzymes may change, with the enzymes transforming into the corresponding isoenzymes or isozymes, as they are then called. Several kinds of biochemical changes have been observed, categorized as follows: (1) transformation linked, (2) progression linked, and (3) coincidental alterations. The first-mentioned enzyme alterations are independent of tumor growth rate, the second relate to growth rate, and the third are not malignancy connected.

For examples of the first category, the enzymes conveniently named PRPP amidotransferase, UDP kinase, and uridine kinase may increase in all tumors, independently of tumor growth rate. On the other hand, the levels of thymidylate synthase, ribonucleide reductase, and IMP dehydrogenase also increase, but increase with the tumor growth rate. (PRPP stands for 5-phosphoribosyl 1-pyrophosphate; UDP, uridine 5'-diphosphate; and IMP, inosine 5'-monophosphate.) All of the aforementioned enzymes are involved in the synthesis and replication of DNA, and whereas some enzymes produce fast growth rates, say, in normal tissue, the rates are different for tumor tissue. What could prove significant would be for certain critical enzymes to act to decrease the growth rates in tumors.

Inhibitors for the foregoing enzymes have been furnished elsewhere (in Appendix D of Hoffman, 1999), with the exception of the enzyme UDP kinase. Interestingly, the substance known as nicotinamide, a vitamin, shows up as an inhibitor for IMP dehydrogenase.

# 4 Starting at the Genetic Level

The main function of normal cells is protein synthesis. Protein is the principal constituent of all cells and of the body's various biochemicals, such as enzymes. Starting with DNA or RNA, protein is the product, and the understanding of the sequence involved is another major achievement of molecular biology or biochemistry.

## DNA, RNA, AND PROTEIN SYNTHESIS

The cellular role of the nucleic acids DNA and RNA is in the formation, or synthesis, of protein, which is by itself a polymer of various amino acids joined together. Whereas the acronym RNA stands for *ribonucleic acid*, the acronym DNA stands for *deoxyribonucleic acid*. The designator "ribo-" indicates the involvement of ribose, a five-carbon sugar with the stoichiometric formula $C_5H_{10}O_5$.

The relationship or sequence involving DNA and RNA in forming or synthesizing protein can be conveniently diagrammed as

$$\text{DNA} \rightarrow \text{RNA} \rightarrow \text{protein}$$
$$\downarrow$$
$$\text{DNA}$$

The first step in this scenario transfers genetic information from DNA to RNA, a step known as *transcription*. In turn, the RNA translates this information and further utilizes it to create protein, via another step called *translation*. Coincidentally, DNA can reproduce itself, or self-replicate, thereby perpetuating the hereditary chain of life. Thus, DNA duplicates or copies itself during cell division, these copies being transferred to the progeny or daughter cells, which inherit all the properties and characteristics of the original cell. An anonymous quote: "People are DNA's way of making more DNA" (Voet and Voet, 1999, p. 1020).

According to the *Academic Press Dictionary of Science and Technology*, for instance, a nucleic acid can be defined as a complex chain of nucleotides of DNA or RNA, as found in chromosomes, mitochondria (cellular regions outside the nucleus), ribosomes (the cellular complexes where protein synthesis occurs), bacteria, and viruses — in short, virtually in all living cells. In the presence of water, DNA, for instance exposes its polar sugar and phosphate groups to water molecules, and creates an acidic condition, denoted by a resulting acidity or pH value of less than 7.0 (Rodwell, in Murray et al., 1996, p.17), hence the designator *nucleic acid* for both DNA and RNA.

A DNA molecule (deoxyribonucleic acid) can thus be classed as a polynucleotide, an immense chain or polymer of subunits called *nucleotides*. And for the record, in DNA a nucleotide is the phosphate ester of deoxyribose linked to a heterocyclic nitrogenous base (Voet and Voet, 1995, pp. 795, 796). A ribose is a pentose, or $C_5$ sugar, whereas deoxyribose denotes the elimination of a hydroxyl group, or OH group, from ribose. The nitrogenous base structures are variously labeled *adenine* (A), *guanine* (G), *cytosine* (C), and *thymine* (T) as they occur in DNA, whereas thymine is replaced by the base *uracil* (U) in RNA. Elimination of the phosphate group yields what are called *nucleosides*. The molecular structure of DNA has gained fame as the *double-stranded double helix*.

An RNA molecule (ribonucleic acid) differs chemically from DNA in that it has ribose sugar residues instead of deoxyribose, and uracil replaces DNA's thymine base (Voet and Voet, 1995, p. 18). Also, RNA is generally single-stranded.

The final conversion product, protein, is an immense chain or polymer formed from the various amino acids synthesized. Relatively smaller chains or polymers are called *peptides* or *polypeptides*.

The genetic information is stored or encoded within this chain or sequence of subunits called the nucleotides. In turn, chromosomes are dense protein–DNA complexes that contain most (99%) of the DNA. The sequence or pattern of subunits is unique to a given individual, and can be used for DNA fingerprinting or typing. A given individual has identical DNA molecules throughout the body, which are passed on to succeeding generations. (There are well-developed chemical and physical procedures for isolating and recovering DNA in the form of a distinct phase, and for further identifying the genetic consequences.)

## THE FUNCTIONS OF DNA

DNA occurs almost exclusively in the eukaryotic (nonbacterial, notably mammalian) cell nucleus, whereas RNA is located in the surrounding region, what is called the *cytosol* or *cytoplasm* (Voet and Voet, 1995, pp. 8, 918). The cytosolic RNA-containing particles are protein rich, and are known as *ribosomes*.

The polymerization of nucleotides to form DNA and RNA is catalyzed by various enzymes called *nucleases*, which serve in a selective manner (Aktipis, in Devlin, 1986, p. 802). Generally known as *DNases* and *RNases*, listings of various kinds with inhibitors are presented in Appendix E and F of Hoffman (1999a).

There is a constant turnover of protein nucleic acids, signifying both synthesis and degradation (Cory, in Devlin, 1986, pp. 659, 660). Synthesis is in part dependent on the enzyme deoxyuridine triphosphatase (dUTPase), and the Cory reference notes that dUTPase may in fact be a factor in cancer proliferation.

A DNA macromolecule is able to store or encode an enormous quantity of genetic information by virtue of its extensive polynucleotide structure (Aktipis, in Devlin, 1986, p. 798ff). The analogy is to proteins, which are made up of a chain of amino acids joined by what are called *peptide bonds*, to yield the polymer or macromolecule. Thus, there is a similarity between the structures of polynucleotides and proteins, which is a factor in transmitting genetic information between the DNA and protein macromolecules, with RNA serving as the medium or intermediate.

## The Functions of RNA

The cell nucleus is the repository of primary genetic information, as encoded in the DNA (cf., Gray, in Devlin, 1986, p. 872ff). This information must be transferred from the DNA to the protein-synthesizing machinery, which is located in the cytoplasm outside the nucleus. The macromolecules or intermediaries that transfer this information reflect the makeup of the DNA, and by virtue of their chemical composition are called *ribonucleic acids*, or *RNAs*, the transfer process itself being called transcription.

It may be added that RNA comes in different molecular forms, for different purposes, and include what are called *messenger RNA*, or mRNA; *transfer RNA*, or *tRNA*; and *ribosomal RNA*, or *rRNA*. Although RNA is chemically very similar to DNA, it is relatively unstable, being rapidly degraded after synthesis and use.

With both DNA and RNA synthesized or involved in reactions catalyzed by specific enzymes, there are in turn enzyme inhibitors for these enzyme catalysts. Examples are listed for both DNA and RNA in Appendix E and Appendix F, respectively, of Hoffman (1999). The listing is extensive, indicating that the biochemistry is quite involved.

As for inhibitors, some of the more common compounds or substances include antibiotics (as may usually be recognized by their suffixes, such as "-cin," etc.). Although antibiotics are specific inhibitors for certain functions of prokaryotic cells, or bacteria, they may also inhibit biochemical reactions in the eukaryotic cells of mammals, including humans, and can even be toxic, some extremely so.

The alkaloids listed as inhibitors commonly end in "-ine." Many are listed in Appendix E and Appendix F of Hoffman (1999). Alkaloids are inherently toxic to protein synthesis, although some may have beneficial uses, for example, vinblastine, a known anticancer agent for blood-related cancers.

With regard to transcription itself, the process transferring genetic information from DNA to RNA, the enzyme responsible is called *DNA-dependent RNA polymerase*, or *DNA-directed polymerase* (Gray, in Devlin, 1986, p. 889). This occurs in the DNA-containing organelles of all cells. Alternately, the enzyme may be called simply *RNA polymerase* or else *transcripterase* (Voet and Voet, 1995, p. 856).

Substances that block the functions of RNA polymerase therefore inhibit transcription (Gray, in Devlin, 1986, p. 897ff). The best-known inhibitor is probably the antibiotic actinomycin D, ethidium bromide being another. Interestingly, actinomycin D is also considered an antitumor agent, although it is also toxic in other ways, negating its widespread use (Gray, in Devlin, 1986, p. 899). The poisonous mushroom *Amanita phalloides* contains the deadly fungal toxin α-amanitin, which inhibits the enzyme called *RNA poymerase II*, contributing to its poisonous nature.

Translation pertains to the biosynthesis of polypeptides or proteins from amino acids, and is directed by messenger RNA, or mRNA (Voet and Voet, 1990, p. 893). This is manifested as the joining together variously of the 20 common amino acids to form proteins (Voet and Voet, 1990, p. 899ff). These amino acids occur in a soluble amino acid pool and are transferred, obviously, by transfer RNA, or tRNA (Gray, in Devlin, 1986, p. 892). The amino acids are thus transferred to the ribosomes, which are the ribonucleic particles (ribosomal RNA or rRNA) in the cell cytoplasm, where synthesis to proteins proceeds.

## THE UBIQUITOUS ROLES OF PROTEINS

Succinctly stated, proteins are polymers or polymerization products of amino acids, and perform two main functions in mammals, distinguished as dynamic and structural or static (Schultz, in Devlin, 1986, p. 30ff). Enzymes themselves are proteins that function dynamically, serving as the biocatalysts for biochemical reactions. Transport is also a dynamic function, illustrated by a proteinaceous hemoglobin-carrying oxygen entity in the blood and a myoglobin-carrying oxygen entity in muscle tissue, with "globin" signifying a peptide or protein. Iron in the blood is transported by transferrin, here a globulin, or globular-shaped protein. There are proteins in the blood that carry hormones from site to site, and both drugs and toxins may bind to proteins as carriers throughout the body. The proteins that are immunoglobins and interferon guard against bacterial and viral infections. Blood loss is countered by the protein known as *fibrin*.

Hormones themselves may be proteins. Notable examples are the more well-known insulin and the lesser-known thyrotropin and somatotropin (the growth hormone), as well as the ovarian luteinizing hormone and the follicle-stimulating hormone. If of relatively low molecular weight, protein-type hormones are also known as *peptides*, or specifically as *peptide hormones*. Examples listed, as a matter of course, are adrenocorticotropin, antidiuretic hormone, glucagon, and calcitonin. (Generally speaking, a peptide is a molecule with fewer than 50 amino acids, and a protein has more than 50 amino acids. The acids are combined in myriad combinations or permutations.)

Proteins are ubiquitous. Not only are gene transcription and translation carried out by proteins, but other proteins are involved notably in muscle contraction; examples are myosin and actin. Still others, for example, are those called the histone proteins, repressor proteins, and proteins in the ribosomes.

Structural proteins comprise the matrix for bone and ligaments, and include collagen and elastin. They also provide strength and elasticity to the internal organs, and to the vascular system. The protein β-keratin plays a role in the structure of epidermal tissue.

All proteins are initially synthesized in the body from only 20 different amino acids, called the *common amino acids*. Each of these has a specific codon or set of codons in the DNA genetic code, a codon being a group of several bases (e.g., adenine, guanine, cytosine, or thymine) that denotes a single amino acid.

The common amino acids have the general chemical structural formula written conveniently as R-CH(NH$_2$)COOH, where the first carbon (C) is the central or *alpha* carbon, and R is an arbitrary side chain (Schultz, in Devlin, 1986, p. 32ff). The side chain R, a hydrogen atom, the amino group (-NH$_2$), and the carboxylic acid group (-COOH) are all attached to the same alpha carbon. Alternately, the representation may be expressed by the chemical formula R*-CH(NH$_3^+$)COO, where the asterisk denotes that the side chain may also contain different amino or other groups. (The superscripted plus sign denotes a positive charge, and the superscripted minus sign a negative charge; these cancel out, overall.) The nature of the amino acid will depend on the particular side group or side chain R. Structures of the 20 common amino acids are provided in Devlin (1986).

Usually the side chain or group (R) will contain carbon, hydrogen, and oxygen, but may contain nitrogen or sulfur as well. For example, the amino acids methionine and cysteine both contain sulfur. In the case of tryptophan, asparagine, glutamine, lysine, arginine, and histidine, the side chain or group (R) contains nitrogen.

The cellular polymerization of the common amino acids into polypeptides or proteins is catalyzed by enzymes. The linkage of the carboxylic group (-COOH) of one amino acid with the amino group ($-NH_2$) of another will release water, that is, $H_2O$ or HOH. That is to say,

$$-COOH + -NH_2 = -CO-NH- + H_2O$$

As polymerization proceeds, the structure built up becomes increasingly complex, with the possible combinations and permutations involving 20 different acids, increasing exponentially with the number of links.

The demands for protein synthesis differ greatly with the kind of cell (Muench, in Devlin, 1986, p. 926ff). At one extreme are mature red blood cells, which do not have the necessary enzymes and organelles (cellular compartments) for protein synthesis, and die off after about 120 days. Other cells exist in a kind of equilibrium state, having the requisite enzymes for renewing structural proteins as needed. Cells that are growing and dividing require higher levels of protein synthesis. And at the other extreme, some cells generate excess protein for export, for example, pancreatic cells, endocrine cells, and liver cells. These cells are oversupplied with the ribonucleoproteins called ribosomes in the cytoplasm (the part of the cell outside the nucleus), whose function is to biosynthesize proteins. More specifically, protein synthesis occurs in the cell *endoplasm*, designated the inner portion of the cell cytoplasm (the latter, as mentioned, being the part of the cell exclusive of the nucleus).

Aberrations may occur in the regulatory mechanisms of cell growth, the most serious being runaway cancerous proliferations. These can be described in terms of chromosomal changes. Thus, chromosomes may exchange genetic material via a process called *translocation*, whereby there may occur altered genes, called *oncogenes*, in turn responsible for abnormal cell proliferation. The subject is further developed by Avery A. Sandberg in an article appearing in the May/June 1994 issue of *CA — A Cancer Journal for Clinicians*, which lists chromosomal changes noted to occur in different tumors. (It may be presumed that enzymes are involved in these genetic changes, which also brings up the subject of inhibitors for the enzymes that may be involved.)

If these kinds of genetic changes can lead to cancerous cells, it gives pause for thought about tinkering with the genetic code. For example, Jane Rissler and Margaret Mellon, in *The Ecological Risks of Engineered Crops* (1996), warn that the transplanting of presumably desirable genes from one plant species into another may have unexpected and adverse side effects. If this could be the case for plants, then what about animals, and what about genetic manipulations in the human animal?

## GENETICS AS SCIENCE

The standard genetic code constitutes a systematic way of classifying or encoding the DNA molecular makeup in order to instruct the cellular mechanism to form peptides or polypeptides (small proteins) and proteins (large polypeptides). For the record, the makeup of the genetic code comprises permutations in groups of three of the four purine and pyrimidine base residues, that is, adenine, guanine, cytosine, and thymine, designated respectively as A, G, C, and T (Muench, in Devlin, 1986, pp. 918–920). Alternately, the base residue uracil, or U, can be substituted for thymine.

If arranged in groups of three, or triplets, in all possible combinations or permutations, these letter designators furnish the code or blueprint to manufacture any of the 20 common amino acids that combine to form peptides or proteins. Each such triplet is called a *codon*, with a given letter variously appearing thrice, twice, or only once in each triplet.

It so turns out that the number of possible permutations is $4^3 = 64$, for groups of three in terms of these four bases, or base residues. The set, or entirety, of the 64 codons or triplets is known as the *genetic code*, or *standard genetic code*. Furthermore, each ordered triplet or codon constitutes the encoded or blueprinted instructions for the cell to form a particular amino acid. Thus, ordered combinations in terms of the base residues adenine (A), cytosine (C), and guanine (G) can be denoted as ACG, AGC, GAC, GCA, CAG, and CGA. These triplets or codons will instruct the cell to synthesize the amino acids *threonine, serine, aspartate* (or *aspartic acid*), *alanine, glutamate* (or *glutamic acid*), and *arginine*, respectively. These are not the only codons for synthesizing these particular amino acids, however.

More than one codon or triplet signifying genetic instructions may exist for synthesizing each amino acid. This information is provided in terms of a tabulation of the standard genetic code, which is given in most biochemical textbooks. That is, it turns out that the number of codons may be one, four, or six, any one of which may serve to encode the instructions for producing a particular amino acid.

Thus, whereas the formation of some amino acids will be instructed by only one codon or triplet, for example, for tryptophan or methionine, the formation of other amino acids may be instructed by any one of as many as six codons, examples being the amino acids arginine, leucine, and serine. Thus, for arginine, genetic instructions are encoded as any one of the six combinations CGU, CGC, CGA, CGG, AGA, and AGG. Any one of the combinations encodes the genetic instructions for the cell to form arginine.

An example is, say,

UCU CUC UCU CUC UCU C...

which encodes the instructions for producing the peptide chain

Ser–Leu–Ser–Leu–Ser–Leu–...

The convention is that one of the codons or triplets is used as a start signal for protein synthesis, and three for a stop signal. The start signal is AUG, which also serves as the codon for the genetic instructions to produce methionine. The stop signals are UAA, UAG, and UGA, which are the instructions for no known amino acids, and are therefore designated as *nonsense codons*.

The genetic code can be applied universally, except for unique uses in the mitochondria, the cellular organelles or compartments associated with respiration. Accordingly, a better descriptor is that use of the genetic code is widespread rather than universal.

It follows that the array of codons represents the instructions for producing 20 amino acids, the so-called common amino acids. These amino acids are named and symbolized as alanine (Ala), arginine (Arg), asparagine (Asn), aspartate (Asp), cysteine (Cys), glutamine (Gln), glutamate (Glu), glycine (Gly), histidine (His), isoleucine (Ile), leucine (Leu), lysine (Lys), methionine (Met), phenylalanine (Phe), proline (Pro), serine (Ser), threonine (Thr), tryptophan (Trp), tyrosine (Tyr), and valine (Val).

Although a combination of codons or triplets is said to encode a peptide or protein, aberrations may occur, and are viewed as mutations. An example is viruses. Viruses contain an outer coat of protein and as such may contain aberrations, which could potentially cause tumors.

A human DNA molecule may obtain upward of 5 million nucleotides or subunits, and the possible arrangements are near infinite, as per DNA fingerprinting. The chances are near zero that two persons could have matching DNA. If there is no match, the DNA sample cannot be from the same person. It is from somebody else.

The foregoing may or may not be an abstract simplification for exceedingly complex and diverse phenomena. Here, we next briefly remark on the applications, or potential applications, to cancer therapy.

The idea of genetic cancer therapy, of using genetic engineering in cancer treatment, is relatively new on the scene, and is the subject of continuing interest and research. One route would utilize "genetic time bombs" within cells, triggered by the presence of cancer proteins. An example provided is the introduction of a gene-produced bacterial enzyme called *purine nucleoside phosphorylase*, capable of turning a harmless cellular component into a toxic cell-killing chemical. The application would be to localized cancerous cells or cell masses.

Thus, the projected use of gene therapy in the systemic treatment of cancer has been reviewed in an article by Irwin H. Krakoff (1996), published by the American Cancer Society, which first discussed cytotoxic and hormonally active agents, with biological agents (bioactive substances) considered the next big step. In gene therapy, the introduction of tumor suppressor genes would confer genetic resistance. Oncogenes and tumor suppressor genes had previously been reviewed by Robert A. Weinberg (1994) in the same publication, with a listing of cloned tumor suppressor genes provided in the article.

A limited positive result for gene therapy was reported in a news release dated August 31, 2006, courtesy of Science Express Reports. The citation concerned cancer regression after the transfer of genetically engineered lymphocytes. Successes were reported for melanoma patients, though only 2 out of 17, and work is being pursued toward more intense treatments. A contact is Steven A. Rosenberg of the National Cancer Institute.

What are properly called genes becomes a subject unto itself, with an explosion of information available on the Internet and elsewhere. As for gene therapy, there is, for instance, the Human Genome Project. Involved, of course, are those entities called genes, which are carried on, or in, chromosomes, and serve as the basic physical and functional units of heredity. The genes as a whole may be referred to as the *genome* for the organism under consideration. Genes are the specific sequences of bases that encode the instructions for making proteins. In turn, these proteins perform most life functions, and also make up most cellular structures. Genetic disorders occur when these encoded proteins malfunction.

A complicating factor is that genes can move about, or jump about, and even share with other organisms (e.g., microbes), or hide by a process called *transpositioning*, with the mobile genes referred to as *transposons*, and the more stable forms called *plasmids* (Garrett, 1995, p. 225). The result can be radical changes in the organism. It is like a game of Scrabble. (The genetic extension is to polymorphism or pleomorphism, as per the controversial works of people such as Livingston, Rife, and Naessens, cited in Chapter 2.)

Without pursuing the multitude of references about genes, we refer to only one, *Sequence — Evolution — Function: Computational Approaches in Comparative Genomics* by Eugene F. Koonin and Michale Y. Galperin, published in 2003. In Section 4.1, titled "Identification of Genes in a Genomic DNA Sequence," it is set forth that in most multicellular eukaryotes gene identification is a major problem because gene organization itself is so very complex. Thus, the genes are separated by extensive intergenetic regions (which also may be called *introns*), and within the genes themselves there are present numerous introns. (The part of the DNA sequence in a gene that contains the codons specifying a particular sequence of amino acids forming a polypeptide is called an *exon*, and includes the beginning and end of the genetic sequence. A codon, as previously indicated, is a sequence of three nucleotides that specify a particular amino acid.) The reference illustrates a typical distribution of exons and introns in a human gene, in this instance what is called the *X chromosome-located gene* encoding iduronate 2-sulfatase (IDS–HUMAN), characterized as a lysosomal enzyme that removes sulfate groups from heparan sulfate and dermatan sulfate. It may be noted that mutations which produce iduronate sulfatase deficiency will cause a lysosomal accumulation of glycoaminoglycans, a condition known as *Hunter's syndrome*. The coding regions constitute only a minor part of the gene, and the various positions of the exons become significant, with the caveat that the majority of human genes will have alternative forms, with the totality defining the gene expression pattern per se. Accordingly, the reference discusses various algorithms and software tools for predicting gene identification, another facet of these exceedingly complicated endeavors. It becomes, ultimately, an esoteric situation of matching theory to evidence, of making the punishment fit the crime.

There are several techniques utilized for correcting defective genes. Broadly speaking, these include inserting a normal gene into a nonspecific location in the genome (the most common technique), the swapping of an abnormal gene for a normal gene, repairing the gene via reverse mutation, or altering gene regulation.

However, in moving genes about, an agent is required, a carrier molecule or entity called a vector. The most commonly used is a virus that has been altered genetically to carry normal human DNA. Thus, cells such as of the patient's liver or lung can be infected with the viral vector, which transfers the normal human gene into the targeted cells. The viruses used include retroviruses, adenoviruses, adeno-associated viruses, and herpes simplex viruses. (Interestingly, HIV is a retrovirus, and cancer itself is thought to be caused by retroviruses that invade the cell chromosome, as per Part 7 in Hoffman [1999]. The subject is that of proto-oncogenes, "proto-" signifying first or foremost, the basic cause of cancer, with the viruses invading the cell chromosome called *proviruses*.) Other, perhaps less effective, are nonviral methods, including the addition of a 47th artificial human chromosome to the normal 46th.

The subject in turn interfaces with genetic engineering (GE) or genetic modification (GM). As may be surmised, there are unintended and unexpected consequences, including patients who have developed leukemia. In other words, the results can be random as well as targeted, with the possibility that the viruses or viral vectors utilized can themselves cause disease. The misgivings of well-known biologist and microbiologist Barry Commoner are appropriate as presented in the section titled "More on DNA" in Chapter 8.

If what are called the APC suppressor genes in mutant form are implanted in colonic cells, the result is hundreds, if not thousands, of polyps. With further mutations over a period of years, the outcome is the uncontrolled growth of colon cancer cells. The problem is to prevent or eliminate the mutations.

This is being investigated, but has not been resolved. An article by Nicholas Calvino, titled "Integrative Medicine in Colon Cancer," published in the February/March 2004 issue of the *Townsend Letter for Doctors & Patients*, states that chemotherapy is in the main ineffective against colon cancer. The charges against the "War on Cancer" initiated by biologist and Nobel laureate James Watson are mentioned (as also mentioned by Walters [1993]), along with an article addressing the issues published back in 1975 by reporter Daniel S. Greenberg and a follow-up article in the *New England Journal of Medicine*. In turn, Calvino discusses the effectiveness of some alternative treatments, for instance, quercetin and biological response modifiers (BRMs). The latter include what are called protoglycan molecules (PGMs), which are found in the weed *Convolvulus arvensis* and in many other species of the same genus in the morning glory or bindweed family (Convolvulaceae). Other anticancer substances of note include omega-3 fatty acids, embryonic pancreatic enzymes, artemisinin (from the genus *Artemisia* of the family Asteracea or Compositae) and a semisynthetic derivative called artesunate (ART). Also mentioned are folic acid, vitamin A and carotonoids, vitamin C, vitamin D (D3), and selenium. Artimisinin is also reported to act against malaria and other parasitic disorders, as well as cancer, as per articles by Robert J. Rowen, M.D., in the December 2002 and July 2006 issues of the *Townsend Letter for Doctors & Patients*, and as cited elsewhere. It has long been used in Vietnam and China for cancer treatment.

In the same issue of the *Townsend Letter for Doctors & Patients*, veterinarian Alfred J. Plechner takes up the issue of cortisol imbalances associated with cancer in animals. Normal cortisol levels favor the immune system and protect against cancer and other diseases. These normal levels maintain a balance among the various thyroid hormones, and among the antibodies IgA, IgG, and IgM, the first-mentioned being the most abundant and most important.

## DIGESTIVE PROCESSES

The subject of proteins serves to introduce the processes of digestion, and of proteins and the other dietary food types, namely, carbohydrates and fats. Expectedly, enzymes play a major role, and there is a connection with cancer.

### PROTEINS

The digestion of proteins involves the salivary glands, the gastric mucosa, and the pancreas, all which introduce digestive enzymes into the gastrointestinal tract (Chaney, in Devlin, 1986, p. 1135ff). These actions are assisted by hydrochloric acid secreted in the gastrointestinal tract, and by the presence of sodium chloride and sodium bicarbonate.

The synthesized or synthetic proteins previously discussed in terms of the genetic code are not necessarily the same as those that start out as nutritional or dietary proteins. However, digestive enzymes break down dietary proteins into the amino acid pool required for subsequent cell protein synthesis, as has been described. The proteins so synthesized variously become cellular structural components, enzymes and hormones, and blood plasma proteins. The latter are involved in cellular osmotic balances, that is, in ensuring a stable pressure difference across the cell walls. These blood proteins also transport substances through the vascular system, and assist in promoting immunity (Chaney, in Devlin, 1986, p. 1179ff).

For the most part, dietary protein is consumed in excess of normal requirements, and the excess becomes an additional energy source. There are also some proteins, composed of what are called *glycogenic* (glycogen-producing) amino acids, that convert to pyruvate and tricarboxylic acid cycle intermediates, and then to glucose or glycogen, and to carbon dioxide and water. Other proteins, composed of ketogenic (ketone-producing) amino acids, convert eventually to fatty acids and keto acids. (The prefix "keto-" connotes ketones, a class of chemical compounds having a carbonyl [C=O] group, and related to a similar class called aldehydes.) The final metabolic nitrogen-containing end products are urea and ammonia, to be excreted from the body.

Overall, the nitrogen balance involves relating the dietary protein in (that is, N or nitrogen in) to that lost by excretion (nitrogen out), the difference being the net nitrogen utilized (which includes the nitrogen remaining in the body). The part utilized consists of that forming an amino acid pool, plus that used in the body to produce tissue protein and for biosynthetic reactions, and that portion converted to energy. In adults, the nitrogen is normally in balance, denoting a steady-state condition. Growing children have a positive balance, with more nitrogen going in than goes out. A negative nitrogen balance is signaled by injury or illness, whereby the body catabolizes its protein content, notably in the tissues. The ravages of cancer and its chemotherapeutic treatment will produce a negative balance, the wasting away called *cachexia*. (And thus the nitrogen balance can be used as a cancer indicator or monitor.)

Mammals (including humans) require certain amino acids, which are classed as either essential or nonessential. The former are those amino acids that must be obtained from outside the body, whereas the latter can be synthesized within the body.

For the record, the ten essential amino acids comprise the following: argenine, histidine, isoleucine, leucine, lysine, methionine, phenylalanine, threonine, tryptophan, and valine — all of which must be obtained from outside the body.

The 11 nonessential amino acids are listed as follows: alanine, asparagine, aspartate, cysteine, glutamine, glutamate, glycine, hydroxyproline, proline, serine, and tyrosine. They are synthesized within the body, for instance, from essential amino acids. Interestingly, however, hydroxyproline is not one of the 20 common amino acids — the latter being the 20 as established by means of the genetic code.

## CARBOHYDRATES

Dietary carbohydrates are the body's main energy source, and include mono-, di-, and polysaccharides (Chaney, in Devlin, 1986, p. 1156ff). The various saccharides can be viewed as a combination of glucose and carboxylic acids, the polysaccharides being the resulting polymers or polymerization products. Starch is a polysaccharide, and sugars are distinguished as a special case by the ending "-ose." Sugars may exist as so-called monomers rather than polymers, an example being glucose, whereas the polymer is called glycogen. Some examples of carbohydrates are amylopectin from potatoes, rice, corn, bread; amulose from the same; sucrose from sugar cane or sugar beets; trehalose from mushrooms; lactose from milk; fructose from fruit and honey; glucose from fruit, honey, and grapes; and raffinose from leguminous seeds. Digestive enzymes catalyze the conversion of carbohydrates, notably to glucose. If the necessary enzymes are lacking, the carbohydrates prove indigestible or nearly so, an example being leguminous seeds or beans.

Excess carbohydrates not used for energy are converted to glycogen and to triglycerides or fats, to be stored (Chaney, in Devlin, 1986, p. 1189ff).

## FATS

The triglycerides, more commonly called *fats*, not only are used as an energy source but also are used as a part of membrane structure, with the excess stored as triglyceride or fat (Chaney, in Devlin, 1986, p. 1190).

A triglyceride is a chemical compound called an *ester*, which is the product of an alcohol and an organic acid. It may also be called a *neutral fat*, or a *triacylglycerol*. In this particular case the alcohol is glycerol, a trihydroxy alcohol representable schematically by the formula $(HO)CH_2CH(OH)CH_2(OH)$, and the acid component is a so-called *fatty acid*. In nature the combined forms are generally called *triglycerides*, and are of a class of substances called *lipids* (Voet and Voet, 1995, p. 278). Lipids are what are also called fats and oils, which are soluble in organic solvents but sparingly so in water, and also include certain vitamins and hormones. Nonprotein cell membrane components, for example, are mostly lipids.

In the body processes, triglycerides or triacylglycerols are converted to the corresponding fatty acids, which in turn are used for energy or for other biochemical processes (LeBaron, in Devlin, 1986, p. 440ff). Additionally, fatty acids can be synthesized in the body. Some fatty acids are considered essential, known by such names as *palmitic, palmitoleic, stearic, oleic, linoleic, linolenic,* and *arachidonic.*

Lipid digestion is initiated by the enzyme lipase from the pancreas, which causes a reaction with water, that is, causes hydrolysis (Chaney, in Devlin, 1986, p. 1162ff). Digestion is continued by means of liver bile acids. Fatty acids are the final product, in the form of microglobules, or "chylomicrons," which are then absorbed by intestinal cells. Released into intercellular space, the chylomicrons eventually move into the blood system or into the lymph vessels, depending on the globule size. Their ultimate fate, via the liver, is either to become an energy source or to be resynthesized to triacylglycerols for storage as body fat in body tissue (Voet and Voet, 1995, p. 791).

## PROTEASES AND THEIR INHIBITORS

The enzymes called proteases are necessary for the digestion of proteins. A newly proposed treatment for acquired immune deficiency syndrome (AIDS) involves the use of protease inhibitors, and as AIDS is an immunodeficiency disease, with cancer sometimes described in the same way, there may be a connection. (AIDS is by most accounts caused by the retrovirus HIV, and cancer may in some instances be traced to retroviruses.)

All the enzymes involved in the digestion of proteins are, in general, classed as peptidases, being hydrolases that break the peptide bonds in the protein polymers (Hopfer, in Devlin, 1986, p. 1150ff). In turn, this general classification is divided into *endopeptidases* and *exopeptidases*. The former break internal chemical bonds, liberating large peptide fragments, and the latter clip off one amino acid at a time from either the COOH end or the $NH_2$ end of the peptide fragments, and may be so designated. The endopeptidases are also called *proteases.*

As previously indicated, the digestion of proteins is ordinarily considered to occur successively via the gastric, pancreatic, and intestinal stages, as per the respective sources of the digestive enzymes. Gastric juices include proteases of the pepsin family, as well as hydrochloric acid. Pancreatic juice contains a number of protease enzymes such as trypsin, chymotrypsin, and elastase, and some are noted to involve a serine residue, serine being 1 of the 20 amino acids incorporated into protein molecules. Hence, the term sometimes used is *serine protease.*

It is noted in the cited reference that compounds that react or interact with serine will in turn inactivate or inhibit these enzymes. In other words, we are speaking of protease inhibitors, and possibly anti-AIDS and anticancer agents. An example furnished is the formidably named diisopropylphosphofluoridate.

Final digestion occurs in the small intestine, whereby aminopeptidase activity is courtesy of the surface epithelial cells. The end product amino acids enter the portal bloodstream going from the intestine to the liver, for subsequent utilization.

(The portal bloodstream, unfortunately, also carries colon cancer cells to the liver, where they become established.)

The serine proteases include trypsin, chymotrypsin, and elastase from the pancreas, as well as various proteases from other sources, with functions other than digestion (Voet and Voet, 1995, p. 389ff). Thus, the protease known as *Complement C1*, as obtained from blood serum, is said to be connected with the immune response.

An inhibitor for trypsin bears the formidable name *bovine pancreatic trypsin inhibitor* (BPTI) (Voet and Voet, 1995, p. 396ff). It functions to keep trypsin from digesting the pancreas itself. The BPTI structure is said to resemble that of trypsin, the similarity causing a binding that cancels the enzymatic activity of trypsin. Again, we are talking of protease inhibitors.

The foregoing reference further states that protease inhibitors are common in nature, providing both protective and regulatory functions, and protease inhibitors may comprise almost 10% of the about 200 proteins existing in blood serum.

Natural protease inhibitors are found to occur in soybeans and other seeds, and evidently also serve as survival agents, that is, the seeds are rendered indigestible by animals (Boik, 1996, p. 156). The Boik reference further notes that protease inhibitors are said to act against cancer, a particular example being the Bowman-Birk protease inhibitor (BBI) as derived from soybeans. In animal tests, at least, it has been found to act against colon, oral cavity, lung, liver, and esophagus cancers. There is the additional factor stated in the reference that soybeans contain still other anticancer agents, for example, what are called isoflavones and lignans.

(On the other hand, according to a long letter and literature search from the article by Sally Fallon and Mary G. Enig appearing in the July 2004 *Townsend Letter for Doctors & Patients*, to be further noted, soy isoflavones have been found to damage DNA. Of particular interest is the isoflavone genistein, which exhibits estrogen-like effects. However, it also acts as an inhibitor for the enzyme tyrosine kinase, which is involved in the metabolism of cancerous stem cells, as will be set forth in Chapter 10, and thus may in turn have a beneficial effect.)

Further, protease inhibitors are listed in Appendix G of Hoffman (1999), with the possibility that some of these inhibitors and their sources might provide clues toward the treatment of both AIDS and cancer.

In Hoffman (1999), the following statement is made: "Some of the sources noted for various protease inhibitors and proteinase inhibitors include black-eyed peas, lima beans, kidney beans, wheat and rye germ, potatoes, bovine cartilage, bee venom, and viper venom." Human bronchial secretions and guinea pig blood are other sources.

With regard to the previous paragraph, various beans (of the plant family Leguminosae) contain the compounds cyanoglycosides (e.g., laetrile or amygdalin), and also alkaloids, though only in trace concentrations. Wheat and rye (of the plant family Gramineae) also contain trace amounts of alkaloids, and the members of the plant family Solanaceae, or nightshade family, are especially noted for alkaloids. This includes parts of the potato plant, but not the tuber under most conditions. These several species are entered in Hartwell's *Plants Used Against Cancer* (1982b). Bovine cartilage, cited earlier, has been publicized as an anticancer agent, along with shark cartilage, as will be noted elsewhere, as has snake venom. (A listing of available venoms is given in the Sigma-Aldrich catalog *Biochemicals, Reagents & Kits.*)

(On p. 209 of his book *Fresh Air Fiend*, traveler and author Paul Theroux briefly describes a Chinese anticancer pill made of "myrrh, muschus, mastix, and calculus bovis." Myrrh is of course the resin from species of the genus *Commiphora*, such as *C. abyssinica*. Mastix is presumably the resin of the mastic tree, *Pistacia lenticus*. Calculus bovis may be presumed to be a concretion or stony substance found in the gall bladder, kidneys, etc., of cattle, or maybe it is bone cartilage from cattle [recall that shark cartilage has been touted as an anticancer agent]. On the same page, Theroux mentions a potion that was claimed to kill the AIDS virus — 100% in 2 minutes. During a trip down the Yangtze River [on pp. 158, 179], Theroux encountered a fellow passenger named Dr. Ringrose, of Leeds, who said, "We put yogurt on some forms of skin cancer.")

Interestingly, perhaps the latest on the folklore scene as an anticancer agent is the diluted venom of the Caribbean blue scorpion (*Rhopalurus junceus*), as described in a column by Ralph W. Moss in the July 2004 *Townsend Letter for Doctors and Patients*. Called *Escozul*, its use has gained widespread popularity in Cuba. Moss, however, remains a "friendly skeptic," being largely noncommittal. Among other things, the biochemical mechanism or explanation for its supposed efficacy has not yet been provided, and the clinical results seem questionable.

## PROTEIN DEGRADATION RATES

Cells are involved in a continual life and death process. This is a process not only of synthesizing proteins but of degrading protein to the component amino acids, with protein lifetimes varying from a few minutes to several weeks or more (Voet and Voet, 1995, p. 1010ff). The turnover gets rid of abnormal or harmful proteins, and controls cell metabolism by eliminating unnecessary enzymes and regulatory proteins. In fact, controlling the rate of protein degradation is as important as controlling the rate of synthesis. The connection with destruction of cancer cells is obvious.

As an example of aberrant behavior, a synthetic hemoglobin was observed to have a half-life of only about 10 minutes, whereas normal hemoglobin in red cells lasts about 120 days and is therefore probably the cytoplasmic protein (protein pertaining to the cell cytoplasm) having the longest lifetime.

The rate of degradation of normal cell proteins depends on identity, with the most rapidly degraded being those proteins of the enzymes that confer important metabolic controls.

Nutritional and hormonal conditions also affect the rate of protein degradation, whereby nutritionally deprived cells degrade protein more rapidly as a means of supplying nutrients for critical metabolic processes. Interestingly, increased degradation rates are countered by antibiotics, but which may act to block protein synthesis at the same time. The possibility is therefore inferred that antibiotics may not only block the degradation of cancer cells, but their formation as well.

The lifetime of a cytoplasmic protein (the protein outside the cell nucleus) is determined by its N-terminal residue, that is, by the identity of an end or terminal amino acid group. The notation is that cytoplasmic proteins terminating in Met, Ser, Ala, Thr, Val, Gly, and Cys residues tend to be more stable, with half-lives of about 20 hours; those ending with Ile, Glu, Tyr, and Gln residues have half-lives of about 10 to 30 minutes, and those with Phe, Leu, Asp, Lys, and Arg end residues have half-lives of about only 2 to 3 minutes. Those with segments of Pro, Glu, Ser, and Thr (called *PEST proteins*) are also rapidly degraded.

It is extremely important to know, therefore, whether the proteins in cancer cells are different from those in normal cells, especially with regard to the terminal amino acids. As a rule of thumb, however, cancer cells are said not only to be slow growing, but slow dying, and mimic the normal cells from which they originate.

## THE INFLUENCE OF ANTIBIOTICS

Antibiotics are known to be protein synthesis inhibitors (Voet and Voet, 1995, pp. 1002–1004). "Antibiotics are bacterially or fungally produced substances that inhibit the growth of other organisms." Some inhibit biologically essential processes, such as DNA replication (e.g., the antibiotic novabiocin), transcription (e.g., rifamycin B), and bacterial cell wall synthesis (e.g., penicillin). Most act to block translation in prokaryotic cells, that is, in bacterial cells. Many are medically significant, some well-known examples being streptomycin, chloramphenicol, and tetracycline. Another is diphtheria toxoid (formaldehyde-inactivated toxin), used for immunization against the deadly disease. There may be toxic side effects, however, or disease-resistant bacterial strains may emerge.

The bacterial selectivity of antibiotics pertains to an interference with prokaryotic protein synthesis as distinguished from eukaryotic protein synthesis (Muench, in Devlin, 1986, pp. 936, 937). As has been indicated, however, some of the antibiotics are too toxic for clinical use, although useful in studying protein synthesis.

Although within the general category of chemotherapy, the subject of antibiotics as anticancer agents has not been of pressing interest. Two exceptions are the closely related daunomycin and adriamycin (Voet and Voet, 1995, pp. 862, 863). Utilized in the treatment of certain human cancers, these particular antibiotics have been judged valuable chemotherapeutic agents. They bind to DNA, inhibiting both transcription and replication (but, unfortunately, for normal cells as well as cancerous cells). Moreover, the antibiotic actinomycin D inhibits nucleic acid synthesis, that is, protein synthesis per se. Effects such as these are why some antibiotics are regarded as too toxic to be used for the intended antibiotic purposes.

In further confirmation, there are antibiotics prominently listed in Appendices E and F of Hoffman (1999) as inhibitors for enzymes involved in DNA and RNA processes. With regard to cancer treatment, however, a search of Medline indicates that most antibiotics are used against bacterial infections incurred during cancer treatment. An exception involves studies at the M.D. Anderson Cancer Center of the University of Texas, located in Houston. These studies utilized actinomycin D and doxorubicin, both said to be known anticancer agents, in conjunction with the mitotic inhibitors vinblastine and Taxol. (The latter two are from plant extracts, and inhibit cell division or mitosis. The first-mentioned is derived from the Madagascar periwinkle [as is another alkaloid called vincristine], the latter from the yew tree of the

Pacific Northwest.) Encyclopedic references comment that the antibiotics doxoru-bicin, daunorubicin, bleomycin, mitomycin, and dactinomycin are all antineoplastic or anticancer agents, but are mostly too toxic for antibiotic use (and perhaps are too toxic to be used as anticancer agents, a case again of adverse side effects).

In a book by Abayami Sofowora titled *Medicinal Plants and Traditional Med-icine in Africa*, published in 1982, mention is made of Madagascar periwinkle (*Catharanthus roseus*) as having long been used in folk medicine in many countries, notably as a treatment for diabetes (Sofowora, 1982, pp. 86, 87). Its discovery as an antileukemic agent is traced to a group of Canadian scientists, dating from 1955 to 1960. A listing of antitumor agents is furnished as follows, listing plant name, country, and active ingredient (Sofowora, 1982, p. 131):

| | | |
|---|---|---|
| *Brucea antidysenterica* | Ethiopia | Bruceantin |
| *Catharanthus roseus* | India | Vincristine, vinblastine, vindesine |
| *Cephalotaxus fortunei* | China | Harringtonine, homoharringtonine |
| *Daphne mezerium* | Several | Mezerein |
| *Heliotropium indicum* | India | Indicine-$n$-oxide |
| *Jatropha gossypiifolia* | Costa Rica | Jatrophone |
| *Maytenus buchananii* | Africa | Maytansine, etc. |
| *Podophyllum peltatum* | U.S. | Podophyllotoxin glycosides |

This information was taken from WHO document No. CAN/TRM/AI. In praise of ethnobotanists, on the same page, Sofowora mentions that selecting anticancer plants on the basis of folkloric information increases the chances of success by a factor of two.

It may be noted that in Joseph W. Bastien's *Healers of the Andes: Kallawaya Herbalists and Their Medicinal Plants* it is stated that when plant species are claimed to be folkloric anticancer agents, about 20% show significant effectiveness (Bastien, 1987, p. 97). For this reason, it is recommended that the information gathered worldwide should be correlated for commonality. In this regard, the species *Plan-taago tomentosa* (of the family Plantaginaceae), also called llantén (or plantain), has been found by James Duke to be one of the three most heard-about plants for cancer cures (Bastien, 1987, p. 64). The other two are *matico* (*Piper* sp.) and *calaguala* (*Polypodium angustifolium*, or fernroot). The most common general purpose herbal used is called *bilyea* (*Psorlea pubescens* of the family Leguminosae), which is related to the breadroot (*Psorlea mutisii*) and used as food by many North American Indians.

Garlic is also a medicinal used by the Kallawaya herbalists, and it is mentioned that crushed garlic contains the powerful bactericidal agent allyl allylthiosulfinate (allicin), which is formed by the interaction of the enzyme allinase with the substrate $S$-ethyl L-cystein sulfoxide (Bastien, 1987, p. 102, n. 6). Bastien in turn supplies the results of an experiment on mice. Thus, in mice infected with sarcoma, injection either of the enzyme allinase or the substrate $S$-ethyl L-cystein sulfoxide (alliin) alone had no effect, all animals dying within 16 days. However, in infected mice treated with both the enzyme and the substrate, the animals were still alive after 6 months. Allicin is therefore the active anticancer ingredient, as will be emphasized especially in Chapter 5.

(Chemistry of these garlic-derived compounds is detailed in Chapter 3 of *Garlic: The Science and Therapeutic Application of* Allium sativum *L. and Related Species*, edited by Heinrich P. Koch and Larry D. Lawson. More limited information is presented in Hoffman [1999], p. 67, 372ff. The nomenclature for the compounds varies.)

The Kallawayas are a Bolivian tribe of the Aymara nation in the Province Bautista Saavedra, Department of La Paz. Incidentally, the foregoing book by Bastien was published in 1987 by the University of Utah Press, whereby it can be commented that Utah's medical school was once involved in the "creosote bush as a cancer cure" controversy.

Vinblastine and vincristine are only two of the many alkaloids found in the Madagascar periwinkle, or rosy periwinkle. Called *Vinca* alkaloids, the original genus name being *Vinca* as per the species *Vinca major* and *Vinca minor*, the more accepted plant classification is now the genus *Catharanthus*, with the Madagascar periwinkle designated as the species *C. roseus* of the family Apocynaceae.

The preface of Joel L. Swerdlow's profusely illustrated *Nature's Medicine: Plants That Heal*, published in 2000 under the imprimatur of the National Geographic Society, provides some insights about the effectiveness of these and other plants, notably against cancer. Thus, Swerdlow's physician brother Paul was diagnosed with acute myelogonous leukemia, a cancer of the bone marrow, for which no drugs worked, although the *Vinca* alkaloids worked against acute lymphatic leukemia, or childhood leukemia. His brother's death led Swerdlow to research the medicinal plant situation, not only in Madagascar, but worldwide. Mention is made that, although Madagascar has more than 10,000 known plant species, only the rosy periwinkle has contributed a drug approved by the FDA. More than this, although it is said that 25 to 50% of prescription drugs in the industrial world are derived from plants, these sources originated from times past. Thus, "no new drug has come out of the Amazon forests beyond those based on plants brought to Europe by the conquistadores and their successors more than 300 years ago."

(Swerdlow's book is not the only foray made by the prestigious National Geographic Society into the world of, shall we say, alternative medicine. For example, there was Lonnelle Aikman's *Nature's Healing Arts: From Folk Medicine to Modern Drugs*, published back in 1977. Much later came the illustrated *Desk Reference to Nature's Medicine*, published in 2006.)

In fact, possibly with one exception, no new modern drug (that is, FDA approved) based on Native American folklore has surfaced. As for Ayurveda, the ancient medical system of India, it has contributed only one. China's massive folkloric pharmacopoeia has contributed only two. Further, the FDA has approved fewer than a dozen plant-based drugs during the past 40 years.

(Speaking further of Ayurvedic cures, Bruce Chatwin furnishes an anecdote on pages 327 and 328 of his best-selling book of recollections, titled *What Am I Doing Here*. It seems that a certain English Member of Parliament, or MP, was in the hospital about to die from a blood clot approaching his heart, but wanted to live until the next Saturday when his racehorse was running at Longchamps. Unfortunately, the horse had been kicked and could not run. But the MP exclaimed that he would have known what to do — namely, feed the horse a couple of pounds of onions. His doctor, remembering an ayurvedic cure, asked the MP if he ever ate onions. The MP replied that he hated them, but the doctor said he was going to feed him 2 lb, anyway. Which he did, force-feeding them down the MP's throat. "The clot dissolved, and the man lived." It so turned out that the chemical compound carrageenan is contained in onions, and which was found to be a powerful antico-agulant, conceivably with the potential to transform heart surgery. Unfortunately, as was commented, onions are not patentable.)

Accordingly, Swerdlow traveled to Madagascar for a first-hand acquaintance with how the local plant life and native healers might contribute to modern medicine. Traveling around the island in a four-wheel drive with Nat Quansah, an ethnobotanist whose specialty was Madagascar's medicinal plants, contact was made with a certain Phillippe Rasoanaivo, a pharmacological researcher who was trained in the West. The latter knew a native healer in the isolated far south of the island who had a plant treatment for cancer called *omamiadana*, or "killing little by little." The healer furnished some leaves, which were in turn forwarded to a laboratory in Switzerland, where they were found to be "extremely effective against cancer." In a follow up visit, the healer refused to furnish any more leaves. However, some more leaves were picked by the party, presumably from the same plant species, but which proved to be ineffective. It was thought that there was some variable that could be detected only by the healer, which affected the plant's medicinal properties.

(A number of factors may affect plant bioactivity: the time of year, stage of growth, even time of day, as well as the particular plant parts and the geographic locale. Conceivably, the makeup of the soil may enter, as has been observed for the vitamin and mineral content of a plant or crop.)

This reluctance of native healers to reveal their secrets is encountered in other areas of the world, as Alex Shoumatoff reported in *The Rivers Amazon*. Maybe this protectionism is similar to the behavior of modern physicians (M.D.s), who resent any invasion of their turf. And, as Swerdlow notes, this kind of vagueness turns off pharmaceutical companies from investing money in the search. (Not to mention that plant-derived substances may not be patentable, and the host countries in many instances now claim the rights. They too have awakened to some of the advantages of capitalism.) Nevertheless, Swerdlow's foray and subsequent forays among native healers spurred him to further explore the possibilities of plant-derived medicines, and inspired him to write the book.

We cite one more incidence as set forth in Swerdlow's first chapter, about the herb mugwort (apparently *Artemesia vulgaris* of the family Compositae or Aster-aceae), as published in a 1998 issue of the *Journal of the American Medical Association*. It was reported that if a bit of it was allowed to smolder on the little toe of pregnant women (and removed before it got too hot), the fetus would move to a head first position from the dangerous breech position. It was, in fact, the ancient Chinese practice to burn mugwort at a certain acupuncture point to cause the fetus to move to the head-first position. "It is bizarre" said the then editor of the *JAMA*, but according to Swendlow, studies verified the ancient practice.

In *Head Hunters of the Amazon*, F.W. Up de Graff reported that a member of the expedition came down with a severe toothache (Up de Graff, 1923, p. 246). He wrote that the local medicine man was consulted, who first went through a series of rituals, to no effect. But then came the real cure. A live piece of charcoal was held in the patient's open mouth, upon which was sprinkled some powdered leaves (species unknown), so that the fumes from the leaves passed around the sore tooth. "The pain left him and never returned." On another occasion, Up de Graff was bitten by a fly that deposited an egg that grew into a grub worm. The medicine man asked for a cigarette, then blew the smoke through a wad of cotton. Applying the cotton, and performing some incantations, out came the worm, presumably owing to the tar and nicotine deposited in the wad of cotton.

(The medicine man wields much power, but his career is generally short-lived, as Up de Graff explains on pages 244 to 246. For he lasts only as long as his prophecies are not too far wrong; otherwise, if he makes a bad guess, he is sacrificed forthwith. Medicine men, however, were familiar with quinine and a number of other natural drugs, some known to modern science and some not. But in general, medicine men do not take kindly to cures made by the rival white man and his medicines — and it can be advantageous to make oneself scarce posthaste, as Nicholas Guppy reported in a chapter on Medicine Men in his book *Wai-Wai: Through the Forests North of the Amazon*. Guppy, incidentally, was the grandson of the well-known ichthyologist for whom the tropical fish was named.)

In David Attenborough's *Zoo Quest to Guiana*, in a chapter titled "Spirits in the Night," a séance is described in which the medicine man summoned all sorts of rustlings in the attempt to cure a patient, the headman — with Attenborough even recording some of the goings-on. No medicinal potions were administered, however, and Attenborough concluded, "As far as we knew, the headman's health did not improve."

Peter Mathiessen speaks of a Captain C in his book *The Cloud Forest*, the captain swearing as to the efficacy of Indian medicines. He claimed to have been cured of a number of severe fevers (Mathiessen, 1966, p. 56). Mentioned as a plant of medicinal use was *oche*, a poison used on arrows, and an ingredient of tranquilizer pills.

## DNA REPLICATION AND ALTERATION

In DNA replication, there is the parallel synthesis of more DNA. The enzymes involved are known as *DNA-directed DNA polymerases*, or simply *DNA polymerases* (Voet and Voet, 1995, p. 1021). That is, DNA directs its own replication (Voet and Voet, 1995, p. 854). Various DNA polymerases are listed in Appendix E of Hoffman (1999), as well as inhibitors for each. The enzyme called *RNA-directed DNA polymerase* is listed in Appendix F along with inhibitors. (This enzyme is also called *reverse transcriptase*, or RT, and is the enzyme distinguishing the retroviruses, such as HIV in AIDS, and the Ebola and Marburg viruses — and maybe cancer-causing viruses.)

Enzymes involved in replication not only include what for various reasons are designated DNA polymerases I, II, and III, but what is known as DNA gyrase, as well as others such as helicases and *DNA ligases* (Voet and Voet, 1990, pp. 952–957). Prokaryotic (bacterial) DNA is understood to have its own mechanisms for replication, but the mechanisms for eukaryotic (animal or human cell) DNA replication are more complex. This is evidenced by the fact that the DNA polymerases involved can in turn be broken down variously into versions designated $\alpha$, $\beta$, $\gamma$, $\delta$, $\epsilon$, a further indication of the complexity of the subject.

DNA alterations consist of the repairs, recombinations, and other modifications that may occur in DNA, as follows. In turn, there may be a connection with cancer.

## DNA Repair

Whereas DNA contains the nucleotide base thymine, RNA contains the nucleotide base uracil instead, and the reason is that the base cytosine, also present in both DNA and RNA, will convert to uracil, which would then cause a nucleotide mismatch if uracil had originally been present in the DNA (Voet and Voet, 1995, p. 1049). And such mismatches mean that mutations would occur. However, if any uracil shows up in the DNA, it is normally converted or excised by the enzyme uracil *N*-glycosylase, to be replaced by cytosine. (Uracyl *N*-glycosylase is also involved in DNA replication.) In other words, nature hopefully can correct itself at the DNA level.

The question here is that if the correction does not occur, will the cells then become mutagenic and, therefore, cancerous? This may mean that the enzyme uracil *N*-glycosylase may have been inhibited by some agent or another, and cancer may be the result.

(A footnote provided in Hoffman (1999) states that an entry for uracil *N*-glycolase could not be found in either Jain [1982] or Zollner [1989, 1993]. The closest similarity was uracil-DNA glycohydrolase in the latter. The four inhibitors listed for the latter enzyme are 6-aminouracil, 5-azauracil, inhibitor protein, and uracil. The latter, uracil, may act as an inhibitor by virtue of being in the particular reaction or else by being chemically similar to a reactant or product, as may the other inhibitors. As noted earlier, uracil is naturally present in RNA, although there is the possibility of an excess, or another source.)

Agents such as UV radiation, alkylating agents, and cross-linking agents have been observed to cause DNA damage in the bacterium *E. coli* (Voet and Voet, 1990, p. 1051ff). This in turn produces cellular changes in *E. coli* called the *SOS response* — signifying an emergency, so to speak. The affected cells cease dividing and act instead to repair the DNA damage. It is further noted in the reference that some *E. coli* with mutant genes have their SOS response permanently turned on. Some very complicated procedures are modeled in the reference for controlling the SOS response.

The question, of course, is that if the prokaryotic cells of the bacterium *E. coli* act in this way, under what circumstances will damaged or cancerous eukaryotic cells (animal or human cells) also act to repair themselves in the same manner?

## Carcinogens and the SOS Response

Cancer-causing agents, or carcinogens, can induce an SOS response in bacteria, and cause mutations, and there is a strong correlation between mutagenesis and carcinogenesis (Voet and Voet, 1995, p. 1051). Further information is provided in the reference for identifying chemicals that may be carcinogenic, which is the purpose of what is known as the *Ames test*.

In brief, a special strain of the bacteria *Salmonella typhimurium* is used in the Ames test for mutagenicity. This bacteria cannot synthesize histidine, a requirement for growth, and therefore does not grow in its absence. The bacteria are placed in a culture medium lacking histidine, but containing a suspected mutagenic or carcinogenic agent. If mutagenesis occurs because of the added agent, some of the bacteria revert and are then able to synthesize histidine, and are observed to grow.

Among the previously unsuspected carcinogens found via the Ames test is the compound with the chemical name *tris*-(2,3-dibromopropyl)phosphate, but commonly called *Tris*, as has been noted. Once used as a fire retardant on children's sleepwear, it unfortunately can be absorbed through the skin. Among other uses, it was even used in Japan as an antibacterial agent in food.

Other unsuspected carcinogens have been uncovered in food, for example, in alfalfa sprouts. And the potent toxin called aflatoxin $B_1$, as found in molded peanuts and corn, is one of the most powerful carcinogens known. Charred foods are also a source of carcinogens, namely, from the conversion of nitrogen-containing proteinaceous organics to adverse inorganic nitrogen compounds. There are, in fact, specialized technical volumes that list literally thousands of carcinogenic chemical compounds.

## DNA RECOMBINATION

By DNA genetic recombination is meant the exchange of segments between different DNA molecules, which is a way of introducing foreign DNA into the recipient's chromosome (Voet and Voet, 1995, p. 1053ff). The segment may come from another chromosome, from a plasmid (another, or foreign, DNA molecule), or from a virus. (A plasmid, simply put, is a DNA molecule distinct from that of the chromosome replicated by the cell.)

The inferences are obvious. DNA genetic recombination can be a conduit for the formation and spread of cancerous cells.

What is called DNA recombination repair is the replacement of a damaged segment of a DNA strand by a corresponding segment from an undamaged strand. In *E. coli*, at least, both these processes have been observed to be mediated or regulated by an enzyme (which is named RecA protein, and further identified as a 38-kDa nuclease).

## DNA METHYLATION

The introduction of a methyl group ($CH_3$- or -$CH_3$) into the nucleotide base residues, for example, into adenine and cytosine, will interrupt eukaryotic gene expression not only in bacteria but in mammals also (Voet and Voet, 1995, p. 1065ff). How this is done is not yet known, but it is presumably catalyzed by enzymes called methylases, with the methyl group furnished by some methyl donor such as *S*-adenosinemethionine. The degree of DNA eukaryotic methylation varies with species, tissue, and the position along the chromosome. Furthermore, the aberration seems to be self-perpetuating.

As emphasized by Hoffman (1999), the inferences are obvious. Methylation could lead to the formation of cancerous cells. Not only this, but the origins of different kinds of cancers can be explained by the fact that methylation varies with species, tissue, and position. And the methylation pattern will be inherited, being maintained in succeeding generations of cells. It can be added that enzyme inhibitors for methylases may be a key to controlling cancer, such as may occur via methylation.

## CHEMOPREVENTION

The National Cancer Institute (NCI), part of the National Institutes of Health (NIH), promotes what is called *chemoprevention*. Articles about the program surface here and there. Its purpose can be traced at least as far back as an editorial in the September 20, 1990, issue of the *New England Journal of Medicine*, describing ongoing and proposed efforts. Titled "Coming of Age — the Chemoprevention of Cancer," and written by Frank Meyskens, among the citations were clinical tests using beta-carotene and isotretinoin, the latter classed as a retinoid compound.

(Whereas *beta-carotene* brings to mind carrots, the word *retinoid* ordinarily indicates a resinlike substance. Resins generally are found in plants, for example, in chaparral or creosote bush. Here, however, it indicates a chemical derivative of retinol, more commonly called vitamin A, a prominent component of carrots. Carrots, not coincidentally, are a folkloric agent against cancer.)

Among the other chemopreventive agents selected for study were folic acid, vitamin C, and vitamin E, with a mention of the huge number of possibilities merely from dietary or food sources. From these many possibilities, the NCI set up a decision-making protocol to select the most promising candidates. At the time, several large-scale projects were already under way, which involved some 100,000 subjects. The ongoing and long-term decisive results are awaited.

Whereas folic acid already has a track record of sorts as a cancer chemopreventive, at least for cervical cancer, no clear conclusions could be drawn about beta-carotene and isotretinoin. The dosage level of beta-carotene may have been overly high, thus interfering with other necessary nutrients. On the other hand, isotretinoin was found to prevent the formation of secondary tumors, and potentially may work against the formation of primary tumors as well.

In the course of the work, the NCI decided on plans for using intermediate markers or indicators for the course of genetic, biochemical, and immunologic functions. This avoids the long waiting period for incipient cancers to grow. (Even more decisive would be a protocol of clinical tests for patients already suffering with cancer, for example, in cancer clinical research centers.)

Many articles continue to be written about work under way, published in various journals, and written by NCI staff and by researchers under NCI sponsorship and funding by various institutions. As one example, the American Cancer Society (ACS) published a review article in the January/February 1995 issue of *CA — A Cancer Journal for Clinicians* written by Greenwald, Kelloff, Burch-Whitman, and Kramer, all of the NCI. The authors observed that the specific chemopreventive agents in fruits and vegetables were yet to be determined. An outline was furnished of selected NCI clinical trials with candidate chemopreventive agents, and in addition, a short list is provided of known or suspected oncogenes and tumor suppressor genes.

Further samplings of NCI articles follow. For starters, there is a series of introductory articles by Michael B. Sporn and others of the NCI staff, which were published fairly early on, circa 1991–1993, with more technical articles to follow. In an article titled "Carcinogenesis and Cancer," Sporn, for instance, views cancer as an ongoing molecular and cellular process, requiring treatment before it is fully developed. In short, cancer should be "controlled."

As for vitamin A (here called *retinol*) and its synthetic analogs (here called *retinoids*), they serve to maintain a hormonelike control over cellular behavior. It is further noted that retinoids exhibit an ability to arrest or reverse carcinogenesis, that is, cancer formation. And retinoids act merely as physiological agents rather than cytotoxic or cell-toxic agents — the latter category comprising most conventional chemotherapy drugs.

Whereas retinol and its esters (which are the forms of vitamin A in foods) are toxic at higher intake or supplement levels, synthetic analogs may avoid this toxicity, examples being derivatives of retinoic acid. A compound known as *13-cis-retinoic acid* has been noted to reverse premalignant lesions in the case of certain kinds of cancer.

(Certain retinoids may prove of value in the treatment of epithelial cancers [cancers in body cavities], although vitamin A itself may never be useful as it only slowly converts to the more bioactive retinoic acid. Beyond this is the fact that vitamin A can accumulate in toxic levels in the liver, a problem avoided with retinoic acid [Chaney, in Devlin, 1986, p. 1203].)

For more on retinoids, a review article by Michael B. Sporn and Anita B. Roberts (1991) lists the effects of retinoids on the transforming growth factor denoted $\beta$ (TGF-$\beta$). This particular growth factor consists of a family of genes and peptides (or low-molecular-weight proteins), their purpose being to regulate normal cell differentiation (or cellular changes) and proliferation. There is apparently a connection between retinoids and TGF-$\beta$, by which retinoids act against cancer growth and even against oncogenes, the cancer-causing genes.

Sporn also writes about the controversial drug tamoxifen in a paper titled "Chemoprevention of Cancer," published in 1993. (Used against estrogen-related cancers of the breast, blocking the estrogen receptors on cancer cells, tamoxifen citrate is regarded as one of the less toxic chemotherapy drugs. Nevertheless, it has some adverse side effects, and those listed include eye damage, mental confusion, gastrointestinal problems, skin photosensitivity, bone pain, bleeding, blood problems, and liver damage.) Accordingly, it is then emphasized that the chemoprevention of cancer should use only noncytotoxic nutrients or pharmaceutical agents, their purpose being to enhance the body's intrinsic physiological mechanisms of cancer protection. This is as opposed to conventional chemotherapy, whose purpose is to destroy cancer cells (and unfortunately kill normal cells as well). Chemoprevention in this context is therefore aimed at blocking carcinogenesis in normal cells, and blocking the incipient growth of premalignant cells.

It is emphasized in NCI's own definition of the word, that chemoprevention is not directed at curing cancer after the cancer has developed. Its purpose is strictly preventive, although the theories and therapies may be applicable even to developing cancers. Anticancer agents may also be useful in chemoprevention.

In a 1994 research paper by Anzano et al., the use of a vitamin D analog is described (whereas other studies have used a vitamin A analog). Directed at the inhibition of breast cancer in rats, the study first utilized a specific, tumor-causing chemical, and then the vitamin D analog was fed in combination with the conventional chemotherapy drug tamoxifen. The treatment was described as very effective, at least in reducing the tumor burden. (The word *cure* is avoided.) And it was proposed that vitamin D analogs be called *deltanoids*, corresponding to the vitamin A (or retinol) analogs (called retinoids.)

In another cited research paper by Anzano et al., the agent was 9-*cis*-retinoic acid (9cRA), used alone or in combination with tamoxifen, and directed against breast cancer in rats. The rats were first injected with a specific, tumor-causing chemical and then fed nontoxic levels of 9cRA. Similar positive results were attained, with the note that the use of 9cRA with low levels of tamoxifen was even more effective.

A paper by Waun Ki Hong et al., all of the University of Texas M.D. Anderson Cancer Center, reviewed retinoid treatments. Published in 1995, the paper described the use of retinoids against aerodigestive cancers, which are secondary cancers of the aerodigestive tract, as derived from primary epithelial cancers. (Epithelial cancers, by definition, occur in cellular tissue covering free surfaces or lining body cavities, for example, as cancers of the lung, head, and neck. In one way or another, they are said to account for 35% of the cancer deaths in the United States.) Conclusively, it is noted that positive results are obtained by using retinoids, but retinoid use as a chemopreventive is not yet standard clinical practice.

A subsequent review article by Peter Greenwald of the NCI appeared in the September 1996 issue of *Scientific American*. The subject of vitamin D against cancer remains of current interest, and is described in Chapter 8.

Research on chemoprevention evidently remains in its infancy, but there seems to be a tie-in with folkloric anticancer agents. In stressing chemoprevention, the NCI may have deemphasized research directed toward the cure of fully developed cancers, that is, advanced or metastasized cancers, which, without a doubt, is a much more formidable task.

## COMMENTARY

The preceding biochemical survey covers a lot of diverse scientific information, but relatively few insights are gleaned about controlling or curing cancer. For, in pure science, the applications are secondary, although science itself rests on experiment and observation, and the conclusion most often heard is that "further research is needed." If these kinds of efforts are ever to be useful, then they should be translatable into a cure for cancer, and provide reasons explaining why certain empirical or folkloric treatments or cures work, if they do indeed work.

It is of concern that relatively few naturally occurring substances are listed in the scientific communications. Apart from folic acid and some of its derivatives, few readily recognizable substances appear in the listings for the chemotherapy drugs used as enzyme inhibitors, for example in Appendix E of Hoffman (1999), and the more recognizable may have some unusual primary sources (as evidenced in the catalog of the Sigma Chemical Company). The listings seem to be mainly of exotic or esoteric chemical compounds, which have to be synthesized by a drug company. James Duke's forebodings, in the foreword of Jonathan Hartwell's *Plants Used Against Cancer* (1982b), to be further mentioned, were that the war against cancer was being left to the drug companies.

(Of course, if the substances work, do not have debilitating and life-threatening side effects, and can be mass-produced, who cares? There is an argument also for using the pure chemical, in that some of the myriad biochemicals or phytochemicals in plants or herbs are additional sources of potentially adverse side effects.)

However, the fact remains that no general, systematic, absolute cure for cancer has been found, either within the mainstream or without. If a cure does indeed exist outside the mainstream, the applications have been haphazard and the results random, with no substantive, repeated clinical evidence, at least according to medical orthodoxy. Whether by design or happenstance, the opposition of medical orthodoxy to anything unorthodox has been constant, but the wall of resistance may be crumbling, for alternative medicine is viewed by many as the wave of the future.

# 5 Enzymatic Biochemical Treatment Protocols

## ENZYMES

There are some who would lump enzymes, hormones, and vitamins into one big family, all three being secretions of organs and glands that are necessary for the regulation of life processes. (Most enzyme names end with an "-ase" as a distinguishing feature, and the full name more or less describes the purpose.) An enzyme can be defined as a protein that catalyzes or favors a certain specific biochemical reaction, a protein being a very large molecule made up of amino acids. What are called *isoenzymes* are those that catalyze the same reaction but have different chemical compositions or chemical structures. The reactants for the reaction so catalyzed are generally called the *substrates*.

However enzymes are categorized, a brief chapter on enzyme therapy is contained in Moss's *Cancer Therapy: The Independent Consumer's Guide to Non-Toxic Treatment and Prevention* (1992). According to Moss, the successes have mostly been modest, at least with the few known enzymes tried. The digestive enzyme papain has long been used for external sores, and Moss comments that enzymes taken internally will undergo decomposition in the digestive system, and the only benefits may be digestion related. (If so generalized, then any substance taken internally is liable to be converted to something else — or is it? There is more here than first meets the eye, as some medications are plainly effective, either as is or as digestive/conversion products.) Mention is made of the therapy called Wobe-Mugos (Mucos, GmbH, Gruenwald, Germany). Research in all phases of enzyme therapy continues. A short chapter is also provided by Moss on Coenzyme Q or CoQ10 (or ubiquinone). An important use seems to be in counteracting the effect of chemotherapy drugs.

Walters' *Options: The Alternative Cancer Therapy Book* (1993) contains a short introduction to the subject under the section "Metabolic Therapies," with the statement that proteolytic (protein-digesting) enzymes are believed to dissolve the walls of cancer cells, and that enzyme treatments are widely used in Europe. More specifically, enzymes are used variously in what are called Issels' therapy, in Wheatgrass therapy, in the Gerson diet, in Kelley's therapy, and in Nieper's therapy (Walters, 1993, pp. 86, 147, 198, 207, 216). It is noted furthermore that chemotherapy destroys the body's enzymes, that cooking destroys the enzymes in food, and that enzymes may be involved in the so-called spontaneous remission of cancer (Walters, 1993, pp. 155, 201). Also noted, in the work of Hans Nieper, is that the enzyme bromelain, derived from pineapple roots, will deshield cancer cells, as will beta-carotene (Walters, 1993, p. 222).

As a special case of an enzyme, there is what is called superoxide dismutase, or SOD, which has been used in cancer treatment. Moss (1992) contains a chapter on the subject (with disclaimers), and Walters (1993) mentions it several times. Its main effects are other than catalytic, however, in that it evidently serves as a free radical scavenger, and as an internal source for hydrogen peroxide, which is also considered an anticancer agent.

In the proliferation of technical literature available, there is a highly readable account that stands out. It is Francis X. Hasselberger's *Uses of Enzymes and Immobilized Enzymes* (published in 1978, but unfortunately out of print now.) Among the more common proteolytic enzymes or proteases that have been used in cancer therapy are trypsin, chymotrypsin, ficin, papain, bromelin or bromelain, and various fungal proteases, with nonproteolytic enzymes used including deoxytribonuclease, lipase, and extracts from calves' thymus (Hasselberger, 1978, p. 146).

In a chapter titled Enzymes Versus Cancer, Hasselberger traces the discovery in 1934 by Freund, in Vienna, of a "normal substance" that dissolves cancer cells (Hasselberger, 1978, p. 141ff). This mysterious substance is not found in the blood or serum of cancer patients, nor in the urine. In its absence, cancer cells were protected against dissolution by normal serum. Furthermore, when sufficient cancer serum lacking the normal substance was added to normal serum, the cell-splitting ability of the normal serum was lost.

This normal substance was later identified as a cell-splitting enzyme that decomposes proteins, fats, and carbohydrates. Its protective action is inhibited by cholesterol esters such as cholesterol succinate and cholesterol butyrate. (Hence, the exclusion of fats in the diet is apparently well justified.) A low level of proteolytic enzymes seems to indicate a predisposition to cancer, and levels decrease in the sickly and the elderly.

Parallel with, or anticipating these developments, was the work of John Beard (1858–1924), who for 30 years was a comparative embryologist at the University of Edinburgh Medical School, and who wrote a book called *The Enzyme Treatment of Cancer* (Moss, 1992, p. 308; Hasselberger, 1978, pp. 139, 140). Few enzymes were known in those times, and known ones were impure at that, so Beard's contribution on the role of enzymes in cancer therapy did not receive a fair trial. The work has continued, however, notably using pancreatic enzymes, with Beard's theories helping to lay the groundwork.

A therapy was commenced by Gaschler in 1948, using a product called "Carzodelan," which was not active orally and had to be administered in other ways. Not an optimized preparation, the results were unimpressive; but it was a start.

Further work was performed by Dr. Max Wolf, who founded the Biological Research Institute in New York City. In some of his studies, cancer cells in close juxtaposition with normal cells would take over. After a few days the normal cells would die off and decompose, while the cancer cells kept growing. If an enzyme solution was introduced, the cancer cells would first start to grow without restraint toward the normal cells, but would then stop growing, and would in turn shrivel and dissolve. The normal cells, however, showed hardly any effect. A mixture prepared from beef pancreas, calf thymus, plus the plant species *Pisum sativum* (pea), *Lens esculenta* (lentil), papaya, and the crystalline alcohol mannitol was found to be most effective. Mannitol itself does not act as an enzyme but is used as a carrier. The commercial preparation so developed became known as Wobe-Mugos.

(Wolf used enzymes in aqueous solutions in his studies. More modern methods of laboratory investigation entrap enzymes in various substrates, and they are then called immobilized enzymes, as per the title of Hasselberger's book.)

Thus, particular mention was made in Hasselberger's book of the Wobe-Mugos enzyme mixture, which has been in use since 1959 mostly in Germany and Europe (Hasselberger, 1978, p. 145ff). It can be given orally, rectally, or injected into the abdominal muscles, but is most effective when injected directly into the tumor, where it is said to literally dissolve the tumorous tissue. The mixture is also said to act against metastasis, the spreading of cancer cells, and against the side effects of radiation. It is also reported that to be effective, the preparation must be used over a long period of time.

Hasselberger's book was published in 1978. At the time it was commented that in the United States the FDA had given permission for the sale, without claims, of several forms of the Wobe-Mucos enzyme preparation, including a vitamin A mixture. The supplier was listed as the Mucose Pharmaceutical Corporation of Los Angeles, California, evidently no longer extant. Ralph Moss, however, lists several sources for enzyme therapy (Moss, 1992, p. 369). Enzymes and supplies can be obtained from Nutri Supplies, 1020 Stony Battery Road, Lancaster, PA 17601, Ph. 800-999-2700, and from NutriCology, Inc., Allergy Research Group, PO Box 489, San Leandro CA 94577-0489, Ph. 800-782-4274. For the Wobe-Marcos therapy there is Wolfgang Scheef, M.D., c/o Robert Janker Clinic, Fauchklinik fur Tumorerkrankenungen, Baumschulallee 12-14, 5300 Bonn 1, Germany, Ph. 011-49-7291-0, and the Janker Clinic (of Mexico), Eduardo Gallegos, M.D., 1527 Blvd. Sanchez Taboada & Mission San Diego, Suite 101, Zone Del Rio, Tijuana, Mexico 22320, Ph. 011-52-66-842200/157. (The Robert Janker Clinic is also listed in John Fink's *Third Opinion*.) A contact listed for the Beardian pancreatic therapy is Ernst T. Krebs, Jr., John Beard Memorial Foundation, PO Box 685, San Francisco, CA 94101, Ph. 415-824-1067. Another name is Nicholas Gonzalez, M.D., 630 Park Avenue, New York, NY 10021, Ph. 212-535-3993. (Nicholas Gonzalez is also listed in John Fink's *Third Opinion*.) The *Alternative Medicine Yellow Pages* has listings for Enzyme Therapy, and notes in particular Karl Ransberger Medizinsiche, Enzyme-forschungsgellschaft, Alpenstrasse 29, D-8192 Geretried 1, Germany, for pancreatic enzyme therapy. An update on digestive enzyme therapy is furnished in John Boik's *Cancer and Natural Medicine*, which describes Wobe-Mugos therapy and also the Gonzalez and Kelley programs (Boik, 1996, pp. 164–166).

Given the apparent activity of enzymes, it may be wondered why they are not effective almost immediately, as reportedly demonstrated by injection into the tumor, and as was apparently once demonstrated with the serum used for Burton's Immuno-Augmentive Therapy (Walters, 1993, p. 61). Or at least in as short a time frame as reported for Rife's bioelectric therapy (Walters, 1993, p. 269). However, this is apparently not the case.

One enzyme in particular is evidently well established in a particular cancer treatment. This is ʟ-asparaganase for acute lymphoblastic leukemia, or ALL (Moss, 1992, p. 307; Hasselberger, 1978, p. 1521ff). The enzyme is found in high concentrations notably in the blood of guinea pigs and the South American steppe hare or agouti, and is therefore known as the guinea pig enzyme. Although not totally successful, this treatment reportedly works to a degree for this form of leukemia; it has not been of use for other kinds of cancer.

Differences in physical properties between normal and cancerous cells have been reported (Hasselberger, 1978, pp. 143–145). Thus, whereas cancer cells show much "stickiness" but a low level of adhesion, normal cells show a high level of adhesion but a low level of stickiness. By adhesion is meant that the cells tend to cling together and not migrate or drift away, whereas stickiness is the tendency to attach to a new surface or location.

Hence, there is the tendency for cancer cells to migrate and "stick" to another part of the body, that is, to metastasize, forming new cancers. Another property of enzymes, therefore, is that they reduce the stickiness of cancer cells, thereby reducing the hazards of metastasis. The use of x-rays (or radiation) and chemotherapeutic agents has been observed to increase the stickiness, thus providing an explanation for the metastases that occur with these treatments.

Moreover, cancer cells apparently have a deficiency of positively charged calcium ions, and consequently have an overall negative electrical charge, which increases as the malignancy grows. Membrane defects near the cancer cell nucleus were also noted, which has a bearing on the use of enzymes against cancer.

It is commented that cancer cells do not proliferate rapidly, as is the popular conception. Rather, cancer cells merely die off less rapidly than normal cells. For with normal cells, cell proliferation is offset by an equal number of cell deaths, which ensures a stable cell population; but this is not the case for cancer cells.

Hasselberger provided many more examples of the uses of enzymes, including a chapter titled "Enzymes in Medicine," in which it is advanced that enzymes may counteract viruses.

There is a section titled "Respiration" that indicates how complicated the processes of glycolysis can be (Hasselberger, 1978, p. 16ff). The overall metabolism of glucose is the means by which energy is normally supplied to the body cells, as has been previously described.

The importance of glycolysis merits further review. Thus, the sequence or sequences of the overall metabolism of glucose first involves a number of steps, as detailed in Chapter 3, via what is called the "Embden–Meyerhoff–Parnas pathway of glycolysis." Each step in the pathway is catalyzed by a different specific enzyme, starting with glucose in the form of its polymer, glycogen. The initial sequence of steps involves the formation of pyruvic acid. Prominently involved are the substances ATP and ADP (adenosine triphosphate and adenosine diphosphate), which convert back and forth, introducing or removing phosphate ions into or from the glycolysis pathway.

The glycolysis pathway is a prominent reaction sequence featured in texts and treatises on biochemistry and microbiology, according to the previously cited Chapter 3, and an abbreviated version is also sometimes presented, for instance, by Boik (1996). To reiterate, the primary product of glycolysis is pyruvic acid, $CH_3COCOOH$, which may also be represented as the pyruvate ion, or $CH_3COCOO^-$. The pyruvic acid or pyruvate further reacts to form carbon dioxide and water, or else forms lactic acid or the lactate ion. The former route is a feature of what may be called aerobic glycolysis; the latter, of anaerobic glycolysis. It may be recalled that normal cells behave aerobically, and cancer cells for the most part behave anaerobically, as discovered by Otto Warburg in the 1920s.

Both the routes mentioned earlier pertain to cell metabolism, which broadly speaking connotes any biologically inspired reaction sequence. Most usually, however, the term applies to oxidative or exothermic reaction sequences involving energy sources such as glucose or glycogen, and the expression of primary metabolism is more definitive, as distinguished from secondary metabolism.

As has also been mentioned in Chapter 3, if sufficient oxygen is present or available, the pyruvic acid or pyruvate is oxidized in what is called the "Krebs tricarboxylic acid cycle," which involves additional steps, each step in turn catalyzed by a specific enzyme. It is sometimes simply called the *Krebs cycle* after its discoverer, H.A. Krebs, or the *tricarboxylic cycle*, or else the *citric acid cycle*, as citric acid or citrate (citric acid being a tricarboxylic acid) is formed as an intermediate — not to mention others such as succinic acid, fumaric acid, and malic acid, or succinate, fumarate and malate. (The terms *citrate, succinate, fumarate, malate, lactate*, etc., are more generic, because the compounds may exist in the form of the corresponding salts, and could conceivably even exist as the ester. The acid form could, of course, be referred to, for example, as hydrogen citrate, etc., and may be partly dissociated in aqueous solution to form the citrate ion.) Water and carbon dioxide are released as net products. The cycle is sustained in that part of the oxygen converts part of the products back to the original state, a process catalyzed by enzymes containing a molecule called flavin and by proteins called cytochromes, but which may also be called enzymes. It may be mentioned that vitamin B2 is also known as riboflavin.

(The foregoing and the following illustrate how complex chemical reactions can be. Chemical reactions are never as simple as their stoichiometric conversions (that is, the material balances) would indicate. All kinds of intermediates and complexes are formed, and competing reactions also occur. [We can distinguish between chemical conversions and chemical reactions, in that a conversion is the overall sequence of individual reactions, presumably known, or unknown — and perhaps can be more aptly described as a chemically reacting system in chaos. Otherwise, the terms are used interchangeably.] In truth, even the simplest conversion will probably never be fully understood. Catalysts, naturally present or added, further complicate the picture. Catalysts affect not only reaction rates but also the very nature of the conversion itself; that is, the intended reaction may not proceed without the catalyst.)

Under low oxygen availability, pyruvic acid, say, is instead reduced to lactic acid, the end product in cancer metabolism uncovered by Warburg. (As stressed before, the enzyme pyruvate dehydrogenase controls the oxidation rate to produce $CO_2$ as an end product; an inhibitor for this enzyme would then favor the production of lactic acid. The enzyme lactate dehydrogenase catalyzes the production of lactic acid; an inhibitor here would then favor oxidation. A difficulty is that cancer cells to a degree also undergo aerobic or oxidative glycolysis.) The conversion of lactic acid back to glucose (or glycogen) in the liver completes this particular cycle, known as the Cori cycle.

A problem is that if an inhibitor or poison is found for any one of the enzymes involved, how will it affect the other enzymes in the conversion sequence? That is, although enzymes are selective, enzyme inhibitors are not. In particular, anything that interferes too much with the tricarboxylic acid cycle acid is probably to be avoided, as respiration is vital for normal cell metabolism. It is all part of a subject area called *metabolic enzyme inhibitors*, with published papers and treatises to match, which grows exponentially and becomes evermore complex. If the objective of science is to simplify, this is not the case here and so maybe science is not necessarily the place to look for a cancer protocol.

(Interestingly, polypeptides can be regarded as enzyme inhibitors as per Dr. Stanislaw Burzynski's antineoplastin therapy, and this may be the role of other nitrogenous compounds. The peptide bond is formed by joining one amino acid with another such that an amine group (or say, the -$NH_2$ group) of one reacts with the more acidic hydroxyl group (or -OH group) of the other, to split off water as HOH. A continuation of the process creates a polymer, which may be called a *polypeptide*. In this way, the extra-large peptide polymers called *proteins* are built up. The extrapolation is to all kinds or combinations of amino acids in the form of peptides or polypeptides that could be enzyme inhibitors against cancer. Given the numbers and permutations, the possibilities are near limitless. Many peptides are commercially available for testing and application, for example, in the Sigma-Aldrich catalog *Biochemicals and Reagents*. Further information and small synthesis samples are available via *PEPscreenTM: Custom Peptide Libraries for Screening Applications*, as per Sigma Genosys, one of the Sigma-Aldrich family of companies.)

A route to some degree of simplification is to examine the further conversion of the intermediate product pyruvic acid. Pyruvic acid (which may also be called acetyl formic acid) is one of the many derivatives of propanoic acid, sometimes called propionic acid. Specifically, pyruvic acid is 2-oxo-propanoic acid, with a chemical formula that may be written as $CH_3COCOOH$, or simply $C_3H_4O_3$. At body temperatures pyruvic acid is a liquid, and is infinitely soluble in water. It is significant that if glucose or glycogen is converted to pyruvic acid, hydrogen is left over. That is, based on a half mole of glucose, say,

$$1/2\ C_6H_{12}O_6 \rightarrow C_3H_4O_3 + 2\ [H]$$

Whether the hydrogen is formed as molecular hydrogen $H_2$, or, say, active atomic hydrogen [H], or further reacts with something else to form a compound, may be immaterial, as ultimately hydrogen is either oxidized or else further reacts anaerobically with pyruvic acid conversion products or in supportive reactions. It may be assumed to be formed indirectly, and manifests itself by causing a chemical reduction in other component species.

If oxidation occurs, as in normal cell metabolism, the overall oxidation of pyruvic acid and coproduct hydrogen can be viewed as

$$C_3H_4O_3 + 2\ [H] + 3O_2 \rightarrow 3H_2O + 3CO_2$$

There are a number of steps involved in the Krebs tricarboxylic, or citric acid, cycle, and oxygen is not added directly to the pyruvic acid but enters later in the cycle. In fact, pyruvic acid or pyruvate is first changed to oxaloacetic acid or oxaloacetate, then into other consecutive reaction products, some of which in turn react to give off $H_2O$ and $CO_2$ and ultimately regenerate oxaloacetic acid to continue the cycle. Besides this, there are other supportive reactions taking place, making the cycle a very complicated affair indeed. Overall, there is a net loss of pyruvic acid, however, as $H_2O$ and $CO_2$ must be produced and discharged from the cycle somehow. New pyruvic acid or pyruvate is continually formed from glucose or glycogen.

On the other hand, if the hydrogen further reacts with the pyruvic acid, then a reduction occurs to form lactic acid by the overall stoichiometric conversion, simplified as follows:

$$C_3H_4O_3 + 2[H] \rightarrow C_3H_6O_3$$

That is, in terms of the chemical formulas,

$$CH_3COCOOH + 2[H] \rightarrow CH_3CH(OH)COOH$$

This conversion would denote the lactic acid formed according to the Warburg theory. Even here, the reaction takes place indirectly as the result of a supportive reaction that introduces hydrogen.

Furthermore, the latter conversion reaction, the hydrogen reduction of pyruvic acid to lactic acid, or pyruvate to lactate, would be the controlling step in the metabolism of cancer cells. It is catalyzed by the enzyme lactate dehydrogenase, as previously noted, and if an effective inhibitor or catalyst poison can be found that is selective to this particular step, it could conceivably suppress the metabolism of cancer cells.

There may be more to it than this, however, as it may also involve oxygen deprivation, as occurs in muscle tissue during intense exercise, where there is a buildup of lactic acid. This brings us to the role of oxygen and oxidants vs. antioxidants, and just what all is going on in the body and the bloodstream. (For instance, in chemotherapy, anemia occurs as a side effect. Is this not compromising the aerobic metabolism of normal cells in favor of the anaerobic metabolism of cancer cells?) It may be noted that the inhibition of glycosis by the presence of oxygen is called the Pasteur effect; the inverse, the inhibition of oxygen uptake by glycolyis, is sometimes called the Crabtree effect (e.g., Aisenberg, 1961, p. 159ff).

These considerations illustrate why an absolute cure for cancer is so elusive, for there are so many partially offsetting factors that are not fully understood. This is why a cure may probably have to precede understanding, and be a happenstance, an exercise in serendipity, like the discovery of antibiotics. (If we had waited until we completely understood the action of antibiotics, we would still be waiting, for a subject is never closed. Each answer leads to another question.) And this is why the aborigines of Amazonia, say, are just as likely as modern medicine to have a cure, if not more likely.

## ENZYME INHIBITORS

The use of selective enzyme inhibitors against cancer cell metabolism conceivably may prove to be the ultimate attack against cancer, for most cancer cells undergo what may be called anaerobic glycolysis. This first involves a series of ten steps, each catalyzed by a particular enzyme, in which glucose or blood sugar is converted to an intermediate compound called pyruvic acid or pyruvate. The pyruvic acid or pyruvate is in turn converted to lactic acid or lactate as the final product. This latter conversion is catalyzed by one or another forms of the enzyme lactate dehydrogenase. Normal cells, on the other hand, undergo what may be called aerobic glycolysis, in which the pyruvic acid or pyruvate is ultimately oxidized to yield carbon dioxide and water in the subsequent sequence of steps called the tricarboxylic acid cycle, also known as the Krebs cycle or the citric acid cycle. These series and sequences may be collectively termed *cell metabolism.*

As described in Chapter 3, although other processes occur simultaneously, such as glutaminolysis and a very limited aerobic glycolysis, the predominant conversion supporting cancer cell metabolism is anaerobic glycolysis. Lactic acid or lactate is the final product, and is in turn reconverted to glucose (or its polymer known as glycogen) in the liver. The premise here is that if a suitable enzyme inhibitor or blocker can be found for lactate dehydrogenase, this would disrupt cancer cell metabolism and lead to cancer cell death. The germ of this idea was broached, for instance, by Donald Voet and Judith G. Voet in their treatise on biochemistry, which was first published in 1990 (Voet and Voet, 1995, p. 557): "Attempts to understand the metabolic differences between cancer cells and normal cells may one day provide a clue to the treatment of certain forms of this devastating disease."

This idea was given substance in the author's paper titled "Enzyme Inhibitors for Cancer Cell Metabolism," published in the May 1997 issue of the *Townsend Letter for Doctors & Patients.* (This periodical, subtitled *The Examiner for Medical Alternatives*, is published by Jonathan Collin, an M.D.) Among the inhibitors listed for lactate dehydrogenase are urea, arsenite, oxalic acid or oxalates (e.g., from spinach, rhubarb, wood sorrel, etc.), fatty acids, mononuceotides (e.g., from sweet potato roots), 2-hydroxy-3-butanoic acid (from bakers yeast), EDTA (the chelating agent ethylenediaminetetraacetic acid), gossypol (from cottonseed), serotonin, and still other compounds or substances, some of which may be of questionable or overt toxicity.

Allicin as a lactate dehydrogenase inhibitor is noteworthy. It is an ephemeral compound released when raw garlic is crushed or chewed. The half-life is said to be only 4 hours, so it cannot be routinely obtained in capsule or pill form, although its garlic-derived precursor can be thus obtained, with allicin released during assimilation.

A primary requirement is that any substance or compound used as a lactate dehydrogenase inhibitor should at the same time be nontoxic for other body functions, especially of the liver and kidneys. It may be noted in this context that most substances or compounds tend to be nonselective, that is, they may inhibit more than one enzyme. This nonselectivity produces the so-called adverse side effects. The encompassing term is cytotoxicity, or "cell toxicity," indicating that the substance is toxic in some degree to all cells. In fact, this is the main problem with conventional cytotoxic chemotherapy: all body cells are affected, some more than others. A conclusion in some quarters is that conventional cytotoxic chemotherapy has been judged ineffective for solid tumors, although it may work against blood-related cancers. Moreover, it predominately affects the fast-growing cells of the immune system and gastrointestinal tract, the slower-growing cancer cells being least affected. It may ultimately act against such vital organs as the heart.

Other potential enzyme inhibitors include the class of compounds known as alkaloids, which are most often distinguished by a certain nitrogen-containing ring structure. These compounds may vary from the mostly benign to the deadly toxic, depending also on dosage and other factors. They are found in plants, and are thus known as *phytochemicals*, or *plant chemicals*, the former designator being more commonly used. Some are known anticancer agents — for example, against blood-related cancers — and others remain in the offing.

It is observed that a variety of alkaloids occur in many garden-variety foods, although in trace amounts. This may partly explain why vegetarian diets are on occasion said to be active against cancer, and have been noted even to cure cancer.

Also mentioned in the previously cited article is the finding that vitamin C, or ascorbic acid, has been found to destroy cancer cells, as Linus Pauling said. Translation to an effective cancer cure apparently remains controversial, at least to medical orthodoxy and the public.

## ENZYME INHIBITION IN MODERN MEDICINE

Modern medicine is increasingly based on the use of enzyme inhibitors, although they may be synthetic as well as natural. As has been stated, the biochemical processes in the body are controlled by enzymes, which are of a proteinaceous nature, and act selectively as catalysts for the myriad biochemical reactions in the body. Almost without exception, there is one particular enzyme for each biochemical reaction. These enzymes are inhibited, blocked, controlled, modulated, or regulated by still other proteinaceous substances, or by other chemicals or biochemicals, which are uniformly called *enzyme inhibitors*. (A few even act as promoters.) Interestingly, a given inhibitor usually acts against more than one enzyme, producing side effects, which can range from the innocuous to the deadly serious.

Notable examples of enzyme inhibitors include the many antibiotics that block certain vital functions in bacteria, but which in controlled doses are not toxic to humans (although there are some antibiotics that are too toxic to use, including some that even kill cancer cells). Bacterial cells, called *prokaryotes*, are fortuitously different from mammalian cells, called *eukaryotes*, and respond differently. The use of fluorides to prevent dental caries is another example, the fluorides acting as inhibitors for certain critical enzymes in oral bacteria, as well as facilitating a beneficial interaction with the dentine at the tooth surfaces. (And, as sometimes warned, if ingested these fluorides can also act as inhibitors for other enzymes within the body.)

The use of chemotherapy drugs against cancer cells is another prominent example. These drugs or chemicals interfere with certain enzymes in cellular

DNA/RNA/protein synthesis, but unfortunately are nonselective. That is, they act as inhibitors against all kinds of body cells, acting against some more than others, sometimes even more so than against cancer cells. Among the cells severely affected are those of the bone marrow, resulting in iron-deficient anemia, for which the common chemo drug 5-FU, or 5-fluorouracil, is notorious. There are ill-advised attempts to remedy this form of anemia by prescribing inorganic iron supplements, notably ferrous sulfate, itself described as toxic in the *Physicians' Desk Reference* or *PDR*. The body's iron demands are preferably met, however, by subtler processes of assimilation from food sources.

In fact, in a monograph chapter by Mathew Suffness and John M. Pezzuto, from the National Cancer Institute and the University of Illinois College of Medicine, respectively, it is flatly stated that conventional chemotherapy is ineffective against solid tumors (in Hostettmann, 1991, pp. 72ff, 116). There are some successes with blood-related cancers such as leukemia, which is a different proposition. Also, a sometimes-mentioned report from the Harvard University School of Public Health, sometimes called the "Cairns report," concluded that conventional chemotherapy is grossly overused. The descriptor "palliative" fits the circumstance, the dictionary definition connoting a hiding or cover-up; that is, a treatment that does not cure.

(Although chemotherapy may be said to keep the cancer from spreading further, there are also indications reported that it may in itself result in the cancer metastasizing. In this regard, it has been observed that cancerous cells have the property of breaking away from their origins more readily than do normal cells, to become entrained in the body fluids, but at the same time have a stickiness for locating at new sites, which very possibly may be further intensified by invasive procedures. This seems a catch-22 situation, as is so often the case. And inasmuch as cancerous cells are normal cells gone awry, the number of potential kinds of cancer may be estimated at from 100 or so to more than 300, with some estimates as high as 600, as previously stated.)

Even the controversial cyanic anticancer substance known as *laetrile*, or *amygdalin*, is thought to be detoxified by a particular enzyme or enzymes in normal cells that is not ordinarily present, or in sufficient concentrations, in cancer cells. The answer is not clear-cut, however, and laetrile remains suspect, if effective at all. More than this, there are certain other food enzymes that may cause laetrile to give off deadly hydrogen cyanide or hydrocyanic acid, or HCN, itself an enzyme inhibitor that acts against bodily processes, notably respiration. (Deadly cyanide, incidentally, is listed as an inhibitor for tyrosinase, the enzyme involved in melanoma.)

It is emphasized in John Heinerman's *The Treatment of Cancer with Herbs* (1984) that although laetrile is sometimes viewed favorably as a cancer treatment, due to enzymatic action it can interact with some other foods to produce HCN internally and cause cyanide poisoning. Specifically forbidden is using laetrile tablets with such "health foods" as nuts, bean and alfalfa sprouts, fresh fruits (peaches), and other uncooked foods found in salads (lettuce, celery, mushrooms), which are high in hydrolytic enzymes that can cause the release of cyanide (Heinerman, 1984, pp. 175,176). Never mix these foods with laetrile!

(The idea has been advanced that the action of cyanide from cyanogenic glucosides such as laetrile or amygdalin is related to the absence or presence of an enzyme named rhodanase. This enzyme catalyzes the conversion of cyanide and thiosulfate or thiosulfinate to the less harmful thiocyanate and sulfate. Cancer cells are said to be characteristically low in this enzyme, and the cyanide thereby destroys the cell, whereas normal cells are high in this enzyme, providing a means of detoxifying the cyanide. There is also the thought that as thiosulfate or thiosulfinate are involved in the conversion of cyanide, the presence of these sulfur compounds may be required to protect normal cells.)

For perhaps a last word, it is said that amygdalin or laetrile will release cyanide in the stomach by the action of the enzyme β-glucosidase, also called emulsin (Smith, in Amdur et al., 1991, p. 277). Not found in mammalian tissues, such enzymes occur in normal human intestinal flora, or gut flora. "For this reason, amygdalin is about 40 times more toxic by mouth than by intravenous injection." Thus amygdalin or laetrile "could be given safely by parenteral routes." (The term *parenteral* signifies routes other than oral administration.)

The reference furnishes a diagram for the biochemical management of cyanide poisoning, as yet imperfectly understood. The basis is the fact that cyanide apparently blocks electron transfer in the cytochrome system, and the electron-carrying iron porphyrin pigment protein involved in cellular respiration may be blocked by the injection of sodium nitrate. The reference also provides three other routes for counteracting cyanide poisoning. The most controversial is the use of amyl nitrate by inhalation. A qualifier is that the cyanide is loosely bound, and may be released to again cause cyanide poisoning.

Another permanent cyanide detoxification method involves the intravenous injection of sodium thiosulfate. The thiosulfate contains a loosely bound sulfur atom that can convert cyanide to thiocyanate by the action of the ubiquitous enzyme rhodanese (thiosulfate-cyanide sulfurtransferase). The much less toxic thiocyanate is excreted via the urine. Rhodanese occurs in both the liver and in skeletal muscle and produces a detoxifying action even in the absence of thiosulfate.

The third method involves using oxygen to supplement the second method, with the explanation that the enzyme rhodanese is not affected by oxygen. It should be added that artificial respiration with 100% oxygen should be instituted immediately if respiratory difficulty is observed (Rumack and Lovejoy, in Amdur et al., 1991, p. 933).

Thus, laetrile or amygdalin injection may or may not be an effective anticancer agent, and has both proponents and detractors. In any event, if cyanide poisoning should occur, there are means for remediation.

The danger, of course, is that the principal action of cyanide is to block cell respiration, causing the victim to suffocate, which generally occurs faster than the accompanying cardiac arrest, also an effect.

However, as distinguished from the aerobic metabolism of normal cells, cancer cell metabolism is in the main anaerobic and does not invoke the carboxylic acid cycle, dependent on oxygen and fundamental to cell respiration, as set forth in Chapter 3 for glycolysis. Thus, respiration of the cancerous cell is excluded from consideration. Hence, from this standpoint, the anticancer claims for amygdalin or laetrile can be viewed as missing the mark. That is, under this interpretation, cyanide would affect aerobic normal cells but not anaerobic cancerous cells.

(However, amygdalin or laetrile conceivably may act against other critical enzymes, for instance, possibly against tyrosine kinase as involved in the metabolism of intractable cancerous stem cells, as described in Chapter 10.)

Cyanide is found in many common household items, such as rat and pest poisons, silver and metal polishes, photographic solutions, and fumigating products (Rumack and Lovejoy, in Amdur et al., 1991, p. 933). Sodium and potassium cyanide can be readily purchased as chemicals, and are used in bulk in gold mining and the attendant separation or purification operations.

Hydrogen sulfide has the same kind of adverse action on respiration as hydrogen cyanide. Although most persons can detect the burnt-almond odor of hydrogen cyanide gas, and can initially detect the rotten-egg odor of hydrogen sulfide gas, the latter quickly deadens the olfactory nerve, so that hydrogen sulfide is especially insidious and deadly.

In turn, gases and vapors may be classified in various ways, depending on the kind and degree of toxicity (Gordon and Amdur, in Amdur et al., 1991, p. 389). Thus, there are irritants, such as ammonia and sulfur dioxide; simple asphyxiants, such as nitrogen and methane; chemical asphyxiants, such as carbon monoxide, hydrogen cyanide, and hydrogen sulfide; central nervous system depressants, such as aliphatic and chlorinated hydrocarbons, and also acetone, ether, and benzene; neurotoxic agents, such as carbon disulfide, mercury vapor, *n*-hexane, and methyl butyl ketone; hepatoxic and nephrotoxic agents, such as carbon tetrachloride and chloroform; blood-damaging agents, such as nitrobenzene; bone-marrow-damaging agents, such as benzene and trinitrotoluene; and carcinogens, such as vinyl chloride and 2-naphthylamine.

For more on chemical carcinogens there are two notable references: *CRC Handbook of Identified Carcinogens and Noncarcinogens*, and Irving Sax's *Cancer Causing Chemicals*, both published in the early 1980s. The EPA, of course, is the main governmental source.

Electromagnetic radiation occasionally surfaces as an alternative treatment for cancer, with its efficacy debated or else discounted. Suffice to say, if there is an effect, it conceivably may be as an enzyme inhibitor, which will in turn relate to intensity and wavelength or frequency.

Among the names that have been prominently cited for electromagnetic therapy, or radiotherapy, is the previously mentioned Royal Rife, whose work is the subject of two books by Barry Lynes (*The Cancer Cure That Worked! Fifty Years of Suppression* and *The Healing of Cancer*). Rife's results evidently have not been duplicated, at least in the opinion of medical orthodoxy. If this line of investigation is to prove productive, among the variables to be zeroed in on are wavelength or frequency and intensity, as suggested earlier. In essence, the problem becomes that of whether or not radiation of a certain kind and degree can serve as an enzyme inhibitor for cancer cell metabolism.

We see again from the foregoing that the major difference between the metabolic pathways of normal cells and cancer cells has been known since the 1920s, as discovered by biochemist Otto Warburg of Germany, who later received a Nobel Prize for other work (in fact, two Nobel Prizes). Thus, normal cells convert glucose or blood sugar (or the glucose polymer called glycogen), eventually to carbon dioxide and water by oxidation (terminating via what is variously called the Krebs, citric acid, or tricarboxylic acid cycle). The $CO_2$ and $H_2O$ end products are the same as would occur from conventional combustion, whereas cancer cells eventually produce lactic acid or lactate, with no terminal oxidative cycle involved.

(The energy release for the conversion of glucose to lactic acid or lactate is very low as compared to that for the conversion to $CO_2$ and $H_2O$ which occurs in normal cells. Whether this comparatively low energy release is merely symptomatic or whether it could somehow be changed so as to turn a cancerous cell into a normal cell has evidently not been studied. Here again, a selective enzyme or enzyme inhibitor may be the key.)

As has been indicated, the entirety of the former sequence or pathway for normal cells may be conveniently referred to as aerobic glycolysis. The latter, corresponding sequence for cancerous cells can be referred to as anaerobic glycolysis, with no oxygen involved. In lieu of the Krebs oxidative cycle, the final and distinguishing step for the latter conversion route is catalyzed by one form or another of an enzyme called lactate dehydrogenase. Furthermore, and most significantly, there are known enzyme inhibitors for this step. Some of these inhibitors are in fact of herbal or plant origin (such as allicin, released from garlic via the action of a certain enzyme in the garlic). Very likely there are many more as yet uncovered or studied. The subject was further amplified in the previously cited paper by Hoffman titled "Enzyme Inhibitors for Cancer Cell Metabolism." Another paper dealing with other routes involved in cancer cell metabolism is by Anthony G. Payne and titled "Achieving Oncolysis by Compromising Tumor Cell Metabolism," which appeared in the December 1996 issue of the *Townsend Letter for Doctors & Patients*.

As an aside, the Helping Hands Society of London was presumably to investigate this approach, particularly with regard to inhibiting lactate dehydrogenase as a means for stopping cancer in its tracks. Along these same lines, it is a continuing and oft-mentioned proposal herein that cancer clinical research centers (CCRCs) be established in the United States as the means for testing and implementing this route and other alternative treatments, to be conducted under expert supervision — whenever possible, on an outpatient basis. (A potential problem with any medication, natural or synthetic, is that a patient may prove hyperallergic and even go into anaphylactic shock. The latter denotes hypersensitivity to a previously encountered antigen, and can cause respiratory distress, even failure. Immediate professional attention is required, notably via administration of some form of adrenaline, say epinephrine, with Benadryl® being a commercial version.)

At the same time, a unified theory is required to explain how and why a particular treatment, or any treatment, should be effective, especially enzyme inhibitors against cancer cell metabolism. Otherwise it all becomes more of an exercise in futility; for example, there are the many herbal remedies proposed that apparently have no basis in substantiated fact other than somebody or another's word for it, is usually second or third hand, that is, is entirely anecdotal, and is as likely as not to be wishful thinking.

(The American Institute for Cancer Research in Washington, D.C., is another organization with an open mind, looking for new approaches for solving the cancer problem.)

## ENZYME INHIBITORS FOR MELANOMA

The inhibition of the enzyme tyrosinase may very well be a key to the control of melanoma, and some of the known inhibitors include common substances. Thus, vitamin C, among other common and uncommon substances, has been listed as an enzyme inhibitor for tyrosinase in M.K. Jain's *Handbook of Enzyme Inhibitors, 1965–1977* (1982). In addition to ascorbic acid (vitamin C), these other substances include the following: halide ion (e.g., from the chloride of common salt, or from iodides and fluorides); butyric acid (from rancid butter); lactic acid (the end product of cancer cell metabolism, found naturally in sour milk products); oxalic acid (ordinarily considered toxic, although it occurs naturally in rhubarb and wood sorrel, etc.); formic acid (a component of ant stings); tyrosine itself; and deadly cyanide (which is a chemically bound component of laetrile), as found in almonds (notably bitter almonds), in apricot seeds, and in certain legumes such as beans, etc., although the heat from cooking may drive off the cyanide content.

(Interestingly, there is another enzyme called tyrosine kinase that is purported to be involved in the metabolism of intractable cancerous stem cells, as set forth in Chapter 10. A number of natural substances are supposedly inhibitors for this particular enzyme (also given in Chapter 10). This listing may include the soy isoflavone genistein. Jain's handbook, being dated, does not mention this particular enzyme.)

Injections of a yucca/alpine sunflower extract, as developed by now-retired University of Wyoming chemistry professor Owen Asplund, have been reported to be used successfully in Switzerland against melanoma, and presumably may act as an enzyme inhibitor. Incidentally, the injections are given in the stomach area, which slows down the assimilation of a potent vaccine, as was practiced with the old rabies vaccine.

## DIET

There is a popular hypothesis that a vegetarian diet reduces cancer incidence. Thus, remote peoples who are vegetarians, such as the Hunzas of the Himalayas and certain Mongolian tribes or societies, are said to have a very low or even nonexistent occurrence of cancer. This conclusion is tempered by the fact that the ancient Eskimos, who survived as meat eaters, also may have had a low cancer incidence.

(This dichotomy has been commented upon by Vilhjalmur Stefansson, who explored and lived in the Canadian Arctic starting in 1906, himself subsisting on an all-meat diet over lengthy periods. He believed that a mixed diet is the source of the trouble, always keeping the digestive system and its intestinal flora off-balance. However, regarding the health of these people, we note Marla Cone's article "Dozens of Words for Snow, None for Pollution," which appeared in the January–February 2005 issue of *Mother Jones*. The oceanic currents are such that pollutants become more concentrated in the Arctic Ocean, including notably mercury and chlorinated hydrocarbons such as PCBs. Thus, the marine life is impacted, and in turn the Inuit, who subsist on the bounty of seals and whales. The further consequence is that pregnant and nursing Inuit mothers pass this toxicity on to their offspring.)

In passing, we again mention medical anthropologist John Heinerman's book *Spritual Wisdom of the Native Americans*, published in 1989. He observes that the Indian tribes of the American Southwest have a very low cancer incidence (Heinerman, 1989b, pp. 133–135), as do the Indian tribes in northwestern Ontario.

Feedlot meat animals are commonly fed or injected with various chemicals, hormones, appetite stimulants, antibiotics, and sedatives, with residues showing up in the meat product that may be cancer causing (Walters, 1993, p. 143). Cows, as another example, may give leukemic milk, not to mention the various infections that may derive from cancer-causing microbes or viruses.

Also, the bacterial flora action in meat eaters' intestines can produce carcinogens, a process intensified by the consumption of fats. A result is that, as has been sometimes reported, the cancer incidence for those who eat meat, poultry, dairy products, and eggs is several times greater than for vegetarians.

Enter, therefore, the subject of diet and nutritional therapies.

*Prevention Magazine* once published a volume titled *The Encyclopedia of Common Diseases*, with a section devoted to cancer, and the chapters at the end of the section described several alternative treatments for cancer, including diet. These chapters included the Gerson Treatment, Insulin as per the Beale Treatment, Krebiozen, the Drosnes–Lazenby Treatment, and the Koch Treatment. Not much is heard about some of these therapies today, though at the time many successes were reported, and intriguing lines for research laid out.

The Gerson Therapy is regarded as an early forerunner in alternative dietary cancer treatments. Developed by Max Gerson, M.D., who wrote a book about it titled *A Cancer Therapy: Results of Fifty Cases*, published in 1958, the treatment has survived harassments, with an office in California and a clinic in Mexico. The diet essentially consists of drinking copious quantities of fresh vegetable juice from organic sources, coffee enemas for detoxification, and maintaining high potassium ratios as compared to sodium. A healthy liver was viewed as vital. The usual alternative medicine references have a chapter on the Gerson diet, and Walters, in particular, is skeptical about the high survival rates claimed for the Gerson Therapy (Walters, 1993, pp. 193, 194). Independent follow-up investigations report a recovery rate of the order of only 5%. If most patients seem to do well at the clinic, when they go home it is another story; the diet protocol is difficult to sustain at home.

The Gerson regimen is similar to most diets promoting good health, and to some that claim to be anticancer diets.

The chapter on the Koch Treatment in *The Encyclopedia of Common Diseases* illustrates the usual proceedings in harassing an alternative therapy out of existence. The Koch Treatment involved a substance called glyoxylide, which was believed to convert cancer-causing poisons into antitoxins that would eliminate the cancerous condition. In spite of positive testimony from and about patients who apparently had been cured, Dr. Koch was prosecuted by the FDA and a permanent injunction was made against Koch Laboratories. It is impossible to tell who may have been right and who may have been wrong. This is why a strong underlying and all-encompassing theory is necessary for explaining how alternative therapies work, backed by large-scale impartial clinical evidence.

It has been observed that lower food intake inhibits the developmental phases of cancer cells (Williams and Weisberger, in Amdur et al., 1991, p. 151), which is corroborated by medical folklore.

Additionally, it has been stated in the Williams and Weisberger reference that a restricted food intake "reduces the incidence of all neoplasms, but especially in endocrine-sensitive organs, and increases overall longevity."

## DIETARY EXTREMES

Vilhjalmur Stefansson, the famous explorer and chronicler of the Canadian Arctic, found that a person could survive very well on a strictly carnivorous diet if enough fat was present. The notable example was that of the Eskimos, and it was also concluded that no vitamin-C-containing fruits or vegetables are necessary, the diet being sufficient in itself. Or else a person can survive and do very well on a strictly vegetarian diet. According to Stefansson, it is the omnivorous diet, of meat along with vegetables and fruits, that apparently causes trouble, with sugar intake prominently mentioned.

His views and observations were first set forth in *Not by Bread Alone*, published in 1946, and later in an expanded version retitled *The Fat of the Land*. He makes the point that intestinal bacteria or flora that flourish on a mixed diet cannot survive on an all-meat diet, nor are they needed (Stefansson, 1956, p. 56). The same goes presumably for an all-vegetarian diet, as practiced for example by the Hunzas of Asia, who evidently do not need the particular intestinal flora required for an all-meat diet or a mixed diet.

Furthermore, Stefansson indicates that salted meat is a prime cause of scurvy, but that fresh or dried meats are sufficient in themselves to prevent scurvy. (The Eskimos dislike salt, and Stefansson himself was able to kick the habit.) He also was keen on fats as a hot-weather diet for the tropics, noting that the Eskimo dress is so warm and their dwellings are so well heated that they think they are in the tropics, anyway. He writes that cannibalism is motivated by the need for meat and fat, although others think it is a cultural matter. For one thing, vegetable fats or oils are readily available in the tropics, for example, the coconut palm and assorted nuts.

It may be mentioned, however, that Eskimos eat fresh berries in the summer months (Stefansson, 1956, p. 94). The North American Plains Indians usually mixed berries with pounded dried meat (or jerky) and fat to make (berry) pemmican, a wintertime staple stored in wrappings of rawhide, or parfleche. Otherwise, (plain) pemmican consisted of pounded meat only, mixed with fat. The Eskimos apparently made only the latter kind, relying instead on meat (with fat) exclusively during the winter months. Their entire vitamin needs were presumably met via meat.

(Stefansson devotes the last half of his book to pemmican and its history and variations, and its limitations and controversies, starting on page 178 in *Fat of the Land*. The debate is summarized in his concluding chapter, as of the date of publication.)

In the late 1950s or early 1960s there was a book published and promoted titled *Calories Don't Count*, which emphasized fats. For their trouble, the authors were prosecuted and convicted for fraud. Apparently no one referenced Stefansson's observations about the Eskimos. Nowadays, it seems, anything goes.

In another book, *Cancer: Disease of Civilization?* Stefansson recounted his experiences starting in 1906, whereby he initially found that the more remote or Stone Age Eskimos never had cancer. Only on acquiring the food habits of Western civilization did cancer appear, as well as tooth problems. The same remarks can be made for a vegetarian diet. An interesting aside is that circa 1840 it was reported that Paris had four times the cancer incidence as London (Stefansson, 1960, p. 28). The discrepancy was not explained except to suggest that perhaps Paris was four times more civilized than London! Attempts by Stefansson to obtain further information about cancer incidence in these and prior times were unsuccessful.

In a chapter titled "The Twentieth Century Forgets the Nineteenth," Stefansson quotes from John Cope's *Cancer: Civilization and Degeneration*, published in London in 1932. "Experimental cancer research has, in short, become so isolated and entrenched that, without being aware of it, the researcher now almost instinctively regards those who criticize his opinion, question his authority, or adopt other methods of working, not as fellow workers, but as amateurs, as 'outsiders,' or even as positive enemies .... " The situation hardly seems to have changed.

In a later chapter about the Hunzas titled "A Cancer-Free People of Asia," Stefansson cites the findings of Sir Robert McCarrison, who was stationed in northern India and studied the Hunza during the period 1904–1911, and was favorably impressed. (In succeeding years there were others, however, who were not.) The Hunzas were lactovegetarians, reportedly with amazing life spans. In a succeeding chapter on prevention, based on the Hunzas (and the Eskimos), it was concluded that cancer-free health could be attained in three key ways.

The first key is that in the months before birth, there should be a healthy mother eating healthy foods. The second key is prolonged breast feeding. The third key is to utilize fresh and raw foods with a minimum of processing (Stefansson extends this to include meats for an all-meat diet.)

It was also observed by Stefansson that a low cancer occurrence correlates directly with low appendicitis, constipation, and corpulence. At the same time, other diseases are avoided, which include arthritis, asthma, beriberi, caries (dental), colitis, diabetes, duodenal ulcers, epilepsy, gallstones, gastric ulcers, hypertension, night blindness, pellagra, rickets, and scurvy.

This sounds familiar in these modern times.

Thus, there is the suspicion that such diseases as hypothyroidism and diabetes correlate with cancer incidence. (Hypothyroidism denotes lower thyroid activity, and diabetes indicates lowered insulin activity, and thus could as well be called *hypoinulinism.*) For instance, in a book by Broda O. Barnes, M.D., and Lawrence Galton, titled *Hypothyroidism: The Unsuspected Illness*, it was indicated that transplanted cancers seldom "take" unless the thyroid gland is first removed, and Dr. Barnes found that his patients who underwent thyroid therapy had a far lower rate of cancer occurrence than expected (Barnes and Galton, *Hypothyroidism: The Unsuspected Illness*, pp. 242, 245). It may be added that the immune system will destroy transplanted cells — normal or cancerous — unless it is suppressed. And evidently the immune system is suppressed by the absence of thyroid activity (in terms of thyroxine, the hormone released by the thyroid gland). The effect of hypothyroidism in compromising the immune system against infectious diseases was, in fact, a major thesis of the book.

With regard to diabetes, and insulin levels, the glycolytic pathway is regulated or modulated by two opposing pancreatic hormones, namely glucagon and insulin. An increase in the activity of the one decreases the activity of the other. It turns out that glycolysis (via the action or reduced action of the enzyme pyruvate kinase) is inhibited by reduced insulin activity, or by increased glucagon activity — that is, by the diabetic condition (Blair, in Venziale, 1981). Moreover, the nonessential amino acid alanine supports the inhibition of pyruvate kinase by enhancing glucagon activity at the expense of insulin activity, and has been denoted a biomarker for anaerobic glycolysis. It may be added that anaerobic glycolysis is the principal pathway for cancer cell metabolism (Guerra et al. 1993). There is the inference, therefore, that alanine and insulin levels may be indicators for, and may even be involved in, cancer progression or regression, and this implication has been suggested in cancer studies.

(The distinguishing conventions are that hormones are secreted from glands, whereas enzymes are formed in cells. In the endocrine glands, such as the thyroid, pituitary, adrenals, and pancreas, the secretions are made internally, directly into the bloodstream. In the exocrine glands, such as the salivary glands, the secretions are introduced externally, exiting through a duct. Inasmuch as glands have cells, the distinction may be viewed as only a convenience.)

As Stefansson indicated, there is an empirical correlation between cancer and many other diseases. Undoubtedly, many effects are interrelated or counterposed in the overall complexity of the body's biochemistry. Although this complexity may certainly be acknowledged, cancer victims would undoubtedly settle for a simple and inexpensive cure or control.

## IRON IN THE DIET

An ubiquitous fact of life is inorganic iron in the diet, consumed intentionally but mostly unintentionally. It is found on the label of many or most prepared foods, generally as reduced iron, indicating the reduced, or ferrous, state as opposed to the oxidized, or ferric state. Moreover, it commonly appears in many multinutritional supplements, and is routinely prescribed for patients who test, or appear, anemic, presumably to counter so-called iron-deficient anemia. The conventional wisdom is that various ferrous salts — namely, the sulfate, gluconate, fumarate, succinate, but also others — act against iron-deficiency anemia, although toxic effects are acknowledged (Hillman, in Hardman et al., 2001, pp. 1323, 1325). It should be emphasized that iron-deficiency anemia is different from vitamin-B12 - and folic-acid-deficient anemia, or pernicious anemia. There is also what is called sickle cell anemia, caused by a mutant hemoglobin (Voet and Voet, 1995, pp. 123, 124). It is prevalent in African countries, but it has been observed and confirmed that the sickle cell trait confers resistance to malaria. In fact, there are various other abnormal hemoglobins (Voet and Voet, 1995, p. 235). For example, *thalassemias* (from the Greek word *thalessia*, for sea) commonly occur in the regions surrounding the Mediterranean Sea (Voet and Voet, 1995, p. 1146).

Now, the *Physicians' Desk Reference* classifies inorganic ferrous sulfate as being toxic, but it is the iron source most commonly added to dietary supplements. Further, it is doubtful if inorganic iron actually corrects iron-deficiency anemia, and its poisonous nature ensures diarrhea as the body tries to rid itself of the toxin. The ubiquitous use of ferrous sulfate and other ferrous salts in multivitamins and enriched flour remains unfathomable, except maybe that this is an easy and profitable way to get rid of the stuff, a by-product from, say, sulfuric acid manufacture based on iron sulfide.

Addressing the toxic effects more fully in a chapter "Clinical Toxicology," the five phases of iron toxicity have been described (Rumack and Lovejoy, in Amdur et al., 1991, p. 937). The first phase, lasting from 30 minutes to 2 hours after ingestion, is characterized by lethargy, restlessness, the vomiting of blood, abdominal pain, and bloody diarrhea. Necrosis of the gastrointestinal tissues occurs. In the second phases there is an apparent recovery, followed by the third phase, occurring 2 to 12 hours after the first phase. Shock, metabolic acidosis (acidity of the blood and tissues), cyanosis (bluish appearance of the skin), and fever are the symptoms. In the fourth phase, occurring 2 to 4 days after ingestion, hepatic (liver) necrosis may be evidenced. The fifth phase, occurring from 2 to 4 weeks after ingestion, is characterized by gastrointestinal obstruction, a result of changes in the gastric tissue involving scarring and healing. Thus, "oral ingestion of iron is a potentially fatal occurrence." The ingestion of 30 mg/kg of body weight is cause for alarm and hospital admission. A counteractive procedure is the use of a stomach pump, and possibly a detoxification agent such as deferoxamine, or desferrioxamine, may be used, although this is controversial.

(A dosage of 30 mg/kg is about 1300 mg per 100 lb of body weight. However, doses smaller than this set value can presumably also be cause for alarm, because of dosage frequency and cumulative dosage considerations.)

Another name encountered for an iron-chelating agent is Desferal. Naturally occurring substances that have been cited as counters include flavonoids, such as quercetin and baicalin.

Incidentally, the iron-scavenging agent desferrioxamine B, or desferrioxamine B mesylate, is derived from a growth factor called coprogen (Bohonos, in Swain, 1972, p. 181; the term *coprogen* is not in common everyday use, but will show up in a few references on Medline or Medscape.) For the record, the term *growth factor* denotes a specific substance that must be present in a growth medium to permit cell multiplication, and hence there is a connection with cancer. These growth factors are polypeptides, such as c-sis (*PDFG* gene), *IL-3* gene, and *EGF* gene, that are encoded by a family of genes; and some are cancer-inducing proto-oncogenes. On the other hand, there is the well-known tumor-suppressor gene denoted as *p53* that has been found to be altered in certain kinds of carcinomas and sarcomas.

(Interestingly, the anticancer agents or antineoplastons as used in the Burzynski therapy are mainly polypeptides. And polypeptides were involved in the anticancer therapy described in Stephen S. Hall's *A Commotion in the Blood* (1997a), cited elsewhere. There are myriad different polypeptides, however, for the combinations and permutations of the amino acids in a proteinaceous molecular chain are almost without end, as Hall spells out. However, some are beneficial, and some are not.)

Iron overload, in the extreme and sometimes deadly form called hemochromatosis (or hemachromatosis), may be chronic or acute. The word is that many people already have iron overload in their blood. Information can be found on the Internet, for example, at the Web site of the Iron Overload Diseases Association, Inc., at 433 Westwood Drive, North Palm Beach, FL 33408, 561-840-8512. Another resource is the Hemochromatosis Foundation, POB 8569, Albany, NY 12208-0569, 518-489-0972. Iron overload has been associated with bacterial/viral infections, for instance, and it had been found that iron may cross the brain's blood barrier, resulting in problems ranging from the neurological to the psychological, including Alzheimer's and dementia. The more usual means of lowering iron overload is to withdraw blood via a phlebotomy, although the chelating agent know as EDTA (ethylenediamine-tetraacetic acid) has also been cited as a means, interfacing with the subject of chelation therapy. The latter is a therapy provided notably by members of the American College for the Advancement of Medicine, or ACAM, who are in the main M.D.s or D.O.s.

As for the disposition of iron in the blood and what part ends up as hemoglobin and what part does not, in the *Encyclopedia of Chemistry,* fourth edition, there is a section "Iron" (in "Biological Systems"), with a subsection "Iron Absorption." An estimate furnished is that a (normal) male weighing 155 lb (about 70 kg) will have about 3.5 g of iron. About 64% of this is hemoglobin in the peripheral blood, and 2.5% in the bone marrow. Four percent is present as myoglobin, which is also involved in oxygen transport and storage. Another 13% exists as ferritin, and 16% as hemosiderin, both being storage forms. Very small amounts occur in the cellular cytochrome and in the enzyme catalase.

Iron is absorbed directly into the blood mainly in the ferrous state. It is taken into the intestinal mucosa cells and converted to ferritin, which is the combination of a protein with iron, and may be called a metalloprotein. After the cell becomes saturated, the ferritin is transferred to plasma. Previously thought to be absorption limiting, such has been found not to be the case. Some substances such as vitamin C enhance absorption; others such as phosphates and carbonates form insoluble iron compounds and reduce absorption.

Upon entering the bloodstream the iron is immediately bound by a plasma protein denoted as a $\beta_1$-globulin, called *transferrin (siderophilin)*. The transferrin-bound iron is utilized for hemoglobin formation via reticulocytes.

The following quote is provided from the cited reference. "If a small amount of ionized iron is injected intravenously, it is bound by this transferrin, which may be completely saturated. If the binding limit is exceeded, ionized iron exhibits toxic effects." In other words, it can be said the body's bloodstream is not meant to tolerate extraneous iron, meaning iron overload.

Iron losses are about 1 mg daily through various excretions. It is noted that iron storage occurs in the form of ferritin and hemosiderin in the reticulo-enothlelian  cells of the liver, spleen, and bone marrow, and in the parenchymal cells of the liver.

Hemoglobin is the respiratory protein for the red blood cells, and contains about 94% protein (globin) and 6% heme, which has the molecular formula $C_{34}H_{32}FeN_4O_4$. Each molecule combines with one molecule of oxygen to form oxyhemoglobin.

Medscape, for instance, furnishes abstracts (and articles) about dietary iron and cancer. The Web site http://www.ironoverload.org/hippocrates.html, in an article titled "The Shocking Truth About Iron" dated Nov–Dec 1995, described a case of a lady who had been on iron supplements for years, and whose liver became swollen; the subsequent biopsy was clean, "except that it was brimming with iron."

Medical laboratories can ordinarily analyze for iron levels. A fact sheet from the Iron Overload Diseases Association speaks of total iron binding capacity (TIBC) and serum iron (SI). Dividing the SI by the TIBC gives the percentage of transferrin saturation (TS), for which the normal range is said to be 12–45%. (A higher value, say, 60%, involves an increased cancer risk, and an increased mortality risk.) The same blood sample can be used to determine serum ferritin, whose normal range is 5 to 150. The normal range for serum iron is a nominal 40–155, measured in $\mu$g/dal (micrograms per decaliter). A value of, say, 200 $\mu$g/dal is cause for concern, with some authorities favoring a lower value of about 5, provided it is feasible.

In the aforementioned fact sheet, mention is made of iron-loading anemia, which signifies low hemoglobin.

Turning now to chemotherapy, one of the misconceptions about it is that its disastrous side effects are just temporary, being easily reversible after stopping the therapy — that is, if it is ever stopped. The patient, however, only recovers very slowly, and incompletely, from some of the more obvious side effects, with other hidden side effects not showing up until years later — perhaps along with a reemergence of the cancer. As one example of the convoluted thinking that goes on, the patient may be prescribed a lot of inorganic iron such as ferrous sulfate to counteract the anemia. The iron itself causes gastrointestinal problems at the least, however, without any positive effects against anemia. If the patient is ever able to overcome the anemia, it will be in other ways, for example, from natural foods containing organic iron, a little bit at a time.

In any event, a cancer patient undergoing conventional cytotoxic chemotherapy, and who develops iron-deficiency anemia, may wish to question the doctor's prescription of large or massive doses of ferrous sulfate. (Thus, in the case of colon cancer, say, would an intestinal blockage be due to the cancerous mass or due to an excessive ingestion of ferrous sulfate?)

The addition of iron in the form of ferrous sulfate to so many foods is partly due to the influence of the chemical industry, for instance, paralleling the production of sulfuric acid from ferrous sulfide or pyrite, FeS. Normally, the once-conventional air-roasting of pyrite ore yields sulfur dioxide as the main product, which is further converted catalytically to sulfur trioxide which, when dissolved in water — or into recycled dilute sulfuric acid — further forms sulfuric acid, $H_2SO_4$, sometimes considered the backbone of the inorganic chemical industry. This once-common industrial process was compromised by the combustion of elemental sulfur obtained via other means, notably from underground sulfur deposits using the Frasch process involving the injection of superheated steam, and from sour crude oils or natural gas containing hydrogen sulfide. In any event, the roasting of pyrite in excess air will also yield iron oxide as red ferric oxide, $Fe_2O_3$ in a concentrated form as the other product or coproduct (and which itself is a common-enough constituent of the Earth).

Alternately, on roasting FeS in the presence of limited air, the first product is ferrous sulfate. (Ferrous sulfate occurs as the mineral *melanterite* or "copperas," from the atmospheric oxidation of native pyrites.) However, on roasting with further air, it converts to ferric oxide plus sulfur dioxide and sulfur trioxide, depending upon the reaction conditions.

However, when more purity is desired, the route is to heat pure iron with dilute sulfuric acid to yield ferrous sulfate and evolve hydrogen. (The evolved hydrogen can in turn be used to reduce ferric oxide back to ferrous oxide, which reacts with sulfuric acid to form ferrous sulfate.) All this and more is set forth in the multivolume *Encyclopedia of Chemical Reactions*. Other details are furnished, for instance, in F. Sherwood Taylor's classic *Inorganic and Theoretical Chemistry* (1939) and J.W. Mellor's *A Comprehensive Treatise on Inorganic and Theoretical Chemistry* (1922–1937).

## GARLIC AND ALLICIN AND OTHER SULFUR-CONTAINING COMPOUNDS AS ANTICANCER AGENTS

There is renewed interest in garlic and its compounds owing to their anticancer, antibiotic, and heart-beneficial properties. Of prime significance is the fact that the organic sulfur compound called allicin is formed from the vegetable garlic by the action between the inherent compound alliin and the enzyme allinase, both naturally present in garlic, and allicin has been listed as an inhibitor for lactate dehydrogenase, the main distinguishing enzyme for cancer cell metabolism (e.g., Hoffman, 1997, 1999a). Garlic itself is a folkloric treatment against cancer. A few brands of garlic tablets claim an equivalent allicin content, for example, Garlicin®, Garlique®, and Garlinase®. The allicin is formed after ingestion, as the tablets contain a dry, powdered mixture of alliin and allinase, and are sealed away from moisture until use.

For a review of the subject, see a chapter called "Chemoprevention of Gastrointestinal Cancer in Animals by Naturally Occurring Organosulfur Compounds in Allium Vegetables," written by Michael J. Wargovich, Hiromichi Sumiyoshi, and Allan Baier, in *Vitamins and Minerals in the Prevention and Treatment of Cancer*, edited by Maryce M. Jacobs. The cancer-inhibiting effects of garlic and garlic-derived agents, particularly diallyl sulfide (DAS) and S-allyl-cysteine (SAC), and also garlic oil, were of special concern. Allicin, however, was not discussed as such.

(Vegetables of the genus *Allium* include the onion. The eye-watering property of onions is due to a gaseous compound named thiopropanal S-oxide. This sulfur compound is formed and released when onion cells are disturbed, causing a particular enzyme to contact an indigenous sulfur compound, yielding thiopropanal S-oxide. Do any or all of these onion-derived compounds have anticancer properties? Another interesting angle, previously described, is that onions contain carrageenan, a chemical compound that is a powerful anticoagulant, as described on page 328 of Bruce

Chatwin's *What Am I Doing Here*. Ingestion of a couple of pounds of onions was said to have dissolved a life-threatening blood clot; but, unfortunately, onions cannot be patented.)

In the same volume, in a chapter by Carmia G. Borek, the antioxidant role of selenium and vitamin E, and vitamin C, is discussed, a fact that is now common knowledge. A chapter by Richard F. Branda on the effect of folic acid deficiency indicates that low levels are found in cancer patients, but, contrarily, increasing folic acid intake may accelerate tumor growth. Accordingly, research on folic acid antagonists as chemotherapeutic agents is under way, although folate deficiency may influence the spread of cancer; altogether, a mixed bag. In a chapter on potassium vs. cancer by Maryce M. Jacobs and Roman J. Pienta, epidemiological and follow-up studies have shown that increased potassium intake decreases cancer risk, whereas increased sodium increases cancer risk. Even more important than levels is the potassium to sodium ratio — the higher the better. Also noted is that potassium levels are higher in normal tissues than in cancerous tissues, with the possible exception of leukemic bone marrow. It was concluded, however, that potassium-rich diets appear to be of questionable merit in curing malignancies.

For more about the medical aspects of garlic, there is the volume *Garlic: The Science and Therapeutic Applications of* Allium sativum *L. and Related Species*, second edition, edited by Heinrich P. Koch and Larry D. Lawson. A list of 2580 references is appended, 2240 of which deal with garlic. A chapter on "The Composition of Garlic Cloves and Processed Garlic" by Larry D. Lawson contains tables listing the general breakdown of the composition of garlic cloves, and provides a bar chart illustrating that garlic has many times the sulfur content of other vegetables, and nearly four times that of onions, broccoli, and cauliflower. Interestingly, apricots have about as much sulfur as the latter three. A more detailed account is presented in the first edition of Hoffman's *Cancer and the Search for Selective Biochemical Inhibitors* (1999a), some of which is paraphrased as follows.

There are nearly 40 organic chemical compounds in garlic, known or anticipated, not including vitamins and minerals. Probably the most significant is alliin and its conversion to allicin by the action of the enzyme allinase (or alliinase), and also compounds called the γ-glutamylcysteines, which are precursors of alliin. Alliin itself has no antibiotic activity per se unless converted to allicin, and allicin is the parent compound of the diallyl sulfides, the characteristic odor-producing compounds. Allicin belongs to a class called thiosulfinates (THS). Its precursor alliin is formed from still other compounds, as indicated, and there are complex pathways for the biogenesis of garlic's indigenous sulfur compounds, starting initially with the sulfate ion (Lawson, in Koch and Lawson, 1996, pp. 72–75). The precursors for alliin in mature plants are concentrated in the bulbs, but in premature plants most may be found in the leaves and stems.

Dried garlic has a sulfur content of 1.0% of its dry weight, and the dried product is about 35% of its fresh weight (Lawson, in Koch and Lawson, 1996, p. 41). About 72% of the sulfur compounds consist of alliin, allicin, and the two principal K-glutamylcysteines. The known sulfur compounds in garlic comprise about 86% of the sulfur content.

Of prime interest are the thiosulfinates, which include allicin, or diallyl thiosulfinate, with the formula $CH_2=CHCH_2–SS(=O)–CH_2CH=CH_2$, for which several optional scientific names exist (Lawson, in Koch and Lawson, 1996, pp. 40–42). The stability of allicin depends on the temperature and solvent and is generally longer than the half-life of a few hours that is sometimes reported. At room temperature, the reference states that pure allicin has a half-life of 16 hours, and in water a half-life of 30 to 40 days. At a temperature of 70°C, allicin in water (ice) had no change in 2 years, but the pure compound had a half-life of only 25 days at the same temperature.

Cooking affects garlic's sulfur compounds in that heat inactivates enzymes (Lawson, in Koch and Lawson, 1996, pp. 68, 69). Thus, allinase (or alliinase) becomes inactivated by cooking, which prevents the formation of allicin and other thiosulfinates. Boiling unpeeled whole garlic cloves for 15 minutes completely deactivates allinase, although there is a small amount of alliin converted owing to the cloves bumping into each other during heating. The small allicin content is in turn converted to diallyl trisulfide for the most part, with smaller amounts of the di- and trisulfides also produced; thus, even boiled garlic can produce garlic breath.

The thiosulfinates (e.g., allicin) are very reactive, combining with reducing agents and undergoing spontaneous reactions in various solvents and media (Lawson, in Koch and Lawson, 1996, pp. 59–65). The reaction products are more stable than the thiosulfinates but still contain the thioallyl groups (S-allyl) or thiomethyl groups, and are active components in garlic oils.

At room temperature the thiosulfinates (e.g., allicin) convert to various diallyl and allyl sulfides, etc., which may be accelerated by heating. Pure allicin itself is an unstable oily liquid, lasting less than 20 hours at room temperature (equivalent to say a half-life of a few hours, as has been reported). The decomposition products include various organic sulfides, and it is also been observed that allicin is very reactive with the amino acid cysteine.

Thus, allicin has been found to inhibit a large number of enzymes *in vitro* if they contain cysteine at the active sites, but otherwise very few (Lawson, in Koch and Lawson, 1996, p. 65). The reference further states that "many of the explanations given for the biological effects of garlic focus on the ability of allicin to react with sulfhydryl enzymes," whatever the latter may be. Moreover, allicin was found to act against cholesterol and triglyceride synthesis.

Whether or not lactate dehydrogenase contains cysteine at the active sites is apparently not known; still, allicin has been reported to inhibit this particular enzyme, according to the later edition of Zollner's *Handbook of Enzyme Inhibitors* (1993).

In Koch and Lawson (1996), in a chapter "Therapeutic Effects and Applications of Garlic and its Preparations" by Hans D. Reuter, Heinrich P. Koch, and Larry D. Lawson, there is a section on "Anticancer Effects." The beneficial role of garlic in treating cancer is traced back to ancient times, and is backed by recent epidemiologic studies. Statistical studies confirm that cancer occurs least in countries where garlic and onions are consumed. Examples cited include the French Provence, Italy, the Netherlands, the Balkan countries, Egypt, India, and China. A specific citation (1936) elicits a cancer-inhibiting action for leek or *Allium* plants, for reasons unknown. The beneficial stimulation of gastric secretions and the restoration of intestinal flora may be involved. Thumbs up were given for black or green tea to be taken along with garlic.

Clinical trials against advanced cancer are apparently in abeyance, although one study was at least reported (Reuter, Koch, and Lawson, in Koch and Lawson, 1996, p. 176). Conducted in Russia, a garlic juice preparation was injected both intravenously and intramuscularly. There were 35 patients involved, with various cancers of the lung, cervix, stomach, lower lip, mammary gland, and larynx, and one patient had leukemia. Of the 35 patients, 26 were said to show positive results of varying degree, but complete healing did not occur.

A more impressive case, reported in a 1993 issue of the journal *Neurochirurgia*, was that of a man whose pituitary gland had shrunk by half on a regime of 5–7 g of fresh garlic daily over a 5-month period. This was said to be an anomaly as this kind of cancer had been found to regress only by the use of chemotherapy or surgery.

The intravenous or intramuscular dosages of garlic juice administered in the previous cases were only over a relatively short period. If administered over a period of months — as with conventional chemotherapy — the results could have been dramatically more favorable. Furthermore, the allicin content was not monitored, which can vary greatly with the degree of freshness.

The reference emphasizes that, on an epidemiologic basis, garlic consumption correlates with a reduced risk for cancer, especially gastrointestinal cancer (Reuter, Koch, and Lawson, in Koch and Lawson, 1996, pp. 176–178). This was confirmed by what was called the "Iowa Women's Health Study," where garlic was found to be the only food that showed a lowering of cancer risk. The foregoing study did not include onions, but other studies conclude that onions and other *Allium* species lower the gastrointestinal cancer risk. Another study, in the Netherlands, however, showed garlic supplements (tablets) to be ineffective against stomach, colon, rectum, lung, and breast cancer risk. The reference notes, however, that there are garlic supplements and there are garlic supplements.

Early *in vivo* experiments (1913) showed that garlic and its compounds acted against tumors in mice, with similar results obtained by others (Reuter, Koch, and Lawson, in *Garlic*, pp. 178–186). Not only could tumor growth be inhibited, but alliin as freshly obtained from garlic bulbs and directly injected into rat sarcomas, resulted in reduction and dissipation. Similar results were obtained for intramuscular injections. Others, however, reported otherwise. On the other hand, allicin deactivated ehrlich ascites tumor cells, and also deactivated cells of Yoshida sarcoma (a mammary tumor). Other examples are described in the reference, with the note that fresh garlic neutralizes cancer cell virulence without compromising the immune response, whereby animals at least become immune to untreated tumor cells.

A further discovery is that garlic and other vegetables contain a polypeptide of unknown structure that acts as an enzyme inhibitor (Reuter, Koch, and Lawson, in Koch and Lawson, 1996, p. 179; Lawson, in Koch and Lawson, 1996, p. 79). Certain polypeptides are assumed or presumed to possess anticancer activity, as per the Burzynski therapy.

Moreover, topical applications of garlic oil, which contains allyl and diallyl sulfides, were found to inhibit skin cancer (Reuter, Koch, and Lawson, in Koch and Lawson, 1996, p. 180).

The anticancer action of garlic may be due to thiosulfinates (of which allicin is the main example) that inhibit proteolytic enzymes in human malignancies (Reuter, Koch, and Lawson, in Koch and Lawson, 1996, p. 181). Also, garlic extract inhibits pyruvate dehydrogenase (involved in the formation of pyruvic acid or pyruvate), thereby interrupting cellular respiration, which may or may not be desirable. Anyway, the authors conclude that "enzyme inhibition may thus be generally considered as the mechanism whereby the active components in garlic exert their tumor-inhibiting effect."

As for the inhibiting action of garlic oil, onion oil, and diallyl sulfide on skin cancers, there is evidently a beneficial action on epidermis cells. As for stomach and colon cancer, it is advanced that the antimicrobial effect of the thiosulfinates in garlic inhibits some of the less desirable gut flora. Other findings are repeated as follows:

- The Ames test has been used to demonstrate that garlic has antimutagenic properties.
- Garlic has been found to interfere with cell division or mitosis.
- The selenium and germanium compounds present in garlic may have an anticancer effect, although it is suspected that the concentrations are too small.

There are other mechanisms advanced in the reference for the anticancer action of garlic and its sulfur-containing compounds. And still other beneficial findings are furnished in the reference. Future studies should include clinical trials with humans (for example, as mentioned in Hoffman, 1999, p. 377).

The foregoing brings up the matter of whether there are any toxic properties, and it has been found that there are acute, subacute, and chronic toxicities (Koch, in Koch and Lawson, 1996, pp. 221–224). Thus, allicin and *Allium* plants, including onions, become markedly hepatotoxic when administered in large doses over a long period. Diallyl sulfide administered intravenously (in alcohol) at high dosages produced cardiac arrest in frogs. Also, rabbits were found to contract myosis (contraction of the pupil of the eye), blood pressure drop, and increasing heart rate.

Aqueous garlic extracts given to rats intraperitoneally, increased lactate dehydrogenase activity in the liver, which, interestingly, may signal carcinogenesis.

Diphenylamine is a compound occurring in onions but not garlic, and is said to have nephrotoxic (kidney-toxic) properties. Garlic oil, for instance, was found to be lethal for fasted rats, but not for fed rats.

For less technical information about garlic's medicinal properties, there is John Heinerman's *The Healing Benefits of Garlic: From Pharaohs to Pharmacists* (1993). Another volume for the general reader is Stephen Fulder's *The Garlic Book: Nature's Powerful Healer* (1997). The latter makes mention of garlic as an anticancer agent, and describes some of the studies undertaken with garlic and its compounds that turned out positive. In fact, over 100 studies have been carried out involving cells, animals, and tissues, and the consensus is that garlic, garlic oil, allicin, the sulfides, and other garlic compounds are anticancer agents, and also protect against DNA damage. The caution, nevertheless, is that garlic serves as a preventive, not a cure.

In many Third World countries, notably in China, garlic is regarded as a cancer preventive. For example, two neighboring counties in China were compared, where the people in the one county ate about six cloves a day, and in the other, none. In the former, the stomach cancer incidence was about 3.5 per 100,000 population, and in the latter about 40 per 100,000, or over 10 times greater.

Fulder adds the well-known fact that garlic is not only an antibiotic, but serves to cleanse the body of toxic heavy metals. Cysteine, for example, is specific to removing lead, and even mercury, and in Bulgaria there is a commercial garlic preparation called Satal for these purposes. Additionally, garlic provides a way to cleanse the body of food additives and solvents.

Fulder declares that garlic is eminently safe, which its daily consumption by millions of people confirms; 20 g or 7 cloves of garlic per day is the standard, although 20 cloves per day has no ill effects; similarly for garlic oil. Only at levels of 300 to 500 cloves of garlic are toxic effects produced.

An interesting article by Eric Block of the State University of New York, Albany, appeared in the March 1985 issue of the *Scientific American*. Titled "The Chemistry of Garlic and Onions," it confirmed many of the previous references and noted that extracts from both garlic and onions are not only antibacterial and antifungal, but are also antithrombotic — inhibiting the aggregation of blood platelets into thrombi, a process also involved in fibrin. The beneficial effects of garlic can be traced back to Egypt's Codex Ebers, circa 1550 B.C. Another item of interest is the mixture sometimes known as Four Thieves Vinegar, composed of garlic macerated in wine. The concoction was said to make gravediggers immune to an outbreak of plague that occurred in France in 1721. It is still available under the name *vinaigre des quatre voleurs.*

Onions are also discussed by Brock, who notes a close chemical relationship with garlic and with alliin, but onions possess a variant that brings tears to an onion slicer. And if garlic and its compounds are anticancer, so is onion.

Lastly, we cite Joseph Mitchell's *Up in the Old Hotel*, a collection of stories about past events in and around New York City and its offshore waters. These stories originally appeared mostly in *The New Yorker* circa the 1930s and 1940s, and Mitchell's reportage was described in the *Chicago-Sun Times* as "so vivid, so real, that it comes out like fiction of the highest order." In a chapter titled "A Spism and a Spasm," Mitchell introduces a garrulous old street preacher named James Jefferson Davis Hall, an ordained Episcopal priest who had migrated from Alabama to New York City. Hall's dinner consisted of "an onion, a bulb of garlic, and a head of cabbage, all raw." No information about well-being, sickness, or lifespan was furnished.

However, Mitchell has a series of chapters about Old Mr. Flood, who was 93 years and intended to live to 115. Mr. Flood's diet was composed of finfish and shellfish, which was not only good to eat, but "an elixir." Mr. Flood hung around the Fulton Street fish market, a whiff of which he said would knock a cold in its tracks. He also told about an old dray horse that was surreptitiously fed oysters and became uncontrollable. In fact, for the few in the know, horse racing was occasionally fixed, reportedly by feeding one of the horses a batch of oysters ahead of time.

Speaking further of garlic, in a brief section about laetrile, garlic is disparagingly cited as an alternative health product in T. Colin Campbell's *The China Study*, as assisted by Thomas M. Campbell II (Campbell, 2005, p. 252). Mention is made of pangamic acid, various bee concoctions, and of zinc supplements, which also may have no apparent benefit.

(Mention was made that animal studies have shown laetrile to be ineffective against cancer, but *in vivo* animal tests generally employ mice, which are simply different from the human animal, as are cattle, etc. And even human individuals vary because of biochemical individuality.)

In fact, the aforementioned study is generally against vitamin supplements per se, with the possible exception of vitamins B12 and D (Campbell, 2005, pp. 94, 95, 215, 228, 229, 242, 269, 270, 288). Vitamins A, C, and E are also given short shrift. It is emphasized that the nutritional supplement industry, as well as the pharmaceutical industry, makes huge profits. Thus, natural foods are considered the ultimate source of vitamins and minerals.

(The counterargument can be made, however, that if supplements make the individual feel better, or mitigate the symptoms of an illness, why put them down? Thus, in times past, it was argued that scientific studies showed that the bumblebee could not fly — but fly it did. The argument can also be made that natural foods may be low in vitamins or minerals, say, from depleted soils, and may also be contaminated with pesticides and the like. The claims and opposing claims are not likely to be resolved any time soon, if ever.)

*The China Study*, however, documents an epidemiologic investigation of major importance and magnitude. As the study was conducted among the Chinese, the population was more or less homogeneous, without any other nationalities or races that could introduce genetic aberrations. It should be emphasized, moreover, that the study was not directed toward cures but, rather, toward what should be the healthiest lifestyles, or in other words, toward what may be called prevention or chemoprevention, but with the emphasis on natural food sources rather than pharmaceuticals.

In Chapter 4 of the book, the variations in cancer rates among these Chinese counties are set forth, and they vary massively (e.g., Campbell, 2005, p. 71). Thus, for all cancers the comparative rates for males (M) varied from 35 to 721 and for females (F) from 35 to 491. Other variations are as follows: nasopharynx: (M) 0–75, (F) 0–26; esophagus: (M) 1–435, (F) 0–286; stomach: (M) 6–386, (F) 2–141; liver: (M) 7–248, (F) 3–67; colorectal: (M) 2–67, (F) 2–61; lung: (M) 3–59, (F) 0–26; breast: (M) to, (F) "0"–20. These wide variations provided dramatic means for comparison and correlation — in terms of environmental/lifestyle factors rather than genetics.

The second chapter of the book introduces the subject of proteins, and whereas animal proteins have heretofore been considered the ideal source, the study concludes otherwise: there are vegetable proteins that are more desirable, especially the lowly peanut (a legume, sometimes called groundnut). This source is compromised by the moldy presence of aflatoxin (AF), a known carcinogen. Analyses showed high levels in commercial peanuts, but not in the whole peanuts as usually bought. The thought was that the high-grade peanuts were sold whole for consumption as is, obviously the less desirable (and moldy) peanuts were made into commercial peanut butter. (A potential solution, of course, is to grind your own peanut butter from high-grade whole peanuts as found in health food stores.)

In the book's third chapter, titled "Turning Off Cancer," the correlation is made with protein type, and it was found that the protein casein occurring in cow's milk could be carcinogenic, whereas the wheat protein gluten was much less so. Soy protein was also more beneficial. Moreover, the presence of aflatoxin in these proteins contributed markedly to cancer initiation and growth.

In Chapter 4, "Lessons from China," the connection is made between animal fat consumption and increased cancer rates. A section on fiber stresses its importance. And as for antioxidants, the colorful vegetables signify their presence, including the anticancer carotenoids. Complex carbohydrates are beneficial, as opposed to the refined variety, including the ubiquitous refined sugars. The Atkins Diet of high protein consumption is pummeled, as is the South Beach Diet to a lesser extent (Campbell, 2005, pp. 95–97, 223).

The Nurses' Health Study is characterized as generating much confusion and misinformation (Campbell, 2005, p. 272ff). This critique is directed mostly toward the Nurses' Health Study findings that dietary (animal) fat and fiber did not relate to breast cancer risk. For still other criticisms of the nurses' study, consult Chapter 14 of the book.

The concluding chapters have the following titles: "The 'Science' of Industry" "Government: Is it for the People?" and "Big Medicine: Whose Health Are They Protecting?"

Signals of cancer formation include blood clotting times or coagulation disorders, as set forth by John Boik in *Cancer and Natural Medicine: A Textbook of Basic Science and Clinical Research*, for they can be related to angiogenesis, the formation of a vascular support system for tumor growth — the network of arteries, veins, and capillaries within the tumor (Boik, 1996, p. 25). The Boik reference also mentions clinical tests in China using garlic preparations on advanced cancer patients, with considerable improvement, but apparently no cures (Boik, 1996, p. 29). It did not specifically bring up the subject of allicin or other garlic compounds as inhibitors for lactate dehydrogenase.

## ABERRATIONS

There is the qualification that enthusiasm for a particular substance or substances should be tempered by the fact that the processes of digestion and assimilation may affect the biochemical nature of ingested substances. Of course, if it works, it works.

One of the mysteries is why some patients recover, whereas others do not, not only in the case of cancer, but with other diseases as well, or even regarding the effects of toxins. There is indeed a difference in the biochemical demands among individuals. Thus, it has been established that the vitamin requirements for different individuals will vary widely, sometimes by orders of magnitude.

A common-enough problem, moreover, is that in testing bioactive agents, what works *in vitro* may not work *in vivo*, or vice versa. And similar divergences may occur for clinical tests, which may not agree with the results of laboratory or animal tests. These kinds of discrepancies are noted, for instance, in the chapter by Suffness and Pezzuto in Volume 6 of the previously cited *Methods in Plant Biochemistry* (Hostettmann, 1991).

Also, there is the well-known fact that the bioactivity of a given plant or herbal species varies with the geographical location, the season, even the time of day, and with the plant part, for example, leaves vs. stems vs. roots. Moreover, in marketing, substitutions may occur, by design or by accident, for plant identification can be tricky.

Another puzzle is that some substances, in low dosages, may act as anticancer agents, whereas in larger dosages they may in themselves become cancer causing.

## IMMUNITY

Another line of investigation that is being actively pursued is to try to make a person's immune system recognize and destroy cancer cells. This work is described by Stephen S. Hall in the April 1997 issue of the *Atlantic Monthly*, and later in a book that deals mainly with melanoma. Ordinarily, in a given individual, cancer cells closely mimic the normal cells from which they originate, and cannot be distinguished by the individual's immune system, no matter how healthy it is. (However, cancer cells introduced from another person would be immediately recognized and killed off, for the same reason that organ transplants are rejected unless the immune system is suppressed.) The desired action is similar to that which occurs with what is called a "major histocompatibility complex," or MHC molecule. This molecule will transport an antigen from the cell interior to the cell surface, which in turn serves to activate the immune system. The immune system, comprising the T cells or white blood cells or lymphocytes, then perforates and destroys the cell. The trick is to determine the one particular antigen, from the huge number of possibilities, in the cancer cell that will trigger the immune system.

Interestingly, in the above-described work the immune-stimulating antigen was eventually found to be a certain peptide chain of nine amino acids.

Among the recent developments in bioactive plant medicines is the preparation, purification, and use of the juice from the Venus flytrap, *Dionaea muscipula*, of the family Droseraceae, or Sundew Family, which Charles Darwin called "the most wonderful plant in the world." This usage has been described by Morton Walker in the November 1997 issue of the *Townsend Letter for Doctors and Patients*. The preparation, with the trademark name Carnivora®, was discovered by Helmut Keller of Bad Steben, Germany, and is purified in a patented process developed by Carnivora Forschungs GmbH of Nordhalben, Germany. Used against cancer and other diseases, its main active constituents are plumbagin and hydroplumbagin-glucoside. It is said to act via the immune system, and a listing of immune system biomarker tests is provided that monitor the patient's response.

Still another recent development that has been publicized concerns an enzyme called human telomerase (with the accent on the second syllable). It has been discovered that the core of this enzyme contains a protein that controls enzymatic activity, and is thought to be the basic, molecular-level cause of virtually every kind of cancer, and at the same time may be central to the aging process. The normal function of human telomerase is to maintain cell health during cell division, that is, to keep the cells "young," but not too young. If this enzyme is overactive, however, the effect is to overdo it and the cells proliferate unchecked, leading to the cancerous condition. There is evidently a balance in that too active an enzyme leads to cancer, and too inactive an enzyme leads to premature aging. Telomerase is said to keep the dividing cells healthy by rejuvenating the chromosome tips, or telomeres, which become frayed from cell division. Otherwise, the telomeres atrophy, and the cell dies. This is a catch-22 situation. And the 64-dollar question is, what substances act as regulators or modulators, or inhibitors or promoters, for this particular enzyme or protein?

(At the Whitehead Institute for Biomedical Research in Boston, research by Matthew Meyerson indicates that a gene called human Ever Shorter Telomeres 2, or *hEST2*, is responsible for making a component of telomerase. It may prove to be a key agent in causing uncontrolled cellular growth.)

Telomerase is chemically similar to the enzyme named reverse transcriptase, also called RNA-dependent DNA polymerase (or RNA-directed DNA polymerase). This latter enzyme is a distinguishing feature of retroviruses, examples being HIV, said to be the source for AIDS, and the Ebola and Marburg viruses. Still other immunodeficiency diseases are believed to be caused by retroviruses, and sometimes cancer is added to the list. (Conversely, however, the ordinarily occurring enzyme known as DNA-dependent RNA polymerase, or DNA-directed RNA polymerase, has also been implicated in cancer formation.) The anticipation is that biochemical modifications in such drugs as AZT, used against AIDS, could produce anticancer drugs that act against overactive human telomerase.

(There are at least a couple of researchers who do not accept current thinking on AIDS and its treatment with AZT, namely, Peter Duesberg and David Rasnick of the University of California, Berkeley. They maintain that the AIDS virus, or HIV, is a harmless passenger virus, and the disease is instead caused by recreational and therapeutic drug use. Furthermore, AZT is in itself toxic, and in actual fact does not prevent or control AIDS, in itself producing the symptoms of AIDS as well as other adverse side effects. All this serves to demonstrate that medical research is by no means clear-cut, is possibly biased, and can be as controversial as any other endeavor.)

## CANCER MARKERS

The November 7, 1997, issue of *Science* contained a series of news items and articles furnishing an update on the cancer situation. The genetics of cancer and how it can be detected and monitored was discussed, which has a bearing on telomerase.

A highlighted section described the disablement of *p53*, the tumor suppressor gene that prevents viral DNA replication (*Science*, November 7, 1997, p. 1057). This is accomplished by means of adenovirus, which is a human respiratory virus. By removing the viral gene that disables *p53*, it was reasoned that the virus would selectively infect only cells in which the *p53* was nonfunctional — that is, cancer cells. It is necessary that the virus be injected directly into the tumor, as if injected into the bloodstream, the immune system would eliminate the virus. The application will consequently be of less use for metastasized cancers.

In another news item, the conclusion is again reached that animal studies are of limited value, as humans and animals react differently to drugs (*Science*, November 7, 1997, p. 1041). Animal studies mostly result in "good mouse drugs rather than good human drugs." Even xenografts, which involve transplanting human tumor cells into mice, are unreliable.

The subsequent articles take up such matters as origins, genetic testing for risk, detection by nucleic-based acid methods, oncogene transcription factors, genetic approaches in the discovery of anticancer drugs, environment and cancer, and chemo-prevention.

An article of special interest in the issue, by David Sidransky titled "Nucleic Acid-Based Methods for the Detection of Cancer" (*Science*, November 7, 1997, pp. 1054–1058), is concerned with these methods as markers for the detection and assessment of tumor burden in cancer patients. The underlying premise is that cancer involves the clonal evolution of transformed cells in which there is an accumulation of mutations, which are either inherited (germ line) or acquired (somatic). These mutations occur in critical proto-oncogenes and tumor suppressor genes. The genetic alterations can in turn be used to detect cancer cells in whatever samples are taken, with DNA serving as the substrate or reactant. Not only can DNA survive under adverse conditions, but its concentrations can be amplified by polymerase chain reaction (PCR) techniques, reducing the amount of sample required to a minimum. Although mutations in oncogenes and tumor suppressor genes can be used as markers, DNA changes can also be used, which involves changes in DNA repeat sequences called *microsatellites*. The procedure is called *microsatellite analysis*, and it detects microsatellite instability.

It is mentioned also that the presence of the enzyme reverse transcriptase may serve to furnish a marker. (This enzyme is otherwise known as RNA-directed DNA polymerase, and is the enzyme distinguishing retroviruses.) The conversion of iso-lated RNA to cDNA, is involved followed by amplification, a process designated as reverse transcriptase-PCR, or simply RT-PCR.

Telomerase, described as a ribonucleoprotein enzyme that extends the sequences at the chromosomal ends (telomeres), is another strong candidate for a marker. It is active in over 90% of primary human tumors, but for the most part is inactive in normal cells. (As noted earlier, however, in limited or inactive amounts it produces no changes, but in excess it leads to cancer, that is, unregulated cell growth.)

In a section on "Sensitivity and Specificity," the reference states that a problem in finding and monitoring cancerous cells in a clinical sample is that they are far outnumbered by normal cells. Furthermore, this will vary with the organ and with the individual. For example, the test for identifying bladder cancer cells in urine, where 50% of the DNA may be from sloughed-off tumor cells, may not apply to the identification of lung cancer in sputum, where only 0.2% or less of the DNA may be from tumor cells.

In a subsection titled "Early Detection," it was observed that oncogene or tumor suppressor gene mutations, namely, for *ras* or *p53*, are found in the drained body fluids of cancer patients. (The acronym *ras* as in *ras* genes stands for rat sarcoma,

i.e., rat sarcoma genes, the transforming principle in retroviruses causing rat sarcomas. Known as a family of transforming genes, *H-ras* pertains to the Harvey sarcoma
virus and *K-ras* pertains to the Kirsten sarcoma virus.) Furthermore, the *ras* mutations occur in colon cancer during tumorigenesis, whereas *p53* mutations most
usually occur in invasive tumors. Another possibility for markers are what are called
*APC* mutations. (The acronym *APC* stands for antigen-presenting cell). Found in
about 70% of colon adenomas, they are the precursors for colon cancer.

As for the effectiveness of microsatellite markers, in a set of tests on urine
samples, over 90% of bladder tumors were found. And as telomerase is expressed
selectively in almost all primary cancers, it is viewed as a promising molecular
marker for detecting cancer.

In a subsection titled "Tumor Burden," the reference notes that molecular markers can also assess the migration of tumor cells, both locally and into the bloodstream.
Thus, as a side effect of surgery, tumor cells often spread beyond the surgical margins
and may not be detectable by light microscopy methods. For instance, in a study
based on *p53* mutations, it was found that tumor cells migrated beyond the surgical
borders in approximately half the patients. Even after follow-up radiation treatments,
about one third of the patients had a recurrence, often developing new tumors next
to or within the cancerous area. Furthermore, for colorectal and lung cancer patients
who were observed to have apparently disease-free lymph nodes, tumor cells were
nevertheless found by these methods of analysis.

In addition to spreading locally, malignant cells can also spread by metastasis;
that is, the cells enter the bloodstream and are carried to other organs, to grow there.
As the serum or blood of cancer patients contain large amounts of circulating DNA,
blood samples can be analyzed for mutations and alterations. Thus, in the case of
patients with head and neck squamous cell carcinomas (HNSCC), 29% of the 21
patients tested had DNA mutations or alterations in serum or plasma. For small-cell
lung cancer patients (SCLC), 71% of another 21 patients tested had alterations or
mutations.

In a tabulation provided in the reference, the following cancer types were listed,
with the kind of clinical sample used and the corresponding genetic marker:

| Head and neck | Saliva | *p53*; telomerase |
|---|---|---|
| Lung | Sputum | *ras*/*p53*; ras, microsatellites |
| Colon | Stool | *ras*; telomerase |
| Pancreas | Juice | *ras*; ras |
| Bladder | Urine | *p53*; microsatellites, telomerase |

In the case of chronic myelogenous leukemia, routine analyses are made of
whole blood and bone marrow to determine the degree of abnormal transcripts
derived from cancerous or neoplastic cells. In this way, a marker is provided for the
progression or regression of the disease. The technique has also been applied to
patients with solid tumors. The use of tyrosine hydroxylase transcripts has been
found to correlate with micrometastatic bone marrow disease in neuroblastoma, and
tyrosine transcript levels are known to relate to the progression (or regression) of
melanoma. Other substances detectable include prostate-specific markers, notably

the prostate-specific antigen (PSA). The detection of micrometastatic disease, however, has not as yet proved conclusive for such tumor types as primary breast, gastric, colorectal, lung, and at times, prostate cancer.

(What are called Bence Jones proteins are said to be a standard marker for multiple myeloma, this being cancer of the marrow in the spinal column. And what is called Electroacupuncture According to Voll, or EAV, or called by still other names, is said to detect disease by the electric current between acupuncture points. Another possibility lies in the domain of biofeedback devices, where changes in the blood pressure, heart rate, galvanic skin response, skin temperature, respiration rate, etc., can be monitored — even by touch. These devices are approved by the FDA. Other encompassing names are bionetic detection and energetics medicine, and in addition to monitoring other diseases, there is the possibility of indirect correlation with the progression or regression of cancer. Among the firms marketing such devices is Physix, Inc., of Houston, Texas. Still other devices may lie in the domain of electromagnetic or magnetic effects, and a manufacturer's name here, for example, is Tools for Exploration, San Rafael, California.)

In an additional subsection titled "Adjuncts to Cytology and Histopathology," the reference takes up the use of needle aspirates that are used in the cancer diagnosis for suspected masses in various organs. It is difficult, nevertheless, to distinguish benign or preneoplastic lesions from overt cancer. These needle biopsies may yield to telomerase as the criterion. As an example, telomerase was detected in all of 11 thyroid follicular carcinomas, but in only 8 out of 33 when the follicular tumors were benign, and normal thyroid tissue never had any. Extrapolation has been made to breast cancer. Cervical cancer, which is almost entirely associated with human papilloma virus (HPV) infections, may be detected by these methods in lieu of the Pap smear. When a patient exhibits only a metastatic lymph node, it is sometimes difficult or impossible to locate the primary tumor, a problem that potentially may be resolved by these methods.

Even if these tests using serum nucleic acid markers may not yet be satisfactory for early tumor detection, the reference concludes that they "may provide useful information on tumor burden and response to therapy."

The fact that the enzyme telomerase is associated with tumors suggests a means for treating cancer, by utilizing inhibitors for telomerase (a complicating factor is modulation, as some telomerase is vital to prevent premature aging). This is also true for the enzyme tyrosinase, as associated with melanoma, and as indicated elsewhere. Very possibly the inhibition of reverse transcriptase (RNA-directed DNA polymerase) may not only act against cancer, but against such retroviruses as HIV (the AIDS virus), and the Ebola and Marburg viruses (which is why cancer is also called an *immunodeficiency disease*.) This is all speculation, of course.

Telomerase has not yet made the enzyme/enzyme inhibitor handbooks, nor the Sigma catalog *Biochemicals and Reagents for Life Science Research* (Sigma-Aldrich, St. Louis, MO). However, a number of inhibitors are listed in the handbooks of enzyme inhibitors for RNA-directed DNA polymerase, including several antibiotics such as actinomycin.

A new development denotes the different mitochondrial structures and functions of normal cells and cancerous cells, as reported by Serge Jurasunas (of Holitherapias

Institute, Lisbon, Portugal) in the August/September 2006 *Townsend Letter for Doctors & Patients*. (Mitochondria are the subcellular organelles that produce cellular energy via the formation of ATP, or adenosine triphosphate.) The article speaks of breaks in the mitochondrial DNA (MTDNA) traceable to oxidative stress from free radicals and possibly to chemotherapy itself, which can lead to cellular defects, mutations, and cancer. The formation and renewal of MTDNA involves the enzyme mitochondrial polymerase (and the inhibition of this enzyme can be viewed as one more factor in this complex scenario).

Although not spelled out as such in the article, presumably the determination of diminished concentrations of cellular-formed ATP, in one way or another, directly or indirectly, furnishes a measure or marker for cancerous activity. The counter to this ATP reduction, by whatever means, will provide a key to the control of cancer. Thus, the article stresses the role of SOD, or superoxide dismutase, as a most important endogenous (or indigenous) antioxidant enzyme in defending against oxidative free radicals. It is noteworthy that SOD has in previous accounts surfaced as an anticancer agent (Moss, 1992).

## HIGH-TECH VS. LOW-TECH

As far as an immediate cancer cure is concerned, this line of investigation will unfortunately require much "further study," a familiar-enough refrain. Fundamental research seems more and more like guaranteed employment and a self-perpetuating bureaucracy, a business rather than a calling. It can be added, moreover, that antibiotics, say, were discovered and utilized before it was fully known how they worked. This is why medical folklore is so important. Too often, however, the emphasis is on high-tech and its high costs, which can seem like putting the cart before the horse.

As for inexpensive low-tech, independent laboratory studies have shown that vitamin C does indeed destroy cancerous cells, as Linus Pauling said. The subject was surveyed for instance by Gary Null, Howard Robbins, Mark Tanenbaum, and Patrick Jennings in the May 1997 issue of the *Townsend Letter for Doctors & Patients*.

This introduces the question as to whether other vitamins may in some way act against cancer. A possibility apparently universally recognized is the B-vitamin folic acid, at least for some cancers, and which, interestingly, is chemically related to the commonly used cytotoxic chemotherapy drug 5-FU or 5-fluorouracil, a drug about which Ralph W. Moss has plenty to say, not much of it good, in *Questioning Chemotherapy*. An entire volume has been devoted to several aspects of the continuing subject of vitamins and their effect, titled *Vitamins and Minerals in the Prevention and Treatment of Cancer*, edited by Maryce M. Jacobs, and previously cited.

(A reminder is that translating *in vitro* laboratory results to *in vivo* clinical procedures, such as for vitamin C, can be elusive, requiring that the most effective dosage methods, levels, and frequencies be established, which, expectedly, will vary with the individual. What works in the laboratory does not necessarily work clinically, and vice versa. Of utmost utility would be a near-instantaneous and noninvasive clinical test to indicate or monitor whether cancer cells are proliferating or regressing in the patient. That is, is the particular anticancer agent or method of treatment proving successful? If not, try another option.)

As is so often implied, can it be that there would not be enough profits in utilizing something as simple, say, as vitamin C, and are egos also involved? Whatever the truth, the cancer patient is the loser.

## FOOTDRAGGING ON USING ENZYME INHIBITORS

The reluctance to pursue the aforementioned line of investigation on enzyme inhibitors is a subject in itself for investigation. In this regard it may again be mentioned that Donald Voet and Judith G. Voet, in their massive treatise titled *Biochemistry*, noted that differences between cancer cell and normal cell metabolism should be further studied, because it might lead to a cure (Voet and Voet, 1995, p. 595).

Work has been done using the chemical compound hydrazine sulfate — apparently with mixed success — as an inhibitor for the reconversion of lactic acid or lactate in the liver to glucose or glycogen, via the Cori cycle, which completes the recycle. (This treatment is sometimes called the Gold therapy, after Joseph Gold, M.D., of the Syracuse Cancer Research Institute, Syracuse, NY.) Evidently, a buildup of lactic acid or lactate would suppress its further formation, and thus act against metabolism. There are a lot of things going on, such as cancer cells undergoing glutaminolysis, or still other conversions or cycles, whereby cancer cells try to sustain metabolism. The controlling cancer metabolic step, however, is probably the production of lactic acid or lactate, and its inhibition is therefore front and center.

(Glutaminolysis in tumor cells has been discussed by E. Eigenbrodt, P. Fister, and M. Reinacher in *Regulation of Carbohydrate Metabolism*, Vol. II, Rivka Beitner, Ed., pp. 141–179. Moreover, it is worth reiterating that in experiments on rats it has been reported that anaerobic glycolysis, overall, may occur at 20 times the rates of aerobic glycolysis, as has been reported by Robert A. Harris in *Textbook of Biochemistry with Clinical Applications*, Thomas M. Devlin, Ed., p. 353. It may be assumed that anaerobic glycolysis is controlling.)

Also, peptides, or polypeptides, are potential enzyme inhibitors against cancer. These are relatively short chains of amino acids that are considered low-molecular-weight proteins. There are myriad peptide combinations, as stressed elsewhere, some of which are available commercially from supply houses such as Sigma-Aldrich of St. Louis, whose catalog also lists various enzymes, test kits, and assorted chemicals and biochemicals, etc.

The controversial Burzynski therapy may again be mentioned, as well as what is called the Naessens 714X therapy; the latter may or may not involve peptides, but probably not. Similarly, as the single most active ingredient in a well-publicized alternative therapy, shark cartilage is said to contain polypeptides; here again, the reviews of its effectiveness are mixed. The book that apparently started it all was *Sharks Don't Get Cancer* by I. William Lane and Linda Comac. Whatever else may be said, shark populations have been hard hit. It may be noted that the Sigma catalog lists bovine cartilage but not shark cartilage.

(Rather than peptides, a nitrogen-containing camphor compound is the reputed substance injected in the Naessens 714X therapy, trimethylbicyclonitraminoheptane chloride. It is not listed in the Sigma-Aldrich catalog. Other sources list the ingredients merely as camphor, ammonium chloride and nitrate, sodium chloride, ethanol, and water — with the possibility of a chemical conversion occurring. Camphor itself is an oxygenated hydrocarbon having a complicated ring structure, with the stoichiometric formula $C_{10}H_{16}O$, and the chemical name d-2-camphanone. Classed as a terpene ketone, it is obtained from the wood and bark of the camphor tree, an evergreen with the scientific name *Cinnamomum camphora* of the plant family Lauraceae or Laurel family. Originally native to China and the Far East, it is now grown in other parts of the world where the climate is suitable, for example, southern California. Interestingly, the species *C. cassia* provides common cinnamon, and the genus is well represented in Hartwell's *Plants Used Against Cancer* [1982b]. According to Cordell's *Alkaloids* [1981], members of the plant family Lauraceae also contain alkaloids.)

Another proposed therapy involves the destruction of internal parasites, said to be the cause of cancer, but here again the reviews are not encouraging. Parasites, however, are the cause of many diseases, especially tropical diseases, and all the causes for cancer, direct or indirect, are certainly not known, so it is possible that they cause cancer. The parasite responsible is said to be the human intestinal fluke, *Fasciolopsis buskii*, in conjunction with propyl alcohol. This was set forth in a book by Hulda Regehr Clark titled *The Cure for All Cancers* (1993). Instead of chemical parasiticides, such folkloric deworming agents as wormwood (*Artemisia absinthium*) — which itself has a checkered past — are recommended. In further comment, the previously mentioned fluke species is said by microbiologists to be rarely found in humans, and what Clark calls "cancer" is not necessarily cancer in the conventional sense.

The subject of parasites and cancer continues to be a topic of some interest, however. The German doctor Hartwig Schuldt, M.D., in an article titled "The Study of Malignancy: A Summary Report from 27 Years of Research," which appeared in the December 1997 issue of the *Townsend Letter for Doctors & Patients* provided a mechanism, but gave no details of therapy save to say that "energy medicine" is involved, which is another name for various alternative therapies, including electric and magnetic fields, herbs, acupuncture, etc. Going back in time, there was a series of books by J. Jackson Clarke, the last of which, *Protists and Disease*, was published in 1922. Clarke was senior surgeon to the Hampstead and North-West London Hospital, and surgeon to the Royal National Orthopaedic Hospital. He was particularly interested in cancer. In a chapter on "Cancer-Bodies," protozoa are described as appearing in cancers, though protozoa are said not to be peculiar to cancer (Clarke, *Protists and Disease*, 1922, p. 92). Clarke further speaks of parasites found in the examination of pathological cancer sections (Clarke, 1922, p. 183ff.). Clarke earlier had written a series of books titled *Protozoa and Disease* (published in four parts, 1902–1915), in which he had mentioned protozoa as a cause of cancer (Clarke, 1912, Part III, p. 66). In any case it is evidently a direction that modern medical research has for the most part not pursued. In herbalist Hanna Kroeger's (1997) book on cancer, *Free Your Body of Tumors and Cysts*, fungi as well as viruses are said to cause cancer.

The conventional wisdom is to avoid what has not yet been scientifically proved. The counterargument is that medical orthodoxy refuses to conduct tests in an impartial manner, preserving its own impregnability. Consequently, alternative treatments mostly remain in the realm of folklore, anecdote, and hearsay (or heresy). However, and whatever the case, if the processes involved cannot be explained in a basically scientific and objective manner, then it cannot be determined whether the therapy actually works or whether someone is fudging, misrepresenting, or manipulating the facts of the matter, or else lying. These remarks of course apply even more if there is money to be made.

(Ralph Moss took up the subject in the April 2006 issue of the *Townsend Letter* in his column titled article "Unmasking a 'Cure'." This pertained to court actions regarding a source marketing a "clinically proven" medicine — evidently Camptosar®, or irinotecan or CPT-11. This is a known drug used against colorectal cancer, but which is not dramatically effective and, moreover, is highly toxic. Attempts at verification from doctors cited on the Internet site Cancer Cure proved nonproductive. In the same article, Moss mentioned a report on mammography dealing with the very real dangers in breast cancer screening and biopsy, and which received kudos from Professor Samuel Epstein, M.D., of the University of Illinois and Joel M. Evans, M.D., of the Albert Einstein College of Medicine.)

The Sigma catalog lists tyrosinase, the enzyme involved in melanoma. As mentioned elsewhere, among the inhibitors listed in the handbooks of enzyme inhibitors are ascorbic acid, or vitamin C, halide ion (the halides being chlorides, notably, but also fluorides, bromides, and iodides), butyric acid (a component of rancid butter), lactic acid (the final product of anaerobic glycolysis, as occurs in cancer cell metabolism, and a component also of sour milk and buttermilk), oxalic acid (e.g., as found in rhubarb and in wood sorrel), formic acid (a component of ant stings), even tyrosine itself, and toxic cyanide ion. And, as has been indicated, alpine sunflower/yucca extract may possibly serve as an enzyme inhibitor for tyrosinase.

There are numerous therapies or treatments described in such books as Moss (1992) and Walters (1993). Some of these treatments (including those of folkloric origin) utilize substances containing known enzyme inhibitors for one or another of the steps involved in glycolysis or cell metabolism. This may be substantiated by examining the two handbooks on enzyme inhibitors that have been published, and have been repeatedly cited.

# 6 The Alternative Scene

## AN INTRODUCTION TO ALTERNATIVES

A few remarks are in order in support of some of the alternatives previously listed and commented upon. These remarks do not constitute recommendations or even suggestions, but are intended for consideration only. It may be stated again that anticancer action does not necessarily constitute a cure, remission being the preferred word.

Thus, attention can be drawn to such therapies as megadoses of vitamin C, Essiac tea, shark cartilage, and elimination of parasitic invaders. More will be further described in the subsequent sections. We particularly recall the works of Ralph W. Moss (1992, 1998), *Cancer Therapy: The Independent Consumer's Guide to Non-Toxic Treatment and Prevention* and *Herbs against Cancer: History and Controversy*, both of which furnish the pros and cons.

Among the most recently discovered contributing causes of cancer are fungi and their chemical constituents. Interestingly, a fungus is sometimes thought of as a bacterium or vice versa, or a plant, or however classified, a phenomenon that could be called *pleomorphism*. Fungi, strangely enough, may sometimes serve as remedies. Inasmuch as a fungus may at times be regarded as a bacterium, this brings up the subject of gut flora or bacteria. They have been identified as including cancer-causing agents and producing biochemical carcinogens that are transported to other parts of the body. On the other hand, species of bacteria have been used as anticancer agents, as in producing Coley's Toxins. More than this, there are other members of the gut flora that have pronouncedly beneficial effects. They consist of perhaps 400 species of friendly microorganisms sometimes referred to as *probiotics*. (An authoritative work on gut flora or microflora is by Rowland [1988]. See also Hoffman [1999a], pp. 205–219).

As for vitamin B and C deficiencies and cancer, *The Complete Book of Vitamins*, by J.I. Rodale et al., published back in 1966, mentions the Gerson diet in the treatment of cancer and the importance of the liver (Rodale et al., 1966, pp. 450–509).

The role and efficacy of plants and herbs and of alternative medicine will be discussed in the following text. It may be commented, however, that medical ortho-doxy will remain skeptical, if not hostile, unless biochemical (or biological) expla-nations can be provided for the beneficial action of these alternative therapies. (This is further complicated by matters of financial reward and of saving face.) But even here, these biochemical explanations are not necessarily the last word.

Nevertheless, theories or hypotheses furnish a means to more closely relate cause and effect, which are often separated by a very long time interval in the case of cancer, thus introducing ambiguities and speculations. That is, the cause, or causes, of cancer and its subsequent onset cannot necessarily be related, at least by obser-vation alone. Also, the cancer occurrence and its remission or cure cannot usually be conclusively related, whatever the treatment used. This could mean that there may be too many other variables or parameters introduced during an excessively long interval between cause and effect, whether we are speaking of cancer origins or cures.

## SOME ALTERNATIVES, INFORMATION SOURCES, AND ASSESSMENTS

All kinds of ongoing information about therapies against cancer and supportive organizations can be found on the Internet, so it is hardly necessary to be too specific. Nevertheless, we proceed as follows, naming a few notable organizations and sources that may or may not still be in existence, as the listings necessarily become dated, even at the moment of writing.

There are networks providing for or advising about unorthodox therapies, with many of the reference sources carried in books and articles here and there. For example, in Moss (1992), there are references interspersed within the text and at the end in a section titled "General References," as of the date of publication. (Moss presently publishes a newsletter titled *The Moss Reports* and has a monthly column in the *Townsend Letter for Doctors & Patients*.) Richard Walters' *Options: The Alternative Cancer Therapy Book* contains much information about therapies and sources, as of the date of publication, 1993. *Alternatives in Cancer Therapy: The Complete Guide to Non-Traditional Treatments* by Ross Pelton and Lee Overholser is another source of information, as of 1994.

The latter book was endorsed by Linus Pauling. (Ross Pelton has a Ph.D. and is a pharmacist who has served as administrator of the world's largest holistic hospital offering alternative cancer therapies, the Hospital Santa Monica in Rosarita Beach, Mexico.) We cite again *An Alternative Medicine Definitive Guide to Cancer*, published in 1997. Also worthy of mention is a slightly earlier exposé and exposition, *The Healing of Cancer* by Barry Lynes, published in 1989, dealing with the work of Royal Rife and his radio frequency generator.

The reference work *Alternative Medicine: The Definitive Guide* has sections "Where to Find Help" and "Recommended Reading" at the end of each chapter, including the chapter on cancer. The reference work *An Alternative Medicine Definitive Guide to Cancer* describes many or most of the "mainstream" alternative therapies. All are listed in its references. Such institutions as the M.D. Anderson Cancer Center in Houston keep a file on alternatives. Much more can be found on the Internet.

(There is also a cancer hotline, 800-422-6237, an NCI-supported service located at various points around the United States. This can be used to obtain information about conventional treatments, that is, the accepted protocols and publications of medical orthodoxy.)

The question, of course, is how to sort it all out. Ideally, we are looking for the absolute cure or cures for each and every individual and for all kinds of cancers, not merely some statistical betterment such as a brief increase in average life spans. We are not so interested in qualifiers. We are inundated with information but not with absolutes. Epidemiology, or the study of the distribution of diseases among and throughout populations, is, for instance, usually more of academic interest, that is, after the fact. Here, we are looking for cures, if we dare use the word — that is, the "magic bullet," the kind of action displayed by antibiotics against bacterial infections.

(Such information as a particular therapy increasing life spans by a few months seems inconsequential. We are thinking in terms of an increase measured in years, even decades, or a lifetime. Unfortunately, there is no comprehensive database by which comparisons can be made in some way or another, not only for alternative therapies, but also for orthodox treatments. It seems a subject that is out of bounds, although Moss [1992] ventured that there did not seem to be much difference between the averaged results of alternative and mainstream treatments. There are even opinions, presumably backed by hard evidence, that no treatment at all is equally effective. A worldwide tour by the investigator Lerner [1994] was, at best, inconclusive. Any successes outside the norm are sure to be challenged from one quarter or another.)

Simply stated, there is as yet no single, well-defined treatment, acceptable to all parties, professional and nonprofessional. Moreover, considering the diversity of the many alternatives, the wide spectrum of approaches, and the lack of corroboration, there is probably no way to set up an orderly means of testing and evaluation that will be satisfactory to all parties. More than this, how can such a life-threatening and devastating disease be subjected to controls? After all, each patient is entitled to be cured, absolutely, not to serve as a reference point or placebo or guinea pig during some sort of test program. The problems and difficulties seem insurmountable, if not hopeless. Nevertheless, these problems must be met head on and this book addresses this goal.

Speaking further of placebos and double-blind clinical trials, where some of the patients receive a placebo and no one is supposed to know who is getting what, not even the doctors, there is the more modern outlook that no one should receive a placebo. That is, the methods of statistical analysis can be used to show the effectiveness of a treatment or therapy. In this way, all the patients receive the treatment.

As has been mentioned, back in 1976, *Prevention Magazine* published *The Encyclopedia of Common Diseases*, compiled and edited by the staff. In the section on cancer, a reiteration of the treatments includes the Gerson Treatment, Insulin (called the *Beale Treatment*), Krebiozen, the Drosnes–Lazenby Treatment, and the Koch Treatment. The Gerson Therapy, previously described, involves drinking fresh vegetable juice from organic sources, coffee enemas, and a diet with high potassium or sodium ratio. The conclusions about the Koch Treatment, for example, remain in limbo, having been shut down by the FDA. These are only two out of the multitude, of which some of the more interesting will be further described subsequently.

(The FDA itself continues to come under fire from time to time, as in an article by James Bovard in the January 1995 issue of the *American Spectator* and his book *Lost Rights: The Destruction of American Liberty*. There was an article by Peter Brimelow and Leslie Spencer in the February 13, 1995, issue of *Forbes*. Some other works are Herbert Burkholz's *The FDA Follies: An Alarming Look at Our Food and*

*Drug Administration* and Dr. Samuel S. Epstein's *The Politics of Cancer Revisited*, published in 1998.)

The public deserves to know what works and what does not, and the degree of the in-between successes, as obtained from a fully independent and impartial appraisal. The public needs this information right now, this very day, as do the practicing medical doctors, literally in the trenches, who require the imprimatur of sanctification. Whether or not promising alternative treatments can infiltrate the body remains speculative, however; there arise the usual problems of egos, power, and money. If medical orthodoxy comes up with a solution first, it is by definition okay, but not so for an outsider. The question is complicated by the necessity of clinical trials and by factors like who will be the patients, who will administer and conduct the trials, and judge the results.

Somehow, the status of alternative cancer therapies is akin to the role played by Australian nurse Sister Elizabeth Kenny in the treatment of polio. Her ways of assisting polio patients were more or less all that was available at the time, although often vilified, until the Salk and Sabin vaccines appeared on the scene. (With the qualifier that most new polio cases are now said to be caused by the vaccine itself.) Thus, we await the magic bullet for cancer, which may be unsuspected, but whose discovery may be fortuitous, as with penicillin and other antibiotics. No one would have anticipated that there could be such destroyers of infection as penicillin, though their existence and use were apparently known in native folklore medicine. Such may be the course for a cancer cure, that is, some native plant remedy may already be in existence, only awaiting discovery by modern medicine. Combining serendipity and purpose, someone might come up with an effective, universal vaccine.

Alternatives apparently abound for cancer treatment, and though by no means infallible, they are begrudgingly starting to be recognized by some in the medical establishment, if only by way of the back door. For an isolated instance, such orthodox treatments as chemotherapy may in turn be replaced or augmented by immune therapy or immunotherapy, biochemical treatments, etc. Investigations into the use of hormonelike substances such as for interleukin-1, interleukin-2, etc. is undercontinuing, even most often discouraging. The subject is in flux, to say the least. Maybe the unorthodox is starting to merge with the orthodox or vice versa.

Furthermore, the average practicing physician is neither a researcher nor a specialist. He or she is merely following the body of established recommended procedures. Apart from conforming to the conventional wisdom, these procedures also protect them legally. The research is done elsewhere, in research hospitals and research institutes, some even in what are called *teaching hospitals*. But the research performed has not been up to the task at hand. Maybe the research has been on the wrong track, maybe too scientific minded, and needs to take more advantage of folklore and native lore, especially of the plants, herbs, and their medicinal qualities.

Thus, John Heinerman contributed *Spiritual Wisdom of the Native Americans, Healing Secrets of the Maya: Health Wisdom from an Ancient Empire,* and *Health Secrets from the Ancient World.* Unfortunately, some of his books are out of print and difficult to find. Whether or not the answers will be found in books such as these is unclear, for there are no impartial clinical trials either to substantiate or to disprove the kind of information provided as yet.

The family physician or the specialist, practicing on the front lines, is also at the forefront in receiving the blame for failed therapies. For the conventional cancer treatments of surgery, radiation and chemotherapy at times seem more like palliatives or placebos, to make it look as though something is being done, or at least to postpone the inevitable. It is the expediency of delaying intractable facts. It is like a catch-22 situation; it's too bad if you do and too bad if you don't.

Surgery has long had the reputation for sometimes causing the cancer to metastasize or spread, and it now turns out that radiation and chemotherapy are also suspect, either causing new or secondary cancers, or the primary cancer to reappear more aggressively and virulently than before.

The reluctance and resistance to seek new or unconventional or alternative therapies, therefore, seems incomprehensible. If no one else is pushing, the family physician and the specialist should both be raising Cain instead of perpetuating the charade, for it is they who are blamed. On average, these physicians start early in the morning and quit late in the evening. But they do not have a clue about how to cure cancer, only to treat it. If this is not so, then why are well over a half million victims dying of cancer every year, averaging one death per minute? These data suggest that cancer could overtake heart diseases as the number one killer.

The conventional treatments are generally judged successful if the patient does not die right away, the 5-year remission being the standard for speaking of a cure. So it may presumably be conceded that sometimes conventional therapies work, especially so for surgery, if it can be performed in time. To recall an old saying, in this context, "Even an anosmic hog will find an acorn once in awhile."

All this is at the expense of the billions spent on conventional cancer treatments and everything that goes with it. But it shows no improvement in overall survival rates. Instead of speaking of the cancer industry, somehow "medical welfare" seems equally appropriate for both the research and the practice. A fear has been instilled, which sends the victim rushing to organized medicine for assistance, a fear that is justified, considering the inadequacy of medical orthodoxy in combating cancer.

The interlocking network that exists between orthodox medicine and the financial world is spelled out in Clarence Mullins' prominently cited book *Death by Injection: The Story of the Medical Conspiracy against America*, particularly, in the early chapters and notably in the chapter titled "Profits from Cancer." Both the American Medical Association (AMA) and the drug companies are involved. The Rockefeller interests are prominently mentioned, as well as the ties with the Memorial Sloan-Kettering Cancer Center (MSKCC).

In the aforementioned and other references, treatments are discussed using everything from megadoses of vitamin C through herbal remedies to shark cartilage to radiotherapy. The following is a brief review and overview of further information about a few of these therapies, many of which are plant derived. Most are described in the previously mentioned reference sources.

## Vitamin C

About megadoses of vitamin C against cancer, Chapter 19 of Linus Pauling's book, *How to Live Longer and Feel Better*, may be consulted. More information is provided in *Cancer and Vitamin C: A Discussion of the Nature, Causes, Prevention, and Treatment of Cancer with Special Reference to the Value of Vitamin C* by Ewan Cameron and Linus Pauling. An update is *Vitamin C and Cancer* by Abram Hoffer, M.D., Ph.D., a former associate of Pauling's.

A megadose used to be considered about 25–30 g of vitamin C per day, but now massive doses, up to 150 g per day, are given intravenously.

It can be further remarked that, at Pauling's insistence, vitamin C was once tested on terminal cancer patients at the Mayo Clinic and found ineffective. Pauling's rebuttal was that the patients had previously been subjected to chemotherapy, which destroyed their immune system. (The debilitating effect of chemotherapy on the immune system is now part of medical folklore.) In response, a second testing was conducted on patients who had not been previously treated with chemotherapy. The results again were that the vitamin C so administered was not effective. In common with other quandaries, the definitive resolution and answer await. There are such matters to be clarified as methods of administration, dosage levels, frequency, length of treatment, and bias.

Speaking of bias in Medline and its database, the U.S. National Library of Medicine (NLM), there is an editorial "Medline Bias" on pages 122 and 123 in the August/September issue of the *Townsend Letter for Doctors & Patients*. It was written by Andrew M. Saul, assistant editor of the *Journal of Orthomolecular Medicine* and the author of a number of books on natural healing, cited at the end of the editorial. Saul notes that certain journals are excluded from coverage, including the *Journal of American Physicians and Surgeons* and the *Journal of Orthomolecular Medicine*. As for the exclusion of the latter, which over the years had contained valuable information from Linus Pauling, for example, about vitamin C against cancer, Saul emphasizes that Pauling's publications in other journals were well represented on Medline.

An article noted in the *Life Extension* Web site, dated September 13, 2005, is from the *Birmingham Post*. Titled "Vitamin C Cancer Hope," it leads off with the statement that new research suggests that high dosages of vitamin C injected into the bloodstream may be effective against cancer. For instance, it has been found that vitamin C in the ascorbate form has killed cancer cells in the laboratory, although the dosages were so high that IV injection would be required. This seemingly contradicts earlier negative results, but the earlier trials were with oral dosages, although trials in 1970 with both oral and IV ascorbate hinted at an anticancer action.

In a recent study led by Dr. Mark Levine of the NIH, laboratory studies that simulated high clinical infusions of vitamin C were performed, employing nine cancer cell types and four normal cell types. It was found that in five of the cancer cell lines, there was a 50% decrease in survival, whereas normal cells were not affected. In studies on lymphoma cells – noted to be especially sensitive to vitamin C – these cells were either directly destroyed or else rendered inactive. Additional tests indicated that cancer cell growth was reduced by at least 99% with exposure to vitamin C.

The effective dosage used in the particular experiments was cited as less than 4 mmol. That is, 0.004 gmol, which would be 0.704 g as ascorbic acid, having the formula $C_6H_8O_6$ with a molecular weight of 176 although this figure was not projected relative to human body weights. It was further stated that this level is not achievable orally, but is readily achievable by IV infusion.

However, in addition to Pauling's and Hoffer's annotated successes, this writer can give a first-hand report of a case in which a 37-year-old person was diagnosed with leukemia, but rejected chemotherapy and instead went on a regimen of self-administered megadoses of vitamin C. The vitamin C was in the form of time-release capsules containing the powder or crystals, totaling 25 to 50 g intake per day. After his white blood cell (WBC) count had gone ballistic, it then showed a steady decrease, and at the age of 63 years, the count is still decreasing with continued vitamin C intake. And all the while, the person led a full, active, and productive life.

(As an aside, it may again be remarked that Gary Null et al. once did a literature search on vitamin C and the treatment of cancer, which was published in the *Townsend Letter for Doctors & Patients* dated June 1997. The limited research results were impressive. Nowadays a person only has to go to Medline or its equivalent, or to the Internet, to be inundated with information on this subject. The need, of course, is for discernment. Thus, one can narrow the search choices; for example, the work of A. Hoffer [2000] can be searched under the subject of "orthomolecular treatment of cancer.")

Vitamin C is suspected of being an antiviral agent, although this is an issue not yet fully resolved (Hoffman, 1999, p. 49). Anyway, it is noted to act against the common cold (caused by a virus) as per Linus Pauling's work. It has also been noted to enhance the utilization of folic acid by one or another biochemical conversions, and inasmuch as folic acid is considered an anticancer agent, so may vitamin C.

(Substantiation of Linus Pauling's findings about vitamin C's action against flu and the common cold is furnished in a letter appearing in the January 2005 issue of the *Townsend Letter for Doctors & Patients*. From Thomas E. Levy, M.D., JD, of Lakewood, Colorado, the letter is titled "Vitamin C and Severe Influenza: A Case Report." Dr. Levy makes the following initial statement: "While the scientific literature has abundant information of the ability of vitamin C to cure a number of viruses considered to be incurable [references cited], I feel it is always of benefit to health care practitioners who are still reluctant to freely give large doses of vitamin C to hear of yet another dramatic case report." The patient was in such a bad condition that a house call was necessary, and the first IV used 1000 cc of lactated Ringer's solution, a standardized solution of sodium, potassium, and calcium chlorides, with 50 g of sodium ascorbate. Small doses of calcium gluconate, magnesium sulfate, and a complex of B vitamins, excluding B12, were added to the IV bag. The dosage was administered over a 3-hour period, followed immediately by 6 g of glutathione to complete the infusion. The same regimen was repeated over a course of 6 days, with the last three given at the clinic. Recovery was ongoing and more or less complete after the fourth infusion, but two more infusions were given to ensure that no relapse occurred, which can happen when high dosages of vitamin C are discontinued. The patient was instructed to continue with oral dosages of vitamins C, E, and A, and also bioavailable B vitamins.)

Biochemically, vitamin C can be viewed as an enzyme inhibitor. Thus, as a matter of record, in Appendix Z of Hoffman's work (1999a), the following enzymes or substances are listed as inhibited by vitamin C and/or its derivatives, with some being of potential interest and some not: adenylate cyclase, Na,K-ATPase, catalase, catechol *O*-methyltransferase, ferredoxin-NADP reductase, glucose-6-P dehydrogenase, lipase, fatty acid oxygenase, peroxidase, cAMP phosphodiestase, tyrosinase, and urea levels; ascorbate-2-sulfate sulfhydro, dehydro-ascorbic acid; β-acetylhexosaminidase; *o*-aminophenol oxidase, β-glucuronidase, GTP cyclohydrolase I, hydroxymethylglutaryl-CoA reductase, and lactoylglutathione lyase.

Based on *in vivo* experimental results reported, vitamin C can also be viewed as an inhibitor for the key enzymes involved in carbohydrate metabolism or glycolysis, including lactate dehydrogenase, which is involved in cancer cell metabolism (Hoffman, 1999, p. 395). The inference is that vitamin C is an anticancer agent, as advanced by Pauling and Hoffer.

In the October 2004 issue of the *Townsend Letter for Doctors & Patients*, Ralph Moss provides an update about vitamin C in his monthly column "The War on Cancer." He cites the work of Kedar N. Prasad, a professor of radiology at the University of Colorado Health Sciences Center, Denver. This work is also cited in Moss (2000). In test tube or *in vitro* experiments, vitamin C was shown to inhibit the growth of cancer cells. The theory is that normal cells closely regulate the minute uptake of an antioxidant such as vitamin C, rejecting any excess, whereas cancer cells do not have this capacity and can accumulate high levels that will cause cell death. Moss in turn reviews the work of Ewan and Cameron (1993), and clinical results at the Mayo Clinic that purported to show it ineffective. However, on further examination of the protocol used, the supplement oral dosages used did not reach high enough levels. Whereas some practitioners administer up to 100 g (4 oz) per day IV (such as physician Abram Hoffer, M.D., Ph.D., of Victoria, British Columbia, and Hugh Riordan, M.D., of the Center for the Improvement of Human Functioning International (CIHFI) at Wichita, Kansas. Moreover, high IV dosages of vitamin C have become a common practice among complementary and alternative medicine (CAM) physicians. (Dr. Riordan died on January 7, 2005, but his work will be carried on. An obituary by Ralph W. Moss appeared in the February/March 2005 issue of the *Townsend Letter for Doctors & Patients*.)

In an article by Reagan Houston in the July 2005 *Townsend Letter for Doctors & Patients*, the work of Abram Hoffer and other physicians is reviewed for different cancers, giving the remarkably higher success rates. Dr. Hoffer's vitamin regimen is included, and daily dosages as high as 100,000 mg (100 g) or even 200,000 mg have been used. Vitamin C as sodium ascorbate can be used as an alternative to ascorbic acid, and IV use is recommended.

Similarly, in the December 2005 issue of the same periodical, an item on page 18 has the title "Intravenous Vitamin C is Selectively Toxic to Cancer Cells." This was confirmed by researchers at the NIH and was reported in an article published in the *Proceedings of the National Academy of Sciences*. The Bio-Communications Research Institute (BCRI) in Wichita, Kansas, has published some 20 scientific articles on the subject, notably in the *British Journal of Cancer*, in 2001. Hugh D. Riordan, M.D., was the principal investigator at BCRI, and the work done by him and his associates using vitamin C parallels and follows that of Linus Pauling and Abram Hoffer in orthomolecular medicine.

In fact, other studies have now shown that IV vitamin C gives much higher blood concentrations than oral dosages, and blood plasma concentrations are 60 times higher. Although clinical trials are always difficult to set up, some have been under way at the University of Kansas Medical Center, under the direction of Jeanne A. Drisko, M.D., and sponsored by the Cancer Treatment Research Foundation. It has been found that most patients need 75–100 g per day to get the plasma vitamin C concentration to a satisfactory level that is toxic to the cancer cells but not to normal cells. WBC and platelet counts, as well as other markers, are used as indicators for possible toxicity. A reference provided is Jeanne Drisko, M.D., Associate Professor and Program Director in Integrative Medicine, Functional Medicine and CAM, University of Kansas Medical Center, Kansas City KS 66160, 913-588-6208, jdrisko@kume.edu.

From time to time, reports surface in the media that megadoses of vitamin C are not safe, and they slam vitamin C in general. The fact that high-dose vitamin C is safe has been further confirmed, as reported in the August/September issue of the *Townsend Letter for Doctors & Patients*. This latest study was funded by the Lincoln Family Foundation and conducted jointly by the University of Nebraska, the University of Puerto Rico Medical Sciences Campus, and the CIHFI, a nonprofit organization founded by Hugh Riordan, M.D., in 1975. The study is a continuation of what is called the *RECNAC II* project. (RECNAC stands for CANCER spelled backwards. Phase I clinical trials were carried out at the University of Nebraska Medical School Hospital, and Phase II clinical trials are under the auspices of the NIH.)

Lastly, but importantly, in a chapter titled "Chemical Carcinogenesis," the following cited authors note that vitamin C inhibits carcinogenesis in the stomach by blocking the formation of nitrosamines from the nitrosation of amines (Williams and Weisberger, in Amdur et al.,1991, p. 146). This is aside from the usual view of medical orthodoxy that vitamin C has no special therapeutic effects other than the alleviation of scurvy (e.g., Marcus and Coulston, in *Pharmacological Basis of Therapeutics*, pp. 1568–1571).

## ESSIAC TEA

About the apparently well-known folkloric herbal remedy called Essiac tea, there is *The Essiac Report: The True Story of a Canadian Herbal Cancer Remedy and of the Thousands of Lives it Continues to Save*, by Richard Thomas. President Kennedy's physician, Dr. Charles A. Brusch, became involved in Essiac research and testing, and is reported to have used it alone to heal his own cancer of the lower bowel. Gary L. Glum has written *Calling of an Angel* and furnishes instructions for making and using Essiac tea. The herbs used are thought to be as follows (Boik, 1996, p. 160): *Arctium lappa* (butdock root), *Rheum* sp. (Indian rhubarb), *Rumex acetosella* (sheep sorrels), and *Ulmus fulva* (slippery elm bark). The active ingredients in the Essiac herbs are thought to be rhein, emodin, high-molecular-weight polysaccharides (sugars and starches), and possibly arctigenin (a lignan). Rhein and emodin are anthroquinones, which display antitumor activity but are also cytotoxic, or cell-toxic (Boik, 1996, p. 117).

An article in the September 25, 1995, issue of *Maclean's Magazine*, written by Patricia Chisholm and titled "Healers or Quacks," noted that in a 1989 Health Canada Bulletin, a trial carried out in 1982 by 112 Canadian doctors found Essiac to be of no benefit, and the National Cancer Institute (NCI) judged similarly in 1983. As for the efficacy of the Essiac tea, it should also depend upon whether the plant sources are of the correct species and are suitably active. This, therefore becomes a quandary within a quandary.

Ralph W. Moss (1998) has a chapter with much information that furnishes both the pros and cons in an even-handed manner.

From time to time, advertisements appear in various health-related magazines for Essiac, for example, in the March/April 1995 issue of *Natural Health*, from ESSIAC International, Ottawa, Ontario, Canada, Tel: 613-820-9311. Also, later on, in the August/September 2006 issue of the *Townsend Letter for Doctors and Patients*, p. 71: www.essiac-canada.com, or POB 365, Lake Worth, FL 33460, 561-585-7111.

(And while we are at it, in the same issue of *Natural Health*, on a back page under "Tomato Warning!" was the information pulled from a copy of the *Journal of the AMA* that the average age of the 40 M.D.s listed in that issue's obituaries was 58 years, as compared to the population as a whole that averages 74.9 years. Thus, a person on the average could gain about 17 years just by not being an M.D. The health enthusiast Linus Pauling lived 93 years. The argument is reminiscent of the furore once created within the American Chemical Society (ACS) when some statistics were brought up showing the average life span of a chemist to be shorter than the population as a whole.)

An additional source for Essiac herbs is the Herbal Healer Academy, HC32 Box 97-B, Mt. View, AR 72560, Tel: 501-269-4177. The herbs, in this instance, were said to be burdock root (*Arctium*), sheep sorrel (*Rumex*), slippery elm (*Ulmus*), and turkey rhubarb root (*Rheum*). All are listed in Hartwell (1982a, b). (According to this herbal source, Clark's *The Cure for All Cancers* (1983) seemed to be a best-seller, although there was dissent about its effectiveness.)

Incidentally, Essiac tea was named after Nurse Renée Caisse of Canada — her last name spelled backwards — and is said to be derived from the herbal lore of Indian tribes in the Canadian North. (And though Essiac tea tastes pretty good, chaparral tea is anything but good; the plant is not called the creosote bush for nothing. So some folks have opted for chaparral pills, tablets, or capsules.)

## SHARK CARTILAGE

For information about shark cartilage, I. William Lane and Linda Comac have written *Sharks Don't Get Cancer: How Shark Cartilage Could Save Your Life*. The thesis is that taking shark cartilage in sufficient doses will cut off the blood supply to cancerous growths. The earlier dose of 30 g of cartilage per day has been replaced by 1 g of cartilage per 2 lb of body weight. Other figures are about 100 g per day for a 150 to 160 lb person (Boik, 1996, p. 164). Smaller doses are said to be less effective or ineffective. Tests have been conducted variously at MIT, in Japan, and at the NCI, all of which seem inconclusive.

The antiangiogenesis or antivascularization effects of cartilage are attributed to enzyme inhibitors called *collagenase inhibitors*, notably tissue inhibitors of metalloproteinases or TIMPs (Boik, 1996, p. 162). Besides shark cartilage, bovine cartilage is considered to be an important source. As an added note, the active ingredients are said to be in the form of polypeptides (relatively short-chain protein molecules composed of amino acids linked together), which are able to pass through the digestive system and enter the circulatory system (Boik, 1996, p. 164). Burzynski therapy, frequently mentioned herein, uses certain polypeptides as enzyme inhibitors in the treatment of cancer. Enzymes and enzyme inhibitors are an important topic, as already introduced in Chapter 3, in particular with regard to glycolysis pathways, the metabolic processes by which the body converts a glucose energy source to energy and end products, by-products, and intermediates.

(According to Nieper therapy, a primary goal of cancer treatment is to eliminate sodium from the system [Walters, 1993, p. 220]. Thus, Dr. Hans Nieper, an M.D. in Hanover, Germany, noted that cancer patients have an excess of sodium in their blood, whereas sharks and other deep-sea fish do not get cancer because they recycle seawater back into the ocean, eliminating sodium.)

Progress has been periodically updated and also discounted (e.g., "Shark Therapy" by Catherine Dold in the April 1996 issue of *Discover*, and "Holistic Medicine" by Susan Crabtree in the September–October 1996 issue of *The National Times*, first published in *Insight*.) Oncologist Charles Simone, formerly with NCI and now located in New Jersey, was supported by the then Office of Alternative Medicine (OAM) of the NIH to check the efficacy of shark cartilage. (Simone once treated Ronald Reagan and Hubert Humphrey for cancer, using nutritional therapy.) As suspected, sharks may become an endangered species, maybe to no avail.

## COMPOUND-X

There is a persisting rumor that the Plains Indians know more about a mysterious, secretive, and potent formulation, which (for lack of a better term) can be referred to as *Compound-X* or *CompoundX*. This is supposed to cure cancers, externally and internally, no question about it, and no questions asked. It is presumably some kind of a fast-acting herbal mixture, and it is rumored that a pharmaceutical company once obtained the rights to the formula. But now, there is a difficulty in its availability. If the Plains Indians know about it, however, one can assume that all tribes are aware of it, north to south and east to west, being a part of the mystical connection. But all this information is hearsay, and therefore suspect. Nevertheless, the speculation is reinforced that there indeed may be a magic bullet for cancer "out there."

Further inquiry reveals that some of the original work on Compound-X was carried out in the early 1980s by Professor Frank Stermitz of the chemistry department at Colorado State University and by others in veterinary science, including Dr. Kenneth Larson. The substance was tested on animals, apparently unsuccessfully. However, John Heinerman mentioned in it *Healing Animals with Herbs*, published in 1977. Again, it should be reminded that what works or does not work on animals, may or may not work for humans and vice versa. Also, the response in individual humans will vary.

(In the foreword to Heinerman's book, he describes a sheep that had a malignancy in and around the mouth. It cured itself by eating from a patch of comfrey [*Symphytum officinale* of the plant family Boraginaceae]. Comfrey is listed under its scientific name as an anticancer agent in Hartwell's (1982) compendium. The manner in which comfrey is described as dissolving the sheep's cancerous growth suggests the action of proteolytic plant enzymes. Unfortunately, comfrey contains pyrrolizidine alkaloids (PAs), and its continued internal use can lead to serious consequences.)

It is said that Compound-X, was, or is, formulated principally from bloodroot, that is, from a powder of *Sanguinaria canadensis* (of the family Papaveraceae), with zinc chloride added to form a caustic paste. Whereas a degree of success was obtained with skin cancers on horses, the substance was said to have had no effect on internal cancers in animals.

A second version of Compound-X might or might not be formulated using chaparral or creosote bush *(Larrea tridentata)*, and redroot has also been mentioned as an ingredient. (Redroot is most usually the species *Lachnanthes tinctoria*, although according to *Webster's Third*, it may also be of the genus *Ceanothus* and sometimes pertains to bloodroot *or S. canadensis. The Random House Dictionary* states that the name may apply to any of several other plants that have red roots, notably alkanet or *Alkanna tinctoria*, pigweed or *Amaranthus retroflexus*, and New Jersey tea or *Ceanothus americanus*, which also underlines a difficulty in dealing with herbs: substitutions may have been made.) There was a company formed at Riverton or Lander, Wyoming, presumably connected with Vipont Pharmaceuticals and was bought out by a Nevada company. Evidently, much research was conducted, with clinical tests in Italy and Costa Rica (Heinerman, 1984, p. 129), and maybe in Portugal. Incidentally, the Riverton/Lander area of northwestern Wyoming is near the Wind River Indian Reservation of the Shoshone and Arapaho.

It can be mentioned that an advertisement for Compound-X appeared in the March/April 1995 issue of *Natural Health* on page 143 and in other magazines. It was then available from Spirit Technologies Inc., P.O. Box 8033 NH, Reno, NV 89507-8033, Tel: 800-320-4884.

## BLOODROOT

A herb previously mentioned is bloodroot, which has a track record of potent anticancer properties (Walters, 1993, p. 96). It is in fact a component of the Hoxsey therapy for skin cancer treatment and has been used by others. For instance, much earlier, in the 1850s at Middlesex Hospital in London, a Dr. J.W. Fell prepared a paste of bloodroot extract, zinc chloride, flour, and water. Applied to external cancerous growths, it was said to destroy the growth in 2 to 4 weeks. "In the 1960s, various teams of doctors reported the complete healing of cancers of the nose, external ear, and other organs using a paste made of bloodroot and zinc chloride, a mixture virtually identical to Hoxsey's." Incidentally, Hartwell's listings (19821) for *S. canadensis* or bloodroot comprise numerous entries. It should be noted, however, that bloodroot is also regarded as poisonous (Hardin and Arena, 1974, p. 69;

Muenscher, 1939, p. 98), though sometimes not quite so much (Kingsbury, 1965, p. 82; Kingsbury, 1964, pp. 152–153). It contains the alkaloid sanguinarine.

Salves for cancer are apparently common enough. Walters supplies several information sources, including some based on Indian remedies (Walters, 1993, p. 94).

For the record, Hoxsey's herbal mixture for internal cancers included the following (Moss, 1992, p. 161; Walters, 1993, p. 97): potassium iodide, cascara (*Rhamnus*), licorice (*Glycyrrhiza*), red clover (*Trifolium*), burdock root (*Arctium*), barberry (*Berberis*), stillingia root (*Stillingia*), pokeroot (*Phytolacca*), prickly ash bark (*Zanthoxylum*), and buckthorn bark (*Rhamnus*). All are listed in Hartwell (1982), and some occur in other herbal remedies for cancer. It has been commented that "orthodox scientific research has by now identified antitumor activity" in most of the plants used by Hoxsey (Walters, 1993, p. 97).

In Brown (1875), a paste of bloodroot and zinc chloride was specified as a cauterizing agent for local cancers (p. 346). Reapplication was continued until the entire cancerous mass was dead; then it would slough off. Brown noted that the juices of poke, laurel, bloodroot, and yellow dock also served the same purpose.

## CONDURANGO

Dr. Brown, cited in the preceding text, wrote at the time that a new plant had been recently brought into notice that would revolutionize the treatment of cancer. The plant was called *cundarango,* or *condurango* (*Equatoria garciana*). Brown tried it in several cases, and it worked. The plant is also called the *condor vine* and is native to the Andes Mountains of South America. It occurs in the mountains surrounding the city of Loja, in southern Ecuador, on the western slope at around 4000 to 5000 ft elevation (Brown, 1875, pp. 74–75). Its medicinal properties were discovered accidentally when an Indian woman tried to poison her husband, who was suffering from a painful cancer. It was subsequently introduced into practice by a Dr. Eguiguren, brother of the governor of the province of Loja. Hartwell (1982) has a listing, where it is variously called cundurango, or condurango, with the scientific name *Equatoria garciana* or *Gonolobus condurango*, of the family Asclepiadaceae. Hartwell notes its usage starting in 1871, with considerable documentation between 1871 and 1911. Otherwise, it seems to have disappeared from the scene, though the South American herb pau d'arco (from *Tabebuia* spp. of the family Bignoniaceae in Hartwell) is now a commonplace herb.

## CAT'S CLAW

Still another plant from South America, occurring in the upper reaches of the Amazon in Peru and in Central America, has been under study since the 1970s. It is called *cat's claw,* or *uña de gato,* and is a spiny shrub or small tree. The scientific name is *Pithecolobium Unguis-cati* of the family Leguminosae, with the genus spelled *Pithecellobium* in Hartwell (1982). Some remarkable cancer cures are attributed to drinking a tea made from the plant. Cat's claw has been made available from health food sources in the United States and is said to have very low toxicity levels, at least in the dosages used. Six alkaloids have so far been found in the plant, some of which apparently stimulate the immune system. That is, the alkaloids, being poisonous, may in small amounts act to enhance the functions of the WBC and macrophages (large blood cells) to destroy harmful microorganisms and foreign substances. Hence, this is a possible role for alkaloids (in very small amounts), for example, as used in homeopathy. (Most alkaloids have a unique nitrogen-containing ring structure, which will be further examined.) Moreover, used along with chemo-therapy, cat's claw is said to ameliorate the side effects. More than this, there are other compounds in cat's claw that may have benefits of a different kind and may explain its strong antioxidant and antiacid indigestion properties.

## PARASITES

Another unorthodox conviction is that cancer is caused by internal parasites. Hulda Regehr Clark wrote a book about it, with specifications for herbal treatment, titled *The Cure For All Cancers* (1993). The claim is also made that these herbs act against HIV and AIDS. One of the herbal ingredients mentioned is the alkaloid-containing wormwood (*Artemisia absinthia* of the family Compositae) as per Hartwell (1982b). In small dosages, it is apparently safe enough, but in large dosages it is toxic, a familiar characteristic of alkaloids and other poisons. As its name implies, worm-wood is a folk remedy against intestinal parasites, used in "deworming." One or another of the species of wormwood (genus *Artemisia*) is a component of vermouth, and another species is used in absinthe. The use in absinthe, presumably to enhance the effects of the alcohol, is the most notorious. (Its use in absinthe has since been outlawed.)

In turn, considered among the latest acknowledged contributing causes of cancer are fungi and their chemical components, which, strangely enough, may sometimes serve as remedies. A fungus may at times be regarded as a bacterium; which again brings up the subject of gut flora or bacteria. They have been identified as cancer-causing agents, producing biochemical carcinogens that are transported to other parts of the body. On the other hand, bacterial species have been used as anticancer agents, as in producing Coley's Toxins.

Interestingly, back during the beginnings of the 1900s, British physician J. Jackson Clarke had contributed *Protozoa and Disease* (1912) and *Protists and Disease* (1922) (the term *protists* signifying the unicellular organisms now collec-tively called *Protista*, which consist of both protozoans and unicellular plants). This will be discussed further in a later chapter.

## RABIES

Though not directly linked with cancer, either as cause or cure, the deadly rabies virus merits special consideration, especially as it may involve the immune response. And there may or may not be herbal remedies. In brief review, the following information is restated.

As previously mentioned, in an article in the August 1961 issue of *Arizona Highways*, Dr. Joseph G. Lee described the use of rue against rabies by the Papago Indians. Dr. Lee in turn speaks of a rapport between the Indian medicine man and the patient. He observes that the rapport is more useful than method, though no one knows just what "rapport" consists of. He states that there is magic and mystery in it, and its absence leaves words of logic and wisdom fruitless and sterile. He then describes the case of an Indian woman who was badly bitten and chewed by a rabid coyote. The coyote was killed and its head sent in for analysis at the Arizona State laboratory, where rabies was confirmed. The woman refused the Pasteur treatment and instead was treated by the village medicine man. Her wounds healed rapidly, and she never ever showed any symptoms of human rabies. This Indian treatment was never determined as it is being kept a secret. Dr. Lee observes that indeed something must have been done, for there have been too many other similar cases.

Dr. Lee further states that the Papago Indians of northern Sonora cut and burn crosses on their dogs' foreheads after the dogs have been bitten by a rabid animal. This is part of the medicine man's treatment. Furthermore, in Sonora and on the southern Arizona reservation, the Papagoes undergo some sort of strange treatment, about which the only thing outsiders know is that it begins "with the drawing of a circle."

Alma R. Hutchens' *Indian Herbalogy of North America* cites herbs that, according to medical folklore, are said to act against hydrophobia or rabies, some of which are in common with Heinerman's listing. In addition to rue, there is mention of balsam fir, beech tree, echinacea, henbane, Jimsonweed, rue, skullcap, St. John's wort, and tansy. Jimsonweed and henbane contain the alkaloid hyoscyamine, as do some other members of the family Solanaceae, or nightshade family. The family Solanaceae, incidentally, is well represented in Hartwell (1982b).

As mentioned, Heinerman documents the use of elecampane root (*Inula helenium*) in several successful rabies cases (Heinerman, 1977, pp. 61–65) is documented. The active ingredient is said to be inulin, or inuline, a polysaccharide also found in other plants, such as the dahlia and Jerusalem artichoke. The herb rue (*Ruta gravolens*) is likewise emphasized as being an old remedy for the prevention and cure of rabies (Heinerman, 1977, p. 55), which is in agreement with Dr. Lee's previously mentioned remarks. The herb yarrow (*Achillea millefolium*) when used with calamint (evidently one or another mint species of the genus *Clinopodium* or *Calamintha*) is also cited as being good for curing rabid conditions (Heinerman, 1977, p. 61).

According to the ancient Greek philosopher Aristotle, garlic (*Allium sativum*) is a cure for hydrophobia, and the Greeks also are reported to have used horehound (*Marrubium vulgare*) as an antidote for the bite of a mad dog, which may have something to do with its common name (*The Rodale Herb Book*, 1974, pp. 450, 468). Another herb is mentioned in Arnold and Connie Krochmal's *A Guide to the Medicinal Plants of the United States*. It is purple echinacea (*Echinacea purpurea*), also known as purple coneflower (Krochmal, 1973, p. 91). There is also mention of a particular lichen in medical folklore. (Lichens, incidentally, are a symbiosis of two kinds of plants growing together, a species of fungus and a species of algae, each supporting the other.) Thus, the dog lichen, *Peltigear canina*, was so named because eating it was supposed to cure rabies.

The rabies virus and its disease remain an enigma, with occasional flare-ups, and large-scale controls are sometimes successful, such as the spread of vaccine-injected food pellets, which have been used to inoculate susceptible predators in the American Southwest. Rabies could be a deadly scourge of the American Frontier, affecting both Indians and the white interlopers (Hoffman, 1999a, pp. 270, 271), and it remains a scourge in Africa. General George Crook's *Autobiography* and the account by Bourke (1950) should be consulted. Interestingly, Dodge (1882) noted that rabid skunks seemed not to bother the native American Indians and instead preferred the white man. However, rabid wolves were deadly toward the Indians.

A peculiarity is that, for two persons bitten by the same rabid animal, one may contract the disease and the other may not, possibly due to a difference in the activities of the immune system. Another complication is that the virus can remain dormant, even for a period that can last years. The virus can also be airborne, as in bat caves, where animals placed in cages have been demonstrated to contract the disease, and on a few rare occasions, human cavers have also contracted the disease as well. The spread may very well be by dust particles containing saliva and fecal matter. Another problem is the fungus causing histoplasmosis (a disease of the reticuloendothelial defense system, resulting in fever, anemia, and emaciation). The subject of rabies is further discussed by Colin Kaplan, G.S. Turner, and D.A. Warrell in *Rabies: The Facts*, second edition (and in Hoffman, 1999a, p. 266ff). It may be added that the rabies virus belongs to the family Rhabdoviridae, which comprises RNA viruses, but which do not contain the enzyme reverse transcriptase, the distinguishing feature of retroviruses.

In Moss (1992), the subject of interference between viruses is studied. He notes that a harmless virus can be used to negate the effects of a lethal virus. In experiments on mice infected with a rabies strain, the death rate could be reduced from 50% to 15% by injecting a harmless avian encephalitis virus (Moss, 1992, p. 441).

Lastly, it may be mentioned that bats are apparently the only mammals that can survive the rabies virus. Although other animals such as skunks are carriers, the rabid populations eventually die out. Such is not the case with bats, as a few cave explorers have inadvertently found out. This sort of viral immunity may ultimately have application in cancer prevention and treatment.

All things said, it is certain that most of us no doubt would prefer to put our trust in a modern version of the Pasteur treatment.

## MORE ABOUT THE PLANT WORLD

In reviewing alternative cancer remedies, the primary emphasis is on plants and herbs, where the baseline authority is Hartwell (1982), cited on numerous occasions. Hartwell, who was a chemist with the NCI, tracked cancer folklore back to the beginnings of recorded history. The aforementioned volume consists of over 700 pages, with approximately 3000 species entries from 1430 genera in 214 different plant families.

For an introduction to the history of herbalogy and some of the early treatises, there is *The Rodale Herb Book*, edited by William H. Hylton (1974). In the Western world, it is noted that the impetus started during the Elizabethan Age, though herbal tradition started much earlier in China. More details are contained in Barbara Griggs' *Green Pharmacy: The History and Evolution of Western Herbal Medicine* (1991), which provides an update, including trials and tribulations with the FDA and AMA. For these and other reasons, herbal medicine is kept off balance and is compelled to wage an uphill battle.

In this context, we are talking mostly about plants and herbs. Moreover, the terms *plants* and *herbs* are used synonymously, though the earlier implications were that the term herbs inferred condiments. More broadly, a herb can be described as a plant used for medicinal, savory, or aromatic purposes. If from the tropics, the word spice is favored for aromatic purposes, so the term herb is more a connotation for the north temperate zone. It also implies that the plant is herbaceous, that is, nonwoody. The catchall term *plant* will cover everything, woody and nonwoody, tropical and nontropical, and the component parts thereof, including the leaves, stems, twigs, limbs, trunk, bark and inner bark, rhizomes, and roots, as well as the flower and the resulting fruit with its shell, peel or covering, its seeds, meats, or kernels.

A problem with the medicinal use of plants and herbs is that substitutions can occur, inadvertently or on purpose. In addition, the herbal activity of a given species may vary with the geographic location, the season, and sometimes even with the time of day. Furthermore, the bioactive substance will usually concentrate in a particular plant part, such as the leaf or root, although it may occur in a much lesser degree throughout the plant

Another problem with plants and herbs is that there are many chemical constituents present, some of which are more bioactive than others. It becomes difficult or impossible to discern the action of each chemical constituent, which is compounded by the fact that the chemical compositions may vary from plant to plant, and from plant part to plant part, depending on a number of factors. Only if the pure compounds are isolated and tested can a consensus be reached. This is an argument in favor of synthetic drugs, in that quality control can be maintained, and controlled testing can be performed. All of these can become a monumental task.

Interestingly, plants that are the most bioactive and potentially useful as medicines are usually also the most poisonous. The description "poisonous and medicinal plants" denotes this symbiosis. Among the more poisonous constituents is the class of nitrogenous compounds called *alkaloids*, some of which can be toxic in the extreme.

To commence with a specific instance, Ernest T. Krebs, Jr., a biochemical researcher studying a class of compounds called *nitrilosides*, of which the commercial substance called *laetrile* is a refined form, famously maintained that these compounds act against cancer. They also counteract other diseases such as sickle cell anemia (e.g., D.W. Harper and M.L. Culbert, *How You Can Beat the Killer Diseases*). To a small degree, raw, confectionary almonds contain this type of compound, also called *amygdalin*, and medical folklore maintains that a fistful a day will help keep the cancer away.

Bitter almonds have a higher (and more deadly) amygdalin content. In fact, it is said that Napoleon met his final end as the result of being given an elixir containing the oil of bitter almonds, as set forth in the concluding chapter of Alan Schom's biography *Napoleon Bonaparte*. This *coup de grace* was the climax to being systematically and chronically poisoned by arsenic added to his medicines.

Raw nuts, in general (as distinguished from peanuts, which are legumes), contain amygdalin to a limited degree. In particular, peach and apricot kernels contain amygdalin in a more concentrated form and are ordinarily not to be recommended as a medicinal substance or otherwise. However, Jonathan V. Wright, M.D., in *Dr. Wright's Book of Nutritional Therapy*, figures that three or four peach or apricot kernels per day should be okay for an adult (Wright, 1979, pp. 425, 426). For more input, however, consider the case of the Hunzas of Central Asia, as described in the following text.

The most notable instance of pronounced dietary use of apricots, particularly, is by the Hunzas and their neighbors, the Nagers, who are located along the Hunza River in the recesses of the northwestern Himalayan massif, part of the Karakoram Range. In a book titled *Horned Moon: An Account of a Journey through Pakistan, Kashmir, and Afghanistan*, by Ian Stephens and published in 1955 by the Indiana University Press, a visit to these peoples is documented. Stephens describes the remarkable role of apricots in the local village economy, although other fruit crops are also grown, namely apples, pears, peaches, cherries, and mulberries (Stephens, 1955, pp. 169, 170). Whereas the other fruits are planted conventionally, apricots are planted as if they were potatoes. A principal crop, they grow to abundant perfection in the climate and soil, and create an extraordinary scenic effect when in bloom.

Stephens adds that the ripe flesh of the apricot fruit is eaten both fresh and dried, but the kernel is the most important of all. It is eaten as it is, like a hard almond, or else it is ground into flour for bread and cakes, which Stevens pronounced delicious. The kernel also produces valuable oil, and experts have judged that the kernel is exceptionally nutritious. Stephens subsisted on apricot kernels in his travels and notes that on one such journey, apricot kernels along with some raisins were his only diet.

He attributed the vigorous health of these people to the apricot factor in the diet and possibly something in the water. Stephens describes visiting with one elderly man of firm handclasp and brisk step, whose knowledge of Kashmir history confirmed his stated 97 years. Stephens said that the man looked no more than 65. He also added that the endurance of the Hunzawals (and Nagerwals) on mountain expeditions was simply astounding and was noted by some to be far superior even to that of the Sherpas of Nepal.

In another book about the Hunzas, by Allen E. Banik and Renée Taylor, published in 1960 and titled *Hunza Land: The Fabulous Health and Youth Wonderland of the World*, farming and food are discussed. Various grains, fruits, and vegetables are listed in the diet, with nuts restricted to walnuts. Goat milk provides butter and cheese (with some cheeses aged for up to 100 years). It is noted that meat is scarce, and principally is mutton. Eggs are imported only for the wealthy and the royal family. Chickens are viewed with suspicion, as they scratch up seeds and crops. (As has previously been noted, the Navajo avoid chicken and chicken products, or used to, and had the lowest natural cancer incidence in the United States, exclusive of the radiation-induced effects from uranium mining.)

Apricot trees are allowed to grow for at least 50 years, after which they are cropped to about 20 ft off the ground, and continue to grow and produce for another

50 years. The tree trunks match forest trees in size, and the fruit yield is prodigious. Apricot trees are, in fact, regarded as valuable property and a measure of affluence, and are passed down as an inheritance.

The apricot flesh is very sweet, with the seed kernels regarded the best part of the fruit, tasting sweet and oily, very much like almonds. (It may be noted that the apricot is of the genus *Prunus* of the plant family Rosaceae, as are peaches and almonds.) Apricot oil is squeezed out under pressure from the ground flour or meal and looks much like olive oil. A spoonful may be taken as needed, and the oil is also used for deep-frying. Other uses include external applications, and it is also mentioned that the oil will even shine silverware. (The preceding information indicates that the apricot kernels are utilized raw, without roasting.)

Finally, it may be mentioned from other sources that apricots are high in sulfur content (Koch and Lawson, 1996, p. 39). Although apricots contain perhaps only a fourth of the sulfur content of garlic, they nevertheless rank equally with onions and broccoli. And garlic, notably, is regarded as a folkloric anticancer agent, as are the cruciferous vegetables (of the mustard family, with the scientific name Brassicaceae or Cruciferae. The name is derived from the fact that the flowers are in the shape of a Greek cross).

For a diametrically opposite view, there is John Clark's *Hunza: Lost Kingdom of the Himalayas*, published in 1956. Clark, a geologist who taught at Princeton, traveled to these parts to do some prospecting and survey the mineral potential, establish a school, etc. He took along a considerable supply of medicines. Clark spent 20 months living among the Hunzas, as noted in his preface, adapting into their ways and outlook, their scarcities, at the same time introducing improvements, only some of which they would accept.

In a chapter titled "The Healthy Hunzas Come to the Doctor," Clark describes some of their ailments and some of his successes at cures. He had a parade of patients, facing over 60 on his fourth day (Clark, 1956, p. 66). Many of the problems were with sores, common types of problems that had arisen during the previous 3 years and were left untreated, and which fortunately yielded to antiseptics and antibiotics (Clark, 1956, p. 68). Clark treated over 5000 patients during his time there, with some dying in spite of treatment, and some beyond help, but with most responding.

In a chapter titled "Gardens and Gardening," Clark observed that the Hunza diet was deficient in oils and vitamin D, as a result of which they have soft teeth, with about half the population exhibiting barrel chests and rheumatic knees, the mark of subclinical rickets (Clark, 1956, p. 205). He offers the sarcasm, "Happy healthy Hunza, where everyone has just enough!" Nowhere, apparently, does Clark mention the long life spans usually attributed to the Hunzas.

About apricots in the Hunza diet, a dish of walnuts and apricot nuts was mentioned as a food item (Clark, 1956, p. 73). In a description of the terrain and the desperate efforts to provide cultivation, Clark calls the Hunzas land-starved people, in spite of visitors writing about Hunza as the land where everyone has "just enough" and where there are no poor (Clark, 1956, p. 202). He indicates that the climate is ideal for apricots, mulberries, and grapes. The Hunzas themselves are good horticulturists, having practiced the art of grafting apricot trees for some 1600 years.

They have at least six local varieties to choose from, to furnish strong roots and the most desirable cuttings for grafting (Clark, 1956, p. 203). The children climb the trees and shake down the ripe fruit, which unfortunately becomes contaminated on the ground, bacillary dysentery being the result.

Clark compares this practice with that in America, where apricot trees are cut down when they become too high for ladders, usually after about 35 years. However, as also mentioned by Stephens and by Banik and Taylor (1960), in the preceding text, the Hunza trees are allowed to grow for 50 years, then cropped about 15 to 20 ft. from the ground, to grow for another 50 years, meantime producing huge yearly crops. When finally cut down, the trees, which have grown as large as forest trees, make for beautiful lumber, suitable for wood carving.

It is stated that the apricots are eaten fresh or dried, and the seeds are cracked open to yield the almondlike nuts. The dried fruit is sweet and soft, but it does not keep well, though it lasts through the winter. It is also mentioned that the sweet apricot nuts are eaten as is, but the bitter apricot nuts are ground, followed by squeezing out of the highly poisonous apricot oil, which is used for fuel in saucer lamps equipped with a cotton wick.

A rash of very sore stomachs among the Hunzas prompted Clark to investigate (Clark, 1956, p. 181). It was found that the Hunzas were flavoring their wine with bitter apricot oil, so Clark tried some himself and wound up with a terrible stomach ache. It was concluded that those "who use prussic acid for bitters must expect a little gastric distress."

Further concerning apricot kernel toxicity and about sweet vs. bitter varieties, a computer search of the information base AGRICOLA turned up an article titled "Toxicological, Nutritional and Microbiological Evaluation of Tempe Fermentation with *Rhizopus oligosporus* of Bitter and Sweet Apricot Seeds," by G. Tunçel, M.J.R. Nout, L. Brimer, and D. Göktan, variously of Ege University, Izmir, Turkey, the Agricultural University, Wageningen, the Netherlands, and the Royal Veterinary University, Frederiksberg, Denmark. The dish called *tempe* is prepared from fermented soybeans, for example, by using the fungus *Rhizopus oligosporus*. Depending on the variety, the seeds left over are suitable for either edible or bitter oil. The article is mainly concerned about the details of leaching and fermentation, and of amygdalin content and toxicity, but illustrates the fact that both sweet and bitter varieties of apricots exist, as also noted for almonds. Furthermore, maybe a spoonful of the oil once in a while is nontoxic, and as for its use in cooking, it may be remarked that heat destroys the cyanic content, as with beans.

Another, later observer of the Hunzas was George B. Schaller, who wrote *Stones of Silence: Journeys in the Himalaya*, first published in 1979. Schaller took the new Karakoram Highway, which runs up into and through the Hunza country, following stretches of the old Silk Road, breaching the Karakoram Range and then down into the Sinkiang Province of China. Schaller could find no differences between the Hunzas and people of the other valleys and asked a local official about the reported long life spans of the Hunzas. The official scoffed at the very idea (Schaller, 1979, p. 87).

There is a long history of using these kinds of cyanic substances for tumors or cancers, dating back to the ancient Sumerians and Assyrians (Heinerman, 1984,

p. 171ff). It was found in prune pits and juniper berry extracts, which are still used as sources. In the early seventeenth century, the English herbalist John Gerarde (or Gerard) noted the use of apricot and peach pits for these purposes. Heinerman further states that, in the Civil War, a Confederate surgeon, Dr. Francis Peyre Porcher, said that the hydrocyanic acid (HCN) in peach pits was the active agent in treating cancerlike infections. Heinerman further writes that the famous English poet Shelley asked for "prussic acid or essential oil of almond," such was its recognized medicinal value at that time.

More about almonds and the almond tree, *Prunus amygdalus*: There are two main subspecies classification: the sweet almond (*dulcis*) and the bitter almond (*amara*). The almond, incidentally, is closely related to the peach and will hybridize with it. Additionally, there are many cultivated varieties of the sweet almond, as well as of the peach. The sweet almond is our everyday kind of almond, used as a food or confectionery source, whereas the bitter almond is utilized for industrial purposes, for example, as a source of chemicals. The seed kernels of both the sweet and bitter subspecies contain a high percentage of oil, but the oil from the bitter almond will hydrolyze to produce poisonous HCN (also called prussic acid), as well as the chemical benzaldehyde. The benzaldehyde provides the characteristic almond flavor and aroma, whereas the HCN gives the bitter taste. This also holds true for peach and apricot kernels. Though the bitter almond is sometimes mentioned as providing the more effective route for cancer treatment, as are peach and apricot kernels, the latent coproduction of HCN makes their use seem somewhat like the game of Russian roulette. Thus, normally, there is a distinct preference for the sweet almond.

(The thermal decomposition of almonds or related seed kernels, such as those of the apricot or peach, even apple seeds, produces the characteristic burnt-almond odor of benzaldehyde, with the other component [hydrogen cyanide] being odorless [this is a favorite clue in murder mysteries]. Accordingly, apple seeds should not be eaten in any great quantity. They have a bitter taste anyway. [Though as an aside, apple sauce made from the core will be naturally sweet, and the seeds can be separated out.] Though the hydrogen cyanide is poisonous, hydrogen sulfide is supposed to be even more so. Hydrogen sulfide has the well-known characteristic smell of rotten eggs and sewer gas. It is also a component of sour crude oils and natural gases, along with other types of objectionable sulfur compounds such as mercaptans. There is even the possibility that hydrogen cyanide may occur naturally in some crude oils and natural gases, as the ingredients are all there, including nitrogen. An insidious property of hydrogen sulfide is that only a small amount will dampen the olfactory sense, and a person may remain unaware of the level of exposure, with fatal consequences.)

Perhaps the use of HCN or its kin could be regarded as some sort of primitive chemotherapy, as compared with modern and generally accepted orthodox practices such as the injection of the chemical called 5-FU or 5-fluorouracil as an anticancer agent; this chemical is also sufficiently poisonous in its own right. One of the questions to be answered is whether HCN and its kin are specific to cancer, whereas synthetic chemicals such as 5-FU are known to be nonspecific, indiscriminately killing healthy cells as well as cancerous ones. This is a reason for the local or topical application of chemicals onto the cancer mass itself.

Naturally occurring laetrile and its derivatives are by no means the only historical possibilities for plant materials that act against cancer. The French botanist Jean Louis Berlandier (1980), in his travels through northeast Mexico and southwest Texas during 1826 to 1834, observed pastures where grew the herb of cancer (*yerba del Cancer*), allegedly a specific against cancerous afflictions.

(The name *yerba del Cancer* applies to species of several genera, in this particular case to *Lythrum californicum*. In Hartwell (1982), several species of the genus *Lythrum* are noted as having been used in decoctions for cancerous ulcers, external cancers, cancer of the lip, and cancer in general. The genus and species are of the family Lythraceae.)

University of Wyoming chemistry professor Owen Asplund is one of those who have studied the antitumor effects from the extracts of native plants. His work, carried out in the early 1980s, has resulted in an extract from the yucca plant being clinically tested in Switzerland and Mexico. Evidently, the thrust is against the skin cancer known as melanoma or skier's disease. (Asplund's work was mentioned by Heinerman [1980,1984].)

Also at the University of Wyoming, pharmacy professor Emery W. Brunett has worked on compiling an information data bank of old remedies, folk remedies, American Indian remedies, and other sources. Similarly, at the University of Wyoming, English professor Silvestor J. Brito worked on surveying the folk medicine of Mexico, but treatments for cancer were not included.

Another former University of Wyoming pharmacy professor, Steve Gillespie, has investigated herbal remedies in conjunction with the Herb Research Foundation at Boulder, Colorado, which is affiliated with the American Botanical Center at Austin, Texas. (Hanna's Herbs at Boulder, Colorado, founded by well-known herbalist Hanna Kroeger, remains an ongoing institution.) As for the plants per se of the Rocky Mountains and surrounding areas, the Rocky Mountain Herbarium or Botany Conservatory at the University of Wyoming is a valuable information source. Interest in the medicinal properties of plant substances is becoming widespread, not just in the Rocky Mountain region, but everywhere.

To elaborate more on the plants of the desert Southwest and Mexico, medical anthropologist and herbal authority John Heinerman has written *Aloe Vera, Jojoba and Yucca*, published in 1982, not to mention his many other books.

Such information is part of a growing pharmacopoeia of medically active plants or plant extracts. Years of investigation, assessment, and controversy will no doubt be required to determine usefulness. We are reminded by the foregoing investigations that this is one of the many reasons for not destroying any member of the diverse species bank, as who knows what remedies may yet be found.

In this regard, Hartwell (1982) has already been cited several times. A literature survey, it was published as a book back in 1982, after first appearing as an 11-part series in the journal *Lloydia* during the period 1967–1971. Many of the plants had already become established in medical folklore; other plants were obscure and some, dangerous. Expectedly, a new listing would be even more comprehensive.

Hartwell's compendium in its entirety was originally included as part of a series, appearing as *Bioactive Plants, Volume II*. The first volume in the series was also published in 1982 as *Bioactive Plants, Volume I*, with the title *Medicinal Uses of Plants by Indian Tribes of Nevada* by Percy Train, James R. Hendrichs and W. Andrew Archer. It was originally published by the U.S. Department of Agriculture, Plant Industry Station, Beltsville, Maryland, in 1957.

For the record, the science of classification of living things is taxonomy, and a categorization from the highest level of abstraction (kingdom) to the lowest level or next lowest level (species) comprises the following: kingdom, phylum or division, class, order, family, genus, and species. There may, of course, be subdivisions. Thus, the species may be further subdivided into subspecies, also known as *variations* or *variants*, *races*, or *strains*, etc. (presumably, mutations can also be included as subspecies). For our purposes here, we are interested only in family, genus, and species, and occasionally subspecies or variants.

Known as the *Linnaean system*, after the Swedish botanist Carolus Linnaeus (1707–1778), its practical application to species involves using the Latinized genus name followed by the species designator. This becomes the rigorous scientific name, as distinguished from the several common names that exist. The combination signifies the particular species, and by requiring that the genus be included, the totality becomes manageable in size. (That is, the same spores designator can be used for different genera.) The common custom is to give the combination or couplet in italics, with the first letter of the genus capitalized. The person responsible for discovering or naming the particular species is added, usually in the form of an abbreviation in Roman letters. The abbreviations or names of many prominent early-day botanists show up, for example, as L. for Linnaeus, Ryd. for Rydberg, Nutt. for Nuttall, etc. (With regard to species in the western United States, the names or abbreviations of well-known early-day western explorers show up, such as for Thomas Nuttall, Edwin James, and William Clark.) Additionally, if a variation or variant is involved, this is signified by the introduction of the abbreviation var. followed by the variant name in uncapitalized italics.

For our purposes here, however, only the genus and species designator will be used. An example is the plant whose common name is bloodroot, and whose scientific name is *Sanguinaria canadensis* or *Sanguinaria canadensis* L. (of the family Papaveraceae, or the poppy family), which contains an alkaloid known as sanguinarine. (Not all family names have been provided a common name.)

All the species members of a genus may be specified by giving the genus name, generally followed by spp. or otherwise so designated. A single member of a species is called a *specimen*, and a collection of specimens may be referred to as a *population*. The plural of *genus* is *genera*.

If the family name embracing the genus is not given, it may be looked up in a specialized dictionary or handbook, for instance, in Willis (1973), now in its eighth edition. For common names that may appear in an ordinary dictionary of the English language, the scientific name is almost always given, and the family name may be added as well. If a higher level of abstraction is desired, that is, order, class, or phylum, then a technical exposition may be sought out. Encyclopedias are a good place to start.

We mention in passing that garlic (genus *Allium*, family Liliaceae), as described previously at length, is prominently listed in Hartwell's compendium (1982b). Aloe vera (genus *Aloe*, family Liliaceae) and jojoba (*Simmondsia californica* of the family Buxaceae, whose genus is also classified as the lone member of the family Simmondsiaceae), an evergreen shrub native to the Southwest, are also listed. Its other main claim to fame is as a source for high-quality lubricants, possibly equal to sperm oil. No listings occur in Hartwell for the several species of yucca as such (genus *Yucca*, family Amaryllidaceae), although there are listings for agave (genus *Agave*, family Amaryllidaceae) in a couple of places. Both the yucca and the agave are considered alternately to be of the Agave family, or Agavaceae. Hartwell, however, first lists the genus *Agave* under the family Amaryllidaceae and then under the family Lilliaceae, which indicates that plant classifications may change from time to time.

Certain other southwestern desert plant species are missing in Hartwell. The waxy, candle-making plant candelilla (*Euphorbia antisyphylitica* of the family Euphorbiaceae) is not listed, although its species name indicates some other medicinal properties, and the genus is well represented. The resurrection plant (*Selaginella lepidophylla* of the family Selaginelliaceae), a perennial herb ranging from Texas to South America, is not mentioned. Also, the resurrection fern (*Polypodium polypodioides* of the family Polypodiaceae), a plant of wetter climes, of the southeastern United States and tropical America is missing, although the genus is represented well enough. Both these species are noted for their ability to come alive or "resurrect" after receiving a few sprinkles of water.

Among the later arrivals on the scene is the chemical compound quercetin, which has been identified as a potent anticancer agent. It occurs naturally in foods, notably in fresh vegetables, particularly, in onions, garlic, and cabbage. It is found in the creosote bush (also called chaparral or greasewood) and occurs in the inner bark of the black oak or yellow bark oak, from which its name is derived (oaks being of the genus *Quercus*).

Some of quercetin's potentially useful vs. potentially harmful properties have been reviewed by Alan Gaby, M.D., in an editorial in the May 1998 issue of the *Townsend Letter for Doctors & Patients*. It acts as an inhibitor for the enzyme phosphodiesterase, and hence may possibly act against asthma. Also, it may act against allergies by inhibiting the release of histamine. Quercetin is also an inhibitor for the enzyme aldose reductase, which is involved in diabetic complications. Perhaps most interestingly, it inhibits the enzyme reverse transcriptase (or RNA-directed DNA polymerase), involved in the action of retroviruses such as the AIDS virus or HIV (and retroviruses may also be involved in cancer formation).

Offsetting these potential beneficial uses is the well-documented fact that quercetin produces mutagenicity in cells, which is an indication of oncogenicity or carcinogenicity. Whether there can be some sort of optimum dosage and manner of dosage is evidently not established.

Also there is Taxol, derived from the bark of the Pacific yew, an evergreen tree or shrub, notably of the Pacific Northwest. (Yew wood was once favored by the Indians for bows and other purposes.) If successful, its relative scarcity vs. demand indicates that chemistry will have to come to the rescue, especially the specialty known as *organic synthesis*.

Additionally, there may be various undiscovered or untried plant foods that will have extraordinary nutritional and medicinal benefits. The trail of forager Euell Gibbons, in his advocacy of unconventional food sources, deserves a follow-up. Some were foods of the aboriginals, and others were their medicines. They are a known quantity in the expanding array of plants and herbs available.

As a footnote to the subject of plants and herbs, according to the aforementioned *The Rodale Herb Book*, much of herbal lore is due to Elizabethan Age herbalists John Gerard, John Parkinson, and Nicholas Culpeper. As mentioned in Chapter 1, Gerard wrote *The Herbal, or General History of Plants* (first published in 1597), which came to be known as *Gerard's Herbal*; Parkinson wrote *Theatrum Botanicum* (1640), and Culpeper wrote *Culpeper's Complete Herbal* (around 1649–1653). Culpeper's work was rendered in modern English by Graeme Tobyn, and titled *Culpeper's Medicine: A Practice of Western Holistic Medicine*. Later, in 1834, there was George Graves' *Hortus Medicus*, which has been republished as *Medicinal Plants: An Illustrated Guide to More than 180 Plants That Cure Disease and Relieve Pain*.

The core of this herbal knowledge was due to the ancients, notably the Greek herbalists. Aristotle, for instance, is reported to have had a garden of 300 plants with medicinal properties. Before this, the Ebers Papyrus, circa 2000 years BCE, is said to have noted some 2000 herbal doctors in Egypt. The Old Testament has occasional references to herbal medicine, as does the New Testament. The Chinese in particular have a long-standing tradition dating back to antiquity and even today are considered the world's preeminent herbalists. In turn, the New World that is America had its fair share of native herbal lore and practiced the doctrine of signatures, the same as was done everywhere else. The most notable of the many compilations made in colonial and postcolonial America is that by Philadelphia physician Dr. Benjamin Smith Barton. Titled *Collections for an Essay Towards a Materia Medica of the United States* (Part I, 1798; Part II, 1804), and usually called the shorter *Materia Medica of the United States*, it still serves as an authoritative reference. In 1813, a herbalist named Samuel Thomson selected some herbal compounds and had them patented, thus beginning the era of patent medicine. His efforts were greeted with litigation, for "Then as now the medical establishment didn't appreciate the work of nonestablishmentarians." More details about the subject are furnished in Barbara Griggs' *Green Pharmacy: The History and Evolution of Western Herbal Medicine*. As a result of these and other troubles, modern herbal medicine is in disarray in the United States. Only a very few citations are provided in Griggs' book for the herbal treatment of cancer.

## POISONOUS AND MEDICINAL PLANTS

Although alkaloids are among the most toxic of naturally occurring plant chemicals, or phytochemicals, varying from the fairly innocuous to the extremely deadly, other bioactive classes are also variously present in plant species, such as glycosides or glucosides (notably cyanic glycosides or glucosides such as laetrile), saponins, phenolics, flavonoids, etc. Among the ultimate in toxicity are the vegetable proteins such as abrin and ricin; ricin is derived from the castor bean plant (*Ricinus communis* of the family Euphorbiaceae).

A good reference on poisonous and medicinal plants is Blackwell (1990). The more toxic or poisonous a plant substance, the more bioactive it is judged to be, and potentially more valuable as a medicine, in very restricted, low-level dosages.

Thus, in searching the tropical rain forests for bioactive plants, the presence of alkaloids — determinable by a relatively simple test — is used as the criterion for cataloging a particular plant. The difficulties are formidable, as merely collecting a sample of plant parts like the leaves, stems, and flowers is hazardous and slow work, as described in Chapter 7 of David G. Campbell's *Land of Ghosts: The Braided Lives of People and the Forest in Far Western Amazonia*. As Campbell mentions in his prologue, he and compatriots only studied a small section of the forest, a total of 18 ha, a hectare being an area of 100 by 100 m (or 2.471 acres); it contained more than 20,000 individual trees, each with its own ecosystem of other life-forms and represented about 2000 species, three times as many as in the whole of North America. The totality of all kinds of different plant species in Amazonia is mind-boggling, although it is under assault from slash-and-burn practices, and the point of no return may be in sight. Then there is the problem of getting the vouchers to the proper taxonomic authorities in various universities and identifying and naming the various species, both new and known, but mostly already known. Campbell illustrates this fact with the genus *Inga*, of the family Leguminosae or Fabaceae. The genus *Inga* comprises about 300 different species in the New World tropics and is evidently not noted for any particular bioactive property.

Another modern-day observer and commentator of rain forest remedies is Elizabeth Royte, who wrote *The Tapir's Morning Bath: Mysteries of the Tropical Rain Forest and the Scientists Who Are Trying to Solve Them*, published in 2001. The particular place studied was Barro Colorado Island (BCI), some 6 mi$^2$ in area (or 1564 ha, a hectare being 0.003861 mi$^2$). The island is located in Gatun Lake, which comprises the midsection of the Panama Canal. The BCI and other islands were formed when the River Chagres was dammed in 1910 to create the lake. (The Guacho Island, extending about 166 mi$^2$, is situated at the center of the lake and later became a wildlife sanctuary in 1924.) The research station on BCI was established in 1923, the brainchild of James Zetek, an entomologist of the United States Department of Agriculture (USDA) who had been working on mosquito control in the Canal Zone; it is now administered by the Smithsonian Tropical Research Institute (STRI). Its fauna and flora constitute a rain forest sample in miniature and serves as an outdoor laboratory for successive arrays of scientists and graduate students, with trails running all over the island. (One of the trails was named after the naturalist David Fairchild, who was one of the early researchers on the island. His name surfaces in anticancer plant circles.) One area in particular, around 50 ha, has been studied and detailed extensively. The episode described constitutes the second trip made to the island by Royte, the first occurring in 1990 in the company of the famous sociobiologist E.O. Wilson (whose specialty was ants). More than the rain forest denizens, Royte's book is about the scientists who are involved in searches and observations (e.g., there is a chapter titled "Higher Primates").

Nevertheless, there is some information furnished in the book that merits repetition, although no index is furnished. Thus, the island contains some 1300 plant species, which had been dauntingly catalogued for a herbarium (Royte, 2002, p. 52). Mention is made of the alkaloids that occur in tropical leaves, seeds, roots, shoots, flowers, and fruits (Royte, 2002, pp. 228, 229). These alkaloids include cocaine, morphine, cannabinol (from Indian hemp, or *Cannabis sativa*), caffeine, and nicotine, some of which have serious side effects in mammals. Also mentioned are saponins, which destroy the fat content of cell membranes and cyanogenic glycosides, which will yield the deadly hydrogen cyanide when contacted with certain digestive enzymes. (The reminder is laetrile.) Members of the legume family, such as peas and beans, contain toxic amino acids that interfere with protein synthesis. In fact, there is a particular amino acid known as L-dopa that occurs in the seeds of some tropical plants and is hallucinogenic. Another fact is that 40% of all pharmaceuticals contain at least one component derived from tropical rain forests (Royte, 2002, p. 269). For instance, the anticoagulants used are based on leeches and snake venom. The rosy periwinkle is cited as being antileukemic, and other tropical plants are used against Hodgkins's disease, heart ailments, and arthritis.

It is mentioned that Bret Weinstein, a visiting scientist and bat specialist, who visited the island, had some interesting theories about cancer (Royte, 2002, p. 78, 294). Not a fan of the species concept, he regarded it as a necessary evil, with no agreed-upon single definition, with nature also at variance. The most common criterion for animals is that of interbreeding; if two animals can produce fertile offspring, then they are of the same species. Enter intercrossing, however, and of hybrids — and if they mate ...? Turning to cancer, the body has around 10 trillion cells, each with the potential for producing a runaway cell line (Royte, 2002, p. 301ff). The body's defense is senescence; thus, there can be runaway cell growth countered by retarded cell growth. In other words, there are substances called *Hayflick limits* that will cut off the unregulated growth of any cell line, thus negating tumors. Involved in this process is the telomere mechanism; telomeres are the long, repetitive sequences of DNA located at the end of chromosomes. They serve to protect the chromosome ends such that any failure of polymerase enzymes to copy the chromosome tip does not destroy any important gene. If an erosion of telomeres occurs, as in senescence, the cellular machinery is shut down. On the other hand, there is an enzyme called *telomerase* that serves to elongate telomeres. This enzyme is present in tumors (and in fetal and sperm cells) but not in normal cells. The tradeoff is that the erosion of telomeres signifies aging, but counters cancer growth, whereas the elongation of telomeres signifies cancer growth. The one plays against the other. An obvious question, in this context, that of why the elderly have a greater incidence of cancer.

Some alkaloids are mind altering or hallucinogenic, such as those of the family Papaveraceae or the poppy family, whereas others may adversely affect vital organs such as the liver and kidneys. The most deadly produce cardiac arrest and respiratory failure, that is, near-immediate suffocation. The effect of the alkaloids in curare, used by South American Indians to kill prey, should be recalled. Also high on the toxicity list is the alkaloid aconitine, derived from the roots of wolfsbane or monkshood, for example, the species *Aconitum napellus* of the family Ranunculaceae. It is described as being tried on cancer, in the form of a vodka extract a few drops at a time, in Alexander Solzhenitsyn's *Cancer Ward* (1969). (The results were not described, but its internal use was made illegal in the Soviet Union.) In his Time-Life book *Soviet Deserts and Mountains* (1974), George St. George takes note of expeditions into the mountains to collect roots and leaves and mentions their uses. It is said that a plant-derived liquid or oily substance rubbed on an arthritic joint proves markedly beneficial, and it has been similarly used against gout and as a local anesthetic (Hoffman, 1999, pp. 166, 339).

It may be added that although the poisonous element may be more concentrated in a particular plant part, it may to a degree also occur throughout the entire plant. Furthermore, as has been previously noted, the concentration or activity may vary with geographical location, the season, and even the time of day. Another interesting fact is that all the species of some plant families tend to be intrinsically toxic. For example, species members of the family Papaveraceae all contain alkaloids of one kind or another. The subject is chemical taxonomy, implied in the title of Peter Tétényi's (1970) *Infraspecific Chemical Taxa of Medical Plants*, translated from the Russian.

Hartwell (1982b) and others caution that natural plants may possess toxicity, even serious or fatal toxicity, as presented in the disclaimer to Hartwell's book. "Neither the author nor the publisher makes any medical claims for any herb. This information is compiled from the published literature. Some plants contain deadly poisons and some mentioned herein are extremely dangerous." Well, for that matter, so are some of the synthetic medical compounds produced en masse in the laboratory.

It is almost certain that a bioactive or medicinal plant will be toxic in large doses. It is a distinguishing factor, and hence the dosage levels and frequency are critical, as with foxglove or digitalis. This is the reason objective, open-minded, and impartial clinical studies are so important. The problem is, of course, who decides what works and what does not?

The usual questions asked are: what is effective, what is the safe, optimum dosage, how should this be administered and how often, and how shall this be determined? The documentations from folklore and the distillations of trial-and-error methods that have already been used on real people with some degree of success are recalled instead of the experiments conducted in test tubes, culture dishes, and on laboratory animals. In other words, there has already been a winnowing of sorts.

A number of books deal with poisonous plants, as cited previously in the section "Poisons in Nature," Chapter 1. Among the noted species of current interest are Western yew trees of the family Taxaceae, which contain the poisonous alkaloid taxine (Hardin and Arena, 1974, p. 42). The anticancer drug Taxol, for instance, is derived from the yew of the Pacific coast *(Taxus brevifolia)*.

Incidentally, a yew-related species from China named *Cephalotaxus fortunei* yields a toxic anticancer substance known as *harringtonine* (Griggs, 1991, p. 318). A similar species in the United States is known as *Cephalotaxus harringtonia,* from which is derived the bioactive substance homoharringtonine.

It was noted in Chapter 1 (in the section "Poisons in Nature") that there is a dearth of research into the toxicology of poisonous plants (Kingsbury, 1964, pp. 8, 9). This requires a team effort and a crossover of specialties, to bridge the "artificial chasm" between studies of animals and of plants and between the poisoned and the "poisoner." Inasmuch as biologically active plants tend to be poisonous, the implications are obvious.

We add that the classical Greek word *pharmakon* has a dual meaning, signifying both the poison and the antidote, the sickness and the cure (Girard, 1977, pp. 95, 288). Its action can be good or bad, depending on the circumstance and the dosage. Hence the term "poisonous and medicinal plants." The folkloric statement that the dosage is the poison may apply even to the minute ministrations of homeopathy, as well as the pharmaceuticals. The concomitant action of the immune system should be recalled.

## PLANTS AND HERBS AS AGENTS AGAINST OTHER DISEASES

The subject of treating rabies, a viral disease, brings up the increasingly vital fact that some herbs or plants, such as those containing alkaloids, are potential virucidal or antiviral agents, as well as potential germicidal, bactericidal, or antibacterial agents. The antibacterial category is of special interest, as bacterial strains continue to develop resistance to antibiotics. Some of the same agents or others are noted to be antifungal, and/or antiparasitic, or antiprotozoal. The former category is associated with such widespread fungal diseases as aspergillosis and histoplasmosis, whereas the latter category is responsible for various other diseases, including malaria, one of the great scourges of mankind. Still other plants or plant-derived substances are anthelminthic (acting against intestinal worms) and others are molluscicidal, acting against mollusks. Mollusks are intermediates in the life cycle for the spread of the blood-fluke disease known as *bilharziasis,* or *schistosomiasis*, another tropical scourge. Other agents or compounds may be insecticidal, antimetazoal, antidiabetic, anti-inflammatory, or simply serve as sweetening agents, etc., and it is apparent that the study of bioactive plants should be on the front burner, not only for cancer, but for other diseases.

Called *idiopathic diseases*, where causes or cures are unknown, there are such ailments as arthritis or inflammation of the joints (interfacing with rheumatism, now sometimes referred to as *fibromyalgia*), and Alzheimer's disease. As for arthritis viral causes are suspected, and there are suspicions that Alzheimer's disease may be caused by the subviral particles called *prions*. Prions are also implicated in mad cow disease, or BSE (bovine spongiform encephalopathy), a bovine form of scrapie originally found in sheep. A similar disease, called *chronic wasting disease,* may occur in deer and elk. These are neurological diseases affecting the brain, and in humans they are manifested notably as Creutzfeldt-Jakob disease (CJD) and may include kuru, the New Guinea disease (caused by eating human brains) called the *Gerstmann–Straussler syndrome.*

As previously indicated, in the foreword to Hartwell's compendium (1982b), James Duke, an authority on medicinal plants and plant compounds, had noted that government-supported research on plants as anticancer agents was inexplicably stopped on October 2, 1981, with whatever direction of research pursued to be left to the discretion of the pharmaceutical companies. We are now trying to catch up on this incomplete research.

(In addition to authoring or coauthoring a number of books about bioactive plant species found in North America and around the world, James A. Duke has been especially zealous about cataloguing phytochemicals, or plant chemicals. His works include *CRC Handbook of Medicinal Herbs* [2002], *Handbook of Biologically Active Phytochemicals and Their Activities* [1992], and *Handbook of Phytochemical Constitutents of GRAS Herbs and Other Economic Plants* [1992]. [The acronym GRAS stands for Generally Recommended as Safe.] The list of different chemical compounds in even a single plant species can be astounding. A selection of antitumor chemical compounds or phytochemicals as per the above references is presented in Appendix W of Hoffman [1999]. Other antitumor phytochemical citations may be found in Moss [1988]. For other citations about many of the chemical compounds or phytochemicals found in various herbal plant species, there is Crellin and Philpott [1990], further described in the following section.)

To continue the enumeration of various reference citations, consider the following partial listing: *A Dictionary of Natural Products; Anticancer Agents from Natural Products; Dictionary of Natural Products; Phytochemicals: Mechanisms of Action; Nutrition and Cancer; Phytopharmaceuticals in Cancer Chemoprevention; Plants That Fight Cancer*, etc. It is a sign of changing times and attitudes. The *Dictionary of Natural Products* has a listing of some 190,000 substances, is available on CD-ROM, and is updated biennially.

To put the medicinal use of plants in perspective, although the native shamans are able to cure some fevers, for the most part they are not able to cure their own, very serious tropical diseases, for example, malaria and bilharziasis or schistosomiasis, and instead must rely on Western medicine. One may of course conclude that the best course of action is not to get sick in the first place.

A particularly informative guide to herbal medicine is Crellin and Philpott [1990]. The authors interviewed a long-time Appalachian herbalist named A.L. Tommie Bass, whose practice was the subject of Volume I of the previously cited book. The breakdown is by herbal plant species under their popular names, some of which are more well known to Bass than are others. Initial features include an introduction and a glossary of terms used. For each species, after a section titled "The Herbalist's Account," there is a commentary section by the authors giving details of the pharmacopeia for the plant, namely, the known active ingredients or phytochemical compounds. A historical background is often furnished as a point of reference, going back to such early-day naturalists and herbalists as Gerard (1597), Parkinson (1640), Culpeper (circa 1649–1653), the Bartram's (circa the 1700s), and one or another of the Barton's (circa the 1800s), and others. Although the subject of cancer is mentioned in a number of places, no specific treatment is emphasized other than salves for cancerlike skin conditions. (Interestingly, the periwinkle or *Vinca* or *Catharanthus* species is mentioned as a potential agent against cancer and also diabetes, and it may be added in comment that an insulin/glycogen imbalance may be indicative of cancer.) The remedies outlined are more for general ailment, and include tonics and blood purifiers, laxatives and emetics, astringents, counters for indigestion and diarrhea, and diuretics to counter dropsy. There are no markedly effective antibacterial, antifungal, or antiviral treatment mentioned, although colds, coughs, and chest ailments receive frequent mention (with slippery elm regarded a strong candidate for coughs), as do fevers and the various febrifuges to counter them. Rheumatism and arthritis rate many citations, as do kidney ailments.

(Speaking further of herbal remedies, Charles Kuralt's *On the Road with Charles Kuralt*, published in 1985, has an interesting series of interviews in a chapter on moonshiners, about soaking the right roots and herbs in a jar of "white lightning." Interviewees Maude Thacker and Hamper McBee mentioned that the ingredients might include ginseng root, poke root, rattleroot, and mayapple, with some persons taking this concoction for rheumatism and arthritis. It was also mentioned that such remedies seemed to help only with subsequent increases in dose. "It didn't stop 'em hurting, but they didn't give a damn for hurting then, you know.")

Another look at medical folklore is furnished in Lonnelle Aikman's previously cited *Nature's Healing Arts: From Folk Medicine to Modern Drugs*, published in 1977 by the National Geographic Society. The book begins with citations of some of the folk remedies from the Ozarks, then proceeds to New Mexico, Chinese traditional medicine, and eventually seems to cover the entire subject. Throughout the book, caution is urged regarding herbal medicines and dosages, for the side effects can be deadly. This calls for counsel with a person well versed in herbal medicines and dosages. The subject involved is pharmocognosy; it is a branch of pharmacology that deals with natural raw materials as utilized in pharmaceuticals.

It may be mentioned in passing that comfrey was cited as a folkloric herb with curative powers; but it is not mentioned that toxic PAs are a component (e.g., in Hoffman, 1999, pp. 76, 90). As for alkaloids, among the anticancer agents mentioned are the *Vinca* alkaloids used successfully against childhood leukemia, and the alkaloids scopolamine and hyoscyamine that occur in the mandrake root (and in other plants, such as henbane).

(The terms mandrake and mayapple are used synonymously in the United States, being the plant species *Podophyllum peltatum* [of the plant family Podophyllaceae], which contains the toxic agent podophyllotoxin, which apparently has an anticancer or cancerostatic action [Hoffman, 1999, p. 81]. However, in Europe the mandrake is the species *Mandragora officinarum* of the family Solanaceae and contains belladonna-type alkaloids, namely, tropane or atropine alkaloids that include scopolamine and hyoscyamine. These are noted to have an anticancer action [Hoffman, 1991, p. 144]).

At the time Aikman was preparing her book, she was able to interview Jonathan L. Hartwell, who was preparing the listings for his book (1982b). She was also able to interview Harvard ethnobotanist Richard E. Schultes, called the *Dean of the Plant Hunters*, who had spent many years in Amazonia. (Schultes is prominently profiled in Wade Davis' book *One River*, cited elsewhere.)

Aikman also devotes considerable space to malaria and the discovery of its treatment with quinine, derived from the genus *Cinchona*; the mood-altering drug reserpine, derived from the species *Rauwolfa serpentina,* is mentioned. Other drugs mentioned that are derived from tropical plants include curare and strychnine. Attention is also given to marine life such as the red-tide dinoflagellates and sponges. The latter contain a host of microorganisms of potential interest.

As for other marine life as anticancer agents, an article by Tsu-Tsair Chi in the August/September 2006 *Townsend Letter for Doctors & Patients* describes tests in which sea cucumber extract inhibited several cancer cell lines, namely, gastric, colorectal, lung, liver, breast, and ovarian. The main effect was inhibition of angiogenesis, the proliferation of supportive blood vessels in cancerous tissue. Moss (1998) has a section on anticancer agents from the sea, including a chapter on shark cartilage against angiogenesis, mentioned previously.

Of special note in Chi's article is the discussion of the RTK inhibition of cancer. RTK refers to receptor tyrosine kinases, as the enzyme tyrosine kinase is implicated in the formation of refractory cancerous stem cells, described in Chapter 10, and the search has been enjoined for inhibitors. The article notes that when tumors reach a certain size (approximately 2 mm in diameter), growth factors or proteins are released in overwhelming amounts into nearby tissues, thus initiating angiogenesis. "The growth factors subsequently bind to their RTKs within endothelial cells in the blood cells." This results in activation of otherwise dormant endothelial cells ("endothelial" pertains to the internal cavities of the body). This results in the division and migration of the endothelial cells toward the diseased tumorous or cancerous cells. But for this to happen, a network of new blood vessels must be formed.

Although Aikman's book appears current even today, it can be said that no dramatic breakthroughs have since occurred with regard to cancer therapies. At the time, there was a great deal of interest in the African shrub *Maytenus buchananii* for cancer treatment. Thus, the alkaloids present in the genus *Maytenus*, notably maytensine, have been found to have an anticancer action, particularly against leukemias (Hoffman, 1999, p. 146). However, this has not yet been translated into a successful, commercial mode of treatment. But this has been the case for most plant-derived medicinal prospects.

If the route for synthetic drugs, from inception to approval, is tortuous, expensive, and long-drawn out, then the route for plant-derived pharmaceuticals is definitely so in spades. In the first place, there would be no commercial and financial incentives unless some sort of patent protection can be obtained, which is doubtful for a plant substance unless a derivative can be synthesized (and a process patent also obtained for the synthesization itself). Accordingly, most natural substances are left out in the cold. More than this, a large enough market must be ensured, which is borderline for cancer treatment as compared to that for much more common ailments such as arthritis. There is also the matter of side effects, which can be controlling and which may range from the innocuous to the deadly, for example, asphyxiation and cardiac arrest. Add to this the problem of biochemical individuality, where some persons may not have adverse effects, but others will (which can be expressed in terms of allergic response), and one can appreciate the complexity of the problem.

(Recall that although antibiotics are natural substances derived from fungi, a degree of patent protection has ensued. Although not so for the original antibiotic penicillin, which is a chemical compound of now-known composition and structure, a gift from its discoverers. The use of moldy substances to fight infection dates back to folklore.)

For the reasons mentioned previously, in whole or in part, it is recommended that widespread and convenient cancer clinical research centers (CCRC) or their equivalent be set up, where nonorthodox cancer therapies and substances can be deployed in a clinical environment under the supervision of M.D.s and D.O.s.

## SELECTIVITY

The objective is that the enzyme-inhibiting substance should be selective only against cancerous cells and not normal cells. In other words, it should not have any adverse side effects, that is, it should not act as an inhibitor for other enzymes involved in the vital functions of normal cells. In particular, these substances should neither impair respiration or cardiac activity nor act against the heart, liver, or other life-sustaining organs. These qualifiers are the rationale for seeking out certain foods or food components that are reputed to be normally nontoxic but which naturally contain anticancer agents, such as traces of bioactive alkaloids.

Even some or most of the common garden vegetables and fruits contain trace amounts of alkaloids as well as other potentially beneficial types of compounds. Our daily cups of coffee contain the alkaloid caffeine. Tobacco and some other plants contain the alkaloid nicotine, and there is ongoing research to determine beneficial medicinal properties for nicotine and related compounds, possibly even against cancer. The alkaloid colchicine is sometimes used as a treatment for gout, although it is a drug also used in horticulture to induce mutations in plant species.

(Having mentioned tobacco and nicotine, a report in the August/September 2006 *Townsend Letter for Doctors & Patients* indicated that a hops flavonoid compound found in beer has anticancer properties. The compound is called *xanthohumol*, and research is being carried out at the Linus Pauling Institute at the Oregon State University. This compound and related ones inhibit a family of enzymes called *cytochromes P450* that activate early tumor growth. Still other compounds classified as *prenylflavonoids* are potent phytoestrogens that are involved in postmenopausal symptoms.)

Consumed in low concentrations (which incidentally borders on the subject of homeopathy), these agents occurring in foodstuffs are demonstrably nontoxic to normal cells, but may have the potential to act against cancer cells. (With tobacco, the carcinogens are evidently the tarry substances present, as distinguished from the alkaloid nicotine by itself). Perhaps this is a reason that, in some cases at least, persons have been cured of cancer by following a largely vegetarian diet.

In this context, we may speak of mutations occurring in animals, for example, in fish as a result of the ingestion of pharmaceuticals. The Colorado fish biologist John Woodling is concerned about the extent of weird mutations that occur in fish (mostly suckers) in the streams and runoffs below Front Range sewage plant outlets, according to an article in the November 19, 2004, issue of the *Rocky Mountain News*. The findings show that a brew of pharmaceuticals shows up in the sewage treatment water, which ultimately enters the water chain, especially as water is increasingly recycled. Ultimately, humans could also be affected.

(It has also been found that some weird mutations have sometimes been found in frogs, a sign of some sort of water pollution.)

The extrapolation is to industrial and agricultural chemicals that are not only considered carcinogenic, but may also cause mutations in the animals.

Consider, therefore, caged chickens, feedlot cattle, and "farmed" fish that are mass-produced, whose feed includes a variety of pharmaceuticals to ward off disease and induce weight gain. More directly, this leads to the question of whether physical and mental aberrations, or mutations, could occur in humans who take drugs for their various ailments, over the long-term. (This is in addition to other side effects, benign or serious, including cancer.) Obviously, this is a subject area better ignored — and surely will be.

## THE NITROGEN CONNECTION AND IMMUNOTHERAPY

A common factor of some cancer therapies is nitrogen content, in the body's very proteinaceous makeup and in anticancer agents. This presence of proteinaceous nitrogen in the body is common enough, particularly in the amine or amino form, though not universal. As for the nitrogen content of anticancer agents, this can either be a positive or negative factor, as with alkaloids.

In some instances, the presence of nitrogen is definitely detrimental. Thus, it can be mentioned that another class of nitrogen compounds, the nitrosamines, are regarded as carcinogenic, or cancer causing, in the intestinal tract. These compounds are formed during the cooking of meat, especially overcooking, as in high-temperature broiling. In this case, the hydrogen of the amine form is replaced by NO, which results in a detrimental nitrosamine. Thus, presumably the form of the nitrogen has much to do with whether a substance acts against cancer or promotes cancer.

It may be added that vitamin C has been found to inhibit the nitrosation of amines in the stomach, thus preventing the formation of nitrosamines (Williams and Weisburger, authors of a chapter titled "Chemical Carcinogenesis," in Amdur et al., 1991, p. 146).

Cause and effect actions may be viewed differently, either independent of the immune system or totally related to it. And in the end we may be talking about the very same thing, only in different ways, and providing different explanations. As for the immune system and its purposes, it can be said that helping the immune system is but a way to help the body itself. In other words, it can be declared a truism that if the immune system is effective, the cancer cells will not grow and multiply, and vice versa.

There are five reported orthodox anticancer immune therapies (Walters, 1993, p. 56). These include BCG, interferon, interleukin-1 or interleukin-2, tumor necrosis factor or TNF (necrosis means death), and monoclonal antibodies. The first, BCG (Bacillus Calmette-Guérin), is described as a tuberculin vaccine that stimulates the body to kill cancer cells, and it has been said that it apparently works best when administered with chemotherapy. (However, BCG has entered into mainstream cancer therapy as a treatment against bladder cancer.) Interferon, a family of proteins, is approved for only two kinds of cancer and may prove to be of limited value in others. Both interferon and the interleukins (another family of proteins) have mainly proved to be disappointments. TNF, produced in minute quantities in the body and otherwise expensive, has achieved some dramatic results on mouse cancer. With humans, the side effects include chills and fever. It is thought that TNF is a tumor antibody. Monoclonal antibodies involve gene splicing and are said to act specifically against cancer cells. Still experimental, the word is that they will also be very expensive.

Besides the various orthodox immunotherapies mentioned in the preceding text, there are other therapies that have been taken off the American Cancer Society (ACS) blacklist (Walters, 1993, p. 8). These include hypothermia or heat therapy, cryogenic therapy or cryotherapy, hydrazine sulfate, Coley Therapy, a couple of others called Lincoln Therapy, and Hendricks Natural Immunity Therapy. That is, cancer may be treated by elevating the body temperature, by applying subfreezing conditions directly to the tumor, or by the chemical hydrazine sulfate, by stimulating the immune system with Coley's Toxins, or by still other means. No one therapy seems to be the perfect answer. Authorized clinical trials are under way with other anticancer agents, such as vitamin A. Moss devoted an entire section in his book to vitamins, notably vitamin A and beta-carotene, the B vitamins and carnitine, vitamin C and the bioflavonoids, and vitamins D, E, and K. Some of these vitamins — notably beta-carotene, and vitamins C and E — are known as *antioxidants*, acting against cancer formation. (At the end of the section is a valuable addendum listing medical centers that are doing vitamin research, e.g., the University of Colorado Health Sciences Center, Denver, which is performing clinical studies on vitamin A.)

There seems to be a connection with chemically bound nitrogen and the immune system in one form or another.

According to Stanislaw Burzynski and his Antineoplaston Therapy, the body's nitrogen content is in the form of amino acid derivatives that are said to inhibit the growth of cancer cells (Walters, 1993, p. 17). These substances are thought to form a biochemical defense against cancer by reprogramming the defective cells. The action is different from that of the immune system, which destroys defective cells.

In Naessens' 714X treatment for cancer, the presence or absence of nitrogenous substances in one way or another is considered a contributing factor to cancer formation and also to its successful treatment, respectively. Thus, the treatment or cure involves the injection of camphor containing chemically bound nitrogen into the body's lymphatic system. (The nitrogen-containing camphor compound used is called *trimethylbicyclonitraminoheptane chloride*.) An explanation provided is that if the immune system is working properly, it will negate the agglomerations of cells constantly forming in the body, which can lead to a cancerous condition (Walters, 1993, pp. 32, 33). If the immune system is not functioning properly, the cells will form a tumor, which in turn requires large quantities of nitrogen or nitrogen derivatives for subsistence, and hence depletes the body's reserves. At the same time, according to Naessens' findings, the cancerous cells emit a substance that Naessens labeled the *Cocancerogenic K Factor*, or CKF, which permits the cells to continue to rob the body of nitrogen and destroys the ability of the cells of the immune system to fight off germs or microorganisms and tumor growth. The injection of the nitrogen-bearing camphor derivative called *714X* into the lymphatic system provides the tumor cells all the nitrogen needed, thus shutting down the production of CKT. This allows the WBC, or leukocytes, to resume their normal function of destroying microorganisms and foreign cells.

A similar argument applies, supposedly, to the use of urea, another nitrogen compound. It can be used alone, in mixtures, or in other derivative forms. Another anticancer agent, hydrazine sulfate, contains nitrogen, as also previously noted.

*Antineoplastons*, the active anticancer agents in Burzynski's therapy, are peptides or relatively short-chain proteins, which are formed from nitrogen-containing amino acids. The term *antineoplaston* literally means anticancer. (Burzynski Therapy is also said to use phenyl acetate, otherwise known as a solvent.)

Arginine, also an anticancer agent, is an amino acid containing nitrogen. In fact all amino acids contain bound nitrogen, as implied by the modifier "amino."

In Burton's Immuno-Augmentative Therapy, blood fractions containing proteins are used to restore normalcy to the immune system, with the object of controlling and combating cancer. Being proteins, there is chemically bound nitrogen present, the same as for amino acids. The proteins, in fact, are complexes made up of amino acids.

In *Kelley's Nutritional Metabolic Therapy*, developed by William Kelley, a fundamental cause of cancer is said to be the inability of the digestive system (including the liver) to metabolize proteins (Walters, 1993, p. 205). To make matters worse, the cancer itself has such high metabolic requirements that it takes up much of the body's nourishment. It is advanced that pancreatic enzymes, the proteolytic or protein-digesting enzymes, can be utilized to correct the protein imbalance. Again, we come back to the nitrogen-bearing compounds, even if indirectly, as bound nitrogen is contained in proteins.

(Kelley's therapy was continued and augmented by Dr. Nicholas Gonzalez, who was a New York City physician and successfully treated cancer patients in this way. Dr. Gonzalez also prepared a 500-page study of the case histories of patients who had been on the Kelley program. The study was sponsored by Robert Good, M.D., Ph.D., then president of the MSKCC. Further details are provided in Chapter 18 of Walters, 1993.)

It appears clearer that cancer formation and regression are related to chemically bound nitrogen levels, in one form or another, as distinguished from free, or molecular, nitrogen. (The presence of free, or molecular, nitrogen in the bloodstream leads to the "bends." This is a hazard of diving underwater and breathing compressed air, which forces nitrogen into the bloodstream.)

Moreover, the action of nitrogen is tied up with the body's immune system in one way or another and may be looked at as rejuvenating it. The regression of the immune system is called immunodeficiency.

This leads to some interesting speculations about various plants and herbs as anticancer agents. According to Hartwell (1982b), there are a host of plants that act against cancer in varying degrees. There is speculation about whether these plants and herbs trigger the immune system in a similar manner as the nitrogen compounds. The very fact that these plants are bioactive and are poisonous to various degrees may be the key. In other words, the body's immune system goes into high gear to repel these foreign substances or invaders, the mildly poisonous limited intake or uptake. A higher, more poisonous uptake can of course lead to poisoning per se.

(It may be added in passing that laetrile, or amygdalin, is a nitrogen-containing substance, although cyanic, denotable as -CN.)

At slightly higher or somewhat higher dosages, to be determined, there is also the possibility that a suitably poisonous plant substance will selectively and directly attack the cancer cells. This type of plant-derived chemotherapy is presumably the role of the HCN released from laetrile. These are the situations where dosage levels become critical, so that the effect is not overdone or underdone. A problem for consideration is its effectiveness in certain people and not in the others. There is also the thought that the doses could perhaps be tailored to suit individuals.

Following this line of thought, the bodily reactions to the ingestion of plants or herbs, their extracts, decoctions, or teas, may be a mild fever and the sweats from time to time, the same reactions produced when the immune system acts against such invaders as viruses. And the WBC count may be expected to rise at the same time, again a manifestation that the body is trying to fight off something, the ingested quasi poison and the tumor, at the same time.

At the DNA and RNA level, chemically bound nitrogen is again encountered. These fundamental entities of living matter are composed of the nucleic acids DNA and RNA. They are composed of a phosphorus or phosphate content, sugar, and a nitrogen-containing base. (A general discussion with examples can be found in the *Encyclopedia Britannica* under the headings "Nucleic Acid" and "Nucleotides.") Nucleic acids can be regarded as long-chain compounds or polymers, in which the basic repeating structural unit or monomer is called a *nucleotide*. Thus, a nucleic acid can also be called a *polynucleotide*.

The nitrogen-containing bases are derivatives of three families of heterocyclic compounds called the *pyrimidines, purines*, and *pyridines*. Here, the kinship with amine- or amino-type compounds becomes apparent.

Even the hemoglobin of the blood is a protein and thus has nitrogen content. Another oxygen-carrying component of the blood called *hemocyanin*, a blue copper protein, also has an additional nitrogen group signified by the suffix "-cyanin." Studies at Oregon State University indicate that it stimulates the immune system and acts as an anticancer agent, at least for bladder cancer.

There is also a kinship with viruses and enzymes (or enzyme catalysts), not to mention genes and chromosomes. The nitrogen-containing, proteinaceous nature of all these basic entities is part of the picture. (For example, *coenzymes* are related to vitamins, and the B vitamins contain nitrogen.) Furthermore, when speaking of viruses and genes, we are talking about cellular changes also at the DNA or RNA level. When cancerous cells are produced, the cell genetic code encapsulated in the DNA or the DNA itself has been altered, by the infusion of viruses or by other means. The genetic code is the fundamental entity that tells the cells what to do, to grow in what manner, or to die out. Thus, to eliminate the cancerous condition, a reversal or negation, or superposition or substitution, of this alteration process must occur. And these processes may be induced by other substances or agents, and/or conditions that are yet to be determined, with the remains sloughed off and discharged as body waste.

Furthermore, this reversal or negation, or superposition or substitution, may be effected by the introduction of still other nitrogen-containing substances that, possibly owing to a nitrogen bond commonality, either stimulate the immune system proper or produce an anticancer action on the cell makeup and/or genetic code. This action, moreover, will be at the molecular level, that is, at the DNA or RNA level. Substances that do not contain nitrogen may presumably serve equally well or almost as well.

Another class of nitrogen compounds, the nitrosamines, are regarded as carcinogenic or cancer causing in the intestinal tract. As has been previously mentioned, these kinds of compounds are formed in the cooking of meat, especially in overcooking, as in high-temperature broiling. In this case, the hydrogen of the amine form is replaced by NO. Thus, the state of the nitrogen present in the substance has much to do with whether it acts against or promotes cancer.

Proteins are ubiquitous nitrogen-bearing polymeric molecules formed from amino acids. Thus, not only do they constitute hormones and the myriad enzymes and enzyme inhibitors that control all body reactions including cell metabolism, but they also constitute such substances as antigens, which serve to stimulate the immune system. Not only are proteins involved in the fight against already-established cancers, but in the body's resistance to cancer in the first place. Nitrogen compounds, it seems, are everywhere, for better or worse.

These speculations, no matter how elaborate, most often leave us in the dark. They are, rather, convenient inventions of the mind, although based on experience and observation, and merely provide a way to talk about something we cannot really explain. They are a means to provide a mechanism or model to fit in the facts as they are or might be. Nevertheless, they are most useful as theory, furnishing a starting point for correlating and unifying the information already known and suggesting avenues for further investigation. And, expectedly, these lines of inquiry will open up more avenues than they close. With cancer, all this becomes a serious business indeed.

Among the most bioactive substances are the previously mentioned alkaloids, which have a unique nitrogen-bearing ring structure. Found in many plants, even common garden vegetables, alkaloids may vary in toxicity from the mild to the deadly, as previously noted. Moreover, some have been found to be anticancer agents; for example, the *Vinca* alkaloids vincristine and vinblastine are used against blood-related cancers.

In further comment, it is estimated that up to 10% of the plant kingdom will contain alkaloids, of which some thousands (perhaps 5000) of the alkaloid-containing species have been identified (Woodward, 1985, p. 21; Kingsbury, 1964, p. 19). Nowadays the figure is said to be more like 10,000. Usually the alkaloids are distributed throughout the plant. Excluding cyanide, the main source of toxicity is from the alkaloids. Also, there exist a relatively few polypeptides and amines (polypeptides being long-chain amino acids), which are poisonous as well (Woodward, 1985, p. 22). All the aforementioned are nitrogen-containing compounds. (In fact, as has been repeatedly mentioned, peptides or short-chain amino acids are used in Burzynski therapy, and amine derivatives are also used as anticancer agents, such as hydrazine sulfate and urea, as are organic cyanides, such as laetrile, or amygdalin.) This further brings up the point that perhaps in small or minute or trace-regulated quantities, these kinds of bioactive toxic compounds may trigger or stimulate the immune system.

(Whereas urea is apparently a common chemical, a source for hydrazine sulfate has been the Syracuse Cancer Research Institute, Presidential Plaza, 600 East Genesee St, Syracuse, NY 13202, (315)472-6616.)

## ALKALOIDS AND BIOACTIVITY

Some of the previously mentioned information has been presented in Appendix U of Hoffman (1999), which has reference to Hartwell (1982) and to Cordell (1981). The correlative comparison is by plant families and emphasizes the presence of bioactive alkaloids. Alkaloids by and large contain a unique nitrogen-containing ring structure, with the rest of the chemical structure varying among the many alkaloids, with about 10,000 and more alkaloid compounds presently known. Alkaloids are almost ubiquitous in the plant world, and Cordell (1981) is an authoritative source in this respect. Some have already been marked and utilized as effective anticancer agents, e.g., vincristine and vinblastine for blood-related cancers. These alkaloids are found in the Madagascar or rosy periwinkle, *Catharanthus roseus* of the family Apocynaceae and are also sometimes referred to as Vinca alkaloids of the genus *Vinca* (as in Hartwell, 1982), thus producing a slight confusion in names.

Although there are a few exceptions, alkaloids have a unique nitrogen-containing ring structure that very likely predisposes them to be enzyme inhibitors. This nitrogen ring is positioned so as to cause them to behave as basic or nonacidic compounds, hence their name, and this action is somewhat similar to that of ammoniacal compounds. Additionally, they have pronounced pharmacological properties of different degrees, with some hallucinogenic effects, whereas others adversely affect the body system.

In searching through the tropical rain forests for medicinal plants and testing and screening them for bioactivity, the presence of alkaloids is used as the main criterion. Unfortunately, there can be side effects. That is, the bioactive compounds can also inhibit other vital enzymatic processes. Thus, the common herb comfrey, for instance, contains PAs that cumulatively act against the liver. The alkaloids vincristine and vinblastine, for example, which are derived from the Madagascar periwinkle (genus *Catharanthus*), are clinically used against blood cancers with a degree of success; at the same time they have side effects, indicating cytotoxicity against other body cells.

In fact, many of our most common poisons are alkaloids, usually designated by the suffix "-ine." Examples include strychnine from tropical trees of the genus *Strychnos*, coniine from poison hemlock, hyoscyamine from jimsonweed of the family Solanaceae or nightshade family (it is found in minor amounts in lettuce, and tomatoes are in the same plant family, as are other common garden vegetables such as potatoes), and swainsonine from locoweed (which in laboratory tests has been found to act against cancer, and has been patented as an anticancer drug in Japan). The poisonous extract curare (from a vine also of the genus *Strychnos* and used by South American Indian tribes to tip arrows) contains alkaloids that kill game by asphyxiation, although in small, carefully monitored, doses it serves as a muscle relaxant. The message seems loud and clear, therefore, to try only very minute quantities, as practiced in homeopathy. (Always, it seems, it is a catch-22 situation or playing one thing against another.) This is similar to the case for the deadly aconitine derived from wolfsbane, monkshood, or aconite, which is described by Solzenhitsyn (1969, pp. 228–233), as previously elaborated. Mostly concentrated in the roots, the substance is so toxic that only a few drops of an alcohol or vodka extract could be used. Even this was forbidden by the Russian government. (However, in essentially undetectable concentrations, aconite is a constituent of certain homeopathic remedies.) An authoritative reference on the general subject of alkaloids and their chemistry and properties, and their history and plant sources, is Cordell (1981).

Alkaloids, however, are by no means the only class of bioactive compounds found in nature. As has been indicated, to the listing may be added the glycosides or glucosides, phenolics, flavonoids, saponins, etc., some of which are interrelated or combined with one another. Among the most poisonous are certain vegetable proteins, such as abrin from the colorful red and black jequirity bean found in Africa, which is used for decorative beads and necklaces, also called the *rosary pea* or *precatory bean* (*Abrus precatorius*), as well as ricin from the common castor bean (*Ricinus communis*), which is also used to make colorful beads. The general subject is described by Blackwell (1990). It may be added that ricin is coming under scrutiny as an agent in biological (and ideological) warfare.

## MICROORGANISMS AND IMMUNITY

Microorganisms have been used in cancer treatment. As previously mentioned, Moss includes a chapter about the use of a mixed bacterial vaccine, Coley's Toxins, in the treatment of cancer (Moss, 1992, pp. 407–412). Moss considers the discovery of these toxins a remarkable advance in cancer therapy. Interest has been revived in the use of these toxins, as per information supplied by a frequent contributor, Wayne Martin, in issues of the *Townsend Letter for Doctors & Patients*, to be further described.

Moss has another chapter about the use of MTH-68 vaccine, a unique form of immunotherapy developed by Laszlo K. Csatay, M.D., of Fort Lauderdale, Florida (Moss, 1992, pp. 437–444). It involves the interference between two viruses, which is a well-known phenomenon. One virus interferes with the activities of the other, in one way or another. The situation may also be looked upon as a case where one virus stimulates the immune system to destroy the other less desirable virus, the latter being the cause of the cancerous condition.

Moss further notes that Csatay and his colleagues published a paper describing the effects of 15 harmless viruses on 4 disease-causing viruses in animals. The results included a marked reduction in the death rate in mice from a strain of rabies, from 50% to 15%.

The work continues in this general area, leading to such anticancer agents as interferons, interleukins, and TNFs (Moss, 1992, p. 441ff). It has been found that disease-causing virus strains induce TNF in human WBC, and so may the interferons and the interleukins, but the latter, by themselves, have not worked out. This in turn has led to the development of a live virus vaccine called *MTH-68N*, with encouraging results.

Another pioneer in immunotherapy is the previously cited Josef Issels, a retired M.D. from Germany, whose methods have been called *Issels' Whole Body Therapy* (Walters, 1993, p. 82ff). His work has continued at the Panama City Clinic in Panama City, Florida. Issels' therapy induces a fever, a practice used in Europe for centuries. Modern medicine generally views fever with alarm, as something to be counteracted with antibiotics. By giving a "fever shot" once a month to raise body temperature to as high as 105°F for a couple of hours, the level of disease-destroying leukocytes in the blood is increased. At the same time the lymphocytes generate antibodies that destroy microbes and toxins. For an active fever, the drug Pyrifer is injected, which is made from *E. coli* bacteria. For a passive fever, hyperthermia is induced by ultrashort waves or microwaves with the patient inside a chamber. These and other methods used have been catalogued with success rates as high as 17% for terminal patients. It has been noted that in patients with a fast-growing cancer, this long-term immunotherapy is combined with chemotherapy (Walters, 1993, p. 85).

There are other ways to describe the immune system and its functioning, as has been previously cited. Thus, in the chapter by Walters' (1993) on Revici Therapy, health is regarded as dependent on a balance between lipids (fatty acids or esters) and sterols (fatty alcohols such as cholesterol). But the overall view is that the immune system is an important factor in the cause, as well as the cure, for cancer.

## IN SHORT SUMMARY

The worldwide baseline reference for the many plants or herbs that have been tried against cancer, whether successfully or not and also poisonous or not, is by Hartwell (1982b). Hartwell was with the NCI and in the course of his literature survey identified about 3000 plant species that appeared in medical folklore as potential anticancer agents.

(Another name that surfaces regularly in discussions of the plant or herbal treatments of cancer and other diseases is medical anthropologist John Heinerman, mentioned elsewhere and author of a number of intriguing books about native remedies, some of which are still in print or available. James A. Duke, now retired from the USDA in Bethesda, Maryland, is another name prominently cited.)

Among the bioactive plants so identified is chaparral, or creosote bush (sometimes called greasewood), which is, or has been, used as a native Indian remedy for a number of ailments, but has also been found to cause liver damage and, very likely, kidney damage. It may or may not be a component of the elusive North American Indian-derived substance called Compound-X. Chaparral may also contain redroot (*Lachanthes tinctoria*). Redroot is the colloquial name for other species having red roots and may well be confused with bloodroot (*Sanguinaria canadensis*), a herbal remedy that contains the alkaloid sanguinarine. Animal studies have indicated that Compound-X is ineffective. But effectiveness in animals cannot be correlated to effectiveness in humans.

There are rumors that Compound-X underwent extensive clinical trials in Portugal and elsewhere, as previously indicated, and was once an item of interest to the company Vipont Pharmaceuticals, formerly headquartered at Fort Collins, Colorado. This company was involved in some kind of operation near Lander and Riverton,

Wyoming, not far from the Shosone/Arapaho Indian reservation. (Evidently blood-root or sanguinarine, however, did end up as an additive in a certain brand of toothpaste, as an anticavity agent.) The subject of its apparent use or trial as an anticancer agent seems to be a forbidden topic of discussion, although there is a mail order source that has advertised in some of the health magazines for a "Compound-X." (As with most such substances, the buzzword is "therapy" or "treatment" but not "cure.") Nevertheless, if there are some latent possibilities in this substance or its close kin (and anecdotal stories continue to surface), then some objective, independent, impartial, and unprejudiced clinical testing is in order.

The creosote bush (*Larrea tridentata* or *L. divaricata* of the family Zygophyl-laceae) contains the compound called nordihydroguaiaretic acid (NDGA), which is a well-known antioxidant that was once used commercially, and also contains the flavonoid-like compound quercetin. NDGA has displayed pronounced antitumor activity both *in vitro* and *in vivo*, but controlled clinical tests are in abeyance. Quercetin is sometimes regarded as an anticancer agent. Additionally, there are some 50 volatile oils, including vinyl and methyl ketones, camphor, and limonene, and its amberlike resin contains flavonoids, lignins, saponins, and waxes. Some of these substances or compounds are viewed as anticancer agents, but their individual side effects are not fully documented.

Another North American Indian herbal combination is Essiac, or Essiac tea; its exact biochemical action yet unspecified and its efficacy discounted. The principal herbs are the burdock root (*Arctium lappa* of the family Asteraceae or Compositae), turkey rhubarb or Indian rhubarb root (e.g., *Rheum officianale* or *R. palmatum* of the family Polygonaceae), sheep sorrel (*Rumex acetosella* of the family Oxali-daceae), and slippery elm bark (*Ulmus fulva* of the family Ulmaceae). But only the roots of the rhubarb plants are recommended, as the leaves are known to be toxic. The active ingredients in Essiac are considered to be the chemicals rhein, emodin, high-molecular-weight polysaccharides, and perhaps the lignan arctigenin. Rhein and emodin are anthroquinones and are known to be cytotoxic, or cell toxic. (In turn, all of these herbs are folkloric anticancer agents in their own right and are listed in Hartwell 1982b.) However, as already indicated, a Canadian study by some 112 doctors arrived at negative conclusions for Essiac, as did the NCI.

(A favorable review of Essiac and its anticancer components has been provided by Morton Walker in the December 1997 issue of the *Townsend Letter for Doctors & Patients*. It should also be added that herbal remedies are not standardized as to activity or to ensure the identity of the plant species used, which makes objectivity elusive, if not impossible. Even if the correct herbs or plants are used, the concen-tration of the active ingredient or ingredients may vary widely with the plant parts used, the locale, the season, and even the time of day.)

It may be added that the Hoxsey treatment, which utilizes a number of herbs, includes burdock, a component also present in Essiac. (Although the Hoxsey treat-ment had many followers, and Hoxsey prevailed in the courts, his treatment proved ineffective against his own cancer.)

South American plant species have been touted from time to time as anticancer agents. These include the condor vine or condorango or condurango (*Marsdenia condurango* or *Gonolobus condurango* or *Condorango blanco* or *Equatoria garciana* of the family Asclepiadaceae, or milkweed family), and pau d'arco (*Tabebuia* spp. of the family Bignoniaceae, of which six species are known, with the pulverized bark of the species *T. heptaphylla* probably being found in the health-food stores). The condor vine seems to have disappeared from view on account of its ineffectiveness, but the pau d'arco is still around and whether it is actually a cure for cancer is anybody's guess.

# 7 Surveying Anticancer Plant Substances

## STATUS OF PLANTS AGAINST CANCER

The remarks herein are another reminder of the foreword to Jonathan L. Hartwell's *Plants Used Against Cancer: A Survey* (1982a), written by botanist James A. (Jim) Duke, then of the U.S. Department of Agriculture. Duke's words have become prophetic, and in one way or another have been often cited. Again consider, therefore, the following:

> I view the publication as one epitaph to the cancer-screening program involving the National Cancer Institute with the U.S. Department of Agriculture for nearly 25 years. In a blow to natural-products chemistry in the U.S., the Board of Scientific Counselors, Division of Cancer Treatment, National Cancer Institute, voted on October 2, 1981, to abolish the NCI research contract program concerned with the development of antitumor agents from plants. I fear this signals the end of significant government-sponsored research in the U.S. on medicinal plants, leaving the research to the pharmaceutical firms, who have shown relative disinterest in plant products.

The situation has since turned around, at least in some ways, as efforts continue by both the government and the pharmaceutical companies to further assay plant sources — and whatever else comes to mind.

Hartwell duly emphasizes caution in a disclaimer, as cited previously, that natural plants may have serious or fatal toxicity. "Neither the author nor the publisher makes any medical claims for any herb. This information is compiled from the published literature. Some plants contain deadly poisons and some mentioned herein are extremely dangerous." And similarly it can be said, likewise, for some or many of the synthetic medicinal compounds produced in the laboratory. In fact, any bioactive or medicinal plant will be toxic in large-enough doses, and this is why dosage levels can be so critical. Foxglove, or digitalis, for heart disease is a notable example; it is beneficial in minute amounts, but deadly in larger amounts. It becomes a question of determining the safe dosage and how and how often it should be administered — for which folklore is sometimes an important source.

As previously indicated, at the time of publication of Hartwell's book, Jim Duke cited in the foreword that about 35,000 higher plant species had been screened for activity against cancer. Of these, about 3,000 had demonstrated reproducible activity, a small fraction of these being potential candidates for clinical trials. The search has since been expanded, and continues.

## LAETRILE QUANDARIES

Perhaps the most well-publicized, cussed and discussed, instance of a proposed herbal remedy/cure for cancer is laetrile, which was introduced in the previous chapter. Also called *amygdalin*, it is a class of cyanide-containing organic compounds known as *cyanoglucosides*, or *cyanoglycosides*. A recapitulation follows.

As first promoted by researcher Ernest T. Krebs, Jr., and as previously noted, these kinds of compounds, also called *nitrilosides*, have been claimed to act not only against cancer but against other diseases such as sickle-cell anemia. Raw, confectionary-type or sweet almonds, for instance, contain small amounts of amygdalin, and there is the folkloric recommendation that a fistful a day will help keep cancer away. What are known as bitter almonds, however, contain much larger amounts, and caution is the watchword, as cyanide poisoning is possible. As has been previously indicated, raw nuts, in general, contain some amygdalin, as do even the leguminous fruits known as beans. Peach and apricot kernels are especially notorious, these fruits belonging to the same genus as almonds (*Prunus*), and again the word is beware. Nevertheless, as has also been mentioned earlier , Jonathan V. Wright, M.D., opines that three or four peach or apricot kernels per day are said to be okay for an adult (Wright, 1979, pp. 425, 426). There is always a cautionary note, however, in that fresh foods high in hydrolytic enzymes can cause the release of cyanide, that is, hydrogen cyanide — another name being prussic acid. Similar cautions of one kind or another have surfaced in other quarters.

As may be suspected, the use of laetrile therapy has had some reverberations. A chapter is given to the subject in Pelton and Overholser's *The Complete Guide to Non-Traditional Treatments* (1994). More technical details are furnished in a chapter "Amygdalin" in Moss's *Cancer Therapy: The Independent Consumer's Guide to Non-Toxic Treatment and Prevention* (1992) — plus some inside information about the nuances. Studies were conducted by a Dr. Kanematsu Sugiura from 1972–1977 at the Memorial Sloan-Kettering Cancer Center, at which Moss was the assistant director of public affairs. Dr. Sugiura obtained some positive results, which were not allowed to be presented in a report to the media. Moss followed this up with a media conference of his own, charging a cover-up, and was fired the next day for his pains (Moss, 1992, pp. 269, 270).

In both Moss (1992) and Pelton and Overholser (1994), laetrile mainly gets a good recommendation. Others tend to be somewhat cautious, at least about some of the side effects. Still another point of view is presented by Steve Austin, a naturopathic physician who tracked a group of 18 late-stage cancer patients at Hospital Del Mar in Tijuana (Walters, 1993, p. 194). The treatment consisted of metabolic therapy with detoxification, laetrile, enzyme supplements, mega doses of vitamins, and special vaccines. Inasmuch as all in this group of patients died within 3 years, Austin recommends that cancer patients avoid the laetrile clinics, in spite of an occasional positive anecdote. Apparently seconding the recommendation is Patrick McGrady of CANHELP, who disdained Mexican cancer clinics in general. *Politics, Science, and Cancer*, published in 1980, reviewed the laetrile phenomenon.

Varro E. Tyler, a prominent pharmacologist, has challenged the proposed role of enzymes in the attempt to explain the anticancer action of laetrile (Tyler, 1993,

p. 32; Hoffman, 1999, p. 351). Laetrile advocates base their arguments on the enzyme β-glucosidase, which is perceived as concentrating in cancerous tissue but not elsewhere. This enzyme is purported to decompose any amygdalin or laetrile present to liberate cyanide, which destroys cancer cells. On the other hand, others explain the selective anticancer action in terms of the enzyme rhodanase, as has been spelled out previously (Hoffman, 1999, p. 351). This enzyme as occurs (and concentrates) in normal tissue serves to catalyze the conversion of cyanide and thiosulfate or thiosulfinate to the less harmful thiocyanate and sulfate, thereby protecting normal cells from cyanic action. The confirming experiments are awaited.

On the other hand ... the death of actor Steve McQueen, who had terminal cancer, is sometimes viewed as a refutation for laetrile. However, it is reported instead that he was responding well under treatment, but was persuaded to undergo an operation and died of an embolism (Mullins, 1992, p. 100). Other positive results have evidently been suppressed, for example, at the Memorial Sloan-Kettering Cancer Center, and Mullins recounts the story of the firing of Ralph Moss, who had contradicted the official negative statements. Still others view laetrile as one more treatment among several, the entirety to be tried as a counter to cancer.

(Most recently, there was the death of Mrs. Martin Luther King at a clinic in Mexico, although Mrs. King was evidently a terminal case, and submitted to treatment as a last resort, with the particular alternative treatment used not clearly specified.)

Although there are reported failures in alternative or unconventional treatments — in this case, say, in Mexico — the fact is that more and more U.S. citizens are crossing the border for health care, even for major operations. The costs are so much lower. For instance, consider the border town of Algadonas, across from Yuma, Arizona, where "snowbirds" can get their dental work done for perhaps one fifth or one fourth as much, and by competent professionals. More than this, there is a Dr. Diaz who gives stem cell shots — reportedly sheep stem cells that are reputed to heal almost anyone with almost anything, although cancer was not mentioned. Two second-hand accounts of successes are as follows. One person who suffered from emphysema was helped and as a side benefit could feel circulation returning to his feet, although meat and dairy products are a no-no for 3 weeks afterward. When this person indulged, he came down with a big fiery-red blotch about a foot in diameter in the middle of his stomach area, a common side reaction. Another person who suffered severely from fibromyalgia had no pain after the shots, and was in fact "kicking up her heels."

(Fibromyalgia is a newer word connoting severe muscle pain, as distinguished from the joint pain of arthritis or rheumatism. Other symptoms such as depression and anxiety may also occur, and may include loss of sleep and flu-like symptoms, hence the catchall term *fibromyalgia syndrome*. There is an overlap with symptoms of chronic fatigue syndrome [CFS].)

There is an inference here that a triggering of the immune system may be involved, in that a foreign substance can cause this sort of bioreaction. And such an immune response can lead to beneficial results, if only temporarily, with the consequence that the treatment must be repeated and even intensified. Not only can the patient feel better, but the symptoms can be countered, possibly even the disease itself. This, in a way of speaking, can be viewed as the protocol of homeopathy, where minute quantities of a potentially toxic substance can have beneficial effects. An example is that of a decrepit horse subjected to minute amounts of arsenic in its feed, which imparts a liveliness in spirit and looks. (The trouble is, the dosage must be ever increased, with often-fatal results.) Another example is that of a person exposed to radon gas, say, in an abandoned mine, which seems to impart beneficial health effects. And the Papago Indians of the American Southwest had reportedly used the herb called *rue* (*Ruta graveolens*) against that most terrible viral disease, rabies — and rue is loaded with alkaloids, known for their toxicity. The involvement of the immune response is suspected, in that some very few persons exposed do not come down with rabies, or at least not until much later.

(Interestingly, fever and flu-like symptoms may accompany a triggering of the immune system, as the body attempts to fight off the invader or the aberration, for example, the chills and fever that accompany an attack by the malaria parasite. This regimen is a feature of hyperthermia, the therapy that involves raising the body temperature in the attempt to counter infections, even cancer. And in turn there is hyperbaric oxygen therapy, etc. A question is, as always, are the benefits, if any, temporary or permanent?)

Continuing with cancer, the many anticancer plants and herbs may act in the same way, stimulating the body's immune system, which may act against the cancerous cells and at least give temporary relief. A potential example is, of course, laetrile, not to mention extracts of aconite, the deadly product of monkshood (genus *Aconitum*), which have been used against cancer, as reported by Solzhenitsyn in *Cancer Ward*, and also used against rheumatism as reported in St. George's *Soviet Deserts and Mountains*. (Medical folklore reports that, for starters, bee or wasp stings, or other venoms, have been used against rheumatism.)

The foregoing is complicated by the fact that cancer cells mimic their counterpart, the normal cells, and both are therefore immune from attack by the immune system. (Although a transplant of another person's cells will be attacked — requiring suppression of the immune system using the appropriate drug. This brings to mind that if there are immune system suppressors, there must be immune system enhancers, which may but be substances that trigger the immune response.) If we assume that cancer cells are independent of the immune system, then these cells must be attacked in some other way, namely by interfering with cancer cell metabolism, which is different from normal cell metabolism. In other words, instead of producing carbon dioxide and water as the main metabolic products, cancer cells produce lactic acid or lactate, courtesy of the enzyme lactate dehydrogenase, for which there are known inhibitors or blockers, some from medical folklore. And for the more refractory or resistant cancerous stem cells, the enzyme tyrosine kinase is involved, for which the search is joined for inhibitors.

An unfortunate side effect, in any event, is that many, or most, of these bioactive substances act as poisons in accelerated dosages (becoming the subject area of poisonous and medicinal plants). The argument can be extended to conventional synthetic, cytotoxic chemotherapy drugs. Thus, the British advocate lower dosages, perhaps thus triggering the immune system, whereas the American practice is to use high dosages, literally destroying the cancerous cells, and other cells as well. And, apparently in all cases, the body becomes increasingly resistant to the substance or drug.

Lastly, there is the reminder that going to a clinic in Mexico can also be a crapshoot, and some horror stories are doing the rounds. And in foreign countries there may be no avenue for redress if something goes wrong; moreover, there may be no medical overseer as we have in the United States. Thus, although the American Medical Association and state medical boards can be faulted at times for overprotectionism, they do perform the valuable service of screening for irregularities (including malpractice) in the practice of medicine — even if they sometimes can be adjudged wrong.

In sum, the policy in the United States is caution, whereas in Mexico the practitioner can afford to be more audacious. In the long run, the optimistic expectation is that this give-and-take will reach a consensus benefiting the patient. The pessimistic expectation is that this will never happen. As Southern novelist James Branch Cabell famously wrote, "The optimist proclaims that we live in the best of all possible worlds; and the pessimist fears this is true."

Heinerman (1984) views this substance favorably as a cancer treatment, although it is stressed that owing to enzymatic action, laetrile can interact with some other foods to produce HCN internally and thus cause cyanide poisoning. We therefore repeat the following warning:

> Specifically forbidden is using laetrile tablets with such health foods as nuts, bean and alfalfa sprouts, fresh fruits (peaches), and other uncooked foods found in salads (lettuce, celery, mushrooms), which are high in hydrolytic enzymes that can cause the unintended release of cyanide (Heinerman, 1984, pp. 175, 176). The warning is never to mix these foods with laetrile!

## PLANTS OF THE AMERICAN WEST AND SOUTHWEST

Of special note are some plants from the American Southwest and Mexico, which according to medical folklore have been used against cancer. One in particular goes by the suggestive name *herb of Cancer* (*yerba del Cancer*). It is among the many plant agents listed in Jonathan L. Hartwell's extensive literature survey, the compendium titled *Plants Used Against Cancer: A Survey* (1982a). It is of the genus *Lythrum*, plant family Lythraceae, and the species is *Lythrum californicum*.

Extracts from the yucca plant and alpine sunflower as agents against melanoma were studied by now-retired University of Wyoming chemistry professor Owen Asplund, reported in Chapter 5, Chapter 6, and Chapter 8. The successful clinical application is said to be in routine use in Switzerland, but has not been given clearance in the United States.

Other naturally occurring anticancer agents include the chemical compound quercetin, which is found in fresh vegetables, particularly onions and garlic. It is also a component of the southwestern desert plant called chaparral, or greasewood, or creosote bush (*Larria tridentata* or *L. divaricata*), sometimes considered in its entirety an anticancer agent. Taxol is presumably another such agent, much publicized, and which is derived from the bark of the yew tree or shrub, an evergreen of the Pacific Northwest.

As has been cited, a yew-related species from China named *Cephalotaxus fortunei* yields an anticancer substance known as *harringtonine* (Griggs, 1991, p. 318). In the United States, a similar species called *Cephalotaxus harringtonia* yields homoharringtonine. Both substances are alkaloids, signified by the suffix "-ine." Alkaloids, as previously described, constitute a class of chemical compounds known to be especially bioactive or medically active; they are also generally poisonous. Another product of China, the fungus *Polyporus umbellata*, is said to be a strong anticancer agent.

The search continues, contributing to a growing pharmacopoeia of medically active plants or plant extracts, but which will take years for investigation and assessment. Hence the importance of not destroying any species, as it may be potentially useful, and which is why teams of ethnobotanists are deployed in the tropical rainforests, hopefully one step ahead of decimation. These plants contain biochemical compounds so far undreamed of.

The famous Harvard ethnobotanist Richard Evans Schultes' interests started out among the Kiowa Indians of Oklahoma circa 1936, and moved on to southern Mexico circa 1938–1939. Schultes' primary focus was on hallucinogenic plants, including mushrooms and especially peyote. From there, straying somewhat afield, he entered the Upper Amazon wilderness. His explorations are a major feature of Wade Davis's *One River: Explorations and Discoveries in the Amazon Rain Forest* (1996). During the World War II years that followed, the U.S. government charged Schultes with finding native sources of rubber or latex in the Upper Amazon region, but at the same time, Schultes encountered hallucinogenic plants used by the Indian tribes of the region. A spin-off was the investigation of coca and its refined drug product cocaine.

(A further consequence was that the oft-mentioned Jim Duke secured a sample of coca leaves and had it analyzed, in 1974. It proved to have all sort of salutary components that benefited the health of the native tribes who chewed it, particularly at the high altitudes involved. Also mentioned by Wade Davis is that Coca-Cola imports the crushed leaves after the cocaine has been removed and sold to pharmaceutical companies. The residue containing the flavorful essential oils imparts the "real thing." Not mentioned is whether traces of cocaine remain in the residue, or traces of other alkaloids, for a rule of thumb is that if one alkaloid occurs, there will be others, although in minor or trace concentrations. And furthermore, alkaloids in trace concentrations may not be harmful, and may be beneficial, in that alkaloids occur in some of the common garden vegetables. For one thing, alkaloids have been found to play a role as biochemical neurotransmitters. This is all aside from the fact that caffeine in coffee and added caffeine in soft drinks has become the dominant alkaloid — although presumably relatively benign.)

Having mentioned Wade Davis, we may note that he and compatriots explored some of the same jungle territory as Schultes, including the reaches of the adjacent Andes mountains. Although hallucinogenic plants, both old and new species were found, no anticancer plants were discovered as such, nor were they on the agenda. (For one thing, a hallucinogen works in short order, whereas an anticancer plant may take much, much longer to act — discernibly, that is.) On the other hand, Davis visited a tribe named the Waorani, who were remarkably free of many ailments, including cancer, but not other sicknesses. This was the kind of situation encountered by Alex Shoumatoff in his travels, described in *The Rivers Amazon*, where the native tribes could cure some ailments, but not others, such as the deadly tropical disease leishmaniasis, which may result in the eating away of the facial parts. (This and other serious diseases require Western medicine.) However, it would be informative to find what element in the Waorani culture inhibits the development of cancer.

Wade Davis wrote a couple of other intriguing books: *The Serpent and the Rainbow: A Harvard Scientist Uncovers the Starting Truth about the Secret World of Haitian Voodoo and Zombis*, and *Passage of Darkness: The Ethnobiology of the Haitian Zombie*. It turned out that the culprit was a species (or several species) of puffer fish and its neurotoxins. The extension is to the Japanese delicacy called *fuju* — a form of Russian roulette, whereby if the chef does not appropriately excise the toxin-containing parts from the fish, food poisoning could occur, with even deadly results. The puffer fish is of the family Tetradontidae, and the toxin is called *tetradontoxin* (Hoffman, 1999a, p. 360). Whether there might be a connection with anticancer action is unknown, although toxins and alkaloids have been isolated from various other terrestrial and marine animal species (Hoffman, 1999a, pp. 113, 146). Perhaps the most notable example is the arrow poison from the skin of the colorful Central and South American frog family Dendrobatidae, the particular species being *D. pumilio* and *D. Aratus*. A South American or Asian herb shop, for instance, will carry an assortment of dried animal and insect parts, which would seem completely unsuspected, as remedies for various ailments. It is difficult to confirm their efficacy.

In speaking further of herbal plants and medicines of the American West, the work of Kelly Kindscher titled *Medicinal Wild Plants of the Prairie: An Ethnobotanical Guide* mentions four different plant species as having been used in the treatment of various types of cancer. These are butterfly milkweed (*Asclepias tuberosa*), purple coneflower (*Echinacea angustifolia*), curly top gumweed (*Grindelia squarrosa*), and goat's rue (*Tephrosia virginiana*), as specifically noted in Kindscher's comprehensive study (Kindscher, 1992, pp. 58, 90, 92, 120, 124, 285). Use of the genus *Echinacea* is commonly mentioned in many herbal books as a cancer treatment, among many others. It has of late been touted as a remedy for colds and flu. (Kindscher also contributed *Edible Wild Plants of the Prairie: An Ethnobotanical Guide*, 1987.)

Specifically, there is Charles Kane's (2006) *Herbal Medicine of the American Southwest: A Guide to the Medical and Edible Plants of the Southwestern United States*. Kane is the principal for the Tucson Clinic of Botanical Medicine, P.O. Box 57304, Tucson AZ 85732, 520-731-3379. The very subject of herbal medicines, say, of the American Southwest will score a volley of hits on the Internet, illustrating the fact that there is almost too much information "out there." The quality of discernment is lacking, a charge sometimes leveled at the famous common man's encyclopedia, Wikipedia.

Kane's book mainly avoids the subject of cancer, not listing the subject in the index, though there is a comment under the heading "Creosote Bush." "Although internal use of creosote bush as a cancer therapy is controversial at best, external preparations are useful in resolving a particular form of premalignant squamous cell carcinoma, called actinic keratosis." These are reddish, scaly patches of sun-damaged skin. (A preparation containing the creosote bush compound nordihydroguaiaretic acid [NDGA], called *Actinex*, was called off the market on account of some adverse side effects).

Thus, Kane's book can be perceived as being on the cautious side, although there are many mentions of medicinal uses, and an array of individual compounds, and classes of compounds, is presented for each herb listed. A general comment supplied that pertains to Essiac tea, Noni juice, and other herbal medicinals believed to possess extraordinary curative powers is that there may be "a window of 5–10 years of trendy use, and then they fall by the wayside" (Kane, 2006, p. 16).

In his foreword, herbalist Michael Moore notes that most bulk herbs are gathered in the Third World and Eastern Europe. They may be gathered and dried with care, or by more crude means, and thus buying herbs in a cooperative or health food store becomes a crapshoot — not to mention mix-ups in plant names, and the fact that sunlight and drying may cause the herbs to deteriorate. "So is the herb industry a cheat? Not exactly. No more so than the rest of commercial America." And as for the herbal practitioners, they may be skilled in medicine but not in plant knowledge, or the other way around, and so forth.

Moore speaks of crews of gatherers in flatbed trucks who scouted the smaller roadsides of Missouri and Arkansas for Echinacea. There are similar reports in the media about medicinal plants such as ginseng being overharvested, and the practice of stripping bark from slipper elms, thus killing the trees. He also mentions green herbalists, individuals who know a bit about medicine, botany, and pharmacy, and can identify a plant and know how to prepare it for medicinal purposes. In this regard, Kane has an initial section titled "Format Explanation" that provides guidelines on drying, preparation, and other facets of utilizing herbs.

There is certainly a cautionary note sounded here, given the array of questionable chemical compounds in the various plants, and the adverse side effects. One can wonder who all tried out each herbal in the first place, for whichever and whatever ailments. Do any of these herbs act against cancer? And how reliable is the information from hearsay or folklore? This brings up the matter of regulation and standardization, a not always welcome idea. In Germany there are higher standards for the formulation of herbs, although this is not so much the case in the United States.

Although ConsumerLab.com tests some of the nutritional substances used (as distinguished from herbs per se), and notably those against cancer, as per the report "Product Review of Supplements for Cancer Prevention" — in this instance, green tea, lycopene, and selenium, with the mention that lead was found in some of the substances. (The results for substances containing folate, garlic, isoflavones, vitamin C, vitamin D, and vitamin E had been reported earlier. Newer reviews will deal with garlic, ginseng, probiotics, and CQ10. The organization has also published *Guide to Buying Vitamins and Supplements: What's Really in the Bottle?*, which is available in bookstores, online, or at 800-431-1579. ConsumerLab.com is affiliated with PharmacyChecker.com and MedicareDrugPlans.com)

On the other hand, the American Association for Health Freedom (www.health-freedom.net), and its U.K. counterpart the Alliance for Natural Health, are resisting pending legislation that would regulate dietary supplements. In effect, a prescription would be required, say from an M.D., likely implying a member of the AMA, thus sharply increasing costs but limiting choices. Not only this, but the association notes that the practitioners of alternative medicine are under siege as their medical licenses are often revoked. One thing always seems to lead to another, expressible as catch-22.

Additionally, there are such volumes as Virgil J. Vogel's *American Indian Medicine*, Melvin R. Gilmore's *Use of Plants by the Indians of the Missouri River Region*, Michael Moore's *Medicinal Plants of the Mountain West*, Charles Francis Saunders' *Western Wildflowers and Their Stories*, James Mooney's *The Swimmer Manuscript of Cherokee Sacred Formulas and Medicinal Prescriptions*, Alma R. Hutchens' *Indian Herbalogy of North America* and *A Handbook of Native American Herbs*, Steven Foster's *Forest Pharmacy: Medicinal Plants in American Forests*, and Steven Foster and Rebecca L. Johnson's *Desk Reference to Nature's Medicine*, which includes a section on the Southwest's chaparral, plus citing over 40 other anticancer plants, all with illustrations. This brings up the observation that although there are many citations for anticancer plants and herbs in the literature and in medical folklore, the corresponding documented cures remain invisible. Somewhere and somehow, the subject seems subject to the law of diminishing returns.

## CHAPARRAL

On page 682 of Hartwell's book there is a citation for the species *Larrea tridentata* of the family Zygophyllaceae. This is the common creosote bush, or greasewood, or chaparral of the desertlike regions of the Southwest. It is reported in the penultimate column of Hartwell's compilation that a tea made from the leaves and stems of this plant may cure stomach cancer, liver cancer, leukemia, lung cancer, and kidney cancer. This information is buried in the central files of the National Cancer Institute.

(We may conjecture that this plant may possibly be the principal active ingredient of the mysterious Compound-X, described elsewhere in this book, for example, in Chapter 6. Then again, it may not be, depending on who is making up Compound-X. And if this plant is indeed curative, how in the world can a pharmaceutical company compete with what grows wild and free in the southwestern deserts?)

The definitive monograph was published back in 1977, titled *Creosote Bush: Biology and Chemistry of* Larrea *in New World Deserts*, edited by T. Mabry, J.H. Hunziker, and D.R. DiFeo. A chapter by Barbara N. Timmermann of the University of Texas at Austin is titled "Practical Uses of *Larrea*." She describes the main active chemical component, as NDGA, for short. A plant lignan, it is among other things a powerful antioxidant, and has even been so used commercially. She noted that NDGA sensitizes certain tumor cells to irradiation, and further wrote, with references provided, that:

> NDGA has been shown to have antitumor activity *in vivo* and *in vitro*. It is a powerful cancer antimetabolite producing *in vitro* complete inhibition of aerobic and anaerobic glycolysis and respiration of suspensions of several types of tumor cells including leukemia types. *In vivo*, NDGA combined with ascorbic acid is reported to reduce

tumors in mice. There is one unproven account that NDGA reduced malignant melanoma of the cheek of one patient.

(NDGA, incidentally, belongs to a class of organic compounds known as *quinones*.)

Other active components exist in *Larrea*, including flavones, flavonols, and flavonoids, which also exhibit anticancer activity. Additionally, the phenolic-type compounds present have germicidal properties, which can be interpreted as providing an antiviral action — as does grape juice, for instance, which has also been proposed as a cancer treatment or cure. Furthermore, the whole may be greater than its parts (synergism), and the plant in its entirety may be more active than any of its chemical parts.

In a chapter in *Creosote Bush* (1977) titled "The Natural Products Chemistry of *Larrea*," T.J. Mabry et al. discuss the flavonoids that are found in this unique plant. They include quercetin and kindred compounds. Quercetin itself is recognized as a strong anticancer agent, and is found in many other plants, including fruits and vegetables such as cabbage, even the horse chestnut tree (Moss, 1992, p. 64). It is also regarded as an enzyme inhibitor. Its original recognized source is from the inner bark of the black oak or yellow-bark oak, or quercetron (*Quercus velutina*; hence its name) of the eastern half of the United States. The Indians and settlers made a yellow dye from the inner bark. Bioflavonoids, more well known, are kin to the flavonoids — the vitamin called *rutin* being an example — and are found among other sources in the inner peel of citrus fruits.

There are, however, different species of *Larrea*, the creosote bush. In the work by Percy Train et al. on the Paiute Indians of Nevada, previously cited, another species or subspecies designated *Larrea divaricata* was used by these Indians, but was not mentioned specifically as a treatment for cancers or tumors, but was instead used for other diseases.

(Tea made from creosote bush roots has long been considered an Indian cure for arthritis, as previously reported, i.e., by Virginia Madison in *The Big Bend Country of Texas* and by Charles Francis Saunders in *Western Wildflowers and Their Stories* [Madison, 1955, p. 221; Saunders, 1993, p. 287]. Even an ointment smeared on the affected joints is said to work. It is also called *Yerba hedionda* or *stink bush*, and *hediondilla*, or the *little bad smeller*. It discourages any other plants from growing around or underneath it, ensuring its survival in its arid surroundings.)

Some further explanations about the genus *Larrea* are therefore in order. The necessary information is contained in the initial chapters of the monograph *Creosote Bush: Biology and Chemistry of* Larrea *in New World Deserts*, in separate chapters by O.T. Solbrig and by J.H. Hunziker et al. There are five species, four in lower South America, for example, in Patagonia, and one in the desert Southwest of North America. All contain NDGA. The North American species is more properly named *Larrea tridentata*. It is, however, very closely similar to the South American species *Larrea divaricata*, and they are considered con-species or subspecies of the same plant. Hence the names are used interchangeably. So one is essentially the other, and both can therefore be regarded as having been used in the treatment of cancer.

(In the introduction to the work by Percy Train et al., it was observed that in any Indian community there would be several individuals who were not rated as medicine men but who would have wide medicinal knowledge. These were the type of informants sought, and they would supply most of the information. It was also noted that one did not simply walk up to an Indian and ask for his medicinal plant lore as handed down from his ancestors. This would be met with a blank stare or a "No savvy." The information was closely guarded, not only from the white man, but from other Indian neighbors as well. But the more the interviewer knew of Indian diseases and medicine, the more readily the information was volunteered.)

Walters (1993) devotes an entire chapter to chaparral and speaks of its amazing properties for curing cancers. He quotes a Pima Indian: "This plant cures everything. It is what nature gave us." (Its positive effect on arthritis is noted in Chapter 1.) Walters provides cases of a number of dramatic cures, and concludes with the comment that though this desert shrub remains on the American Cancer Society's Unproven Methods blacklist, it may outlive even the ACS's condemnation.

At the end of his chapter on chaparral, Walters cites Heinerman (1984). Chaparral is one of the many plants or herbs reported to have been used, and used successfully.

(In any event, it is rumored that doctors have been known to prescribe the use of this plant surreptitiously. The use of Chaparral is in fact mentioned in many herbal books as a treatment for cancer. [We capitalize the word to distinguish that it is of the genus *Larrea* rather than one of the many other plants called "chaparral."] Its sale in the United States is banned by the FDA, presumably due to a contaminated batch, as is laetrile for other reasons. The principal active component NDGA was removed from the FDA's "Generally Recognized As Safe (GRAS)" list back in 1970, according to Barbara N. Timmermann in the last chapter of *Creosote Bush: Biology and Chemistry of* Larrea *in New World Deserts*. This, however, is not the case for such poisonous therapeutics as 5-FU [5-Flourouracil], used in chemotherapy.)

Although the sale of Chaparral per se is banned, it evidently may still be used in herbal mixtures sold commercially, for example, Jason Winter's Herbal Tea, which contains chaparral, red clover, and an undisclosed root from a flower, and which is reported to cure or benefit cancer patients (Walters, 1993, pp. 139, 140). Red clover, incidentally, is an ingredient of the Hoxsey therapy.

A formula provided by herbalist Michael Tierra has multiple ingredients (Walters, 1993, p. 139). Its principal components are chaparral and echinacea (or purple coneflower), plus red clover blossoms, cascara sagrada, astralagus, ginseng roots, and other herbs. Another formula supplied has chaparral, echinacea root, pau d'arco, and red clover blossoms. Echinacea root itself is apparently in renewed favor as an anticancer agent.

A recipe for Chaparral tea has been furnished by Arlin J. Brown of the Arlin J. Brown Information Center in Fort Belvoir, VA (Walters, 1993, p. 138). The decoction is prepared by adding a cup of boiling water to 4 oz of chaparral (leaves or stems). After steeping for about 10 min, more boiling water is added so as to make about 2 qt. Seal in a bottle and keep in the sun for 2 days. Three cups per day is the dosage. Brown further notes that taking chaparral tea, or pau d'arco, or Essiac tea alone may not be enough (Walters, 1993, p. 139). Detoxification and immune-boosting regimens should also be followed, by diet and by supplements.

Similarly, Ralph W. Moss (1992) also has a section on chaparral in his book. Along with Walters, he cites noteworthy work conducted at the University of Utah

Medical Center. There is the caution that NDGA may harm the kidneys, apparently a fact long known. In *Alternatives in Cancer Therapy: The Complete Guide to Non-Traditional Treatments*, authors Ross Pelton and Lee Overholser cite a case where high dosages of chaparral caused liver damage, though cutting back on the dosage level solved the problem. In fact, there may be an optimum dosage, neither too small, which may allow tumor growth, nor too large (Pelton and Overholser, 1994, pp. 210, 211). On the other hand, Walters gives it more of a clean bill of health, but with the warning that it can cause an eventual depletion of iron in the body, and its use and that of other herbal remedies should be backed up by a strong nutritional program. The overall comment might be made that there is a trade-off even in the use of herbal or plant remedies, that is, we are always playing one factor against another.

(We add here that as far as inorganic iron supplements are concerned, ferrous fumarate is preferable to ferrous gluconate, which is in turn preferable to ferrous sulfate, the bottom of the barrel. Organic iron sources may be considered the way to go, therefore.)

A computer search of Medline showed that there have been some cases where Chaparral or creosote bush has caused acute hepatitis (inflammation of the liver). The leaves had either been eaten or a tea had been made and consumed over an extended period. NDGA was in some cases thought to be the problem ingredient. (It has been indicated that NDGA may harm the kidneys.) On average, about one case per year was reported. There are of course other sources of hepatitis, such as pathogens from untreated sewage that get into food. Whether the creosote bush itself was the source is not known conclusively, but there was a strong indication that it was. The issue hinges on whether or not there are some pretreatments for creosote bush to be used before human consumption. (According to some roundabout Indian lore, this may very well be the case.)

No mention was made in the preceding reports about whether the Chaparral had been used against cancer, and if so, whether the treatment was successful. Considering the toxicity of conventional chemotherapy drugs, for which hepatitis or liver damage would be only one side effect among several, there is a counterargument for considering Chaparral instead.

It may be noted, furthermore, that the several books on poisonous plants that have been examined did not have *Larrea*, that is, Chaparral, greasewood, or creosote bush listed. For instance, John M. Kingsbury's comprehensive *Poisonous Plants of the United States and Canada* does not mention *Larrea*, as such, or any of its other names. Admittedly, some of these books are aimed more at livestock poisoning than at human poisoning.

(Although some confusion remains about what is to be called chaparral, or greasewood, or creosote bush, the genus of interest is specifically *Larrea*, here a plant found in low southwestern deserts. There are other species called greasewood, e.g., *Sarcobatus vermiculatus* of the goosefoot family or Chenopodiaceae, as found, say, in southern Wyoming, and which contains concentrations of sodium and potassium oxalates, which can act as poisons if ingested in sufficient amounts.)

The University of Utah, previously cited, was involved in conducting studies on Chaparral circa 1970, supported by the National Cancer Institute. According to

Walters, the reported results were mixed (Walters, 1993, p. 96). Walters further notes that Heinerman (1984) pointed out some inconsistencies in the study. Heinerman suggests that, as a result of media publicity surrounding the study, the university medical team became "somewhat upset," and concluded that "the full story about the abrupt halt in the Chaparral research done at the University of Utah Medical Center in 1969 will never be fully known" (Heinerman, 1984, p. 205).

Incidentally, the word is that further experimental work by Jonathan Hartwell and his associates showed that Chaparral did not act against cancers in mice, the standard test for efficacy of treatment. This kind of test, however, is not necessarily the last word. It is only one kind of screening procedure, whereas the actual world is more complicated, calling for clinical tests on humans instead.

John Heinerman goes into considerable detail documenting the case of a Mesa, Arizona man, Ernest Farr, who cured himself of virulent melanoma skin cancer drinking Chaparral tea (Heinerman, 1989b, p. 94). This case is reported in several of the other books cited about alternative treatments for cancer, for example, by Walters (1993). Furthermore, there is at least anecdotal evidence circulating that melanoma has also been cured by using a bit of the tarry extract known as Compound-X on the cancer. The cancer literally comes out by the roots. (Milkweed, genus *Asclepias*, is known to remove external tumors such as warts.)

Other cases using Chaparral reportedly have not always been successful, though the information is not conclusive. Similarly so with other alternative therapies, as well as for the conventional treatments of surgery, radiation, and chemotherapy, sometimes referred to derisively as cut, burn, and poison. The acid test for any treatment is the cure or remission of the deadly threesome: liver cancer, lung cancer, and pancreatic cancer.

## OTHER PLANTS AND HERBS

Many specifics about anticancer plants and extracts worldwide are compiled in Chapter 3, Section 3.3, and in the appendices of Hoffman (1999a). We add peripheral information here. Prominent names of persons involved in collecting this anticancer information include Jonathan Hartwell, of course, plus James A. Duke, Geoffrey A. Cordell (alkaloids), Edward S. Ayensu, Robert A. DeFillips, John Heinerman, and Ralph Moss, to name a very few.

Of special mention is Ralph Moss's informative *Herbs Against Cancer: History and Controversy*, which has chapters on dilemmas in other countries as well as the United States. It does not try to be all inclusive, not having a chapter on either laetrile or creosote bush (chaparral), for instance, which may or may not be referred to as herbs.

In Heinerman (1984), there is a chapter about specific herbs for cancer from around the world. The following is an overview of some of that information. For further details the reader is referred to Dr. Heinerman's book. (John Heinerman, 1984. Out of print. Photocopies at one time could be ordered from the author at P.O. Box 11471, Salt Lake City UT, (801)521-8824. Of course, there is Interlibrary Loan, and used books are available via the Internet from other sources, e.g., Amazon.com.)

The reminder, again, is that the designator anticancer does not signify a cure —
only the possibility, which may be remote or nonexistent. Adverse, even fatal, side
effects are possible.

## South Africa

From South Africa there is oven-heated cactus (*Opuntia maxima*), which was used
with some success internally for large bowel cancer Heinerman, 1984, p. 106. Next,
there was a herbal mixture called the *David Remedy*, consisting of the leaves of the
plant called *maytens* (*Maytenus heterophylla*), the roots and leaves of a plant with
the scientific name *Scutia martina*, and the roots of sanservia (genus *Sanservia*), as
well as other unidentified herbs. This herb *Maytenus* was found to be very active
against several forms of cancer, and its main ingredient, maytansine, was specific
for leukemia.

Another plant or shrub from coastal Zululand is of the genus *Putterlickia*, and
was described as "the world's richest source of a new powerful anticancer chemical,"
which turned out to be maytansine. Another possibility is called the *sausage tree*
(*Kigelia panata*).

As the definitive work, Heinerman cites *Medicinal and Poisonous Plants of
Southern and Eastern Africa* by John Mitchell Watt and Maria Gerdina Breyer-
Brandwijk. Although specific cancer references are not explicitly mentioned, Heinerman and other scientists have deduced a few such as *Senecio serratus*, *Cheilanthes
hirsuta*, *Euphorbia ingens*, *Podaxis pistillaris*, and *Raphionacme hirsuta*. The coauthor and chemist Dr. Maria G. Breyer-Brandwijk said that most of the cancer
treatments cited were for local, rather than internal, application.

## China

In the People's Republic of China, several interesting treatments have been cited.
One is glossy privet (*Ligustrum lucidum*) for animal tumors. Amygdalin, or laetrile,
is derived variously from the dried kernel of the Japanese plum (*Prunus amygdalis*),
the American plum (*Prunus americana*), and the Japanese apricot (*Prunus armeni-
aca*). A reference publication is cited here as well, titled *Herbal Pharmacology of
the People's Republic of China*. The ubiquitous James A. Duke and Edward S.
Ayensu have contributed *Medicinal Plants of China*, published in 1985.

It has in fact been commented by James A. Duke that half of the medicinal
folklore from ancient China has scientific validity. For instance, spiny ginseng (genus
*Acanthopanax*) has been tested clinically against certain cancers as well as for other
ailments, including the side effects of chemotherapy. Another plant called *Tangkuei*
or *Dongguei* (*Angelica sinensis*), which at least at the time of publication of Heinerman's book could be purchased in California, has been successfully used in clinical
trials to treat esophagus and liver cancers. For treatment of the esophagus, it is
combined with elecampane (*Inula helenium*) in equal parts and the decoction is
taken internally (Heinerman, 1984, p. 110). (It is mentioned that elecampane has
been used successfully in the treatment of rabies.) Heinerman goes on to say that
Tangkui used with dandelion root, peach bark, and sarsaparilla herb has proved

tremendously effective on liver cancer. Both liver cancer and cirrhosis of the liver have responded dramatically using Tangkuei, which is one of China's newer cancer herbs. It is reported to be rich in vitamin E, and contains saponins (also called *glucosides*, and which cause a soapy lather), and similar to yucca, ginseng, and sarsaparilla, as well as other chemical compounds, known and unknown.

Heinerman speaks of another promising herb for mass tumor reduction, called *Ho-Shou-Wu* (*Polygonum multiflorum*). An example is provided of the reduction of a brain tumor, permitting the sufferer to lead a normal life.

Courtesy of Dr. Bin Xu from the Shanghai Institute of Materia Medica, who was a visiting professor with the Institute of Cancer Research at Columbia University at the time, a number of other plants or substances that were being screened and tested for anticancer activity are listed by Heinerman. One was an alkaloid derived from the Chinese tree *Camptotheca acuminata*, called *camptothecin*. A derivative is called *10-hydroxycamptothecin*. Both of the extracts containing these substances have proved greatly beneficial for primary liver cancer, cancer of the head and neck, gastric cancer, and leukemia.

We mention again that the plum yew tree (*Cephatolaxus harringtonii*) has yielded extracts or natural compounds called *harringtonine* and *hemoharringtonine*, which have been effective against several forms of leukemia. This was confirmed at the Memorial Sloan-Kettering Cancer Center.

Also mentioned in the aforecited book are colchicine and colchicinamide, derived from the common autumn crocus (*Colchicum autumnale*), also called *meadow saffron*. (Colchicine, incidentally, is used in plant genetics to artificially produce mutations.) The notable use cited is against breast cancer, but gout and arthritis also yield to treatment. It is emphasized that both these alkaloids are potent, and their use requires expert medical supervision. Another plant mentioned is crotalaria (*Crotalaria spectabilis*), from which a toxic alkaloid called monocrotaline may be obtained. This substance also has antitumor properties, but acts against the liver.

(Saffron, derived from the stigma of *Crocus sativum*, of the family Iridaceae, is briefly mentioned as an anticancer agent in Pat Willard's book of the same name [2001] along with some other medicinal properties, about all of which Willard remains skeptical.)

A parasitic fungus named *Grifola umbrellata*, which grows variously on the roots of oak, maple, and mahogany trees contains ingredients with anticancer properties, as does *Poria cocos*, a fungus growing on the roots of old pine trees. Also mentioned are garlic (*Allium sativum*) and the tuber of another herb with the scientific name *Pinella pedatisecta*.

(Another species, found in China, the fungus *Polyporus umbellata*, is also said to be a strong anticancer agent [Griggs, 1991, p. 318]. We note that the use of fungi is intruding into the domain of antibiotics, which are fungus derived.)

Heinerman comments that the Chinese used these herbs along with conventional Western drugs such as are employed in chemotherapy, whereby the herbs reduce the toxic side effects. *Pinella ternata* is an example, for its antivomiting property. Another example is a species of sage (*Salvia miltrorrhiza*), used in conjunction with barbiturates to enhance the tranquilizing effects. Heinerman suggests that herbs be investigated further here in America for their benefits when used with chemotherapy.

A paragraph is given to herbal medicine as practiced in Tibet, with the comment that many of their substances have bad side effects, the same as for conventional chemotherapy. Some of these substances are aconite (*Aconitum ferrox*), which is very poisonous, sweet flag or calamus (*Acorus calamus*), bitumen, and arsenic, all of which require close monitoring.

## Soviet Union

In what was the Soviet Union, or USSR, conventional chemotherapy and radiation employed are the same as elsewhere, but herbs are used simultaneously. One of these herbs is catnip (*Nepeta Cataria*), which helps to reduce the common side effects. Another herb used this way is Siberian ginseng (genus *Eleutherococcus*), which appears to work better than regular ginseng (*Panax ginseng*). The former reduces stress, whereas the latter may cause stress. Siberian ginseng has even been used in space missions for its antistress properties; moreover, it is said to provide protection against solar radiation.

The herb St. Johns wort (*Hypericum peforatum*) has been used to help detect intestinal cancer during x-ray procedures using barium-water enemas. It serves to sharpen the photographic image.

There apparently is a renewed interest in folk medicine by Russian scientists. As a particular example, peony root (genus *Paeonia*) is used successfully as an anticancer agent at many major hospitals in Russia.

## Mexico

Heinerman notes that there is a rich tradition of botanical lore, handed down from the ancient Aztecs and Mayas. Not all the multitude of treatments have survived in time, but agave or maguey (genus *Agave*) has been used for skin ailments. It has been discovered that the saponins (mainly gitogenin and galactose) from the species called the *Schott agave* (*Agave schottii*) will inhibit the growth of skin cancers and intramuscular tumors. A ground-up herb called *Anil del Muerto* or *golden crown-beard* (*Verbesina encilioides*) has been used on skin cancer. The branches from Encino (de la hoja ancha) or Gambell's scrub oak (*Quercus gambelii*) were boiled and the liquid extract applied to skin cancers, followed by sprinkling ground-up bark and acorns. Mashed-up jimson weed or toloache (*Datura meteloides* or *Datura stramonium*) was mixed with butter and applied to skin cancers. Leaves from the fendler globemallow or Yerba de la Negrita (*Sphaeralcea fendleri*) were ground and mixed with warm water and strained, and the patient was given a cupful a day for a week. This was supposed to loosen the tumor, causing it to leave the body. Even if the claims are exaggerated, Mexican scientists have nevertheless found that some of these and other remedies actually work.

## AUSTRALIA

Interest has started to build about the plants used by the aborigines, particularly at the Western Australia Institute of Technology in Bentley. Of about 30 herbs studied, 4 have been used against cancer. The latex of the Australian spurge (*Euphorbia australis*) is used against skin cancers and sores. Another, the snakewood spurge (*Euphorbia hirta*) is used for asthma and lung cancer. Cancer is also treated by a species with the scientific name *Scaevola spinescens*, in which the active ingredients are said to be *furanocoumarins*. In fact, the coumarins have been studied as anti-cancer agents in terms of their diuretic properties, and their beneficial effect on cholesterol, hardening of the arteries, and blood coagulation.

## EGYPT AND ISRAEL

One of the herbs mentioned in the Bible is myrrh, that is, Arabian or Somalian myrrh. It is a gum or resin from a tree that grows in East Africa and Arabia with the scientific name *Commiphora myrra* or *Commiphora abyssinica*. Among its other uses, myrrh is said to have been tried for leprosy and skin cancer, the sores that never heal. It is an active antibacterial agent, and is also being further investigated for its effect on internal as well as external cancers. In parts of the Sudan, honey is sometimes used against cancer. Its high acidity seems to be beneficial, at least in the growth of typhoid-colon bacteria. In Egyptian studies, of eight plants tried, three showed anticancer activity, of which only one was decisive. This was the periwinkle (*Catharanthus roseus*).

Extracts from the periwinkle are already in common use in modern medicine, for example, vincristine and vinblastine, in the treatment of leukemia. Egyptian studies have shown, furthermore, there is an effect on abdominal cancer too. Folklore says that Egyptian onions also are anticancer agents, and studies are under way.

In Israel, interferon has been under study as an anticancer agent, in common with other countries. The same type of interferon-like agent may be bred into plants or herbs such as tobacco, to yield a "herbal interferon," or so-called *N-gene* or *N-factor*, which occurs in the nicotine alkaloids. Besides, species of the genus *Nicotonia*, different varieties or species of *Datura* can be used, for instance jimsonweed (*Datura stramonium*), which have previously been used against cancer. Nicotine alkaloids containing the N-factor show up as well in the common milkweed or silky milkweed (*Aesclipias syrica*). Milkweed, incidentally, is a folklore remedy for cancer. Indian tobacco, of the genus *Lobelia*, also contains alkaloids, notably lobaline, used in helping to break the smoking habit.

The plant or plants called *Lobelia* have a track record in the treatment of infectious diseases, including tetanus and blood poisoning. The Iroquois Indians used *Lobelia syphilitica*, as the scientific name implies, against venereal diseases, maybe even uterine cancer. In the Civil War the species *Lobelia inflata* was used variously as an enema and for snake, spider, and insect bites.

The alkaloid lobeline (as derived from *Lobelia inflata*) bears a striking resemblance to nicotine, and both have similar chemical actions. This may extend to cancer treatment. Heinerman observes that the nineteenth century American herbalist

Samuel Thomson praised the use of *L. inflata* and *L. syphilitica* for an array of diseases, including rabies, measles, and smallpox, and even for removing pimples and warts. He lists other herbs to be used with lobelia, such as capsicum, ginger, bayberry, and sage, as well as goldenseal and comfrey, and peach tree bark and myyrh. Peppermint and spearmint may be added, and catnip too.

Finally, if lobelia will not cure cancer, it may very well stop the spread of cancer, and it is safer than, say, radiation.

## United States

Heinerman states that in the United States more research has probably been conducted on plants with anticancer properties than anywhere else in the world. He cites, in particular, the work of Jonathan L. Hartwell of the National Cancer Institute, which has been frequently referred to in this book. Hartwell began his work in the early 1950s, identifying and studying the chemical agents in podophyllin that produced anticancer activity in mice. Podyphyllin is the resin from the American mandrake, or Mayapple (*Podophyllum peltatum*). In doing a literature search he found that it had been reported some years earlier that the Penobscot Indians of Maine used the resin against cancer. In fact, he discovered that the America *Materia Medica* had recommended the resin for cancer treatment over 100 years earlier, and physicians in Mississippi had been using it as early as 1897. Therefore, he initiated a comprehensive search in both folklore and the technical literature. Over 1000 books from around the world were searched, and at least 500 items of correspondence ensued.

In a subsequent symposium on "Plants and Cancer" the question was posed, "Can folklore be used as a tool in predicting antitumor agents?" The overall answer was of course yes, which included the statement that "the closest relationship seen has been between antitumor activity and plants known to be poisonous."

Heinerman observes that a huge number of plants could be cited, but he presents a limited few excerpted from an article by Dr. Hartwell on "Plant Remedies for Cancer." These are further listed in Table 7.1, for the record, but with no guarantees.

Also mentioned in the Heinerman reference is the use of an extract of St. Johns wort (*Hypericum perforatum*) for hopeless cancer cases. Mention is made of several cases of cancer cured using Chaparral tea (*Larrea divaricata*).

Garlic is given special emphasis, going back to Hippocrates, and later India. France is reported to have a low cancer rate due to eating garlic and maybe drinking red wine as per Chapter 1, and Bulgarian garlic eaters are said to be virtually cancerfree. This bit of folklore was substantiated in the laboratory with mice and other laboratory animals.

Bloodroot (*Sanguinaria canadensis*) is also mentioned as another remedy for cancer. It was used in London hospitals in the nineteenth century by a doctor who had learned of it from Indians living near Lake Superior. It was confirmed in the laboratory that alkaloids derived from bloodroot, for example, sanguarine and chelerythrine, produced tumor reduction in mice.

## TABLE 7.1
## Selected Anticancer Plants Found in the U.S.

| Name | Method of Use |
| --- | --- |
| Alfalfa (*Medicago sativa*) | Combined with flowers from the date tree and an oak tree fungus (*Peniollium crustacaecum*). |
| Woodland angelica (*Angelica sylvestris*) | Root decoction taken orally. |
| Virginia beechnut (*Epifagus virginiana*) | Entire plant chewed for cancer of the mouth and esophagus. |
| Birch (genus *Betula*) | Tea from the shaved bark for abdominal cancer. |
| Black walnut (*Juglans nigra*) | Walnut meat combined with milk and apples, to be taken orally for leukemia. |
| Blessed thistle (*Cnicus benedictus*) | Powdered extract for skin cancer. |
| Blue flag iris (*Iris versicolor*) | Tea from root combined with cobalt sulfate for lymphatic cancer and kidney cancer. |
| Burdock (*Arctium lappa*) | Combined with yellow dock and sarsaparilla in a tea for general cancer. |
| Buttercup (*Ranunculus bulbosus*) | Liquid extract taken for breast cancer and cancer of the uterine cervix. |
| Canaigre dock (*Rumex hymenosepalus*) | Soak bandages in extract and apply to skin cancer. |
| Carrot (*Daucus carota*) | Fresh, raw juice for leukemia. |
| Black cohosh (*Cimicifuga racemosa*) | Extract with unnamed herbs taken for cancer of the tongue and glandular breast cancer. Alternately, with Peruvian bark (genus *Cinchona*) and horsebalm, also called horseweed, heal-all, or stoneroot (*Collinsonia canadensus*). |
| Cockleburr (genus *Xanthium* or *Arctium*) | Tea with yellow dock and sarsaparilla for general cancer. |
| Cranberries (genus *Vaccinium*) | Ground, fresh berry in poultice for skin cancer. |
| Dandelion (*Taraxacum officinale*) | Pills from extract for general cancer. |
| Dogwood (*Cornus florida*) | Baked bark inhalation for breast cancer. |
| Elder tree (*Sambucus nigra*) | Decoction of branches and roots taken for general cancer. |
| Herb-Robert geranium (*Geranium robertianum*) | Extract used for cancer of lung, rectum, throat, prostate, breast, and leukemia. |
| Garlic (*Allium sativa*) | Juice taken orally; cut garlic rubbed on sores. Intravenous injection of vitamins E, F, K, and chlorophyll with oral administration of garlic, peppermint, and brewer's yeast for lung cancer, leukemia, and general cancer. |
| Ginger (*Zingiber officinale*) | For breast cancer, lobelia poultices while taking ginger and baking soda (or hops) orally. |
| Lobelia (*Lobelia inflata*) | Used as poultice. Tea with ginger and soda (or hops) added for breast cancer. |
| Madonna lily (*Lilium candidum*) | Poultices from crushed bulbs and olive oil. Salve from bulbs with pine pitch and deer tallow for lung and breast cancer. Milkweed (genus *Ascelepias*) milky latex for nose cancer. |

**TABLE 7.1 (CONTINUED)**
**Selected Anticancer Plants Found in the U.S.**

| Name | Method of Use |
|---|---|
| Mustard, wild (genus *Brassica* or *Sisymbriam*) | Salve from dried blossoms for skin cancer. |
| Onion (*Allium cepa*) | Juice injections for breast and rectum cancers. |
| Pipsissewa (*Chimaphila umbellata*) | Liquid extract taken for uterine cervix cancer and breast cancer. |
| Pokeroot (*Phytolacca americana*) | Poultices from root. Root mixture taken internally also. For lip cancer and general cancer. |
| Potato (*Solanum tuberosum*) | Extract for subcutaneous cancers. |
| Queen's root (*Stillingia sylvatica*) | Decoction taken for general cancer. |
| Red clover (*Trifolium pratense*) | Tea from blossoms for breast cancer and general cancer. |
| Red oak (*Quercus rubra*) | Salve prepared by evaporating decoction of inner bark. For nose cancer. |
| Sarsaparilla (genus *Smilax*) | Root decoction with other unnamed roots taken for general cancer. |
| Sassafras (*Sassafras albidum*) | Salve and extract from bark taken for general cancer. |
| Sheep sorrel (*Rumex acetosella*) | Evaporate juice for salve. Poultice from crushed fresh plant. Tea from fluid extract. For breast and internal cancers. |
| Sycamore (*Platanus occidentalis*) | Fluid extract for general cancer. |
| Tomato (*Lycopersicon esculentum*) | Juice from ground tops mixed with 95% alcohol or 5% iodine and taken orally. Residue used as salve. For liver cancer. |
| Violet (genus *Viola*) | Tea from dried leaves. Tea also from dried leaves of violet and red clover plus yellow dock root. Also a decoction from flower, plant and root. All for general cancer. |
| Wintergreen (*Gaultheria procumbens*) | Take wintergreen oil with dandelion root. Or the entire root. For general cancer and leukemia. |
| Yellow dock (*Rumex obtusifolius* or *Rumex crispus*) | Root with leaves of red clover and violet. Taken for general cancer. |

*Source:* Adapted from Heinerman, J., *The Treatment of Cancer with Herbs*, BiWorld, Orem, UT, 1980, 1984; as taken from Jonathan L. Hartwell's "Plant Remedies for Cancer," *Cancer Chemotherapy Reports*, 7:19–24, May 1960.

Incidentally, Dr. Hartwell concluded his compendium with the statement that "if there is any hope in a chemical treatment for cancer, it is reasonable to believe that such an agent is as likely to originate from a plant as from pure synthesis."

Heinerman continues with still other developments and information, abstracted as follows.

The herb called periwinkle, which may be any of several genera and species, supplies two compounds used in modern medicine. One of these, vinblastine, is employed for Hodgkin's disease and lymphomas, and is also used on solid tumors. The other, vincrystine, is employed for lymphatic leukemia. Mayapple, or podophyllum, has also been found effective. Periwinkle in itself has, of course, been used as a cancer treatment, as previously indicated.

It was reported that American mistletoe (*Phoradendron flavescens*) and its European counterpart (*Viscum album*) are being studied. The twigs and leaves contain the active components against cancer. An extract also performs as a chemotherapy agent. (Walters, 1993, contains a chapter "Mistletoe," as does Moss, 1992, but under the heading "Iscador." Pelton and Overholzer, 1994, also include a chapter.)

At Brigham Young University, in the department of biochemistry, Dr. John Mangum has been involved in testing juniper berry extract, as well as watercress, chaparral, and yarrow. The crystalline anticancer agent occurs in what is called *savin*, which is obtained from the dried needles.

The work of Dr. Owen Asplund in the chemistry department at the University of Wyoming, cited in Chapter 5, Chapter 6, Chapter 8, and Chapter 9, was reviewed by Heinerman. The fresh flowers of the yucca (*Yucca glauca*) showed anticancer activity against melanoma. (And are now, apparently, being clinically tested in Switzerland and Mexico, as was cited above.) Dr. Asplund has also tested the Alpine sunflower (*Hymenoxys grandiflora*) and the garden variety canterbury bell, or bluebell (*Campanula calycanthema*). The sunflower was found active against melanoma.

Mention was also made by Heinerman of work being done at that time by a firm called the Chemex Corporation, at Riverton and Lander, Wyoming (located in northwestern Wyoming, next to the Wind River Indian Reservation). Tests apparently were being conducted using the creosote bush, or chaparral. Tests had been done on animals in the United States, and encouraging progress was reported for human volunteers in Costa Rica and Italy. (The substance used may be the mysterious Compound-X, as reported in Chapter 6. And the firm may have been Vipont or Viadent rather than Chemex. That is, Chemex was working with yucca plant extracts. In further explanation, Vipont was a large pharmaceutical firm that has been involved in, among other things, marketing a toothpaste containing *Sanguinaria*, or bloodroot, as an antitartar agent. The toothpaste is called Viadent, and Vipont Pharmaceuticals is now owned by Colgate-Palmolive.)

Work at the University of Arizona Health Sciences Center, conducted by Dr. Sydney E. Salmon, focused on tests for determining the most effective treatment for a particular person's cancer. The patient's own cancer cells were used to determine the most effective and least effective drugs.

Among the drugs claimed to minimize the side effects of chemotherapy are Siberian ginseng, lobelia, goldenseal, echinacea, sarsparilla and wild Oregon grape.

For radiation side effects there are liquid aloe vera, Siberian ginseng, kelp, huckleberry leaves, comfrey root and leaves, and chickweed.

The nonessential amino acid asparagine has been found to have strong anticancer properties. It occurs in a variety of plants, including asparagas root (*Asparagus officianalis*), sprouting vetch (*Vicia sativa*), white lupine (genus *Lupinus*), and soybean seedlings (genus *Glycine*). An asparagine derivative acted against leukemia cells in culture tests.

NDGA is also reported upon. The NDGA factor is said to be active against melanoma in many cancer patients.

The comment is supplied that the activity of a herb against cancer may depend on the geographic location. Thus, the root of the herb with the scientific name

*Tripterygium wilfordii* was most active against cancer if obtained from Taiwan, whereas the root from Hong Kong showed no activity.

An extract from the hard, scurrilous blackish knobs from the trunks of the birch tree can be taken to retard the growth of advanced cancers, and to reduce the pain.

The leaves from the myrtle (*Myrtus communis*) make into a tea that is good for diabetes and also acts against cancer. For cancer, comfrey and aloe vera are added. It is said to be active against breast, lung, bone, and glandular cancers.

Heinerman provided some background for the plant testing work that was under way at the National Cancer Institute at the time. (Some of this has been indicated as per Chapter 6 in the description of Hartwell's work.) Starting in 1957, from 2,500 to 4,000 plant samples were screened each year, involving from 600 to 1,500 different plants. The latest cumulative number was about 235,000 plant species and about 108,000 extracts. The testing was against murine (mouse) tumors *in vivo*, or for cell cytotoxicity (cyto- also indicating cell or cellular) vs. the KB (human nasopharynx, or nasal passages) line of cancer cells. Various universities and research foundations were under contract for assistance. As previously noted, the program was discontinued in 1981.

Heinerman also outlines the difficulties encountered in the screening program. Whereas folklore is a relatively easy way to get prescreening, there are such human problems as credibility and secrecy, and such other botanical problems as picking and choosing, and distinguishing between plants.

Another difficulty is that just because a plant fails one kind of cancer test, is not necessarily an indication that it will fail another kind of test. That is, the plants may tend to be selective against different sorts of cancers. This was brought out by Owen Asplund in his work on yucca blossoms against cancer, previously cited. Thus, in the standard leukemia test the yucca did not work. But instead of discontinuing the work at that point, a test was made against melanoma, with strikingly positive results. A paragraph is included in Heinerman's reference, giving Dr. Asplund's remarks.

The screening and testing procedures were also criticized by Dr. Solomon Garb, a professor of pharmacology at the University of Missouri School of Medicine. His criticisms were presented at considerable length.

Other anticancer possibilities include the allelopathic (not allopathic) herbs, which by definition tend to suppress other herbal growth. Included in this category is the black walnut (*Juglans nigra*), in which the most active agent is called *juglone*. It is toxic to bacteria and fungi as well, curing a number of skin ailments.

The sunflower is also an allelopathic plant, and a sunflower extract was found to inhibit the growth of such common weeds as jimsonweed, velvetleaf, johnsongrass, curly dock, red sorrel, ragweed, purslane, smartweed, wild mustard, and lamb's-quarter. (Creosote bush, or chaparral, may be the outstanding example of an allelopathic plant. No other plant can live next to or under a creosote bush.)

The purple sage of southern California is another example, as is the eucalyptus tree, an import from Australia. The common chrysanthemum is allelopathic, even unto its own kind.

Heinerman lists some other medicinal plants that are allelopathic and may prove to be anticancer agents. These include hackberry (*Ailanthus altissima*), giant foxtail (*Setaria faberii*), wormwood (*Artemisia absinthum*), black locust (*Robinia pseudoacacia*), crabgrass (*Digitaria sanguinalis*), goldenrod (*Solidago canadensis*), black cherry (*Prunus serotina*), white birch (*Betula alba*), and yellow dock (*Rumex crispus*).

## GREAT BRITAIN

Heinerman showcases the talents of the famous Dr. Denis Parsons Burkitt of London. Serving in Africa, he discovered a viral tumor in African children, which came to be known as Burkitt's lymphoma. He also uncovered the fact that dietary fiber acts against colon cancer and other intestinal diseases.

Another significant discovery by Dr. Burkitt, previously cited but mostly gone unnoticed by the medical profession, is that just a little bit of chemotherapy goes a long way in reducing cancerous tumors.

During his time in Africa, Dr. Burkitt went on to utilize several new chemotherapy drugs that, as it turned out, worked successfully against a variety of cancers. These drugs included methotrexate, cyclophosamide (also called *endoxan* and *cytosan*), and vincristine. Some of his testimony is provided.

Heinerman's following chapter is titled "Vegetarianism — A New Cancer Diet Scientifically Supported."

Among the items of information supplied is the fact that human feces may contain mutagenic material in varying amounts that may be carcinogenic. Notable among these mutagenic materials are nitroso compounds, which are highly carcinogenic, and which are formed from the nitrogen content of the foods eaten. (Proteins, for instance, contain bound nitrogen in the molecules.) Increasing the fiber intake will have a beneficial effect.

Another interesting item supplied is that reducing caloric intake also reduces the chances for cancer.

Special attention is given to the work conducted by Dr. Chiu Nan Lai of the Department of Biology of the University of Texas System Cancer Center, located at the M.D. Anderson Hospital and Tumor Institute in Houston. Using the Ames bacterial test as an indicator of carcinogenicity, Dr. Lai found that certain chlorophyll-containing vegetables acted against cancer-causing chemical agents. The greener the vegetable, the greater the anticancer activity.

The histidine content of vegetables was used as a measure of chlorophyll activity. (Histidine is an amino acid that will convert to histamine by the action of putrefactive bacteria.) Vegetables were therefore ranked by their histidine content as follows, and apparently the higher the better: Those with a low histidine content included cucumber, celery, iceberg lettuce, and dandelion. Those with a medium histidine content included carrots, leafy lettuce, and endive. Those with a high histidine content included cabbage, parsley, spinach, mustard greens, and broccoli. Dr. Lai also found that wheat, mung bean, and lentil sprouts strongly inhibit carcinogens that require body metabolism, but not carcinogens that do not require body metabolism.

(In this connection, there is what is called *Wheatgrass therapy*, using freshly sprouted wheat with its high chlorophyll content [Walters, 1993, p. 147ff]. It may be mentioned also that there are a number of products on the market produced from grain sprouts, notably barley, including the products called Barley Green® and Green

Magma®. Heinerman notes the place for ground-up alfalfa, or alfalfa meal, as an anticancer agent [Heinerman, 1984, p. 155]. This is an item also sold in health food stores, for example, in capsules.)

Heinerman also reviews the work of Dr. Lee W. Wattenberg of the Department of Laboratory Medicine at the University of Minnesota Medical School in Minneapolis. Dr. Wattenberg provided evidence that selenium-containing diets inhibited cancer in both humans and animals. Other inhibitors included creosote oil fractions (from chaparral), thymine (from thyme), and asparagine (from asparagus and other vegetables).

In further work, Dr. Wattenberg found that phenethyl isothiocyanate and benzyl isothiocyanate added to the feed of mice inhibited chemically induced intestinal and mammary cancers. The cruciferous vegetables cabbage, brussels sprouts, cauliflower, kale, and turnips (of the mustard family, or family Cruciferae, or family Brassicaceae) contain phenethyl isothiocyanate. Watercress, another example, contains benzyl isothiocyanate.

(The prefix "thio-" implies sulfur in the molecular structure. Cyanates are compounds derived from cyanic acid [HOCN]. There is a strong similarity with cyanides, as derived from hydrogen cyanide [HCN]. These would seem to be a parallel here with laetrile, or amygdalin, as used in cancer treatment.)

Indoles are another type of compound encountered in cruciferous vegetables, indole itself having the chemical formula $C_8H_7N$ (indoles may also be formed from the putrefaction of proteins). Note the presence of bound nitrogen in these and other anticancer substances. It was commented that the liver was a vital link, with cancer-inhibiting actions occurring there.

Ground-up alfalfa, or alfalfa meal, was found to be another anticancer agent, particularly for the liver. (It may be commented that capsules containing powdered alfalfa have long been on the market in health food stores.)

Dr. Heinerman furnishes still other evidence about the advantages of a vegetarian diet, such as the fact that cruciferous vegetables reduce the incidence of colon and rectum cancers. At the same time it is cautioned that some other factors may play a part, such as a deficiency in mineral uptake by the body.

A section is devoted to laetrile, which occurs widely in nature, especially in wild fruits. Legumes also contain appreciable quantities, especially in sprouted mung beans and lentils (refer also to the work of Dr. Lai, described earlier in this chapter.) Domesticated fruits, however, have been genetically changed to get rid of the wild, bitter taste, and accordingly are deficient in laetrile. The same goes for corn. This may be one reason why people who subsist on wild fruits and vegetables tend to remain cancerfree.

The chapter is concluded with the compelling story of a Dr. Anthony Sattilaro, who cured himself of a virulent cancer by going on a vegetarian, macrobiotic diet.

Heinerman's penultimate chapter is titled "Traditional and Clinical Therapies for the Treatment of Cancer." It is divided into sections on "Vitamin-Mineral Therapy," "Laetrile," "Hoxsey Therapy," "The Kelley Method," "The Gerson Therapy," 'Essiac," "Comfrey," and "Chaparral." These subjects are also covered in the several other books cited herein, such as Walters (1993), Moss (1992), and Pelton and

Overholser (1994). Some of the more noteworthy or intriguing aspects of Heinerman's accounts will now be described.

Heinerman is a proponent of folic acid and vitamin A from natural sources, vitamin C, selenium, vitamin E, and zinc.

Laetrile has already been covered earlier in this chapter, and we reiterate that consuming laetrile with such foods as nuts, bean and alfalfa sprouts, fresh fruits (peaches), and uncooked lettuce, celery, and mushrooms may lead to cyanide poisoning.

Otherwise, laetrile is regarded as nontoxic, but it should be used with vitamins A and C to be effective. Among those who have researched laetrile is Dr. Harold W. Manner, head of the Department of Biology at Loyola University in Chicago. He observes that laetrile contains cyanide, but so do lima beans, lentil beans, buckwheat, and many other food products. In fact, vitamin B12 is loaded with cyanide. If part of a chemical complex, however, it is not toxic as such.

Hoxsey Therapy discovery dates back to 1840, when Harry Hoxsey's grandfather experimented on a horse, trying various herbs growing around the farm. The compositions have been provided in Chapter 6.

The Kelley method emphasizes coffee enemas and eating almonds. Otherwise it is similar to the Gerson Therapy. A feature of the Gerson Therapy is the use of cleansing formulas. A number of recipes are furnished, though other formulations are available in most health food stores. Mention is made again of the Chinese herb Tangkuei or Dongguei (*Angelica sinensis*) as an anticancer agent, in addition to its other uses. It is combined with other herbs, for which a particular recipe is provided.

Details of the Essiac tea phenomenon are provided, that is, of the career of Renée Caisse. It is stated that the Essiac formula contains six herbs (Heinerman, 1984, p. 198), whereas some other formulations contain only four, as previously described.

In 1896, in Great Britain, comfrey received some publicity as an anticancer agent. A facial tumor was removed by using a poultice of fresh comfrey. Other successes have since been reported, including by taking comfrey as a drink, tea, or salad, or even by using the root in a pudding. (As has been mentioned, in the preliminaries of his book *Healing Animals with Herbs*, Dr. John Heinerman reported the case of a sheep cured of mouth cancer by eating comfrey. Comfrey contains toxic pyrrolizidine alkaloids, however, as also previously noted.) Two formulations of herbal combinations are provided, one for detoxifying drug addictions and the other for cancer. The former uses comfrey root, mullein leaves, spearmint, blackberry root, chickweed, grapevine bark, rosehips, goldenseal, and myrrh. The latter uses comfrey root, leaves, blossoms, red clover, myrrh, yucca, chaparral, wormwood, goldenseal, licorice, and clay or dolomite.

Nor does comfrey (*Symphylum officinale*, family Boraginaceae) receive many accolades from Foster and Johnson (2006). It is noted, however, to contain two primary positive therapeutic constituents: allantoin and rosmarinic acid. Allantoin causes cells to multiply and thereby aids the regeneration of damaged tissues, as in wounds, burns, and sores, and is thus a fairly common ingredient in ointments for skin problems. Rosmarinic acid is an anti-inflammatory agent, and is found in the herb rosemary and in members of the mint family.

Nevertheless, Foster and Johnson emphasize that comfrey also contains toxic pyrrolizidine alkaloids (PAs), as documented in Chapter 6. Although PAs will help stop bleeding, the negative effects outweigh the beneficial, for comfrey has been found to cause liver damage and produce cancerous liver tumors. Despite its long history in herbal medicine, no clinical studies have documented any positive effects attributable to comfrey. Many studies, however, have demonstrated its liver toxicity.

As for rue (*Ruta graveolens*, family Rutaceae), no mention of it is made in the Foster and Johnson reference. As has been noted in Chapter 1, it is loaded with toxic alkaloids, although it is said to have been used by the Papago Indians as a cure against rabies.

A select listing of anticancer plants from around the world is furnished in Table 7.2, derived from Foster and Johnson (2006).

More information is provided about using comfrey in Mark Bricklin's *The Practical Encyclopedia of Natural Healing*, based on work by an English Physician, Charles J. Macalister, M.D., who wrote a book about it, published in 1936 (Bricklin, 1976, pp. 230–235). The most important active ingredient is called allantoin. (As previously emphasized, comfrey also contains toxic pyrrolizidine alkaloids.) Bricklin also supplies information about other herbs, experiences, and uses, including garlic, camomile, peppermint, cayenne, sage, horseradish, catnip, rosemary, and coltsfoot. He advises against using such dangerous herbs or plants as jimsonweed, daffodils, spurge, arnica, wormwood, mandrake, hellebore, squill, poison hemlock (which looks like parsley), tobacco (internally), tonka beans, aconite, white bryony, nux vomica, calabar bean, camphor (internally), ergot, ignatius beans, bittersweet, gelsium, henbane, celandine (externally), belladonna (deadly nightshade), foxglove (source of digitalis), and mayflower. Presumably safe in small amounts are tansy, rue, valerian, lobelia, goldenseal, and bloodroot. Pregnant women should not take pennyroyal.

A short section written by James Duke is presented with the titled "'Quack' Salad and Cancer" (Bricklin, 1976, pp. 249, 250). Based on folklore as per Jonathan Hartwell's findings, and for those who might like to live dangerously, the list consists of absinthe, arnica, atriplex, beet, black walnut, borage, calendula, celery, chicory, chive, chufa, colocynth, crimson clover, crown vetch, cucumber, cumin, flax, garlic, hot pepper, licorice, onion, peanut, poke salad, safflower, salvia, tamarind, tansy, tea, and tomato. No curative claims are made, but over half are said to have compounds that have been useful in cancer treatments.

There is conflicting evidence about chaparral, in particular as per the University of Utah Medical Center. The case of Ernest Farr, who healed himself of melanoma by drinking Chaparral tea, is repeated. Perhaps of special interest is the PDR Cancer Formula developed by F. Joseph Montagna of Portland, Oregon (Heinerman, 1984, pp. 206–207). It contained the following ingredients: Chaparral leaves, bloodroot, red clover blossoms, burdock root, echinacae root, goldenseal root, comfrey leaves, ginseng root, and greater celandine, plus poke, parsley, blue violet leaves, licorice, dandelion root, cayenne, prickly ash, garlic, cleavers, gotu kola, periwinkle, sassafras, agrimony, and ground ivy; in other words, about every herb that has ever been labeled an anticancer agent. The materials were pressed into tablets, to be taken several to many times a day, depending on the severity. (The citation given was

## TABLE 7.2
## Selected Anticancer Plants from Around the World (Adapted from Foster and Johnson, 2006)

| Name | Method of Use |
|---|---|
| Aloe (*Aloe vera* or *Aloe. barbadensis,* family Asphodelaceae) | Leaf extracts exhibit some anticancer properties, but more research is needed. |
| American ginseng *(Panax quinquefolius,* family Araliaceae) | Root inhibits the growth of cancer *in vitro.* Helps treat attention deficit/hyperactivity disorder (ADHD) in children. Most work so far has been done on Asian ginseng. |
| Ashwagandha (*Withania somnifera,* family Solanaceae) | An evergreen shrub of Africa, the Middle East, and India, whose roots, seeds, and leaves have been a part of Ayurvedic medicine in India for thousands of years, for varied ailments. *In vitro* studies show that ashwagandha inhibits the growth of cancers of the breast, central nervous system, lung, and colon. |
| Astragalus (*Astragalus membranaceus,* family Fabaceae) | Stimulates immune system of cancer patients. In Chinese medicine, *huang qi.* |
| Autumn crocus (*Colchicum autumnale,* family Liliaceae) | Corms and seeds are a source for the alkaloid colchicine, which inhibits cell division, that is, cancer. The side effects are severe, negating its use against cancer, although it is sometimes used against gout. Also called naked lady, autumn saffron. |
| Bethroot (*Trillium erectum,* family Liliaceae) | Rhizomes (underground stems) used by Native American tribes against cancerous tumors. |
| Bilberry (*Vaccinium myrtillus,* family Ericaceae) | A native of Europe whose fruits and leaves contain the flavonoids called *anthocyanosides.* These are described as powerful antioxidants that act to scavenge free radicals. Extracts have been found to inhibit the growth of certain kinds of cancers. Also known as *whortleberry, huckleberry, European blueberry.* |
| Bitterleaf (*Vernonia amygdalina,* family Asteraceae) | Native to the more southern parts of Africa, its extracts show powerful antiparasitic, antibacterial, and anticancer properties. It has significant antimalarial activity against the parasite *Plasmodium berghi.* DNA synthesis has been found to be inhibited in breast cancer cells. |
| Bloodroot (*Sanguinaria canadensis,* family Papaveraceae) | Rhizome (underground stem) used by Native Americans against skin tumors and cancerous sores. Rich in alkaloids, known to induce mutations in DNA. Prolonged use in oral hygiene products may be potentially harmful. |
| Cascara sagrada (*Frangula purshiana* or *Rhamnus purshiana,* family Rhamnaceae) | A plant of the Pacific Northwest, used by Native Americans as a laxative. An active ingredient of the bark, emodin, may have anticancer properties. Also called *California buckthorn.* |
| Castor bean (*Ricinus communis,* family Euphorbiaceae) | Native to eastern and far western Africa, its seeds contain the deadly poisons, ricinine and especially ricin. Current research involves attempts to attach ricin molecules to antibodies that in turn bind to cancer cells, thus destroying the cells. (Medicinal castor oil undergoes a detoxifying process to eliminate the poisonous components.) |

**TABLE 7.2 (CONTINUED)**
**Selected Anticancer Plants from Around the World (Adapted from Foster and Johnson, 2006)**

| Name | Method of Use |
|---|---|
| Cat's claw (*Uncaria tomentosa* and *U. guianensis*, family Rubiaceae) | Bark and roots used against cancer in Peruvian Amazon. Also called *una de gato*. |
| Chaparral (*Larrea tridentata*, family Zygophyllaceae) | A native of the American Southwest, and a traditional medicine of Native Americans, a tea made from the leaves and twigs contains the lignan named nordihydoiguaiaretic acid (NDGA). Considered the active ingredient, it has powerful antioxidant properties. The leaf extract of a South American subspecies was in fact found to inhibit cancer growth. In any event, there are reports of liver damage from its use. Definitive human clinical trials await. |
| Chinese rhubarb (*Rheum palmatum*, family Polygonaceae) | The extract, emodin, inhibits cancer cells in mice. Also called *turkey rhubarb*. In Chinese medicine, *da-huang*. |
| Chocolate (*Theobroma cacao*, family Sterculiaceae) | Native to northeast South America, and cultivated worldwide, the seeds contain numerous chemical compounds, the most prominent being the alkaloids caffeine and theobromine. Serving as an antioxidant, there is the possibility of preventing or delaying such degenerative diseases as cancer. |
| Echinacea (*Echinacea purpurea, E. pallida, E. angustifolia*, family Asteraceae) | Used against certain types of cancer; used by the Sioux against rabies. Also called purple coneflower. |
| Elecampane (*Inula helenium*, family Asteraceae) | Used in Chinese medicine against cancer. (It has also been cited elsewhere as a folklore remedy against rabies.) |
| European elder (*Sambucus nigra*, family Caprifoliaceae) | A native of Europe and the northwest coast of Africa, various flavonoids and triterpenes are the most active ingredients. Strong immune stimulating properties signal the treatment of cancer patients with weak immune systems. Studies show a capability to neutralize the West Nile virus. Also called elderberry. |
| European mistletoe (*Viscum album*, family Viscadeae) | Used in supportive treatment of cancer. Stimulates immune system to kill cancer cells. |
| Flax (*Linum usitatissimum*, family Linaceae) | Seed and oil used against colon, breast, and prostate cancers. Also called flaxseed and linseed. |
| Garlic (*Allium sativum*, family Liliaceae) | Originally from central Asia, the bulbs contain allicin, exhibiting antibiotic, antiviral, and antifungal properties, and are said to reduce the risk of certain cancers. |
| Goldenseal (*Hydrastis canadensis*, family Ranunculaceae) | Rhizome (underground stem) and roots used by Native Americans as a cancer treatment. Contains the alkaloids berberine and hydrastine, as used in Chinese medicine against diarrhea. Found to be toxic against cancer cells, fungal cells, and a wide range of bacteria, including *Staphylococcus*. |

## TABLE 7.2 (CONTINUED)
## Selected Anticancer Plants from Around the World (Adapted from Foster and Johnson, 2006)

| Name | Method of Use |
|---|---|
| Gotu kola (*Centella asiatica*, family Apiaceae) | A native of India and southeast Asia, it was traditionally used in Ayurvedic medicine. The most active ingredients are various triterpenoids that affect cells and tissues. In both laboratory and animal studies gotu kola extracts have shown anticancer effects. In Chinese medicine, *luei gong gen*. |
| Happy tree (*Camptotheca acuminata*, family Nyssaceae) | Contains camptothecin, a powerful and toxic anticancer agent. Source for Taxol. In Chinese medicine, *xi-shu*, tree of joy, cancer tree. |
| Hemp (*Cannabis sativa*, family Cannabaceae) | Native to Central Asia, the flowering tops, berries contain flavonoids, tannins, a bitter compound called juniperin, and volatile oil. Leaves, and seeds are biochemically active. An ointment made from the seed was a folk remedy for cancerous ulcers, and a decoction of the root was thought to heal hard tumors. The active narcotic ingredients are tetrahydrocannabinol (THC), cannabinol, and cannabidiol. Also known as *Indian hemp, marijuana, hashish.* |
| Herb-Robert (*Geranium robertianum*, family Geraniaceae) | A bitter, astringent, and fetid smelling native of Europe and Asia, herb-Robert has spread into North and South America, and is considered a folk cancer remedy. Preparations are applied externally to tumors and ulcers. Freshly picked and crushed leaves, when rubbed upon the skin, are said to repel mosquitoes. Fresh extracts are active against vesicular stomatitis virus (VSV), which is in the same family as the rabies virus. Antibacterial effects also occur. |
| Juniper (*Juniperus communis*, family Cupressaceae) | This evergreen conifer is native to the northern temperate regions of Europe, Asia, and North America; and is also cultivated. In Western folk medicine, among other uses, the berries were considered active against certain types of cancer. The berries contain flavonoids, tannins, a bitter compound called *juniperin*, and a volatile oil of myriad constituents. In addition to the berries being anti-inflammatory, there is antiviral activity. |
| Kelp (*Laminaria digitata* and related species, family Laminariaceae) | The native range is along the North Atlantic shoreline, with the blade considered a source of nutritional iodine. There may be weak anticancer effects; however, long usage may have adverse effects on iron, sodium, and potassium absorption. |
| Madagascar periwinkle (*Catharanthus roseus*, family Apocynaceae) | Alkaloids vincristine and vinblastine used successfully against lymphoma and leukemia, and Hodgkin's disease. |

**TABLE 7.2 (CONTINUED)**
**Selected Anticancer Plants from Around the World (Adapted from Foster and Johnson, 2006)**

| Name | Method of Use |
|---|---|
| Maté (*Ilex paraguariensis*, family Aquifoliaceae) | A native medium-sized evergreen tree found along streams throughout South America: in Argentina, Chile, Peru, Brazil, Paraguay, and Uruguay, where it is cultivated. Used widely as a caffeinated medicinal beverage for various ailments, its use may slightly increase the chances of contracting cancer. |
| Mayapple (*Podophyllum peltatum*, family Berberidaceae) | Rhizome (underground stem) used by Native Americans against certain types of cancer. Contains the resin podophyllin, composed of several toxic glycosides, notably podophyllotoxin, and which is active against benign skin tumors such as warts. Two derivatives, etoposide and teniposide, kill cells undergoing division, namely cancer cells. Used variously against testicular cancer, small-cell lung cancer, Kaposi's sarcoma, lymphomas, and malignant melanomas. Also called American mandrake, hog apple. |
| Myrrh (*Commiphora myrrha*, family Burseraceae) | An aromatic shrub or small tree native to northeastern Africa, it has a long history as a healing and rejuvenating herb, e.g., in Ayurvedic medicine. The oleo-gum-resin produced contains terpenes that have been shown *in vivo* to inhibit certain solid-tumor cancers. In Chinese medicine, *mo yao shu*, *mo yao*. |
| Noni (*Morinda citrifolia*, family Rubiaceae) | Various parts used against cancer, but toxicity significant. An evergreen of the pacific islands, Polynesia, Australia, it is also called Indian mulberry, hog apple. |
| Pacific yew (*Taxus brevifolia*, family Taxaceae) | A small evergreen of the Pacific Northwest whose bark is the source for paclitaxel, which has remarkable anticancer properties, notably against ovarian and breast cancers. |
| Pau d'arco (*Tabebuia impetiginosa*, family Bignoniaceae) | Used by Brazilian tribes against cancer. Small doses stimulate immune system, high doses suppress it. |
| Red cinchona (*Cinchona officinalis*, family Rubiaceae) | Used by Amazon tribes against cancer. Also called quinine, Peruvian bark, Jesuit's bark. Has been the remedy of choice for malaria, now making a comeback with the emergence of strains resistant to synthetic drugs. |
| Red clover (*Trifolium pratense*, family Fabaceae) | Used against cancerous ulcers, and against benign prostate hyperplasia (BPH). A component of Harry M. Hoxsey's Red Clover Tonic. The authors review the past controversies, and add the following. "Subsequently, isolated studies have begun to demonstrate some cancer-fighting properties for ingredients in his tonic. Research continues." |

## TABLE 7.2 (CONTINUED)
## Selected Anticancer Plants from Around the World (Adapted from Foster and Johnson, 2006)

| Name | Method of Use |
|---|---|
| Rosemary (*Rosmarinus officinalis*, family Lamiaceae) | A low evergreen shrub native to the coast of the Mediterranean. The leaves contain rosmarinic acid — also found in the mint family, which has antiviral, antibacterial, anti-inflammatory, and antioxidant properties. A dilute extract fed to laboratory animals resulted in nearly a 50% decrease in experimentally induced mammary gland tumors, and the same for colon and lung cancers. |
| Slippery elm (*Ulmus rubra* or *U. fulva*, family Ulmaceae) | Inner bark and ingredient in two widely used cancer treatments, Flor-Essence and Essiac. |
| Thuja (*Thuja occidentalis*, family Cupressaceae) | Young leafy twigs used against some types of cancer. Commonly removes warts. Known as an abortifacient. Also called eastern arborvitae, eastern white cedar, northern white cedar, swamp cedar, tree of life. |
| Yellow dock (*Rumex crispus*, family Polygonaceae) | Native to Europe and Africa, it has spread all over, and the root contains anthroquinones and glycosides, along with various tannins and oxalates, which can be poisonous. It was used in the 1930s as a component of the herbal remedy Essiac, or Essiac tea, but was discounted by medical orthodoxy. Then, in 2004, a mixture of Essiac herbs was shown to inhibit the growth of prostate cancer cells *in vitro*. Subsequent animal studies showed antioxidant, anti-inflammatory, and anticancer activity, but further research is needed. |
| Yellow jasmine (*Gelsemium sempervirens*, family Loganiaceae) | A native wildflower of the southeastern U.S., its medicinal properties were not noted until the mid-1800s, when it was discovered by chance. Its purported beneficial actions were many and varied, including cancer-fighting properties and as a remedy for certain kinds of cancerous tumors. The report of the discovery concerns a Mississippi planter suffering a severe fever, who was fed the rhizomes by mistake. First showing signs of *Gelsemium* poisoning, these effects gradually wore off, and the planter was cured of his fever. Subsequently, *Gelsemium* remedies became popular with what was called the Eclectic school of medicine, which practiced both homeopathic and conventional treatments. Other names are Carolina jasmine, wild woodbine. |

*Source:* Adapted from Foster, S. and Johnson, R.L., *Desk Reference to Nature's Medicine*, National Geographic Society, Washington, D.C., 2006.

F. Joseph Montagna, *PDR Traditional Herbal Formulas*; Portland, Oregon, 1980; Vol. I, p. 39.) Successes were reported and testimonials given. But Mr. Montagna got into trouble by declaring that his remedy was a cancer-cure formula. He was prosecuted and put out of business. He should have been more circumspect and worked within the system. In other words, he should have promoted his formula, say, as nutritional herb supplements.

In a later book, *Double the Power of Your Immune System*, published in 1991, in a section on cancer, Heinerman lists several herbs that help fight cancer. In addition to chaparral, there is goldenseal, pau d'arco, red beets, and garlic. Also mentioned are chlorophyll, diet, and the power of the mind (i.e., attitude). It may be noted that in addition to chaparral and garlic, previously referenced, the three remaining herbs all appear in Hartwell's compilation. Goldenseal (*Hydrastis canadensis*) is listed under both the family Berberidaceae and the family Ranunculaceae. Pau d'arco (of the genus *Tabebuia*) is in the family Bignoniaceae. The inner bark is used, with the name Lapacho appearing on the commercially sold product. The red beet (*Beta vulgaris*) is in the family Chenopodiaceae.

(Heinerman, in emphasizing the role of diet, mentioned in particular a clinic in Tijuana, Mexico, called the East/West Wellness Center, which used nutritional chemotherapy against cancer.)

Heinerman's *The Healing Benefits of Garlic*, published in 1994 and previously cited, contains a section on cancer, where the emphasis is on prevention. Restated, in addition to containing the element germanium or its compounds, which acts as an anticancer agent, garlic is a sulfur-rich vegetable, a class known to be anticarcinogenic. The antiseptic properties of garlic have long been known, and it has been used to combat such infectious or degenerative diseases as leprosy, meningitis, multiple sclerosis, polio, tuberculosis, whooping cough, bronchitis, and even asthma (Heinerman, 1993, pp. 106–112). The Greek philosopher Aristotle wrote about garlic being a cure for hydrophobia, but as with other herbal treatments for this dreaded disease, most, or all, modern victims will no doubt opt for the surety of the Pasteur treatment whenever possible.

Even lowly castor oil (from *Ricinus communis*) gets into the act, being also listed in Hartwell under the family Euphorbiaceae, as does peanut oil (from the species *Arachis hypogaea* of the family Leguminosae), although as a treatment for plantar warts. Peanuts, however, host fungi of the genus *Aspergillus*, which produce aflatoxin, a known carcinogen, and the government keeps an eye on the levels in the peanut crop. (It is possible that roasting the peanuts may decompose the aflatoxin.)

Some further annotations about indigenous plants are provided in *A Guide to the Medicinal Plants of the United States* by Arnold and Connie Krochmal. The citations are given in page order (Krochmal, 1973, pp. 4, 42, 63, 173, 185, 200). These citations include the common pokeweed (*Phytolacca americana*), whose fruit has been found to inhibit in some way or another the division of body cells, which is the basic prerequisite in treating cancers and tumors. Also the root and seeds of great burdock (*Arctium lappa*), the root bark of bittersweet (*Celastrus scandens*), the rootstock of common mayapple (*Podophyllum peltatum*), the bark and branches of Gambel's oak (*Quercus gambelii*) for skin cancer, and the roots of the well-known bloodroot (*Sanguinaria canadensis*), although bloodroot is considered poisonous, though not markedly so. Also, there are several other plants called bloodroot.

A region of the New World, and therefore closer to home, is that area called Neo Tropica, lying between the Tropic of Cancer and the Tropic of Capricorn, which includes the rain forests of Amazonia and Central America. A short description of investigations that have been under way is presented in Chapter 3, Section 3.3 and in Appendix N of Hoffman (1999). It can be described as under intensive investigation, although racing against decimation, and will be further reported on in a subsequent section.

The extensive investigations undertaken in these fecund tropical rain forests, and the meager results so far, illustrate the difficulties in pinning down a cure for cancer from tropical plants, or any plants, as most that is known is from native folklore or hearsay. You are never quite sure which plant species is supposed to do exactly what, if anything; and you are not even sure about which species is which. If an active chemical component perchance is found, it is probably just one of tens or maybe hundreds or thousands in the same species, which may act together synergistically, for the complexity of nature is infinite. Large-scale, controlled impartial clinical studies are lacking, the subject being beyond mainstream medicine, and there is a lack of other possibilities.

This provides a place to start, however, assuming a degree of discernment. And the problem will no doubt remain, as always, of why may the medicine work for some patients some of the time, and not for others at other times? The resolution of this dilemma may lead to a cure for cancer.

Along these lines, a special feature appeared in the *Tulsa World*, September 24, 1995, titled "Wonder Drug? Maybe, Maybe Not." Written by Lou Ann Ruark, it describes the search of a certain W.H. Meade in the thickets west of Bartlesville, OK, north of Tulsa, for a medicinal plant that might cure a fungus that had been on his hand for many years. Meade, then living in Claremore, Oklahoma, would collect plant specimens, make an extract, and try it out, meantime keeping a sample specimen for his records.

After about 20 years of searching, Meade met with success. He refused to further identify the plant, but passed out free samples of the brownish, viscous fluid obtained. "Skin cancers of every type go into remission, rashes disappear as does psoriasis, black moles, the raised, blackened welts caused by childhood strep infections; also tick, mosquito and other insect bites and stings." Meade was given encouragement by some in the local medical community, with the opinion that perhaps 98% of all plants have not yet been checked out for medicinal properties. Karen McMahon, a biological science professor at the nearby University of Tulsa and coauthor of a botany textbook, noted that most plants have not yet been "identified" by science, and the quest continues for new medicinal plants, which "contain chemicals no scientist could dream up." Inasmuch as a plant cannot be patented, about all Meade could do at this time was give samples away.

(It may be mentioned that species of the genus *Asclepias* or milkweed are known to act against warts and the like.)

It can be asked, furthermore, if plants and herbs and nutrition are so successful in some cancer cases, nowadays, or in even some few cancer cases, why are they not successful in all cancer cases? Why has Jonathan L. Hartwell been able to come up with so many plants that are or were perceived as anticancer agents in his literature survey *Plants Used Against Cancer* (1982)? Judging from the number of plants, it would even seem that most of the more common plants have at one time or another been used against cancer, dating back to the ancients. (Though this would be a gross exaggeration, based on the total number of plant species worldwide. Nevertheless, the approximately 3000 plant species listed in his survey as being anticancer is a considerable number.) The medical folklore is impressive, by any measure.

The action of these plant remedies mostly remains mysterious. Why do so many different plant species act against cancer or cancers? Do they in fact act in a common way, or in diverse ways? One obvious conjecture at least is that they somehow trigger an immune response. That is, being bioactive means that they may be called "poisonous" to a degree. That is to say, in our terminology here, "bioactive" and "poisonous" more or less imply the same thing. We could as well use the term "foreign" substance. And by bioactive or poisonous or foreign is also meant that their intake causes adverse reactions in the body, or in another way of saying it, triggers the immune system. In a way of speaking then, all these terms imply more or less the same thing. The body counterattacks the attackers, the (mildly) poisonous or foreign substances being administered in limited fashion. And in doing so, the body itself, activated and with enhanced capability, goes on the offensive with renewed vigor, to counter the cancerous condition at the same time.

Inasmuch as we are here talking of bioactive (or poisonous) plants, we are also talking of only administering small or minute or micro amounts, at least internally. This is the particular expertise of homeopathy, that practice of administering minute amounts of medicinal substances to stimulate the body's protective natural immune system.

(The extension is to the introduction of microorganisms and their toxins to stimulate the immune system as per Coley's Toxins. From there, the extrapolation is to the use of vaccines or serums, as per the Pasteur treatment for rabies. The ultimate goal is preventive inoculation, as for polio.)

We can further ask, were human beings somehow constituted differently in times past? Were their immune systems more active and more responsive to outside stimuli, say from the plant remedies administered? And were the plants themselves, back then, more biologically active?

Has in fact the pervasive use of antibiotics somehow weakened the natural immune system of humans? Have environmental changes (degradations) also changed the human animal, also promoting cancer? And has the vigor of the soil been sapped and compromised by the use of myriad agricultural chemicals, from inorganic fertilizers to pesticides and herbicides? And have genetic changes been incurred along the way, both in the human animal and in plants?

Add to this the fact that we are all biologically and biochemically different — a condition that has been observed and written about by noted biochemist Roger J. Williams, and we can be expected to respond differently to stimuli. It can be expected, furthermore, that the power of the immune system will vary from one individual to another. The solution, therefore, could be to make the necessary adjustments in treatment such that each individual can be made impervious to cancer, both before and after the fact.

No doubt some of the herbal and other remedies are fraudulent, a sales pitch no less. But the same can be said for conventional medicine; no cures are guaranteed. Always it seems, some treatments work for some people some of the time, and at other times they do not. (This scenario is further complicated by con artists and wishful thinking, this being reason enough, apparently, for such monitoring organizations as Quackbusters — but, of course, who monitors the monitors?)

The conventional wisdom is that conventional medicine is somehow more scientific. But to be called science, in the strictest sense, the experiments must be repeatable and the data reproducible. On a given individual, this becomes impossible, as the precise initial conditions can never be reestablished. Only a collection or sampling of individuals can be so tested, with the anticipation that a pattern will emerge. Hopefully, a cure will become evident, which works for most people most of the time. Less than perfect, and not science in the strict sense of the word, it will probably be as close as we can get. On the other hand, this does not prevent us from seeking absolute cures as an ideal; cures, preferably by inoculation and immunization, and that work for everyone, every time.

## STILL OTHER OPTIONS

We have mainly been talking about organic materials, but there is also an array of inorganics to consider, as described further by Moss (1992). Thus, under the category "Minerals," Moss's book has chapters with the headings "Calcium," "Cesium and Rubidium," "Germanium," "Lithium," "Magnesium," "Molybdenum," "Selenium," "Tellurium," and "Zinc." A variety of organic chemicals and such other inorganics as hydrazine sulfate and urea are also discussed, though the latter is generally classified as an organic as it contains carbon. (Urea is synthesized from carbon dioxide [$CO_2$], and nitrogen [$NH_3$], both of which are considered inorganic compounds.)

(One of the early proponents of the notion that mineral deficiencies or excesses influenced cancer were J.I. Rodale and others of *Prevention Magazine*, described in their *The Complete Book of Minerals for Health*, published in 1972. Thus, magnesium deficiencies were prominently mentioned [Rodale et al., 1972, pp. 118, 119, 488, 679], as were problems with iron, salt and iodized salt, fluoridation, and aluminum [Rodale et al., 1972, pp. 163, 334, 335, 348, 360, 394]. In addition to describing the pronounced beneficial effect of eating dried beef liver on stamina, the part played by liver desiccation in cancer was also explored, based on the work of Dr. Sugiura and others, including Bosshardt et al. of the pharmaceutical company Sharp and Dohme [Rodale et al., 1972, pp. 696–698]. An update to the reference is *Prevention Magazine's Complete Book of Vitamins and Minerals*.)

The use of selenium compounds, for instance, is a feature of the Revici Therapy (Moss, 1992, pp. 112, 113; Walters, 1993, p. 45). The Revici Therapy can in a way be regarded as a form of immunotherapy, and can thus be included under the corresponding heading.

Urine has been used as a medicine from ancient times, and from it are derived some of today's useful drugs, including the antineoplastons used in Burzynski's method of cancer treatment (Moss, 1992, p. 361). The principal chemical in urine aside from water is urea. And urea has apparently been used successfully as a cancer treatment, notably by the localized injection of an aqueous urea solution.

A newer development is the use of urea in a mixture, called "Carbatine®," containing urea and creatine (Moss, 1992, p. 372). For the record, creatine is (α-methylguanido) acetic acid, with the chemical or molecular formula $NH_2C(:NH)N(CH_3)CH_2CO_2H$. It is an alkaloid or amino acid found in the muscles of vertebrates. The active nitrogen content is apparently greater compared to that of urea alone. Moss supplies the names of doctors who use urea therapy as well as suppliers for the creatine hydrate and Carbatine.

Another category of substances that comes up often in Moss's book is hormones, natural and synthetic. Hormones have a checkered record, however, being both blamed as a cause of cancer, and sometimes used in the treatment of cancer. This appears to be the case for many courses of treatment, which can act either positively or negatively, depending on, among other things, the dosage levels.

There is, however, a recent interest in melatonin as a treatment for cancer. The chief hormone from the pineal gland, it has vital mind–body functions, as described by Michael J. Norden in *Beyond Prozac*. A neurohormone that acts in tandem with its parent, serotonin, it benefits depression and anxiety and has antiaging properties but, interestingly, it is also being tried as a treatment for cancer, apparently with some success. A computer search of Medline for the year 1995 and later, for example, revealed any number of entries under the subject heading *melatonin and cancer*, with much of the work being done overseas. Thus, for instance, it has been found that low melatonin levels correlate with increased cancer occurrence. Also observed is that melatonin levels decrease in the presence of an electromagnetic field. It has been pronounced a strong oncostatic agent (cancer-stabilizing agent), and is therefore said to prevent the initiation and promotion of cancer. It is noted that plants contain melatonin, some having more than others. Melatonin, moreover, can be obtained as a nutritional supplement.

As for Prozac® itself and other antidepressants, they are coming under fire as causing suicides and violence, and the accumulating evidence to this effect is looking more and more convincing. The FDA is also coming under fire for its imprimatur, with the political influence of the pharmaceutical industry casting a shadow over the issue. Colorado's Columbine High School killers are suspected of using anti-depressants. (If cigarette class-action lawsuits were successful, can judgments against alcoholic beverages and pharmaceuticals be far behind? Stay tuned, as long-term end effect and side effects may be, or are, encountered.) Plant-derived antidepressants include St. John's wort, about which reports are inconclusive. A study sometimes cited is that St. John's wort did not fare any better than a placebo. However, well-known botanist James Duke has remarked that neither did the antidepressant Zoloft®, and adds the counter that St John's wort has indeed shown a measure of effectiveness against depression. (Called *copycat drugs*, other brand names of antidepressants include Luvox®, Paxil®, Celexa®, Lexapro®, Effexor®, Wellbutrin®, Serzone®, and Remeron®. What will complicate the issues is if one or another of these drugs should show some unexpected, beneficial effects, such as being an anticancer agent.)

Thus, consider, for instance, ubiquitous aspirin, which is given a chapter in Moss's book. Studies have shown that aspirin intake may reduce colon cancer risk by some 50%. The effect seems to be enhanced by also taking nicotinic acid (niacin), or vitamin B3.

Walters (1993) divides cancer therapies into biologic and pharmacologic therapies, immune therapies, herbal therapies, nutritional therapies, metabolic therapies,
adjunctive treatments, energy medicine, and the mind–body connection.

In the first category, notably, is a chapter on the oft-mentioned Antineoplaston
Therapy, developed by Stanislaw Burzynski, M.D., whose clinic is in Houston. This
treatment, as has been frequently noted, involves a class of compounds known as
*peptides*, and has shown some remarkable successes. The outpatient treatment is
comparatively expensive, though some health insurance companies will cover it
(Walters, 1993, p. 20). In any event, it is much less expensive than surgical fees and
extended hospitalization. Governmental authorities have had an off-and-on relationship with Burzynski's operations, for example, at one time allowing no new patients
but permitting a continuation of the treatments in progress, with more complete
records required. (Burzynski's work was profiled in an article by Molly Glentzer in
the January 1996 issue of *Good Housekeeping*, and has made the TV circuit.)
Incidentally, Burzynski's compounds are referred to as *enzyme inhibitors*, a fact
noted in Chapter 5.

Another advocate of polypeptides or peptides against cancer is Julian Whitaker,
M.D. (1-800-539-8219). His newsletter *Health & Healing*, Summer 2006, describes
several dramatic recoveries: from prostate cancer, breast cancer, brain cancer, and
lung cancer. Due credit is given to Stanislaw Burzynski, M.D.

Not to be overlooked is vitamin C, as previously described, and  the work of
Cameron and Pauling (1993), and of Hoffer (2000). Separate chapters are contained
in both Moss (1992) and Pelton and Overholser (1994). The controversy over the
Mayo Clinic studies is reviewed objectively, and it is stressed that vitamin C works
only if the immune system has not been damaged by chemotherapy. Moreover, there
is said to be a rebound effect with vitamin C, whereby a sudden stoppage severely
depletes the blood serum levels. The patient should be taken off slowly.

(It may be again added that attention was called to vitamin C deficiencies and
cancer in *The Complete Book of Vitamins*, by J.I. Rodale et al., published in 1966,
as were vitamin B deficiencies, and mention was made of the Gerson diet in the
treatment of cancer, and the importance of the liver [Rodale et al., 1966, pp.
450–509]. An update to the reference is *Prevention Magazine's Complete Book of
Vitamins and Minerals*, cited elsewhere.)

By megadoses of vitamin C is ordinarily meant, say, 25 or 30 g a day. Taken
orally, even this gets to be a chore, and instead of vitamin C as ascorbic acid, the
sodium or calcium salts may have to be used. (Sodium intake should be restricted,
however, as it causes some undesirable side effects, even producing tumor growth
instead of remission.) But here, this is only the starting point. For the dosage levels
are to be increased by increments on successive days until about 150 g per day are
used. This means that IV injection will be required. Furthermore, the services of a
medical practitioner will also be necessary, which complicates matters, even if one
can be found who will go along with this unconventional treatment, and hospitalization. It may be added that this kind of massive vitamin C therapy has also been
tried for AIDS patients, reportedly with some degree of success or life prolongation.

Massive intravenous vitamin C therapy can be regarded as a form of chelation
therapy — the term *chelation* signifying the formation of a chemical complex or

loose chemical compound. Walters, in fact, has a chapter on chelation, which includes information about using vitamin C in megadoses from 20 to 100 g per IV bottle (Walters, 1993, p. 256). Ordinarily, chelation therapy is directed more at removing the plaquelike deposits layered down inside the blood vessel walls, thereby correcting arteriosclerosis, or hardening of the arteries. In consequence, it is said to reduce the possibility of a heart attack and stroke, lower blood pressure, and relieve angina. It has been quoted as being substantially more effective and infinitely less dangerous than heart bypass surgery. The chelating agent used is a synthetic amino acid called ethylenediaminetetraacetic acid (EDTA), which is administered by intravenous drip.

In addition to the plaquelike deposits, the chelating agent also ties up toxic metals such as iron, copper, and lead that may be present, and which can then be removed from the body blood system via the kidneys. This removal also aids cancer inhibition, by minimizing the formation of free radicals from the reaction of these metals with oxygen in the blood. Moreover, Walters notes that chelation therapy has shown some positive effects for such other ailments as Alzheimer's disease, diabetes, emphysema, arthritis, osteoporosis, Parkinson's disease, kidney diseases, and gangrene.

Returning to intravenous vitamin C, the vitamin C may be introduced along with such other vitamins and minerals as vitamin B, zinc, and selenium. It is claimed that vitamin C reacts with copper in the blood to generate hydrogen peroxide, which destroys cancer cells by oxidation. Not everyone is convinced that chelation is as helpful in cancer as claimed, for it may in fact stimulate further cancer growth, as well as remove valuable minerals from the body, and may have other harmful side effects such as overloading the kidneys (Walters, 1993, p. 256). A lengthy study in Switzerland was favorable, however, though there is the opinion that chelation therapy is more for cancer prevention than treatment (*Alternative Medicine: The Definitive Guide*, p. 130).

Another cure or way advanced to control cancer, especially prostate cancer, is called the *macrobiotic diet*, a part of what is called macrobiotics. The diet is described in chapters in Walters (1993), Moss (1992), and Pelton and Overholser (1994). The principal features are no red meat and, instead, whole grains and vegetables.

(A herbal treatment for prostate problems called *benign prostatic hyperplasia* or *hypertrophy* [BPH] consists of the use of an extract derived from the oil of saw palmetto berries. The saw, or sawtooth, palmetto grows in the West Indies and along the Atlantic Coast of North America from Florida to North Carolina. Its use is an old Indian remedy, picked up by the early settlers.)

Following the chapter on macrobiotics, Walters has a chapter "Moerman's Anti-cancer Diet." The beneficial role of an essentially vegetarian diet is pervasive, though Moerman, for instance, also includes various nutritional supplements.

Oxygen Therapy involves the administration of either ozone or hydrogen peroxide (Walters, 1993, pp. 229–239, Pelton and Overholser, 1994, pp. 111–121). The results seem to be mixed, and undesirable side effects can occur (Walters, 1993, p. 238). Apparently the verdict is still out, though the subject merits a special listing of doctors in the *Alternative Medicine Yellow Pages*. Hyperthermia, the application of heat to cancerous tissue, constitutes the next chapter in Walters' book, with mixed conclusions, and is given a special section in the *Alternative Medicine Yellow Pages*. It may work best with other conventional treatments such as chemotherapy.

An update on oxygen therapy pros and cons involves the aforementioned work of Otto Warburg, which can be interpreted as follows: as cancer cells have such a low respiration rate, they would die off if exposed to higher oxygen levels. A counterargument is that tumors grow rapidly in tissues well supplied with oxygen; and also, conversely, depriving tumors of oxygen will not stimulate their growth.

On the other hand, consider what Dr. Warburg said in a lecture to the German Central Committee on Cancer Control presented at Stuttgart on May 25, 1955, and published in *Naturwissenishaften*, *42*, 401 (1955). It was translated and republished as "On the Origin of Cancer Cells" in *Science*, *123*, 309–314 (1956). "Since the respiration of all cancer cells is damaged, our first question is, How can the respiration of body cells be injured? Of this damage to respiration it can be said at the outset that it must be irreversible, since the respiration of cancer cells never returns to normal ..." (This information is courtesy of University of Georgia physics professor Winfield J. Abbe, in an assessment of Warburg's work.) Thus, it can be surmised that Dr. Warburg never said that fully formed cancer cells would revert to the normal state upon oxygen administration. (Nor did he say that adding oxygen would kill off the cancer cells.)

In turn, Dr. Warburg addressed the latency period for transforming normal cells to abnormal ones, expressed in terms of *sleeping cancer cells* as follows: "Since the increase in fermentation in the development of cancer cells takes place gradually, there must be a transition phase between normal body cells and fully formed cancer cells." The result is that "we may have cancer cells which indeed look like cancer cells but are still energetically insufficient. Such cells, which are clinically not cancer cells, have lately been found not only in the prostate, but also in the lungs, kidney, and stomach of elderly persons."

Additionally, Dr. Warburg made the following statement in 1967: "Because no cancer cell exists, the respiration of which is intact, it cannot be disputed that cancer could be prevented if the respiration of body cells could be kept intact." It was recommended by Dr. Warburg that the bloodstream be well supplied with oxygen, that high levels of hemoglobin be kept in the blood, and that the respiratory enzymes be kept at sufficiently high levels, say via the very foods we eat. It is emphasized that these protocols refer to the prevention of cancer rather than to the reversal of fully developed cancer.

However, it may be questioned as to whether the foregoing discussion may, or may not, pertain to selectively destroying or immolating cancer cells.

About the role of the presence or absence of oxygen in cancer formation, further statements of biochemist Otto Warburg are instructive. In perspective, he at one time was director of the prestigious Max Planck Institute for Cell Physiology, Berlin-Dahlem, Germany. Dr. Warburg won a Nobel Prize in 1931 for his discovery of the oxygen-transforming enzyme of cell respiration, an iron porphyrin derivative. He is also recognized for his discovery of the hydrogen-transforming enzymes, and for his pioneering work in photosynthesis. Here we are concerned with his conclusions about the difference between the behavior of normal cells and cancer cells, in that the former are aerobic and the latter anaerobic. His conclusions are apparently still considered controversial in some quarters, and there is evidently much more involved than is evident at first glance. Nevertheless it is a bold theory, striking in its simplicity, and has provided a point of departure for continued investigations.

Additional information about the career and work of Dr. Warburg is presented in the appropriately titled *Otto Warburg: Cell Physiologist, Biochemist and Eccentric*, by Hans Krebs with Roswatha Schmid.

The following quotation is supplied from a lecture "The Prime Cause and Prevention of Cancer," delivered by Dr. Warburg at the 1966 annual meeting of Nobel laureates at Landau, Germany (Mullins, 1992, p. 351; Krebs, 1981, pp. 24, 25):

> Summarized in a few words, the prime cause of cancer is the replacement of the respiration of oxygen in normal body cells by a fermentation of sugar. All normal body cells meet their energy needs by respiration of oxygen, whereas cancer cells meet their energy needs in great part by fermentation. All normal body cells are thus obligate aerobes, whereas all cancer cells are partial anaerobes.... Oxygen gas, the donor of energy in plants and animals is dethroned in the cancer cells and replaced by an energy yielding reaction of the lowest living forms, namely, a fermentation of glucose.

Mullins commented that this concept has never been followed up by the scientific community.

Additional information about Otto Warburg and his work is detailed in chapters of *The Hidden Story of Cancer: Find Out Why Cancer has Medical Science on the Run and How a Simple Plan Based on New Science Can Prevent It*, by Brian Scott Peskin and Amid Habib, M.D., published in 2006.

In Section 2 of the book, titled "The Cancer Answer," emphasis is on the anticancer action of essential fatty acids (EFAs). The (dietary) sources and proportions of omega-3 and omega-6 EFAs are discussed; these substances serve as "oxygen magnets," enabling the cells to absorb more oxygen from the bloodstream, and thus acting against cancer.

Chapter 12 and Chapter 13 furnish quotes from Dr. Warburg, with commentary and the appendices, and establish with references the foundations for the anticancer protocol or plan established in the book.

This brings to mind all the mainstream talk about antioxidants against cancer, even heart disease, etc. It is a protocol discounted in some quarters. Thus, the question is raised: why should oxygen, which is so vital to normal cell metabolism, be eliminated?

There is the need for independent clinics, which can be referred to as cancer clinical research centers (CCRCs), whereby cancer patients can be treated with alternative therapies of their choice, including omega fatty acids, etc. As has been repeatedly indicated, these centers would be under the supervision of (independent) M.D.s and D.O.s, with backup and support by pharmacologists, etc., even herbalists and naturopaths. Given the present situation in this country, such a program may be feasible only in Mexico or Germany, or elsewhere. However, in this regard, it can be mentioned again that the Riordan clinic in Wichita, Kansas, has had reported successes using vitamin C, as has Abram Hoffer in Vancouver, and Coley's Toxins have been given renewed publicity, in particular by Wayne Martin in the *Townsend*

*Letter for Doctors & Patients* and on the Internet. A problem, unfortunately, is that no statistics are available for successes vs. failures along with the mitigating circumstances.

It is imperative that a near-instantaneous, noninvasive biochemical marker be further developed to monitor cancer growth or remission. In this way it can be definitively established whether a particular treatment is proving effective against the cancer, and if not, another treatment protocol can be started.

Work on hydrazine sulfate by Joseph Gold, M.D., of the Syracuse Cancer Research Institute, Syracuse, New York, is said to be based on the "Warburg effect" (Moss, 1992, p. 316). The theory is that hydrazine sulfate cuts off the supplies of new glucose in the liver and thus starves the cancer and stops cachexia, the wasting away that accompanies cancer.

It has been noted that cancer cells use sugar in 10 to 15 times the amounts used by normal cells (Walters, 1993, p. 50), which is inefficient. Moreover, the sugar used by the cancer cells mainly comes from the conversion of lactic acid back to glucose. (Normal cells use sugar from the food eaten.) Furthermore, when the cancer cells convert the sugar to energy, lactic acid is given off as a waste product in the blood, which is recycled to the liver to be converted back into glucose — the vicious cycle. The production of glucose from lactic acid is called *gluconeogenesis*, and hydrazine sulfate, for instance, is thought to shut down the enzyme that favors this conversion of lactic acid to glucose. In a manner of speaking, therefore, we are talking about selective enzyme therapy, that is, of favoring one enzyme or enzyme-catalyzed reaction over another.

As previously mentioned, hydrazine sulfate has been said to inhibit the conversion of lactic acid back to glucose. A more direct way to break the cycle would be the inhibition or negation of the conversion of glucose to lactic acid in the first place, for a lactic acid buildup in the blood can in itself be bad news.

Robert C. Atkins, M.D., made the call that "sugar is the Western world's most frequently consumed carcinogen" (Atkins, 1995, p. 161). Dr. Atkins saw the problems with sugar as more compelling than any cancer-causing effect of fats, and wonders why sugar consumption has not been included in various dietary studies about cancer, and particularly so for colorectal cancer.

The process of *glycolysis* involves the enzymatic breakdown of sugars and other carbohydrates, and its inhibition may thus be a key to anticancer activity (Walters, 1993, p. 135). That is, the partial conversion of glucose to lactic acid by cancer cells would be inhibited. Thus, it has been found that NDGA, as contained in or derived from chaparral or creosote bush, acts as an inhibitor for both aerobic and anaerobic glycolysis, the latter pertaining to cancer cells. This may be the manner in which NDGA acts as an anticancer agent.

Aerobic glycolysis as occurs in normal cells would eventually involve the complete oxidation or conversion of glucose to carbon dioxide and water, yielding energy in the process. That is, in simplest terms, the overall conversion can be written as

$$C_6H_{12}O_6 + 6O_2 \rightarrow 6CO_2 + 6H_2O + \text{energy}$$

Anaerobic glycolysis involves only a fermentation yielding lactic acid and a much, much lesser amount of energy:

$$C_6H_{12}O_6 \rightarrow 2CH_3CH(OH)COOH + energy$$

where the stoichiometric formula for lactic acid, discussed earlier, is $C_3H_6O_3$, the proportions being exactly one-half those for glucose. The reverse of the latter reaction is the conversion of lactic acid back to glucose. Note that at least some energy is produced in the conversion to lactic acid, even though oxygen is not used as a reactant. (That is, comparatively speaking, the heat of reaction for the conversion or fermentation of glucose to lactic acid will be markedly less than for the conversion or oxidation to carbon dioxide and water. This may have something to do with the fact that cancer cells preferentially proliferate.) More details about glycolysis were furnished in Chapter 3.

Sugar, along with fat, protein, and refined cereal products, is credited with causing high rates of colon cancer, which in more "civilized" populations is accentuated by an excess of fecal bile acids and sterol hormones (Moss, 1992, p. 223). Thus, there may be some truth to the adage about starving a cancer, possibly for several reasons, including the breaking of the nutritional supply chain, that is, the glucose/lactic acid linkage.

It may be observed that in talking about the aerobic glycolysis or oxidation of glucose in normal cells, antioxidants presumably would act against this normal process and hence indirectly favor cancer cell growth instead, though antioxidants are supposed to be anticancer agents. Seemingly there could be a contradiction. But then we also note that there is nothing permanent about theories, for we sometimes abandon them whenever the facts do not fit.

Immuno-augmentative therapy (IAT) has been described as perhaps the most well-publicized alternative cancer therapy. Chapters are devoted to IAT in Walters (1993), Moss (1992), and Pelton and Overholser (1994). It was developed by Dr. Lawrence Burton in the 1960s, then a microbiologist/oncologist at St. Vincent's Hospital in New York City. The treatment consisted of daily injections of blood serum made from proteinaceous blood fractions, which may be self-administered. In demonstrations, he was able to make tumors disappear from mice in as short a period as an hour. The machinations that plagued Dr. Burton's work are described in the references. He eventually moved to Freeport in the Grand Bahamas in 1977. Full acceptance in the medical community was never forthcoming, however, and Moss comments that the IAT clinic became a "fairly typical offshore cancer clinic: long on claims, short on scientific documentation."

Michael Lerner is keen on various Chinese therapies, herbal and otherwise, and in particular on what is called *qi gong* (Lerner, 1994, pp 387–393). Qi gong is a psychophysiological therapy, akin to yoga, which is easier described than explained. The explanation involves the mind–body connection.

Even snake venom has been tried. Called *crotoxins*, from the genus *Crotalus*, one of the two genera for rattlesnakes, these are neurotoxins that were found to have some sort of anticancer effect, direct or indirect, but presumably in very small concentrations. The snake in particular was said to be the cascabel, or *Crotalus terrificus*, from Argentina. After creating a minor international incident, and being outlawed in the United States, this particular treatment seems to have disappeared from the scene.

The subject of plant and herbal treatments for cancer, and most of the other options as well, remains mostly a gray area, with as yet no large-scale groundswell of public opinion demanding a no-nonsense, unbiased, definitive resolution, say of Chaparral usage and other alternatives. Most people do not even know that there are alternatives and remain complacent with the status quo, helpless and resigned to fate. The War on Cancer announced in 1971 during the Nixon administration continues to fizzle, with a final, absolute cure for cancer but a distant dream. If as much time, money, and effort had been spent on researching, developing, and demonstrating unconventional cancer therapies as on conventional ones, then there would by now likely be some proven options — options that work without a doubt.

## MYSTIQUE SURROUNDING CANCER CURES

Cancer cures, in common with other cures, have an aura of mystique around them. In this regard we again note that, among other books, medical anthropologist and herbalist John Heinerman has written *The Spiritual Wisdom of the Native Americans* and *Healing Secrets of the Maya: Health Wisdom from an Ancient Empire*, and *Health Secrets from the Ancient World*. From here, Heinerman progresses to more modern times, but there remains a reservoir of knowledge from the past. For a few more, we mention again Heinerman's *Aloe Vera, Jojoba and Yucca*, and *The Healing Benefits of Garlic From Pharaohs to Pharmacists*. Plus *Double the Power of Your Immune System*. There will be the occasion to continue to refer to several of Heinerman's books. Unfortunately, some of his books are out of print and difficult to find.

A persistent rumor regarding cancer cures pertains to the previously mentioned Compound-X — supposedly a mysterious, secretive, and potent formulation originating with the Plains Indians, or maybe southwestern Indians, or even Canadian Indians. It is supposed to cure both external and internal cancers, but it seems no one wants to talk about it, what is in it, or how it works. Presumably it is a herbal mixture of unknown makeup, although Chaparral and bloodroot may be in it. A rumor is that a pharmaceutical company was once interested, and along these lines a certain toothpaste contains bloodroot (*Sanguarine canadensis*) as an anticavity agent.

Further inquiry reveals that some of the original work on a version of something called Compound-X was carried out on animals at Colorado State University, apparently with no positive results. As if in anticipation, however, John Heinerman wrote *Healing Animals with Herbs*, published in 1977.

The examples herein illustrate the ambiguity in pinning down a cure for cancer from tropical plants, or any plants, as what is known is from native folklore or hearsay. You are never quite sure which plant species is supposed to do exactly what, if anything, and are not even sure about which species is which. If an active chemical component perchance is found, it is probably just one of tens or maybe hundreds or thousands in the same species, which act together synergistically, for the complexity of nature can be infinite. Controlled, impartial clinical studies are lacking, the subject being beyond mainstream medicine, and only one of many possibilities. Folklore provides a place to start, however, assuming a degree of discernment.

## MISCELLANEOUS

Heinerman was a proponent of folic acid and vitamin A, and Ralph Moss describes folic acid as having been used against lung cancer and cervical cancer (Moss, 1992, pp. 42–44). More is contained in *Folate in Health and Disease*, edited by Lynn B. Bailey. Another volume of interest is titled *Apricots and Oncogenes: On Vegetables and Cancer Prevention*, written by Eileen Jennings. It emphasizes the two vitamins folic acid and beta-carotene; both are found in vegetables, and the indication is of why folic acid deficiency may be a principal cause of colon cancer and breast cancer. (It may be commented that folic acid is listed as an enzyme inhibitor for certain cancer-causing enzymatic reactions.)

As has also been indicated, John Heinerman's *The Healing Benefits of Garlic*, published in 1994, makes mention of the presence in garlic of the element germanium or its compounds, which act as anticancer agents, as do selenium and some other minerals or inorganic compounds. An early proponent of the idea that either mineral deficiencies or excesses affected cancer was J.I. Rodale and others of *Prevention* magazine, described in their *The Complete Book of Minerals*, published in 1972. Magnesium deficiencies were implicated (Rodale et al., 1972, pp. 118, 119, 488, 679), as were problems from iron, salt and iodized salt, fluoridation, and aluminum (Rodale et al., 1972, pp. 163, 334, 335, 348, 360, 394).

Another interesting, if rare and older, book is by a Dr. O. Phelps Brown, previously cited, titled *The Complete Herbalist: Or, the People Their Own Physicians, By the Use of Nature's Remedies; Describing the Great Curative Powers Found in the Herbal Kingdom*, and published in 1875. Several treatments for different kinds of cancer are mentioned, if not convincingly (Brown, 1875, pp. 74, 346). Brown said he successfully used the bark of a South American plant known as the *cundurango*, or *condor vine* (also spelled condurango; *Equatoria garciana* or *Gonolobus condurango*, of the family Asclepiadaceae) against cancer. Hartwell lists this plant, but subsequent investigations have proved unsuccessful.

Another bioactive plant from South America, occurring in the upper reaches of the Amazon in Peru, is colloquially known as cat's claw, or Uña de Gato (*Uncaria tomentosa*.of the family Rubiaceae). Anecdotal evidence describes some remarkable cancer cures using a tea made from this plant, and it is available in the United States. The action may be due to the presence of alkaloids, but one is not entirely convinced.

### Neo Tropica

The region called Neo Tropica or Neotropica — the part of the New World lying between the Tropic of Cancer and the Tropic of Capricorn — is prime territory for newly discovered plant species, as it includes the rain forests of Amazonia and Central America. As the result of continuing explorations and investigations, a series of monographs exists under the general heading *Flora Neotropica*, as prepared by the New York Botanical Garden for the Organization of Flora Neotropica. Each monograph generally deals with a single plant family. The first was published in 1968, and by 1994, some 65 monographs had been published, an impressive start, but still with a long way to go. Unfortunately, the medicinal properties have not been studied, only the taxonomy.

Interestingly, however, Hartwell's compendium contains species from 30 of the 65 plant families so far studied in *Flora Neotropica*. (Hartwell's listings comprise a total of 214 plant families.)

Thus, the herb known as pau d'arco is included, a common name for one of several trees of the family Bignoniaceae, genus *Tabebuia*. Identification is made in Monograph 25(II), published in 1980 and titled *Bignoniaceae*, by Alwyn H. Gentry (who was later killed in an expedition plane crash). There are six species of *Tabebuia* listed, one being *T. impetiginosa*. However, another named *T. heptaphylla*, which grows in the northeastern coastal regions of South America, is evidently the species whose pulverized inner bark is marketed as pau d'arco. Hartwell lists both, and another named *T. avellanidae*. The name *Tecoma* also surfaces, and Hartwell furnishes the information that infusions have been used against metastasized liver cancer and cancer of the pancreas (two of perhaps the three most deadly cancers, the other being cancer of the lung).

Also in the same monograph is a description for the "cancer tree," *Jacaranda caerulea*. Hartwell lists this species also under Bignoniaceae, as well as a couple of others, *J. brasiliana* and *J. procera*. All are designated antitumor agents.

Another useful volume encompassing the territory is the *Amazonian Ethnobotanical Dictionary*, by James Alan Duke and Rudolfo Vasquez, published in 1994. This is the same Jim Duke, of the U.S. Department of Agriculture at Beltsville, Maryland, who wrote the Foreword to Jonathan Hartwell (1982). Many of the medicinal properties of select species are provided, listing both common and scientific names, and annotated with descriptors POISON and TOXIC wherever they apply. The medicinal uses are as based on folklore.

As for one particular instance, there are the several plants called cat's claw, or Uña de Gato (Duke and Vasquez, 1994, p. 172). The commercially sold herb in the health food stores is named *Uncaria tomentosa*, which comes from the upper reaches of Amazonia in Peru. Its action may be more that of an anti-inflammatory agent. There is another, however, named *Uncaria guianensis* and also called *Uña de gavilán*. It is cited as used by the Columbian and Guianan Indians as an anticancer agent. Both are from the family Rubiaceae. Neither is listed in Hartwell, though another species named *Uncaria sclerophylla* or, elephant's trunk, from Malaya, is mentioned as having been used for callous ulcer.

## SOME FURTHER ALTERNATIVES

Another way to at least control cancer, especially prostate cancer, is called the macrobiotic diet, a part of the general subject of macrobiotics. The diet is described in the usual references. There is to be no red meat and, instead, whole grains and vegetables are included. The analogy to the Gerson Diet, previously described, and other such diets, is obvious.

(Prostate troubles, called benign prostatic hyperplasia or hypertrophy [BPH], are said to yield to an extract from the oil of saw or sawtooth palmetto berries. It grows in the West Indies and up along the Atlantic Coast of North America from Florida to North Carolina; apparently an old Indian remedy, it was picked up by the early settlers.)

Burton's Immuno-augmentative therapy (IAT) has already been noted, with descriptive chapters in the usual references. Involved are daily injections of blood serum made from proteinaceous blood fractions, which may be self-administered. Tumors were said to disappear from mice literally in hours.

Another treatment that did not survive involved radiotherapy, which involves the subject of viral/microbial origins and treatments. Called Rife therapy, it has been extensively commented upon. In reiteration, it was first developed by a scientist/inventor named Royal Rife. A book has been written about it called *The Cancer Cure That Worked!*, by Barry Lynes, and a description is also included in a chapter "Bioelectric Therapies" in Richard Walters (1993). Dating back to the 1930s, Rife constructed what was called an electromagnetic frequency generator. Said to be very effective against cancer, nevertheless he and his associates were put out of business by the medical establishment — and his efforts and results have never been duplicated.

At the same time, as has been noted, Rife developed a powerful light microscope permitting the viewing of live cancer microbes, which varied in size from a fungus to a bacillus down to a virus. Moreover, the microbe was said to be pleomorphic, that is, able to change from one form (and size) to another. The work preceded that of Livingston and Naessens, also previously described.

(It can be added that under different conditions that is, different wavelengths, intensities, and exposures, electromagnetic wave generation can be regarded as a cause of cancer. For example, consider x-rays, microwaves, and power line radiation, not to mention sunlight.)

## SUCCESSES VS. FAILURES

It can again be asked, if plants and herbs and nutrition are said to be so successful in some cancer cases, or in even some few cancer cases, why are they not successful in all cancer cases? A conjecture of course is that these plants or plant-derived substances somehow trigger the immune system, and every individual is different. Furthermore, a person's immune system does not ordinarily recognize that person's own cancer cells. In other words, the cancer cells mimic the normal cells. Only if cancerous cells from another person are introduced does an attack by the immune system occur. This is why immune suppressants must be used for organ transplants. Research is proceeding, however, on how to make cancerous cells recognizable to the person's own immune system. There has been limited success against melanoma, as previously described in the Stephen S. Hall references.

The subject of plant and herbal treatments for cancer, and most of the other options for that matter, can be viewed as remaining mostly a gray area, with as yet no large-scale groundswell of public opinion demanding a no-nonsense, definitive resolution for, say, plant or herbal usage and other alternatives.

As for hard figures for success rates, or remission rates, the facts mostly seem in abeyance. A quote by Patrick McGrady, founder of CANHELP, is perhaps enlightening (Walters, 1993, p. 5ff): "Most alternative therapies are almost totally useless — just like the conventional therapies."

Apparently, the estimates for success vary widely, depending on the particular patient and the type of cancer. A holistic health advocate named Gary Null (author of *Gary Null's Complete Guide to Healing Your Body Naturally*) has investigated this problem over the years, with findings that success rates range from 2 to 20% for terminal cancer. Ralph Moss has also commented on the scene as follows: "My subjective impression is a baseline 4 to 5% five-year remission rate in all of the alternative clinics. Then the figure goes up with less severe cases. If I found a 20% rate of five-year remission, that would be really exciting." An additional comment is that previous radiation and chemotherapy treatments have severely compromised the immune system and normal body functions.

Michael Lerner (1994) reported similar impressions. After traveling worldwide visiting doctors and clinics, Lerner gives the impression that alternative cancer therapies and conventional therapies have about the same overall success rates, although alternative treatments have an element of secrecy and a dearth of records.

Another interesting piece of information is that a study showed that where there was a so-called spontaneous remission of cancer, most of the patients (88%) had made major dietary changes, for example, to vegetarianism (Walters, 1993, p. 3). However, statistically speaking within the totality of cases, Walters makes the observation that the overall survival rates are about the same, with or without treatment.

## BIOLOGICAL RESPONSE

Richard Walters (1993), at the end of the preface of his book, states that there are many sophisticated nonanimal methods that can be used in testing. He quotes a former American Cancer Society president about the problems with animal studies. "My own belief is that we have relied too heavily on animal testing, and we believed in it too strongly. Now, I think we are commencing to realize that what goes on in an animal may not necessarily be applicable to humans." (Or, what does not go on is maybe not applicable, either.) Walters supplied an address for other information about using animals: People for the Ethical Treatment of Animals (PETA), PO Box 42516, Washington, D.C. 20015, (301)770-PETA. (Another similar partisan organization is Physicians Committee for Responsible Medicine [PCRM].)

If biological responses vary from individual to individual, as per biochemist Roger Williams' findings in *Free and Unequal: The Biological Basis of Individual Liberty*, then it can certainly be expected that human responses are different from that of animal responses and vice versa.

(We may wish to exclude identical twins from the comparison, however, whose biological and behavioral patterns are so similar that it gives evidence that maybe we are all genetically preprogrammed as to how we will turn out. For even when separated at birth and raised in totally different environments, unaware of each other, their lives are uncannily similar, sometimes including the diseases contracted, and when.)

There remains the incontrovertible fact that cures have been effected by unconventional as well as conventional methods. For instances of (unexplained) spontaneous remissions, a record is kept by the Institute for Noetic Sciences, Sausalito, California. More or less an anthology, there is *A Cancer Survivor's Almanac: Charting Your Journey*, edited by Barbara Hoffman. One of the many specific examples is the book by Barbara A. Arpante, *The Recovery of a Cancer Patient: A Personal Diary*. Another is Juliet Wittman's *Breast Cancer Journal: A Century of Petals*, describing a chemotherapy regimen that apparently was successful (as of 1993), with a Resources Guide appended. Michael Gearin-Tosh's *Living Proof: A Medical Mutiny*, and his conflict with medical orthodoxy, will be discussed subsequently. Another example is that of Peny Goodson-Kjome of Laramie, Wyoming (since deceased), who wrote up her experiences with cancer in *This Adventure Called Life*. Forsaking conventional treatment, she underwent a spiritual healing in ceremonies of the Plains Indians, and mentions a mysterious herbal mixture, which may be or may not be related to Compound-X. Heinerman (1989), in Chapter 4 of his book *The Spiritual Wisdom of the Native Americans*, writes about sweat ceremonies and their importance, and speaks further of the value of enemas, notably among the ancient Maya. In speaking of the role of religious faith in making decisions, there is *Hope in the Face of Cancer: A Survival Guide for the Journey You Did Not Choose*, by Amy Givler, M.D., herself a cancer survivor.

(In an essay on nutritional therapies, Richard Walters comments that meat animals are force-fed or injected with various chemicals, hormones, appetite stimulants, antibiotics, and sedatives [Walters, 1993, p.143]. The meat products will contain the residues, many of which are cancer-causing. More than this, many of the animals are infected with diseases, but the animals and carcasses get by the inspectors. These infections include cancer-causing microbes. [In a cited example, chimpanzees fed from birth with milk from leukemic cows died from leukemia within the first year.] Even though the tumors may be cut out, the cancer viruses remain in the rest of the meat. Moreover, the cut-out tumors may end up in mixed meats such as hot dogs. In turn, bacterial action in the meat-eaters' intestines can produce carcinogens, and the consumption of fat magnifies the problem. Walters observes that cancer rates for those who eat meat, poultry, dairy products, and eggs are several times greater than for vegetarians, which correlates somewhat with the dietary protocol of the Navajos. Similarly, Heinerman notes the occurrence of mutagenic compounds in human feces [Heinerman, 1984, pp. 149, 150].)

It can of course be suggested that the Navajos may also partake of herbal remedies, and similarly for the Indians of northwestern Ontario, the North American tribes with the lowest cancer rates. (It can be argued as well that cancer is inhibited by the Indians' biochemical makeup or their genes.)

It may be mentioned that there is a considerable opposition to vaccinations from some quarters, which believe they have serious side effects. This includes the vaccination for smallpox. Thus, a doctor has reported that cancer was virtually unknown until compulsory vaccination with cowpox vaccine began to be introduced (Mullins, 1992, p. 132). Maybe by not being vaccinated, native or aboriginal populations escape cancer. The idea deserves further evaluation. The analogy might carry over into the routine use of polio vaccines, derived from monkeys, which have been accused of introducing some strange viruses into the human population, including that causing the lethargy associated with the hippy generation.

(There are other pockets of native peoples who show low or nonexistent cancer occurrences. For instance, there are the Manchurians or Kargasoks, who drink Kombucha elixer or Manchurian tea, also called *Kargasok tea*, in an area of Russia called Kargasok. It is made from the Kombucha fungus, and is a yeast-culture tea that is fermented. It is also now widely used in Japan. The Kombucha fungus itself is a symbiosis of yeast cells and various bacteria. All kinds of benefits are claimed. They stick to a vegetable and dairy diet, and remain cancerfree. Other long-lived peoples can be mentioned, such as in mountainous Caucasia, Yakutia in Siberia, the Poltaya District of the Ukraine, and in Tibet and Spain. John Heinerman describes a past visit to Georgia, where the people are said to live to 110, 120, 130, or even 140 years [Heinerman, 1984, p. 146]. They go by the philosophy that once fresh food is cooked, canned, or in any way processed, the food begins to "die.")

# 8 On Overcoming the Intractability of Cancer

## CELL RESISTANCE AND SOME CONSEQUENCES

Cell resistance is a well-known consequence of cancer chemotherapy, indeed of the overuse of antibiotics, as is increasingly publicized by the media. There was a relevant article on the topic by Sharon Begley in the July 11, 2003, issue of the *Wall Street Journal*. Titled "Cancer Cells Appear To Be Unusually Adept at Dodging Therapies," the article appeared in the "Marketplace" section under the heading "Science Journal." Among the authorities cited is molecular biologist Robert Weinberg of the Whitehead Institute in Cambridge, Massachusetts, who notes the evasive maneuvers of cancer cells, which unfortunately can activate alternative pathways to circumvent a particular therapy. Thus, Lawrence Loeb of the University of Washington, Seattle, addresses genetic instability, whereby cancer cells undergo thousands of random mutations, even in the early stages, some of which will be resistant to standard chemotherapy. And, significantly, oncologist Roy Herbst of the M.D. Anderson Cancer Center in Houston states that for a therapy to be effective, it must target a particular cancer cell pathway whereby "that pathway has to be one of the main ones driving that abnormal cell."

This statement is about cancer cell metabolism, the main metabolic pathway of which is the conversion of glucose or glycogen to lactic acid or lactate rather than to carbon dioxide and water, as occurs in normal cells. Furthermore, the key enzyme for the conversion of glucose to lactic acid is lactate dehydrogenase. Fortunately, a number of enzyme inhibitors for lactate dehydrogenase are known and can be viewed as potential anticancer agents, with others presumably in the offing.

## ALTERNATIVE TREATMENT: THE STATUS QUO

The foregoing remarks specifically lead to those of the Life Extension Foundation's about 1500-page volume titled *Disease Prevention and Treatment*, expanded fourth edition, published in 2003. The contents are arranged alphabetically by subject, with several sections devoted to the latest findings (as of 2003) on cancer and its treatment. The voluminous references are furnished on the LEF Web site (www.lef.org/references).

(On first opening the Web site, the viewer is confronted with a listing of protocols, in terms of a numbering system, e.g., prtcl-022 pertains to breast cancer, prtcl-026 to cancer surgery, prtcl-113 to pancreatic cancer, etc. Further exploration at the Web site under the heading of "Protocols" will yield a listing titled "Cancer Adjuvant Therapies — References: Online References," from which the actual list of references is forthcoming. There is apparently no system for linking each reference to the text proper. This has the advantage of not cluttering up the text, but does not permit ready access to further substantiating information.)

In the section in the text titled "Cancer Adjuvant Therapy," there are listings of substances known to act against cancer, with descriptive information about dosages and successes. For the most part, these substances can be viewed as producing remissions and extending lifetimes rather than furnishing absolute cures. This is embodied in the word *adjuvant*, meaning that which is contributory, helpful, or assisting (although vitamin C or ascorbic acid deserves a special mention in that it has a track record). For the record, the agents or substances in Table 8.1 were listed under the text heading of "Complementary Therapies," in their order of appearance in the volume.

Now apparently out of favor, the cyanogenetic glycoside called laetrile or amygdalin is not listed nor indexed in the aforementioned compilation. However, the Cancer Control Society (2043 N. Berendo St, Los Angeles, CA 90027, 323-663-7801) continues to investigate laetrile as a therapy, along with other alternative therapies, holding an annual cancer convention and publishing *Cancer Control Journal*. The various investigations are well represented by M.D.'s.

(The publisher of the *Townsend Letter* — Jonathan Collin, M.D. — has some good things to say about the Cancer Control Society on pages 7 and 14 of the November 2005 issue. He writes of testimonials from individuals who were expected to die of cancer in weeks or months, but who utilized alternative therapies and survived for 20, 25, or 30 years and more. These therapies have been outlawed in the United States by various means, requiring patients to go to Tijuana, Mexico, and other places for treatment. Moreover, the treatments are a mix of the old and the new, with an emphasis on diet and lifestyle changes, the use of enzymes, vitamins, and minerals, and of chelation and intravenous vitamin C. Treatments cited also include IPT [insulin potentiated chemotherapy], metabolic therapies, herbals, hypothermia, and oxicagave ["oxic" pertaining to a kind of soil, and "agave" to a member of the genus "agave"] therapies.)

Some of these alternative therapies may be compared with some more conventional antitumor agents, as shown in Table 8.2. And in turn may also be compared with some more conventional chemopreventive agents as shown in Table 8.3. The information presented in Table 8.2 and Table 8.3 is taken from a publication of the Sigma-Aldrich Chemical Company titled *Cancer Research: From Carcinogenesis to Intervention: The Right Tools*. Further details are provided for each particular product code in the extensive catalog available from Sigma-Aldrich, a major source of biochemical substances for medical research and practice. The inference here is that there is a degree of merging under way between orthodox medicine and complementary and alternative medicine (CAM), a fact maybe not to be mentioned out loud.

Thus, it may be mentioned that the National Center for Complementary and Alternative Medicine (NCCAM), a division of the National Institutes of Health (NIH), is seeking scientific answers using CAM against cancer, for example, from practitioners and patients. In light of the fact that more than 1.3 million Americans are diagnosed with cancer each year (accompanied by over 0.5 or 0.6 million deaths), all things considered the total cost can be set at $171.6 billion at the time of writing.

---

**TABLE 8.1**
**Tabulation of Adjuvant Cancer Therapies**

Alpha-lipoic acid
Arginine
Carotenoids
Cimetidine (Tagamet®)
Clodronate
Coenzyme Q10 and statin drugs
Conjugated linoleic acid (CLA)
Cyclooxygenase (COX-2) inhibitors
Berberine-containing herbs
Feverfew
Ginger
Green tea
Curcumin
Dimethyl sulfoxide (DMSO)
Essential fatty acids (EFAs)
Garlic
Glutamine
Inositol hexaphosphate (IP-6)
Lactoferrin
Melatonin
MGN
Modified citrus pectin (MCP)
*N*-acetyl-cysteine (NAC)
Resveratrol
Selenium
Silibinin (from milk thistle)
Soy
Theanine
Thymus extract
Vitamin A
Vitamin C
Vitamin D
Vitamin E
Vitamin K

*Source:* From Life Extension Foundation, *Disease Prevention and Treatment: Scientific Protocols that Integrate Mainstream and Alternative Medicine*, expanded 4th ed., Hollywood, FL, 2003. With permission.

---

And the NCCAM director, Stephen E. Straus, M.D., notes that "for millions of Americans, cancer prevention and treatment concerns are not being adequately addressed through conventional medicine. Many are turning outside the medical

**TABLE 8.2**
**Antitumor Agents**

| Product Code[a] | Product Description | Application |
|---|---|---|
| | *Angiogenesis Inhibitors* | |
| A 1477 | Angiostatin K1-3, human, recombinant expressed in *Pichia pastoris* (a yeast fungus) without N-linked glycosylation | A proteolytic fragment of plasminogen that is a specific inhibitor of endothelial cell growth and angiogenesis. |
| D-193 | DL-α-Difluoromethylornithine hydrochloride | Irreversible inhibitor of ornithine decarboxylate (ODC); chemoprotective agent that blocks angiogenesis. |
| E 8154 | Endostatin, human, recombinant expressed in *Pichia pastoris* | Potent inhibitor of angiogenesis and tumor growth; inhibits endothelial cell proliferation. |
| E 8279 | Endostatin, murine, recombinant expressed in *Pichia pastoris* | Potent inhibitor of angiogenesis and tumor growth; inhibits endothelial cell proliferation. |
| G 6649 | Genestein, synthetic | Antiangiogenic agent, downregulates the transcription of genes involved in controlling angiogenesis. |
| G 6776 | Genestein from *Glycine max* (soybean) | Antiangiogenic agent, downregulates the transcription of genes involved in controlling angiogenesis. |
| S 4400 | Staurosporine from S*treptomyces* sp. | Blocks angiogenesis by inhibiting the upregulation of VEGF expression in tumor cells. |
| T-144 | Thalidomide | Selectively inhibits biosynthesis of tumor necrosis factor α (TNF-α); inhibits angiogenesis. |
| | *DNA Intercalators/Crosslinkers* | |
| C 2538 | Carboplatin | Broad-spectrum antitumor agent. Forms cytotoxic adducts with DNA; induces apoptosis. |
| C 0400 | Carmustine | DNA alkylating/cross-linking agent effective against glioma and other solid tumors. |
| C 0253 | Chlorambucil | Alkylates DNA; induces apoptosis of leukemia cells by a p53-dependent mechanism. |
| C 0768 | Cyclophosphamide monohydrate | Cytotoxic nitrogen mustard that cross-links DNA and causes strand breakage. |
| C 7397 | Cyclophosphamide monohydrate *ISOPAC® | Cytotoxic nitrogen mustard that cross-links DNA and causes strand breakage. |
| M 2011 | Melphalan | Forms DNA intrastrand cross-links by alkylation of 5'-(GGC) sequences. |
| M 6545 | Mitoxantrone dihydrochloride | DNA intercalating agent that inhibits DNA synthesis. |
| 0 9512 | Oxaliplatin | Antitumor agent with activity against colorectal cancer; cytotoxicity follows the formation of adducts with DNA. |
| P 4394 | *Cis*-diammineplatinum(II) dichloride (cisplatin) | Forms cytotoxic adducts with the DNA dinucleotide d(pGpG); induces apoptosis. |

## TABLE 8.2 (CONTINUED)
## Antitumor Agents

| Product Code[a] | Product Description | Application |
|---|---|---|
| **DNA Synthesis Inhibitors** | | |
| A 7019 | (±)-Amethopterin (methotrexate) | Folic acid antagonist; blocks nucleotide biosynthesis by inhibiting dihydrofolate reductase. |
| A 1784 | Aminopterin | Folic acid antagonist; blocks nucleotide biosynthesis by inhibiting dihydrofolate reductase. More potent, but more toxic, than methotrexate. |
| B 5507 | Bleomycin sulfate from *Streptomyces verticillus* | Inhibits DNA synthesis and causes cleavage at specific base sequences. Induces apoptosis in a variety of cells; inhibits tumor angiogenesis. |
| C 1768 | Cytosine β-D-arabinofuranoside | Antileukemia agent; selective inhibitor of DNA synthesis. |
| C 6645 | Cytosine β-D-arabinofuranoside hydrochloride | Antileukemia agent; selective inhibitor of DNA synthesis. |
| F 8791 | 5-fluoro-5′-deoxyuridine | Inhibits proliferation of tumors, cell lines or fibroblasts transformed by *H-ras* or *trk* oncogenes. |
| F 6627 | 5-Fluorouracil | Inhibits thymidylate synthetase and depletes dTTP; it forms nucleotides that can be incorporated into RNA and DNA and induces p53-dependent apoptosis. |
| G 2536 | Ganciclovir | In suicide gene therapy of solid tumors, the gene for *Herpes simplex* virus thymidine kinase is delivered to tumor cells and expressed, which in turn activates ganciclovir cytotoxicity. |
| H 8627 | Hydroxyurea | Inactivates ribonucleoside reductase and blocks the synthesis of deoxynucleotides, thus inhibiting DNA synthesis and inducing cell death. |
| M 0503 | Mitomycin C from *Streptomyces caespitosus* | Inhibits DNA synthesis, nucleotide division, and proliferation of cancer cells. |
| **DNA-RNA Transcription Regulators** | | |
| A 1410 | Actinomycin D from *Streptomycin* sp. | Inhibits cell proliferation by complexing to DNA and blocking the production of mRNA by RNA polymerase; induces apoptosis. |
| D 8809 | Daunorubicin hydrochloride USP | Complexes to DNA and blocks production of mRNA by RNA polymerase. |
| D 1515 | Doxorubicin hydrochloride | Binds to DNA and inhibits reverse transcripterase and RNA polymerase. |
| I 1656 | Idarubicin hydrochloride | Antileukemia agent with higher DNA binding capacity and greater cytoxicity than daunorubicin. |

## TABLE 8.2 (CONTINUED)
## Antitumor Agents

| Product Code[a] | Product Description | Application |
|---|---|---|
| | **Enzyme Inhibitors** | |
| C 9911 | (S)-(+)-Campatothecin | Binds irreversibly to the DNA–topoisomerase 1 complex, leading to the irreversible cleavage of DNA and the destruction of cellular topoisomerase 1 by the ubiquitin–proteosome pathway. Induces apoptosis in many normal and tumor cell lines. |
| C 7727 | Curcumin | Potent antitumor agent with anti-inflammatory and antioxidant properties. Potent inhibitor of protein kinase C, EGFR tyrosine kinase, and IKB kinase. Induces apoptosis of cancer cells. |
| 37,762-7 | 2-Imino-1-imidazolidineacetic acid (cyclocreatine) | Creatine analog; decreases the rate of ATP production via creatine kinase and reduces the proliferation of tumor cell lines characterized by high levels of creatine kinase expression. |
| E 1383 | Etoposide | Binds to the DNA–topoisomerase II complex to enhance cleavage and inhibit religation; inhibits synthesis of the oncoprotein Mdm2 and induces apoptosis of tumor lines that overexpress Mdm2. |
| F 2552 | Formestane | Aromotase inhibitor used as an anticancer agent against estrogen-dependent tumors. |
| I 7378 | Indomethacin | Cyclooxygenase 2 inhibitor; has efficacy against colorectal cancer. |
| M 2147 | Mevinolin from *Aspergillus* sp. | Inhibits mevalonic acid production and blocks the isoprenylation and membrane localization of Ras-family oncoproteins and nuclear lamins. |
| S 1438 | Sulindac sulfone | Cyclooxygenase inhibitor. Inhibits the development and induces regression of premalignant adenomatous polyps. |
| T 8552 | Trichostatin A from *Streptomyces* sp. | Histone deacetylase inhibitor that enhances the cytotoxic efficacy of anticancer drugs that target DNA. |
| | **Gene Regulation** | |
| A 3656 | 5-Aza-2′-deoxycytidine | Causes DNA demethylation or hemidemethylation, creating openings that allow transcription factors to bind to DNA and reactivate tumor suppressor genes. |
| A 2385 | 5-Azacytidine | Causes DNA demethylation or hemi-demethylation, creating openings that allow transcription factors to bind to DNA and reactivate tumor suppressor genes. |
| C 9756 | Cholecalciferol (vitamin D3) | Antiproliferative action on breast, prostate, and colon cancer cells. |

## TABLE 8.2 (CONTINUED)
## Antitumor Agents

| Product Code[a] | Product Description | Application |
|---|---|---|
| H 6278 | 4-Hydroxytamoxifen, minimum 70% of Z-isomer (remainder primarily E-isomer) | Metabolism of tamoxifen, which is a potent selective estrogen response modifier (SERM); the *trans* (Z) isomer has efficacy against estrogen-sensitive cancers. The *cis* (E) isomer is an estrogen agonist. |
| M 5250 | Melatonin | Enhances apoptic death of cancer cells; inhibits proliferation/metastasis of breast cancer cells by inhibiting estrogen receptor action. |
| R 1402 | Raloxifene hydrochloride | Selective estrogen response modifier (SERM), may be effective against estrogen-sensitive cancers. |
| R 2500 | All *trans*-retinol (vitamin A aldehyde) | Ligands for both the retinoic acid receptor (RAR) and the retinoid X receptor (RXR) that act as transcription factors to regulate the growth and differentiation of normal and malignant cells. |
| R 2625 | Retinoic acid, all *trans* (vitamin A acid) | Ligands for both the retinoic acid receptor (RAR) and the retinoid X receptor (RXR) that act as transcription factors to regulate the growth and differentiation of normal and malignant cells. |
| R 4643 | 9-*cis*-Retinoic acid | Ligands for both the retinoic acid receptor (RAR) and the retinoid X receptor (RXR) that act as transcription factors to regulate the growth and differentiation of normal and malignant cells. |
| R 7632 | Retinol (vitamin A) | Ligands for both the retinoic acid receptor (RAR) and the retinoid X receptor (RXR) that act as transcription factors to regulate the growth and differentiation of normal and malignant cells. |
| T 5648 | Tamoxifen | Selective estrogen response modifier (SERM), used therapeutically and prophylactically against estrogen-sensitive tumors. |
| T 9262 | Tamoxifen citrate salt | Selective estrogen response modifier (SERM), used therapeutically and prophylactically against estrogen-sensitive tumors. |
| T 22573 | Troglitazone | Antitumor agent; PPAR-$\gamma$ agonist; induces apoptosis via a p53 pathway. |

**Microtube Inhibitors**

| Product Code[a] | Product Description | Application |
|---|---|---|
| C 9754 | Colchicine | Antimitotic agent that disrupts microtubules by binding to tubulin and preventing its polymerization; induces apoptosis in several normal and tumor cell lines. |
| M 1404 | Nocodazole | Antimitotic agent that binds to $\beta$-tubulin and disrupts mitotic spindle function; induces apoptosis in several normal and tumor cell lines. |

**TABLE 8.2 (CONTINUED)**
**Antitumor Agents**

| Product Code[a] | Product Description | Application |
|---|---|---|
| T 7191 | Paclitaxel, semisynthetic from *Taxus* sp. | Binds to β-tubulin and promotes the formation of highly stable microtubules that resist depolymerization, preventing cell division. |
| T 7402 | Paclitaxel from *Taxus brevifolia* | Binds to β-tubulin and promotes the formation of highly stable microtubules that resist depolymerization, preventing cell division. |
| T 1912 | Paclitaxel from *Taxus yannanensis* | Binds to β-tubulin and promotes the formation of highly stable microtubules that resist depolymerization, preventing cell division. |
| P 4405 | Podophyllotoxin | Inhibits microtube assembly. |
| V 1377 | Vinblastine sulfate salt | Antimitotic agent. Inhibits microtube assembly by binding tubulin and inducing self-association; depolymerizes preexisting microtubules. Induces apoptosis in several cell lines. |
| V 8879 | Vincristine sulfate salt | Antimitotic agent. Inhibits microtube assembly by binding tubulin and inducing self-association; depolymerizes preexisting microtubules. Induces apoptosis in several cell lines. |
| V 8254 | Vindesine sulfate salt | Antimitotic agent. Inhibits microtube assembly by binding tubulin and inducing self-association; depolymerizes preexisting microtubules. Induces apoptosis in several cell lines. |
| V 2264 | Vinorelbine (navelbine) ditartrate salt | Potent antimitotic antitumor agent. Low neurotoxicity is related to its higher affinity for mitotic microtubules than for axonal microtubules. |
| | | **Other** |
| A 5376 | Acetylsalicylic acid | Reduces the incidence of colorectal and other solid tumors, perhaps by activating p53-mediated apoptosis. |
| L 0399 | Leuprolide (leuprorelin) | Luteinizing hormone releasing hormone (LH-RH) agonist. |
| M 8046 | Mifepristone | Progesterone receptor antagonist. |
| R 0395 | Rapamycin from *Streptomyces hygroscopicus* | Inhibition of the molecular target of rapamycin (mTOR) mediates the antiproliferative and anticancer activity of rapamycin by blocking the P13K/Akt pathway. |
| T 9033 | Thapsigargin | Cytotoxin that induces apoptosis by disrupting intracellular free $Ca^{2+}$ levels; incorporated into chemotherapeutic prodrug formulations. |

[a] Product codes refer to the Sigma-Aldrich catalog.

*Source:* Adapted from *Cancer Research*, Sigma-Aldrich Fine Chemicals, St. Louis, MO, 2004. A brochure based on a collection of booklets. Sigma-Aldrich also published the annual catalog *Biochemicals, Reagents & Kits for Life Science Research*.

## TABLE 8.3
## Chemopreventive Agents

| Product Code[a] | Product Description | Application |
|---|---|---|
| A 7250 | n-Acetyl-L-cysteine | Antioxidant; increases cellular pools of free radical scavengers. Reduces carcinogenicity of environmental toxins. |
| A 7007 | 5-(5′-Adenosyl)-L-methionine chloride | Methyl donor; cofactor for enzyme-catalyzed methylations; cofactor for DNA methylation. |
| A 7506 | Ascorbic acid (vitamin C), ~ 325 mesh | Antioxidant. |
| A 0278 | Ascorbic acid (vitamin C), 20–200 mesh | Antioxidant. |
| B 2515 | L-Buthionine-sulfoximine | Blocks cellular resistance to chemotherapy by inhibiting $\gamma$-glutamylcysteine synthetase, a key enzyme in glutathione biosynthesis. |
| C 4582 | $\beta$-Carotene, synthetic, min. 95% (HPCL) | Antioxidant or pro-oxidant depending on cellular environment; reduces incidence of many cancers, but enhances lung cancer incidence in smokers. |
| C 9750 | $\beta$-Carotene, synthetic, ~ 95% (UV) | Antioxidant or pro-oxidant depending on cellular environment; reduces incidence of many cancers, but enhances lung cancer incidence in smokers. |
| D 7802 | Daidzein, synthetic | A photoestrogen, recently suggested to play a role in preventing hormone-induced cancers. |
| E 4143 | (–)-Epigallocatechin gallate from green tea, min. 95% | Tumor-inhibiting constituent of green tea; inhibits VEGF-induced tyrosine phosphorylation. |
| E 4268 | (–)-Epigallocatechin gallate from green tea, min. 80% | Tumor-inhibiting constituent of green tea; inhibits VEGF-induced tyrosine phosphorylation. |
| F 7876 | Folic acid | Enzyme cofactor essential for the synthesis, methylation, and repair of DNA. Folic acid supplements may reduce colorectal cancer risk. |
| L 9879 | Lycopene from tomato | Antioxidant micronutrient of tomatoes associated with decreased risk for cancer and cardiovascular disease. Enhances gap junction communication between cells and reduces proliferation of cancer cells in culture. |
| O 5507 | Octadecadienoic acid, conjugated (conjugated linoleic acid) | Potent inhibitor of breast, skin, and colon carcinogenesis and tumor cell proliferation. |
| Q 0125 | Quercetin dihydrate | Antioxidant flavonoid with anticancer activity. Antiproliferative effects on cancer cell lines; reduces cancer cell growth via type II estrogen receptors. |
| R 5010 | Resveratrol | Dietary stilbene found in grapes and peanuts. Potent antagonist of chemical carcinogenesis; androgen receptor antagonist. |

## TABLE 8.3 (CONTINUED)
## Chemopreventive Agents

| Product Code[a] | Product Description | Application |
|---|---|---|
| S 3132 | Seleno-L-methionine | Antioxidant. Administration to cancer cell lines results in apoptic cell death and aberrant mitosis; reduces cancer incidence *in vivo*. |
| 21,448-5 | Sodium selenite | More potent than selenomethionine in reducing carcinogenesis. |
| T 3634 | α-Tocopherol (vitamin E) from vegetable oil, about 1000 IU/g | Antioxidant. |

[a] Product codes refer to the Sigma-Aldrich catalog.

*Source:* Adapted from *Cancer Research*, Sigma-Aldrich Fine Chemicals, St. Louis, MO, 2004.

mainstream to CAM approaches that are affordable and accessible, but largely untested."

In this regard, a number of specialized research centers are slated to address and participate in discussions on these issues, and include the following: the Johns Hopkins Center for Cancer Complementary Medicine; the Specialized Center of Research in Hyperbaric Oxygen Therapy at the University of Pennsylvania; the Botanical Center for Age-Related Diseases at Purdue University; and the UCLA Center for Dietary Supplement Research on Botanicals. These are in addition to other well-known cancer research and treatment centers located around the country, such as the Memorial Sloan-Kettering Cancer Center in New York City, the M.D. Anderson Cancer Center in Houston, the Fred Hutchinson Cancer Research Center in Seattle, etc.

Clinical trials involving people, rather than animals, as patients are under way in a number of areas, including acupuncture, shark cartilage, diet alternatives (e.g., macrobiotic and flaxseed), the Asian therapy called Noni, L-carnitine, massage, electroacupuncture, and mistletoe (combined with the chemotherapy drug gemcitabine).

Further, an NCCAM Clearinghouse has been set up as an information source: POB 7923, Gaithersburg, MD 20898, TEL: 888-644-6226 or 301-519-3153, and for the hearing impaired, 866-464-3615, FAX: 866-464-3616.

Additionally, the Office of Cancer Complementary and Alternative Medicine (OCCAM) of the National Cancer Institute (NCI) is calling for information identifying CAM practitioners who would be willing to cooperate as participants in an NCI survey about CAM approaches to the treatment of cancer. The contact at the time of this writing is: Anne C. Washburn, MPH, Manager, Communications Program, The National Cancer Institute, Office of Cancer Complementary and Alternative Medicine, 6116 Executive Blvd., #600, MSC 8339, Bethesda, MD 20852, TEL: 301-594-9983, FAX: 301-480-0075.

It looks as if things are starting to get serious. Howsoever, an article in the July 2004 issue of the *Townsend Letter for Doctors & Patients* by Marcus A. Cohen — described as "Townsend's New York Observer" — furnishes some of the behind-the-scenes intrigue that has been going on. Prominently quoted is Frank Wiewel of People Against Cancer, located at Otho, Iowa. Basically, Wiewel cites the foot dragging within the National Institutes of Health, even when the NIH is challenged by people such as Senators Harkin and Grassley, both of Iowa. In other words, the NIH apparently remains adamant against alternative medicine and, to put matters in perspective, the cost of the FDA's safety and efficacy requirement studies for a new pharmaceutical drug, plus the necessary clinical trials, now total about 1 billion dollars.

Cohen's column in the August/September 2004 issue of the *Townsend Letter* concerns censorship in the medical arena, and is titled "The Impact of Medical Censorship on Patient Care: Part 1." A prime obstacle in the progress of medicine is the practice of peer review, which stifles innovation. Presumably there will be more articles, much farther down the road, as per the October 2004 and November 2004 issues, which will be described in the following text.

Concerning censorship — including censorship by omission – Ralph Moss's column in the same issue describes his attendance at the 2004 New Orleans meeting of ASCO, this being the American Society for Clinical Oncology. The number of attendees and participants could be called huge, being some 25,000 in all. Moss was most interested in (dramatic) unconventional and out-of-the-mainstream cancer treatments, and in this and other respects he was disappointed, for the theme of the meeting seemed to be, as expressed by a participant, that "little by little, new targeted therapies are helping cancer patients live longer, even if they do not offer miraculous cures.... " Moss's conclusion is that advanced cancer is no more curable today than it was 30 years ago. The subject of CAM or its equivalent received hardly any notice at all, and Moss notes that chemotherapy was apparently the treatment of choice, with the conference a "paean to the surging profitability of the new cancer medicine." Moss further mentions that Andrew Pollack of the *New York Times* made clear that "the ASCO meeting has become the new trading floor of the biotech industry."

("Chemotherapy" is a broad term that can denote both synthetic and natural substances. The inference here is to synthetic, and hence patentable, substances. In other words, there has to be the prospect of making a return on investment, and preferably a large return.)

Moss continues his comments in the December 2004 issue of the *Townsend Letter*, comparing the huge attendance at the 2004 ASCO meeting with the much smaller attendance at the 2004 meeting of the Cancer Control Society (CCS). First mentioning presentations on some of the more conventional cancer treatment protocols of alternative medicine, including Chinese medicine, there were talks about the compound Poly-MVA, notably employed against melanoma, as used by Tony Martinez, M.D., at the "Hope4Cancer" clinic. A shortage of new ideas was noted by Bruce Johnson, M.D., of the Dana-Farber Cancer Institute, Boston. The fundamental medicolegal principle of "freedom of choice" continues to receive unwavering support by CCS. It may be added that Ralph W. Moss received the CCS's yearly Humanitarian Award at the meeting. Earlier recipients include Stanislaw R. Burzynski, M.D., Ph.D., Prof. Samuel S. Epstein, M.D., Josef M. Issels, M.D., and O. Carl Simonton, M.D.

Moss also attended the 2005 meeting of ASCO, which he reported on in the August/September 2005 issue of the *Townsend Letter*. Disappointments were recorded for some of the more prominent anticancer drugs: Avastatin®, PTK/ZK®, Gemzar®, Tarceva®, and Herceptin®. The consensus seems to be that patient lifetimes were not significantly extended. As for costs, the older treatment using 5-FU against colon cancer would cost a patient only about $500 over the patent's lifetime, whereas some of the newer drugs could cost $250,000 per patient, although extending lifetimes. (The descriptor "cures" was not used.)

Further returning to the matter of medical censorship, the October 2004 issue of the *Townsend Letter* contains Part 2 of Marcus A. Cohen's series. Cohen speaks of the dogmatic attitude of medicine, highlighting an article by radiation oncologist Samuel Hellman on a history and analysis of cancer management from the late nineteenth century through the last decade of the twentieth century. Titled "Dogma and Inquisition in Medicine," it was published in the April 1, 1993, issue of the journal *Cancer*. The emphasis was on breast cancer, which "was an orderly disease progressing in a contiguous fashion from a primary site by direct extension through the lymphatic vessels to the regional lymph nodes and then to distant sites." The first dogma was that radical mastectomies were the treatment of choice. This was successfully challenged over a period of time, with the observation that there were two types of breast cancer, one treatable by radiation, and the other more surreptitious, involving hidden micrometastases. Thus the new paradigm or dogma in turn involved adjuvant systemic therapies directed at killing these hidden micrometastases. A quote from Hellman is that "Cancer therapy and its success requires skill, courage, and risk taking (again the risks are the patient's).… The medical oncologist now supplants the surgeon as the central figure in cancer management." This was superseded by a still later dogma, with Hellman an originator, that three kinds of breast cancer can occur, each with its own treatment protocol.

Cohen's second article again takes up the subject of peer review, citing a number of instances, particularly as provided by Dr. David Horrobin in the March 9, 1990, issue of the *Journal of the American Medical Association*. Not only stifling publication, peer review kills the research grant process for the innovative investigator. A way around it is to be oblique, that is, to not actually state what is intended.

Lastly, in his second article, Cohen takes up the case of virologist Peter Duesberg (and David Rasnick) of the University of California, mentioned earlier. Duesberg, among others, does not buy the official line on AIDS-HIV, attributing the illness and its consequences to lifestyle and treatment with highly immunosuppressive chemotherapy. Cohen concludes with the remark, attributed to Horrobin, above, about not knowing whether an investigator is right or wrong: "I do know that he deserves a hearing."

In Part 3, Cohen focuses on the American Cancer Society and its blacklist of alternative therapies. For starters, he cites an article by Andrew Vickers titled "Alternative Cancer Cures: 'Unproven' or 'Disproven'?" in the March/April 2004 issue of *CA — A Cancer Journal for Clinicians*, a publication of the American Cancer Society. Vickers is described as an Assisting Attending Research Methodologist at Memorial Sloan-Kettering Cancer Center. Asserting that "many alternative cancer treatments have been investigated in good quality clinical trials," Vickers states that the label "unproven" as formerly used should therefore be replaced by "disproven." However, soon after the War on Cancer was declared in 1971, a certain high-ranking insider at the National Cancer Institute, Dr. Dean Burk, criticized the same NCI for a "widespread but scientifically unjustified scorn of searches for truly nontoxic efficacious anticancer compounds, as distinguished from merely less toxic, more efficacious anticancer compounds." (Cohen notes that the ACS has included a number of these "truly nontoxic" alternatives on its blacklist.) Burk further criticized the ACS's "Unproven Methods of Cancer Treatment" as unsupported by little evidence other than the usual refrain that, "After careful study of the literature and other information available to it, the American Cancer Society has found no evidence that treatment … results in any objective benefit in … human cancer." It was characterized by Burk as a statement of "zero scientific worth" although of much propaganda value. The ACS blacklist was recently retitled as "Complementary and Alternative Methods," but Cohen remains skeptical, citing ACS's "self-appointed mission — to help set priorities in research and policy."

In turn, Cohen traces the origins of the American Cancer Society to its roots as the American Society for the Control of Cancer (ASCC), originally funded by John D. Rockefeller, Jr. A history has been provided by Ralph W. Moss in his *The Cancer Industry*, and by James T. Patterson in *The Dread Disease: Cancer and Modern American Culture*. Originally composed of the wealthy elite, the ASCC was taken over by a group skilled in promoting charitable fund-raising, to become the American Cancer Society. The ascendancy of the ACS tied in with other scientific and technical advances, but the hope and hype remain unrealized. As a science writer once put it in comparing the development of the atomic bomb and cancer treatment: "The basic principles of atomic fission had been discovered in Germany long before we had laid out a nickel for the Manhattan Project. The basic principles of the insidious biological fission we call cancer, however, are still among the unknowns."

In Part 4, Cohen again takes on the American Cancer Society. He first notes the ACS policy of withholding information about therapies that might prove beneficial to cancer victims, especially those who have intractable forms of the disease. He also notes that the ACS's blacklist is only one avenue of how the society influences cancer care. Thus, its funding campaigns and lobbying for greater government are a way to influence and control cancer research priorities. Furthermore, the ACS employs scare tactics to keep public funding rolling into the ACS, citing what has been called the "weapon of fear." There have also been inflated cancer "cure" rates, thus coupling good news with bad, another way to keep the "money pump" going for cancer research — and a way to keep on the good side of the National Cancer Institute by pushing for ever greater NCI budgets. The War on Cancer was an ACS brainchild, and further swelled the NCI budgets. Nevertheless, there have been critiques by individuals and organizations, within and without, notably by Dean Burk of the NCI and by Ralph Moss, formerly of Sloan-Kettering, and by the Cancer Control Society. Burk noted in particular that the optimistic statements on cure rates by both the ACS and NCI were seldom backed up by statistical or epidemiological data. Back in 1975 article by science writer Daniel Greenberg appeared in the *Columbia Journalism Review*. "Today's patient, who is supposedly the beneficiary of the burgeoning of cancer research that began in the early 1950s, has approximately the same chance of surviving for at least five years as a patient whose illness was diagnosed before any of that research took place." A later review appeared in the May 18, 1996, issue of *The Lancet*, written by Dr. Michael Sporn, who was in charge of chemoprevention at NCI, and who outlined the complexity of cancer, a complexity requiring new approaches to treatment. An article by Dr. Daniel Groopman that appeared in the June 4, 2001, issue of *The New Yorker*, asked, "The Thirty Year's War: Have We Been Fighting Cancer the Wrong Way?" These misgivings were confirmed in interviews with past directors of the NCI. Generally speaking, as per the ACS blacklist, the protocol is to omit or downgrade positive results and amplify negative results.

(One suspects that it will take a dramatic, irrefutable breakthrough in treatment — the "magic bullet" — to turn things around. Given the mindset of organized medicine in the United States, this breakthrough may have to come from abroad, and even then may not be acknowledged.)

It may therefore be observed that some of the substances listed in Table 8.2 and Table 8.3 are employed in what may be called medical folklore, that is, in the arena of complementary and alternative medicine (CAM). A listing is as follows: camptothecin, curcumin, melatonin, vitamin A analogs, colchicines, paclitaxels, several of the vinca alkaloids, and acetylsalicylic acid, as well as ascorbic acid or vitamin C, β-carotene, a certain gallate compound from green tea, folic acid, lycopene from tomatoes, conjugated linoleic acid, quercetin, resveratrol, sodium selenite, and α-tocopherol or vitamin E.

Some further comments include the fact that resveratrol has been extensively studied at the University of Illinois at Chicago, an institution that is said to have the broadest-based chemoprevention drug discovery program in the world. (Information about resveratrol is also provided by Hoffman, 1999a, p. 214). Some 2500 natural substances have been tested under the direction of pharmacy professor John Pezzuto (who is cited elsewhere as coauthor with Mathew Suffness of a chapter in *Methods in Plant Biochemistry*, Vol. 6, *Assays for Bioactivity*, pp. 72ff, 116). This anticancer substance (resveratrol) has been identified in over 70 plant species, notably in red-grape skins (and in red wine), but also in mulberries and peanuts.

As for the action of vitamin C, and the work of Linus Pauling and Ewan Cameron, and of Abram Hoffer, the work of Hugh Riordan is also of special note. Dr. Riordan, of Wichita, Kansas, was recognized as a world leader on the injection of megadoses of vitamin C against cancer. This work is carried out at the Center for the Improvement of Human Functioning International, 3100 North Hillside Avenue, Wichita KS 67219, (316) 682-3100, with Phase I clinical trials at the University of Nebraska Medical School Hospital, and Phase II clinical trials under the auspices of the National Institutes of Health. (The acronym for the center is RECNAC, which is Cancer spelled backwards.)

For additional information, reference may be made to the volume by Life Extension Foundation (2003). It should also be mentioned that this volume has the following chapter or section titles: "Cancer: Overview of Protocols; Cancer Adjuvant Therapies;" "Cancer Chemotherapy;" "Cancer: Clinics Offering Alternative Therapies;" and "Cancer: Gene Therapies, Stem Cells, Telomeres, and Cytokines." There are also chapters or sections titled "Cancer Prevention; Cancer Radiation Therapy;"

"Cancer: Should Patients Take Dietary Supplements?;" "Cancer Surgery; Cancer Treatment: The Critical Factors; and Cancer Vaccines."

Of special interest here is the information presented in "Cancer: Clinics Offering Alternative Therapies." A listing follows:

*Aloe vera (a glyconutrient):* This work is carried out by H. R. McDaniel, an affiliate of Mannatech Inc. The active ingredients of the aloe plant are said to be eight chains of the mannose sugars: glucose, galactose, mannose, fructose, xylose, *N*-acetylglucosamine, *N*-acetylgalactosamine, and *N*-acetylneuraminic acid. A number of enzymes are also involved: endonucleases, hydrolases, esterases, and lipases. Information is furnished for the purchase of Mannatech *Aloe vera* products.

*Bindweed (an angiogenesis inhibitor):* Studies are under way at RECNAC in Wichita, Kansas, concurrent with studies using vitamin C.

*Antineoplaston therapy:* This was developed by Stanislaw Burzynski, M.D., at his clinic in Houston, TX (and as mentioned elsewhere [e.g., in Chapter 5]). Under scrutiny for years, this therapy boasts some amazing success stories for certain kinds of cancer. The current address given in the listing is 9432 Old Katy Road, Ste 200, Houston TX 77055, 713-335-5697. (An update was furnished in the May 2004 issue of *Life Extension* in an article and interview by Terri Mitchell.) It may be mentioned again that antineoplastons consist of peptides, or polypeptides, signifying relatively short chains of various amino acids linked together. (The longer chains are called proteins.) The particular makeup determines the particular activity for a particular function, including serving as an anticancer agent, for example, as an inhibitor for one or another of the critical enzymes involved in cancer cell metabolism.

*Gonzalez cancer therapy:* Developed by Nicholas Gonzalez, M.D. (now deceased), this therapy is described in terms of proteolytic enzymes, and involves diet, supplements, and detoxification. A contact in New York City is Michelle Gabay, RN, at 212-305-9468, with a Web site located at http://www.dr-gonzalez.com/.

*Radio frequency ablation (RFA):* A titanium electrode is directed to the tumor (using MRI techniques) and enough heat is generated to kill the cancerous cells. The NIH has given its imprimatur for this therapy. For further information contact the M.D. Anderson Cancer Center, Houston, at 713-792-2121 or the University Hospital of Cleveland, at 216-844-1000.

This radiofrequency treatment was in some respects similar to that advocated by Royal Rife, as will be subsequently described.

Another up-to-date source of great interest is Morton Walker's *German Cancer Therapies: Natural and Conventional Medicines That Offer Hope and Healing*, published in 2003, which describes the German protocols. It is stated that a fully documented 88% remission rate has been achieved by doctors in clinics all across Germany. (There are, of course, different degrees of remission, as distinguished from "cures.") These innovative treatments include Polyerga® and Carnivora® therapies, and galvanotherapy, hypothermia, induced remission therapy, and the utilization of Hawaiian noni fruit and the mushroom *Coriolos versicolor*. Moreover, unlike in the United States these therapies are perceived in Germany as mainstream medicine rather than CAM.

Polyerga® therapy utilizes porcine spleen extract that is composed of various peptides, that is, of relatively short-chain proteins. It is noted in the reference that the sole U.S. distributor of Polyerga® is European Lifestyle Products, POB 1345, Gibsonia, PA 15944, 724-934-3068.

The reference partially lists what are called biological immune system enhancement agents, as follows: porcine spleen peptides/Polyerga®; antineoplastins (Burzynski therapy); bovine thymus extract; porcine and bovine liver extracts; phytochemicals; crude bacteria; cytokines; shark cartilage; interferons; colony-stimulating factors; glandular and organ extracts; harvested T-lymphocytes; tumor necrosis factors; gene therapy; alkylglycerols/shark liver oil; antiangiogenesis factors; monoclonal antibodies; human breast milk; dimethyl sulfoxide (DMSO); camphor and organic salts/714X® (Naessen's therapy); homeopathic-potentized nucleic acids; Venus flytrap extracts/Carnivora®; Hansi homeopathic activator; chlorella; sea vegetables; green concentrates; aloe vera; amygdalin/laetrile; genus *Astragalus*; cat's claw/uña de gato; genus *Echinacea*; Essiac; flavonoids; garlic; *Ginkgo biloba*; ginseng/*Panax*; oligomeric proanthocyanidin/OPC®; grape seed extract/Pycnogenol®; green tea/catechins; Haelin® 451; Hoxsey herbs; mistletoe/Iscador®; larch arabinogalactan/Larix®, ARA-6®; maitake mushroom/Grifola®; sodium butyrate; hydrazine sulfate; glutathione/Immunocal®; staphage lysate; Dr Pekar's autologous vaccine; Coley's toxins; immunoaugmentive therapy; TVZ-7 lymphocyte treatment; antimycoplasma autovaccine; enerlein/pleomorphic remedies; melatonin; autologous vaccine; pau d'arco/lapacho; modified citrus pectin; silymarin/milk thistle (*Sylibum mariannum*); turmeric; ukrain; urea; BCG, or bacillus Calmette-Guerin vaccine; T/Tn antigen breast cancer vaccine; immunoplacental therapy; and oxygen therapies. A number of these anticancer agents or treatments are described, for instance, by Moss (1992) and Walters (1993).

The drug known as Carnivora® is derived from Venus flytrap (*Dioneae muscipula* of the Sundew family or Droseraceae). Developed by Helmut G. Keller, M.D., of Nordhalben, Germany, the American contact is Dietmer Schildwachter, M.D., of Southern Consultants International, Inc. (POB 16602, Dulles International Airport, Washington, D.C. 220041, 703-430-7789). It has been employed against cancer by the former well-known physician Robert C. Atkins, M.D., of the Atkins Center in New York City. The reference furnishes a lengthy list of 105 remedial substances that act adjunctively against cancer and other diseases, lending aid and support to cancer patients.

It may be added that there is support from the herbal standpoint in terms of *The Complete German Commission E Monograph*, cited elsewhere.

Lastly, it should also be mentioned that the organization People Against Cancer (Otho, IA at 515-972-4444) has for many years sponsored overseas trips to German clinics.

With regard to turmeric, cited earlier as an immune system enhancement agent, and a spice used in curry, curcumin (or turmeric), the bright yellow active ingredient, is an anticancer agent. Thus, it is of great interest that a news item on page 8 in the September 1, 2003, issue of *Chemical & Engineering News* (*C&EN*), a weekly news journal of the American Chemical Society, is titled "How Curry Combats Cancer." The article reports on work conducted at Sejong University, Seoul, by bioscience professor Ho Jeong Kwon and associates in which curcumin was found to act as an inhibitor for the enzyme aminopeptidase N, or APN. (The peptidases are ordinarily involved in the digestion of proteins, including aminopeptidases, as per p. 43 in Hoffman, 1999.) The enzyme APN favors tumor invasiveness and angiogenesis, the growth of blood vessels in cancerous tissue. Curcumin was in fact one of some 3000 substances screened for activity against APN, and was found the most promising. Thus, this inhibition of angiogenesis by curcumin — an inhibition described as direct and irreversible — is an important development, and curcumin is now undergoing Phase I clinical trials against colon cancer. Not only can curcumin be taken orally, there are apparently no adverse side effects.

As a further benefit, a letter from Wayne Martin in the April 2004 *Townsend Letter for Doctors & Patients* observes that curcumin prevents blood clots.

Central to any discussion is the role of enzymes, the proteinaceous compounds that act as selective catalysts for the myriad biochemical reactions that take place in the body and, in fact, in all living organisms. By and large, there is but a single enzyme that catalyzes each particular biochemical reaction, although other substances may be involved. Also central are enzyme inhibitors, each of which serves to block or regulate a certain biochemical reaction, notably those that are disease causing. (And a given substance may act as an inhibitor for more than one biochemical reaction, the phenomenon of side effects or adverse side effects.) The notable examples are the antibiotics, which block certain critical enzymes necessary for bacterial metabolism and structure. Thus, enzyme inhibitors have in fact been described as the basis of modern medicine.

Then, there looms the problem that there is so often a huge time gap between cause and effect, between inception and diagnosis, compounded by the time lag from therapy to cure (i.e., remission), if any. There is the dilemma of whether the therapy protocol is indeed working, or has worked, not to mention what all brought on the cancerous condition in the first place.

## CONTROVERSIES

Sometimes, even Nobel Prize winners are dragged into controversy. Thus, Otto Warburg, who won in physiology-medicine in 1931 for his work on the nature and action of respiratory enzymes and who earlier had elucidated the metabolism of cancer cells, met with objections, as did Albert Szent-Györgyi, who won the Nobel Prize in 1937 for his work on biological combustion, and who earlier had discovered vitamin C. Both have been the subject of books.

According to Macfarlane (1985), there is also controversy about Alexander Fleming's prominence, when most of the work in developing penicillin was done by Howard Florey, assisted by Ernst Boris Chain. Reviewing this controversy, Fleming admittedly discovered penicillin in 1928 and duly reported its action (which may have been erroneous), but let the subject lie dormant for the next 12 years. (Penicillin in its pure state is a chemical compound, and its name is derived from its source, the pencil-shaped fungus or mold genus *Penicillium*.) In the meantime, Howard Florey, an Australian who had come to England on a Rhodes Scholarship, saw the great potential, and he and his associates worked unceasingly to bring it to fruition. Then Fleming stepped in again with "his" penicillin to reap by far the lion's share of publicity, although he ended up sharing a 1949 Nobel Prize with both Florey and Chain. A more popular account is furnished by André Maurois in *The Life of Sir Alexander Fleming: Discoverer of Penicillin* (Dutton, New York, 1959). A more recent account is Eric Lax's *The Mold in Dr. Florey's Coat: The Story of the Penicillin Miracle* (Holt, New York, 2004).

As has been indicated, Fleming's original interest was in lysozymes, as was Florey's. These turned out to be enzymes present in mucus that act against bacteria, as in the mucus secreted in the nose from the mucous membranes. A parallel discovery was that a vitamin A deficiency caused mucous secretions to cease in the intestine, which was then followed by an invasion of virulent bacteria into intestinal tissues (Macfarlane, 1985, p. 161). An item of peripheral interest is that curare, a poisonous mixture of alkaloids derived from plants of the South American genus *Strychnos*, acts against tetanus (Macfarlane, 1985, p. 163).

(The foregoing may be an indirect way in which vitamin A protects against cancer, as intestinal flora or bacteria are associated with the production of carcinogenic substances.)

It was originally thought that penicillin might be an enzyme, but it turned out that it acts instead as an enzyme inhibitor. Along the way, there was a developing interest in using synthetic dyes as antibacterial agents, in particular, one with the trade name Prontosil, which, interestingly, was effective in the body but not in cultures (Macfarlane, 1985, p. 148). The latter is sometimes a problem in assaying bioactive substances (which illustrates inconsistencies that may occur in projecting from *in vitro* to *in vivo* experiments to clinical trials, and back again). The foregoing led to the development of sulfonamides, the first generation of chemotherapy agents, but penicillin proved far more effective against bacteria. Enter Florey, who along with Fleming, incidentally, was highly critical of orthodox viewpoints (Macfarlane, 1985, p. 155). Another fact of interest is that Peter B. Medawar joined Florey's group, and shared a Nobel Prize in 1960 for his work on tissue immunity, which laid the foundations for modern transplant surgery (Macfarlane, 1985, p. 167).

The reference further mentions that it turned out the enzymatic action of lysozymes was to break down an essential polysaccharide $N$-acetyl glucosamine in the bacteria cell wall (MacFarlane, 1985, p.168). Among the oddities later found in testing penicillin was that it was toxic to guinea pigs but not to humans (Macfarlane, 1985, p. 184). Thus if *in vivo* testing with guinea pigs had been tried first, it is very likely that the therapeutic or clinical application of penicillin would have been delayed or abandoned, another example of the perplexities of assaying bioactive substances. As it was, a penicillin mixture was tried clinically at the very outset of testing. Subsequently it was found that the action of penicillin is not against mature cells, but occurs only after they have divided (Macfarlane, 1985, p. 246). The penicillin blocks or inhibits the synthesis of compounds in the young bacteria cells necessary to build the cell walls. The specific enzymes blocked have since been determined — after the fact.

Further information about the discovery and development of penicillin is furnished in *Cures Out of Chaos* by M. Lawrence Podolsky, M.D. A principal bottleneck during the development was growing enough of the antibiotic for clinical trials. This was eventually solved in the United States, but the U.S. developers took the credit, the patents, and the money. Podolsky notes that the English never capitalized on the successes. (Podolsky's book is a highly readable goldmine of other information about the course of medicine.)

It appears that what is needed in the War on Cancer is the unique few with the determination and altruism of Florey and Chain and associates.

It has been mentioned that fewer than half the doctors in the United States have been reported to be connected in some way with the American Medical Association, or AMA — sometimes called a trade union — with the proportion further dropping from a high in years past of about 90%. As cited elsewhere, the subject has been explored by Howard Wolinsky and Tom Brune in *The Serpent on the Staff: The Unhealthy Politics of the American Medical Association*, published in 1994. Perhaps in consequence, the word is that medicine is evolving from "pill pushing" to what is sometimes called alternative or complementary or holistic medicine. Up to now, if an antibiotic or a shot or an operation wouldn't do it, the patient was in trouble — so what are the alternatives?

There continues to be talk of alternative medicine, therefore, with a revolution in the infrastructure, as was anticipated, for instance, by George Howe Colt in the September 1996 issue of *Life*. Thus, as has been noted, medical schools are starting to get on board, offering courses in alternative medicine, with even the AMA advocating that maybe its members should learn more about this phenomenon.

(It may again be noted that in 1992 the AMA published *The Reader's Guide to Alternative Health Methods* which, as previously commented, is said to have used the word "quack" 209 times. And we may add that a doctor's life is not necessarily a bed of roses, and is downright miserable sometimes, what with life-or-death situations, long and erratic hours even without home calls, patient–doctor confrontations, malpractice worries, and trying to keep up with the latest in medicine. The prestige and the pay, as good as it may be, may seem hardly worth it.)

However, in the meantime ... organized medicine considers home treatment — and even house calls — *verboten* and has been succeeded by high tech. Hospitals and medical centers have become gigantic, propelled by the medical insurance industry and government Medicare, not to mention HMOs. But it may be added that the patient still pays the difference between what is charged and what is allowed by insurance. There are a few wags who say that on the average this difference amounts only to what we as individuals would be paying if the country had never heard of medical insurance — private or government. Insurance or not, among the more deadly concerns is a lack of success with treating and curing cancer.

Thus, take the War on Cancer. Since its inception back in 1971, perhaps about $50 billion has been spent on research, with very little to show. (Surgery, radiation, and chemotherapy remain the big three — sometimes called "cut, burn, and poison" — and are at times successful if the cancer hasn't spread or metastasized. Conversely, these treatments in themselves may cause the cancer to spread. Even biopsies are under suspicion.) No sure-fire absolute cure has been found, and the battle plan can be viewed as more of a medical researchers' relief fund, as previously indicated. If this appellation appears outrageous, then where is the cure?

If the preceding assessment seems overstated, consider the accomplishments, or lack thereof, of various federal programs, agencies, or departments, that is, the bureaucracy, and all the machinations that go on, especially if businesses that is, corporations, may be involved. Altruism is not your common, everyday, primordial instinct. (As has been set in concrete, altruism plus some loose change is worth the price of a cup of coffee.) Not to mention that about 15–20,000 articles or publications dealing with cancer enter the literature each year — and still no sure-fire cures. In the meantime, mortality is approaching 600,000 deaths per year, with the case load per unit population said to be increasing with perhaps 1.5 million or whatever new cases appearing annually.

With regard to business volume, the cancer treatment industry can be understated at $100 billion and more per year (or up to nearly $200 billion per year, everything included). There was at one time perhaps $10 billion or so going for cytotoxic (cell-toxic) chemotherapy alone, as supplied in Ralph W. Moss's *Questioning Chemotherapy* (Equinox Press, Brooklyn, NY, 1995, p. 75). Now, double this. If these figures seem out of line, consider that perhaps the 1.5 million new cancer cases divided into, say, $200 billion averages out to $133,000 per case per year. For it is nothing to run up combined medical bills of $100,000 and more, or much more, in hardly any time at all — especially if the patient is insured. It's a veritable gravy train. So, one may ask, outside of the poor patient and the patient's family, who wants a cancer cure, especially an inexpensive, off-the-shelf cure? And such (expensive) treatments as are offered are too often only a palliative, especially so in the case of conventional cell-toxic chemotherapy.

(Later figures indicate that the moneys spent on cancer and its treatment constitute about one fourth of all medical outlays, which as of the year 2000 were an estimated one trillion dollars annually and, in fact, going as high as $1.3 trillion. Not only this, but the death rate from cancer in the United States has been estimated even as high as 750,000 per year, and worldwide at about some 6 million per year. These figures of course revolve around the issue of primary cause vs. secondary cause.)

As has been cited elsewhere, Ralph Moss had previously covered this ground in *The Cancer Industry: Unraveling the Politics* (Paragon House, New York, 1989; a revision of the previously published *The Cancer Syndrome*, Grove, New York, 1980). Later books by Moss noted elsewhere include *Antioxidants Against Cancer* and *Herbs Against Cancer: History and Controversy*. The latter reviews in comprehensive fashion the effectiveness, or lack thereof, of a number of the more-publicized treatments such as Hoxsey therapy, Essiac tea, the so-called grape cure, and still other treatments. Both Hoxsey therapy and Essiac tea, for instance, utilize mixtures of herbs, a protocol advocated in Swerdlow's *Nature's Medicine*. Another "underground" treatment, presumably of American Indian origins and cited herein on several occasions, is that so-called Compound-X, which also uses a mixture of herbs or plants, including most likely bloodroot (*Sanguinaria canadensis*) and possibly goldenseal (*Hydrastis canadensis*) together with maybe creosote bush (*Larrea tri-dentata* or *L. divaricata*), also called chaparral, or greasewood. All three species have been touted as treatments in themselves. The judgment is also mixed, with medical orthodoxy mostly turning thumbs down.

The rise and fall of Harry Hoxsey was detailed in Kenny Ausubel's *When Healing Becomes a Crime: The Amazing Story of the Hoxsey Cancer Clinics and the Return of Alternative Therapies*. (Ausubel also made an award-winning video about Hoxsey and his cancer treatment.) Ausubel detailed information about the machinations that have gone on (and are still going on) within the world of medicine. His book has an introduction by Bernie Siegel, M.D., and is further endorsed by other prominent names: Larry Dossey, M.D.; Mark Blumenthal of the American Botanical Council; Andrew Weil, M.D.; botanist James Duke; Ralph Moss; Samuel Epstein, M.D. All are well-known names in the field of complementary and alternative medicine (CAM).

Ausubel mentions therapies such as Krebiozen, the Gerson diet, Essiac tea, Coley's Toxins, the Hoxsey Therapy, and Stanislaw Burzynski's antineoplastons, etc., a number of which are further described, for instance, by Moss (1992) and Walters (1993). These therapies have all been involved in government-led prosecutions.

(The details of another round of government-led persecutions are furnished in attorney Ellen Brown's *Forbidden Medicine*, about a certain Jimmy Keller, who advocated and prescribed a tonic containing L-arginine, with backup testimonials of its anticancer actions.)

The subject of angiogenesis can be introduced, as per the work of Judah Folkman, M.D., and coworkers. Also of interest is the macrobiotic diet, as per the Kushi Institute, which in many respects parallels the Gerson diet, emphasizing vegetarianism. Of recent vintage is Verne Varona's *Nature's Cancer-Fighting Foods*, and *Comprehensive Cancer Care: Integrating Alternative, Complementary, and Conventional Therapies* by James S. Gordon, M.D., and Sharon Curtin — the latter book also pertaining to an annual conference dealing with the mind-body medicine approach. (Another annual conference or convention about alternatives is put on by the Cancer Control Society, as mentioned elsewhere in this Chapter.)

And not to be overlooked is *Vitamin C and Cancer: Discovery, Recovery, Controversy* by Abram Hoffer, M.D., Ph.D., a former associate of Linus Pauling. In an interview and update in the January 2003 issue of *Life Extension*, Hoffer mentions successes using niacin and vitamin C, a treatment originally used effectively against schizophrenia.

Some more recent books about complementary and alternative medicine include the *Essentials of Complementary and Alternative Medicine*, and a series of volumes forthcoming on *Alternative Medicine® Review, Monographs*. The first-mentioned is edited by Wayne B. Jonas, M.D., former director of the former Office of Alternative Medicine within NIH, and Jeffrey S. Levin.

Another polemic that can be found, this time on the Internet, is under the aegis of *Liberty For All: Online Magazine*, dated February 8, 2002, and titled "The Cancer Racket," by Gavin Phillips. The note is provided that the article was originally published in the February/March issue of *Clamor* magazine under the title "Can You

Trust Your Doctor?" Several alternative treatments are first discussed, which are variously presented by Moss (1992) and Walters (1993). A listing of section headings in Phillips' article starts with three case studies: Royal Raymond Rife, amygada-lin/laetrile, and the Hoxsey remedies. This is followed by background histories and updates for "Mainstream Medicine vs. Alternative Treatments," "The Establish-ment," "The National Cancer Institute," "The American Cancer Society," "The Fed-eral Drug Administration," "The American Medical Association," and "The War on Cancer." The note is appended that references for the article can be found at http://www.cancerinform.org/refs1.html, with more information at http://www.can-cerinform.org/index.html. The author's quote is furnished at the end, that, "I traveled extensively in my mid-20s. I have an eclectic, insatiable curiosity and constantly question conventional wisdom and the so-called experts. I have found both to be severely wanting."

## HEROIC EFFORTS

The work of Judah Folkman and coworkers, notably Michael O'Reilly, pertains mainly to developing antiangiogenetic drugs or angiogenesis inhibitors that suppress the formation of blood vessels in cancerous tissue. A comprehensive presentation of the last-mentioned heroic efforts is contained in Robert Cooke's *Dr. Folkman's War: Angiogenesis and the Struggle to Defeat Cancer*. The drugs angiostatin and endostatin are featured, which were so successful against cancer in mice but much less so in humans. (Shark cartilage, once the object of much hype as an antiangio-genesis agent, has been reported to be mostly ineffective.) The note is furnished that humans vis-à-vis mice constitute a different proposition when it comes to cancer treatment. "It was true, as Dana Farber's Howard Fine had said, that researchers had been curing cancer in mice for fifty years" (Cooke, 2001, p. 280). Nonetheless, in spite of failures, Dr. Folkman's successes were sometimes stunning, as set forth in chapters 15 and 19 of Cooke's book. Beyond this, however, was a positive spinoff in a different direction, namely the use of angiogenesis per se in the treatment of cardiovascular disease, to stimulate blood vessel growth in the repair of heart and legs (Cooke, 2001, p. 309ff). Cooke writes that Dr. Folkman's work "would pay off first and most dramatically in the battle against cardiovascular disease, rather than cancer." However, it has been on hold.

(The statins include what are variously called angiostatins, endostatins, and exostatins. As recounted on page 367 of Hoffman [1999], the term encompasses plasminogen fragments that are precursors to the plasmin occurring in blood plasma and serum, where plasmin is a proteolytic enzyme that dissolves the fibrin in blood clots. In further explanation, fibrin itself is a protein, ordinarily insoluble, that results in a network of fibers. Some later findings are that statin drugs can have undesirable side effects, namely triggering what is called *transient global amnesia*, or TGA, the inability to originate new memory — as well as causing retrograde memory loss. There are also the more common symptoms of disorientation, confusion, and for-getfulness. An authority on the subject is Duane Gravelin, M.D., who has returned to space medicine research at the Kennedy Space Center. More information can be obtained at www.spacedoc.net.)

Another such heroic effort was described in the previously mentioned article "Vaccinating Against Cancer" by Stephen S. Hall, which appeared in the April 1977 issue of *Atlantic Monthly*, and a concomitant book titled *A Commotion in the Blood: Life, Death, and the Immune System*. The work of German physician Alexander Knuth and Flemish-born and American-educated molecular geneticist Thierry Boon is detailed (e.g., and as also described in Hoffman, 1999, p. 313ff). In brief recapitulation, there are involved cell-surface proteins called major histocompatibility complex (MHC) proteins, which serve as "markers of individuality" and relate to the body's recognizing, and the immune system's attacking, extraneous invasive agents such as viruses — and cancer cells. A German lady known as Frau H. developed a rabid form of skin cancer or melanoma, usually fatal, but her immune system somehow could recognize the cancerous cells with "exquisite specificity" and counteract the cancer.

Cell proteins are cannibalized into peptide fragments, which are displayed by the MHC molecules for the T cells of the immune system to examine for abnormality. The abnormal peptide fragments constitute antigens, to be attacked and destroyed by the antigen-specific T cells. The number of possible combinations or permutations is staggering, given the large polymeric or globular makeup of proteins, with the basic peptide fragment found to consist of a chain of only nine amino acids of different kinds. It was the procedure of the investigators to chop up the DNA from the melanoma cells, dividing it into groups or colonies that would conceivably contain the gene encoding of the antigen activating the T cells. Like the needle in the haystack, in one set of experiments, out of 29,000 colonies tested, only 5 contained the gene encoding for an antigen recognized by the T cells. And each such antigen recognized would connote a different cancer vaccine. The results in clinical trials were mixed, but the work continues. Interestingly, certain body substances act as antigens: the enzyme tyrosinase, for instance, involved in melanoma, and the protein mucin, found in certain breast, colon, and stomach cancers. The spinoff may thus be less complicated approaches for attacking and destroying cancer cells.

(An important aside furnished in Hall's book is that the researchers declined to do a biopsy on the cancerous tissue of Frau H., for fear that this might cause the cancer to spread. This kind of cautious approach has been seconded by several Harvard professors, as reported in the British medical journal *The Lancet*, Vol. 357, pp. 1048, 2001. This further citation was furnished on page 22 of the *Townsend Letter for Doctors & Patients*, July 2001.)

It should be emphasized that there are similarities with Burzynski's antineoplastons, which are said to be peptides. Could these certain peptides in fact serve as the particular antigens recognized by the T cells as described above in Hall's book?

## MORE ABOUT COMPOUND-X AND THE LIKE

According to Ingrid Naiman's *Cancer Salves: A Botanical Approach to Treatment*, there are a number of different versions of Compound-X. Naiman's intriguing investigations focus mainly on salves, as the title indicates, which are designated by the adjective *escharotic*, meaning that the substance is caustic in one way or another, producing a chemical reaction with tissue, and thus destroying cancerous tissue. Bloodroot (*Sanguinaria canadensis* of the Poppy family [Papaveraceae]), for instance, is very active in this manner, whereas goldenseal (*Hydrastis canadensis* of the Buttercup family [Ranuncalaceae]) is much less so. Zinc chloride is commonly used as an additive in herbal salves. Naiman furnishes case studies, even photographs, with Appendix A providing information about the various herbs and Appendix B giving recipes for the more well-known herbal combinations. Although not emphasized, it is mentioned that occasionally some of these mixtures have been taken internally, not to mention their use as herbal suppositories or boluses, say, for colorectal cancer.

Bloodroot contains toxic alkaloids, notably sanguinarine; in fact, all the members of Papaveraceae contain alkaloids. Goldenseal also contains toxic alkaloids, notably hydrastine and berberine. These several alkaloids are viewed as anticancer agents, at least to a degree. In fact, alkaloids are among the most bioactive of naturally derived substances, and this bioactivity is in part reflected in anticancer and other disease-countering properties; hence the descriptor sometimes used, "poisonous and medicinal plants." (Thus, it is said that in evaluating the potential medicinal properties of rain forest plants, for instance, a test for the presence of alkaloids is commonly used as an indicator. Most alkaloids have a unique nitrogen-containing cyclic or ring structure, for which routine tests are available.) It goes almost without saying that the word is caution, or extreme caution, in the internal use of such plants.

Escharotic (caustic) plant substances may be found in seemingly unexpected places, for example, in the plant family Bromeliaceae, or the pineapple family. Thus, the juice of the berries from the Brazilian species *Bromelia arenaria* is used for cleansing malignant sores, destroying the tissue at the same time. This information is found in the *Medicinal Plants of Brazil* by Mors, Rizzinni, and Pereira, edited by DeFillipps, and published in 2000. (This adds to the several volumes containing information about medicinal plants from around the world, as abstracted in Hoffman, 1999.) Interestingly, some of the bromeliads, as members of Bromeliaceae are called, may contain digestive enzymes such as bromelin, which are protein digesting and are otherwise known as proteases.

For the record, the few other potential anticancer plants cited by Mors et al. (2000) include the following, with the plant family listed first followed by the genus and species in parenthesis:

Apocynaceae (*Aspidosperma* * *nigricans*)
Apocynaceae (*Himatanthus* * *sucuuba*)
Aracaceae (*Obignya* * *phalterata*)
Aristoclochiaceae (*Aristolochia* spp.)
Bignoniaceae (*Tabebuia imptetiginosa* and *Tabebuia* spp., some species of which are known as pau d'arco and contain the phenylnaphthoquinone anticancer compound lapachol)
Caesalpiniaceae* (*Copaifera officinalis*)
Fabaceae (*Dalbergia* * *subcymosa*)
Santalaceae (*Jodina* * *rhombifolia*)

The pea family Fabaceae is also known as Leguminosae. Of the preceding plant families, only Caesalpiniaceae is not found in Hartwell's *Plants Used Against Cancer*. Of the genus and species, those cited with an asterisk are not found in Hartwell.

Another volume of similar interest is Leslie Taylor's *Herbal Secrets of the Rainforest: The Healing Power of Over 50 Medicinal Plants You Should Know About*, published in 1998. Also for the record, anticancer plants cited are as follows, here in alphabetical order by plant family (the reference lists the common names in alphabetical order). In parenthesis, the genera and species are italicized, followed by the common name. (The sunflower family Asteraceae occurs as Compositae in many references. The plant family Smilacaceae is more commonly known as the lily family Liliaceae.)

Amaranthaceae (*Pfaffia\* paniculata*, suma)
Annonaceae (*Annona\* muricata*, graviola)
Asteraceae (*Achyrocline\* satureoides*, macela)
Asteraceae (*Baccharis genistelloides\**, carqueja)
Bignoniaceae (*Tabebuia impetiginosa, heptaphylla, avellanedae*, pau d'arco)
Celasteraceae (*Maytenus ilicifolia*, espinephra santa)
Melicaceae (*Carapa\* guianensis*, andiroba)
Polypodiaceae (*Polypodium lepidopteris\*, decumanum\**, samambaia)
Rubiaceae (*Uncaria tomentosa\**, cat's claw or uña de gato)
Smilacaceae (*Smilax officinalis*, sarsaparilla)
Solanaceae (*Brunfelsia\* uniforus, grandiflora*, manacá)
Solanaceae (*Physalis angulata*, mullaca)
Sterculiaceae (*Guasuma\* ulmifolia*, mutamba)

Again, the genus and species designators not appearing in Hartwell are cited with an asterisk, thereby indicating newer information. A listing of phytochemicals or plant chemicals as found in each is included in the reference. Representative phytochemicals are also presented by Hoffman (1999), for example, as variously derived from James A. Duke's previously cited *Handbook of Medicinal Herbs*, *Handbook of Biologically Active Phytochemicals and Their Activities*, and *Handbook of Phytochemical Constituents of GRAS Herbs and Other Economic Plants*.

As for the plant family Annonaceae and the species *Annona\* muricata*, or graviola, cited in the foregoing listing, cancer researcher and author Ralph Moss dealt with the subject in his monthly column "The War on Cancer" in the November 2003 issue of the *Townsend Letter*. Exploring the Internet using the search engine Google, he came up with about 12,300 citations. There were many effusive statements about effectiveness, and many sources to order from, but apparently a dearth (meaning none?) of substantiating clinical trails. There were, presumably test tube, studies using various cancer cell lines that found a much greater potency for graviola than for some standard anticancer drugs such as adriamycin. Howsoever, the usual independent consensus, based on experience, is that test tube or *in vitro* studies (or even *in vivo* studies on mice) do not necessarily translate to clinical effectiveness in humans.

In Leslie Taylor's section concerning pau d'arco, there are comments that adulteration or substitutions are often made. Thus, a main anticancer constituent is the compound lapachol, which may be in concentrations of 2 to 7% in true pau d'arco, whereas other related species may have none. Moreover, in the chemical analysis of 12 commercially available products, only 1 showed even trace amounts. Either substitutions had been made, or there was degradation during processing, transport, and storage. And whereas most research studies have been confined to the heartwood, most commercially available products contain the inner and outer bark of the tree, which is stripped at the sawmills from the ten or so species that are logged. The call is for standardized extracts that guarantee the lapachol and naphthoquinone content.

(Regarding standards and standardization, the German government has become involved in herbal remedies, as per the Commission E recommendations published by the German Federal Department of Health. An English translation was in turn published in 1998 by the American Botanical Council, Austin, Texas, titled *The Complete German Commission E Monograph*. It may be added that the American Botanical Council publishes a newsletter called *HerbalGram* and is affiliated with the Herb Research Foundation of Boulder, Colorado. Also, the council has issued a CD titled "Herbal Remedies," as prepared by T. Brendler, J. Gruenwald, and C. Jaenicke. Information is provided for over 600 plants, including further annotations about dosage levels, side effects, interactions, contraindications, reference sources, etc. The foregoing includes traditional Chinese and Japanese medicine. While on the subject, there is also a *Physicians' Desk Reference for Herbs*, companion to the well-known *Physicians' Desk Reference,* or *PDR*.)

Herbal or plant potency is related to the plant parts, geographical location, soil, climate, seasons, even time of day and other factors (such as processing and storage), obvious and not so obvious. Thus, the same species of plant may be, say, ten times more potent in one area than in another. That is, the bioactive constituents may vary markedly in concentration (and composition). This divergence can to a degree be accommodated by the use of subspecie or subspecies (var.), or other designators to be specified. Another consideration is that attempts to isolate and utilize the active ingredients may be counterproductive. Thus, whereas the raw herbal substance itself may be effective, the act of "dereplicating" the plant extracts to yield and isolate what are thought to be the active ingredients may negate the effectiveness (Teresi, 2002, p. 318).

Part One of Taylor's book is titled "Rainforest Destruction and Survival," which contains chilling information about the rate of destruction, and highlights the fact that more than 25% of the active ingredients for anticancer agents come from organisms found only in the rain forest. It is noted that extensive "bioprospecting" is under way in rain forests by over 100 pharmaceutical companies and several agencies of the U.S. government, including the National Cancer Institute. (As has been indicated, the word is that the screening process first looks for alkaloids, among the most bioactive classes of plant-derived compounds.)

Illustrative of the dedication of botanists in finding new plant species is Mulford B. and Racine Sarasy Foster's *Brazil: Orchid of the Tropics*, published in 1945. Confined mostly to the more southerly coastline of Brazil and its immediate interior, circa the year 1939, the Foster's adventurous search was almost exclusively for bromeliads, although occasional mention was made of the profusion of orchids often occurring along the way. (It is noted that whereas orchids by and large give off scents to attract pollinating insects and hummingbirds, the bromeliads depend on intense colorations. There are exceptions, however, such as the bromeliad Spanish moss, which is an air-sustained epiphyte to boot.) Interestingly, trained botanists can merely look at a plant and give the family, if not the genus and species. It may be added that such searches are mainly for identification purposes, to add to the known body of flora; the medicinal properties are another subject, although mostly associated with folklore.

A relevant technical book, published in 2002, is the *Pharmacodynamic Basis of Herbal Medicine* by pharmacologist Manuchair Ebadi. It is described as building a bridge between Eastern and Western medicine. Ebadi's book first introduces some of the more well-known herbs and their purported curative properties, arranged alphabetically using their common names, from aloe vera to valerian, and follows this with chapters on alternative medicine and herbal therapeutics. The latter chapter contains information on many ancient herbs, ranging from agnus castus and agrimony to yucca, some 150 entries in all. Chapter 3 of the book concerns vitamins and diet. Chapter 8 deals with herbal products for AIDS. Chapter 10 takes up the subject of alkaloids, which are described as being nitrogenous, usually of plant origins, are frequently basic in character, and often have a definite physiological action. (It can be added once more that the nitrogen is generally bonded into a ring-type structure, and alkaloids are most usually designated by the suffix "-ine," which is also used as a suffix for other types of compounds, such as amino acids.)

Among the considerations is the fact that many alkaloids are toxic, or extremely so, capable of producing cardiac arrest or respiratory failure, or both, as well as acting chronically (or even acutely) against other organs such as the kidneys and liver. Similar considerations apply to certain other compounds and classes, such as cardioglycosides. These life-threatening actions depend on dosage level and frequency. Some may also act as abortifacients, so pregnant women must be cautious about taking any herbal substance.

More specifically, Ebadi's later chapters take up select plant families, genera, and species, and associated foods, substances, and compounds in considerable detail, including their effects and properties. For our purposes, those noted to have anticancer effects will be emphasized.

Thus, in Chapter 15 on brussel sprouts, Ebadi observes that vegetables and fruits such as brussel sprouts, cabbage, leeks, citrus, herbs and spices, as well as food ingredients such as antioxidant vitamins, flavonoids, glucosinolates, and organosulfur compounds are considered to be potentially antimutagenic or anticarcinogenic. For instance, brussel spouts and cabbage, of the Cruciferae or Brassicaceae family, contain the class of compounds called glucosinolates, which have been linked to anticancer activity.

(Cruciferous vegetables are so called because their blooms resemble a cross, or Greek cross, and contain other compounds of much interest as anticancer agents. Thus, there is a compound in broccoli called sulforaphane that stimulates so-called phase 2 detoxification enzymes. Ordinarily found only in very low concentrations in the mature plant, the sprouts have been found to have much higher concentrations. Another that shows up is chlorophyllin, said to neutralize dietary mutagens. Still another anticancer agent present is called I3C, for indole-3-carbinol. The Life Extension Foundation — publishers of the health journal or magazine *Life Extension* — markets concentrates of some of these reported cancer-fighting substances such as curcumin and lycopene, etc. There is a listing in their catalog under the heading of "Cancer Adjuvant Therapies" CLA or conjugated linoleic acid, I3C or indole-3-carbinol, L-theanine, pecta-sol, phyto-food, pork pancreas enzymes, SE-methylselenocysteine, super CLA W/guarana, ultra soy extract, etc.)

In Chapter 18, Ebadi discusses the antioxidative properties of the spices capsicum, rosemary, and turmeric, along with the well-known antioxidants that are the tocopherols (vitamin E), β-carotene, and ascorbic acid (vitamin C), with the observation that anticancer properties exist.

(Nutritionist Jean Carper, who contributes a weekly column titled "EatSmart" in *USA Weekend*, states that turmeric, a constituent of curry powder, is an anticancer agent. In her column in the November 8–10, 2002, issue, she mentions that turmeric contains high concentrations of the potent antioxidant curcumin. Used successfully *in vitro* and *in vivo* against prostate cancer, the speculation is that curcumin blocks the activation of cancer-causing genes, and may do the same for breast and colon cancers. It is also reported to act against arthritic inflammation, and may have a beneficial effect on Alzheimer's. Other herbs and effects mentioned are ginger for inflammation, oregano against germs, and cinnamon for diabetes.)

Ebadi's Chapter 19 takes up the class of compounds known as carotenoids, which are known to reduce the risk of prostate cancer, breast cancer, and head and neck cancers. Carotenoids are pigments ranging from yellow to deep red, as found in many common vegetables and fruits, including carrots, leading to the present-day recommendation to consume colorful fruits and vegetables.

In Ebadi's Chapter 23, the plant family Compositae or Asteraceae is said to contain members that have antitumor action. Among the classes of compounds present are the sesquiterpene lactones (SQLs), associated with antitumor activity, for example, the substance known as parthenin.

The subject of flavonoids is taken up in Ebadi's Chapter 29, some of which are said to be effective against breast cancer. Various subclasses are listed, and their antioxidant properties are noted, along with their role as enzyme inhibitors. The chemical compound quercetin is singled out as among the most active, and it is commonly found in onion, apples, kale, red wine, and green/black teas. A reduced risk of not only of breast cancer, but also of prostate, lung, colon, and stomach cancers is associated with an increased intake of fruits, vegetables, and soy products.

Other conclusions in Ebadi's book are as follows:

- A chapter on green and black teas notes their antineoplastic or anticancer effect, explainable in terms of antioxidant properties. There is also an apparent effect against various skin cancers.
- Tomatoes are singled out in another chapter, along with the predominant carotenoid compound lycopene, which is a notable tumor suppressant.

- Olives and olive oil are associated with a lower cancer incidence in the Mediterranean area.
- Onion and garlic are notable anticancer foods.
- Saffron, as derived from *Crocus sativus*, is noted to have antitumor effects, presumably due to the presence of caretonoids.

Chapter 55 of Ebadi's book takes up the latest on Taxol® (paclitaxel) as an anticancer agent. It is derived from the bark of the Western yew tree (*Taxus brevifolia* of the family Taxaceae). The same chapter also discusses other cancer chemotherapy agents, including alkylating agents such as nitrogen mustards, antimetabolites such as flurouracil, and natural products such as the vinca alkaloids (vinblastine, vincreistine, and vindesine, which are used against blood-related cancers. (The vinca alkaloids were first derived from the Madagascar periwinkle.) Also, such antibiotics as dactinomycin, mithramycin, daunorubicin and doxorubicin, and bleomycin are considered. (There are still other anticancer antibiotics, but which are too deadly to use.) Other miscellaneous anticancer agents include asparaginase (Elspar), hydroxyurea, *cis*-platinum (cisplatin), carboplatin, procarbazine, and etoposide. Side effects are noted.

Less technical is the *Natural Health Bible*, edited by Steven Bratman and David Kroll (1999), which discusses many of the more common herbs, as well as vitamins and minerals. Significant phytochemicals are also emphasized. Steven Bratman, M.D., has a private practice in Fort Collins, Colorado, and David Kroll is a professor of pharmacology and toxicology at the University of Colorado. The book is part of The Natural Pharmacist Series, whose Web site is www.TNP.com. The title page annotation is that the book is an A–Z guide to 200 herbs, vitamins, and supplements. The subject of cancer is given attention, but only with respect to prevention (reducing the risk) rather than cure (the latter being a touchy subject sometimes and maybe better left alone).

## AN UPDATE ON NEWS AND VIEWS

This section describes relevant books, some of which were already mentioned in earlier chapters. Thus, a book that paralleled Moss's *Cancer Industry*, also titled *Cancer Syndrome*, was Samuel S. Epstein's *The Politics of Cancer* (Sierra Club Books, San Francisco, 1978; Anchor/Doubleday, New York, 1979). Epstein, an M.D., has made several subsequent forays into the subject, including *Preventing Breast Cancer* (Macmillan, New York, 1998). An update is furnished in Epstein's *The Politics of Cancer Revisited* (East Ridge Press USA, Fremont Center, NY, 1998). In the same genre is Robert N. Proctor's *Cancer Wars: What We Know and Don't Know About Cancer* (Basic Books, New York, 1995). Michael Lerner attempted an objective comparison of therapies in *Choices in Healing: The Best of Conventional and Complementary Approaches to Cancer* (MIT Press, Cambridge, MA, 1994). A 1116-page compendium with the premise that cancer can be reversed is *An Alternative Medicine Definitive Guide to Cancer* (Future Medicine Publishing, Puyallup, WA, 1997). In substantiation, information is provided about the treatments and successes of several well-known M.D.s. A catchall buzzword increasingly used is "energy medicine," another name for alternative therapies consisting variously of energy and magnetic fields, herbals, homeopathy, acupuncture, etc.

(The subject of homeopathy is mostly treated with contempt in medical orthodoxy, although some astounding cures are reported, questionable or not. In any event, minute concentrations of sometimes-toxic materials in a tincture or solution [or emulsion or suspension] are used. The particular prescription may be based on the idea of "signatures" in which there is thought to be some kind of similarity, say, physical, between the illness and the herb used. This particular idea aside, there is also the very real possibility that the low-level toxicity stimulates the immune system but without overtly or fatally toxic results. Thus, there is the phenomenon given the technical name *hormesis* whereby environmental contaminants at low or very low levels can act or react or interact favorably with the body. In other words, such toxicity-caused cellular insults stimulate the body's defense system. An example is the use of small amounts of arsenic in the feed to put a spring in the step and a shine on the coat of horses, as described in a chapter of Ben Green's *Horse Trading'* — but which later becomes counterproductive, since increased doses are required, which became toxic. Other examples may be bathing where the water is sulfurous, mineral-laden, or slightly radioactive, or even sitting in caves where there is radioactive radon. The subject is in flux and is, of course, controversial.)

Additionally, Robert N. Proctor has written *The Nazi War on Cancer* (Princeton University Press, Princeton, NJ, 1999). Among the items reported is that Nazi scientists were the first to link smoking and cancer. Other policies and discoveries that predated the rest of the world were healthier workplaces, restrictions against asbestos, pesticides, and food additives, as well as improvements in diet and lifestyles. (Nevertheless, there are reports that Hitler was addicted to sugar and sweets.) This contrasts sharply with the unmentionable atrocities of inhuman medical experiments and the death camps.

Ralph Moss's name continues to surface with regard to innovative cancer treatments. For instance, he was interviewed by Lily Giambarba Casura in the January 1998 issue of the *Townsend Letter for Doctors & Patient*. Among other things it was mentioned that Moss's newsletter *The Cancer Chronicles* has been switched entirely over to the Internet, and in fact Moss has written *Alternative Medicine Online: A Guide to Natural Remedies on the Internet* (Equinox Press, Brooklyn, NY, 1997). This takes some of the chore out of searching the Internet for information about cancer, for instance.

A review of the cancer situation according to the medical establishment was carried in the November 7, 1997, issue of *Science*, published by the American Academy for the Advancement of Science, or AAAS. Consisting of both news items and technical articles, it is in many ways a review of the same, as indicated on the editorial page. A criticism leveled in this issue of *Science* is that there has not been a sufficient emphasis on chemoprevention. Nevertheless, within all the commotion, the indication is that some important work is going on — if it can only be carried to fruition, that is, to a cure.

Another news item confirms that animal studies are of limited value, in that humans and animals react differently to drugs. It is the old story that *in vitro* results cannot necessarily be translated to *in vivo* results, which in turn cannot necessarily be translated to clinical results. A homily provided is that animal studies have resulted in "good mouse drugs rather than good human drugs." Even xenografts, which involve the transplantation of human tumor cells into mice, are unreliable.

A reading of the preceding series of news items and articles indicates that the investigations are mostly limited to synthetic chemicals rather than plant-derived substances, with pharmaceutical companies being heavily involved. However, if biotechnology is a business proposition, it is nevertheless a risky one. The statistic is supplied that for 1400 biotechnology companies located in North America, fewer that 50 products have been successfully commercialized. The quote is added that biotech is "one of the worst investments on the street."

As far as cancer treatment per se is concerned, the trouble is that no one still knows exactly what is "best." The remark continues to be made in the preceding news items that the best available strategies for tumors are to "poison them, burn them, or cut them out." Unfortunately, these treatments are overtly invasive — so-called blunt instruments. And furthermore, as Michael Lerner stated in his book *Choices in Healing*, after examining the cancer therapy situation worldwide, no positive, sure-fire, absolute cures were found, alternative or otherwise. Although alternative or complementary therapies sometimes work, and conventional therapies sometimes work, especially if the cancer has not metastasized, nothing can be guaranteed. A similar conclusion may be reached in reading the books by Moss or Walters, where the emphasis, necessarily, is on treatments, not cures. Although some cures are described, if that is the word, failures are also noted. What is needed, obviously, is a near-absolute cure, which may very well be of a biochemical nature, that is, will involve the biological and chemical reactions or interactions occurring in the body. In particular, we're speaking of the metabolism of cancer cells compared to normal cells, and of the selective inhibiting effect of certain substances on cancer cell biochemistries, without adverse side effects.

Without belaboring the point, there are also credibility problems within the scientific and bureaucratic communities, as spelled out in Rodney Barker's *And the Waters Turned to Blood: The Ultimate Biological Threat* (Simon & Schuster, New York, 1997). Barker's book is about the coastal marine dinoflagellate called *Pfiesteria* or *Pfiesteria piscicida*, of the same family as the "red tides," which are of a different species named *Gymnodinium breve*. The book is also about this marine organism's discoverer, JoAnn Burkholder of North Carolina State University, and of her trials in trying to do something about this lethal threat. This particular marine organism, in its metamorphic state existing more as either plantlike or animal-like, not only kills fish and shellfish, but adversely affects humans. Thus, skin contact with its toxins produces lesions and a sloughing off of tissue in the fashion of a brown recluse spider bite. Furthermore, there is a neurotoxic effect upon breathing the vapors, which causes memory loss and confusion, with the eventual possibility of death, directly or indirectly. Besides being responsible for extensive fish kills, it is a serious health hazard to the fishermen involved. Burkholder's subsequent investigations seemed to be blocked from every angle, notwithstanding widespread public and media interest, and considerable support from some of her peers. Burkholder, how-ever, at times looks at the situation philosophically, borrowing from one of the Nick Adams stories by Ernest Hemingway (Barker, 1997, p. 113). The death of a scientist was described by a colleague as a terrible loss to science. To which the scientist's son responded, "Oh, science took it very well."

This immense dollar outlay for cancer treatment is no doubt good business, and good for business, part of the gross national product or gross domestic product, whatever it is called and however it is calculated. Alternative herbal or plant-derived treatments are discouraged in the United States, no doubt as undesirable competition, unlike in Europe, where alternative treatments are used successfully. (In Swiss medicine, as previously noted, an alpine sunflower/yucca extract is used routinely and successfully against melanoma, a line of research initiated by now-retired University of Wyoming chemistry professor Owen Asplund.) And there is inside talk of musical chairs among the personnel of the Food and Drug Administration, the National Institutes of Health (home of the National Cancer Institute), and the drug or pharmaceutical companies, not to mention the involvement of the world financial community. Given this kind of institutional and financial clout, there is absolutely no prospect of an investigation by Congress or the administration; nor even a serious look by mainline investigative journalism, nor airings by TV talk programs, considering that companies or corporations own so much of the media, and in turn have interlocking connections with other segments of industry and finance.

Among the venoms — whether or not of interest in anticancer studies — a mention of brown recluse spider (BRS) bites (or envenomations) brings to mind that this, along with other ailments and treatments, can be searched on the Internet. Thus, for example, there is the site http://www.emedicine.com/EMERG, which lists "bites, insect" — and, more specifically, as topic 547.htm. The author is Thomas Arnold, M.D., of the Louisiana Poison Control Center at Louisiana State University, with a host of prominent M.D.s serving as editors. Several modes of treatment are listed, with due note taken of side effects: antibiotics, such as dapsone (Avlosulfone); corticosteroids, for example, methylprednisolone (Solu-Medrol) and prednisone (Deltasone, Orasone, Meticorten); and antihistamines, such as diphenhydramine (Brenadryl). There are several species of brown recluse spiders, the most commonly associated with what is called *necrotic arachnidism* being *Loxoscleles reclusus*. The venom is said to contain at least eight active components, including the enzymes hyaluronidase, deoxyribonuclease, alkaline phosphatase, and lipase. The enzyme most responsible for the necrotic action is specified to be sphingomyelinase D (SMase D), also called phospolipase D. There has been a proliferation of related Internet sites.

The venom of the brown recluse spider (or fiddleback, or violin spider) is listed in the *Handbook of Pest Control* by Arnold Mallis (cited by Hoffman [1999], p. 187). Authorities who have also been cited include Collis Geren of the University of Arkansas and Gary W. Tamkin, M.D., of the Highland General Hospital, Alameda Medical Center, Oakland, California, and the University of California, San Francisco. Particular mention of these "flesh-eating" toxins is made here as they may be of potential use against skin cancer, as may similar biological agents.

Thus, noteworthy is the sap or juice from members of the genus *Asclepias*, or milkweed, of the family Asclepiadaceae, as indicated elsewhere, and which contains alkaloids (e.g., Hoffman, 1999, p. 505). Traditionally, such tissue-destroying chemicals as phenol (carbolic acid) have been used to selectively remove warts (although stump water, as was prescribed in Mark Twain's *Huckleberry Finn*, may presumably be disregarded). Compound-X, described elsewhere, is said to successfully remove skin cancers. Also, there is the (internal) use of yucca plant extracts against melanoma, as developed by retired University of Wyoming chemistry professor Owen Asplund, which has been described several times elsewhere.

Significantly, insect bites may in themselves be a potential source of cancer, even bee stings (Hoffman, 1999, pp. 187, 273–278). Thus, the toxins injected conceivably could be a cause of cancer, as may insect-carried viruses, as some insects carry large numbers of viruses. Plant and insect viruses may in fact be related, the latter perhaps evolving from the former, as set forth in Australian R.A.F. Matthews' authoritative volume *Plant Virology*. (Suspicions are aroused, therefore, about potential insect/plant origins for the Marburg and Ebola viruses, and crossover to humans, for the animal/human crossover is a feature of influenza, and maybe of AIDS.) German cancer specialist Hans A. Nieper, M.D., in the November 1997 issue of the *Townsend Letter for Doctors & Patients*, wrote that "insects such as ants can carry enormous loads of viruses within themselves."

(We mention again Nieper anticancer therapy as profiled, for instance, by Richard Walters [1993]. Described as a complex nutritional and metabolic therapy, it variously involves vitamins, minerals, laetrile, animal and plant extracts, pharmaceuticals, and vaccines such as that called BCG, for bacillus Calmette-Guérin, a weakened strain of tuberculosis bacillus. The latter has entered medical orthodoxy as a treatment for bladder cancer.)

Another consideration is that an insect bite or a plant exposure may trigger an allergic reaction, even deadly anaphylactic shock, which may require the immediate administration of a histamine-countering drug such as epinephrine (adrenalin) or Benadryl®.

Of note is a study about glutathione (GSH) as an inhibitor for the enzyme SMase, or more specifically, *N*-Smase, as may be connected with cancer cell behavior. Glutathione is a normal body component, which can be described as a peptide — that is, a short-chain protein — and which contains sulfur, denoted by the "thio" in its name, and by the symbol "S." The technical article or paper is titled "Inhibition of the Neutral Magnesium-Dependent Sphingomyelinase," by Bin Liu and Yusuf A. Hannun of the Department of Medicine and Cell Biology, Duke University. (A deficiency in the enzyme sphingomyelinase, or Smase, is generally associated with liver and spleen enlargement, and mental retardation.) The article was published in the *Journal of Biological Chemistry*, Vol. 272, No. 26, dated June 26, 1997, and can be found at the Web site http://www.jbc.org. The tests were conducted *in vitro* using Molt-4 human leukemia cells.

(Another treatment, unusual, is called the Modified Stun Gun Treatment. It is briefly mentioned at the Internet Web site http://www.highway60.com/mark/brs/medical.htm. The enzyme sphingomyelinase D is described as disrupting cellular membranes, with various other enzymes in the venom used acting as foreign antigens, triggering the victim's immune response, and thereby contributing to necrosis.)

Mention of sphingomyelinase further brings up a study conducted at Lund University in Lund, Sweden. A thesis or dissertation by Erik Hertervig, abstracted in 2000, the title is "Alkaline Sphingomyelinase: A Potential Inhibitor in Colorectal

Carcinogenesis." The abstract concludes that "The enzyme may be important in cell growth regulation and its reduction may facilitate the development of colorectal cancer." The particular Internet site is listed as http://eprints.lub.lu.se/archive/00005505/ — or the article can be found by searching with the keyword "sphingomyelinase."

## CANCER DIRECTIVES

We next introduce, or reintroduce, other and various aspects of cancer, its causes and its treatment. (The word *cure* is apparently a no-no in official circles. However, we would settle for at least a 99.9999+ percent remission rate.) For the record, much of this ground is covered elsewhere and by Hoffman (1999). Along the way, it may again be emphasized that the death rate is about one death per minute in the United States alone, which would be equivalent to about 525,000 deaths per year. The grassroots organization People Against Cancer supplied a figure of 750,000 deaths for 1998. Worldwide, the death rate is more like 6 million (or more) per year. These figures will revolve around the issue of primary vs. secondary causes of death.

As has been noted, the biogenesis of cancer may be expressed in terms of oncogenes, the genetic entity involved in the transformation of a normal cell into a cancerous one. The overall process may be called *carcinogenesis*, or *oncogenesis*. The induction of oncogenes may be from viruses, radiation, or chemicals (carcinogens). In the case of viruses, for instance, a virus may invade a chromosome, causing a transformation of the genetic material into an oncogene. The inference is that viral causes may be more pervasive than formerly thought. Prominently mentioned are retroviruses, or RNA viruses, the same category as the AIDS virus or HIV, and the Marburg and Ebola viruses.

In addition to animal viruses, which may cross the species barrier, there are also insect viruses and plant viruses, as well as bacterial viruses — also called bacteriophages (which "eat up" the bacterial cells). There is the possibility or probability, not only of mutations, but of interactions — for example, plant viruses may have evolved from insect viruses. Given the destruction of the tropical rain forests and the attendant land convolutions, the prognosis is that all kinds of strange viruses are emerging. There is the consideration, therefore, that such emerging viruses as the Marburg and Ebola may have nonanimal origins. Several books have dealt with these and related concerns, for example, *Boston Globe* science writer Madeline Drexler's *Secret Agents: The Menace of Emerging Infections*, published in 2002. Another is *The Killers Within: The Deadly Rise of Drug-Resistant Bacteria*, by Michael Shnayerson and Mark J. Plotkin, which takes aim first at hospitals, and then at the larger medical community. It has been observed that violent sandstorms occurring in the Sahara, notably those called the *hermatten*, may result in sand particles being carried on westerly winds clear into the western hemisphere. Thus, in a chapter titled "The Winds," authors Marq de Villiers and Sheila Hirtle document this fact in *Sahara: A Natural History*, where it is also noted that wind-borne pathogens can cause the toxic oceanic bloom called *red tide*, as well as illnesses in humans. It may thus be concluded that fungi, bacteria, and various viruses are also so carried, with the potential of causing cancer as well as other diseases. So it is with wind storms in general — another variable or parameter for the epidemiologists.

An intriguing and thought-provoking book by Amherst biologist Paul W. Ewald, published in 2000, is *Plague Time: How Stealth Infections Cause Cancers, Heart Disease, and Other Deadly Ailments*. In a chapter "Malignant Growths in Our Backyard," Ewald names some of the viruses known to cause or suspected of causing cancer. These include human papillomaviruses, which are associated with sexually transmitted diseases, and can ratchet from a relatively mild form, producing warts, into a deadly form (Ewald, 2000, p. 94ff).

Another bit of information furnished is that it was known back in the 1940s that a bacterium caused ulcers, and a cure could be effected using antibiotics (Ewald, 2000, p. 98ff). Somehow, this knowledge was not utilized, and was not employed until the mid-1980s, when other investigators made the same discovery. Now the antibiotic ulcer treatment is routine.

Diseases transferred by pathogens crossing the species barrier are referred to as zoonoses, and the zoonotic diseases very likely include Ebola and AIDS (Ewald, 2000, p. 103ff). This leads us to the link between breast cancer and retroviruses (other sources consider retroviruses to cause cancer). Evidence of retroviruses has been found in cancerous breast tissue but not in surrounding normal tissue. Moreover, the viral sequences are indistinguishable from those for the mouse mammary tumor virus. And the geographic distribution of breast cancer correlates with that for the distribution for the virus's primary host, *Mus domesticus*, the common house mouse. A cosuspect is the Epstein-Barr virus, found disproportionately in human breast cancers.

Speaking further of breast cancer, well-known author Barbara Ehrenreich has some forceful comments in an article in the November 2001 issue of *Harper's Magazine*. The article is titled "Welcome to Cancerland: A Mammogram Leads to a Culture of Pink Kitsch," and some of cancer victim Ehrenreich's telling comments are highlighted in the article. Regarding the breast cancer culture, which ranges from personal experiences and grassroots organizations to corporate sponsorship and celebrities: "In the breast cancer culture, cheerfulness is more or less mandatory, dissent a kind of treason." Furthermore: "The cult turns women into dupes of corporations that produce carcinogens and then offer toxic pharmaceutical treatments."

More on mammography is furnished by Malcolm Gladwell in "The Annals of Technology" in the December 13, 2004, issue of the *New Yorker*. Things are not always as they are seen in the x-ray pictures, for there is the further matter of the interpretation of the images. The assorted lumps and bumps, or tumors, appearing may or may not be cancerous. Additionally, there is the matter of calcium deposits that are simultaneously created, which may or may not indicate a cancerous condition. (The source of the calcium is not specified in the article. However, on page 64 of Hoffman (1999), intracellular calcium is reported to bind with the eukaryotic protein called calmodulin, producing an interaction with certain enzymes to cause cell proliferation, as in a tumor.) In controlled experiments with qualified radiologists, their interpretations were quite diverse (Gladwell, 2004, p. 76). All this can tend to leave those involved in a quandary — to treat or not to treat, with the qualifier that mammography itself is only a screening process, and not a treatment.

Commercial meat products contain a wide assortment of viruses, as well as bacteria. Interestingly, in a letter to the *Townsend Letter for Doctors & Patients*, April 2002, frequent contributor Wayne Martin reassesses the role of meat in the incidence of colorectal cancer, which becomes near zero for vegetarian diets — a conclusion reached by others. Martin cites an editorial that appeared in the April 27, 1974, issue of *The Lancet*, the prestigious British medical journal. Titled "Beware of the Ox," the article stated that the incidence of colon cancer is proportional to the amount of beef consumed in the human diet. In the same letter, Martin mentions cimetidine, trade name Tagamet®, as an effective anticancer agent. (Its nominal function is to reduce stomach acidity.) Thus, cimetidine is said to inhibit both T-suppressor cells and the immunosuppressive action of histamine. The drug is also said to allow cancer-cell-killing lymphocytes to invade malignant tumors.

Martin further discusses the use of cimetidine against cancer in a letter in the *Townsend Letter for Doctors and Patients*, July 2003. Other anticancer agents discussed in the same letter include dipyridamole, which is said to prevent cancer cells from attaching to the walls of arteries and veins, thus blocking metastasis (and also acting against strokes). Another mentioned is the well-known herbal remedy digitoxin, an ingredient of digitalis, ordinarily used to treat congestive heart disease. Still another is azelaic acid, also called nonanedioic acid or 1,7-heptanedicarboxylic acid (chemical formula $HO_2C(CH_2)_7CO_2H$), which may inhibit the enzyme tryosinase, which is suspected of causing or advancing certain cancers. Also cited is coumadin, better known as the rat poison warfarin, which is noted to dissolve the fibrin that ordinarily coats and protects cancer cells from the immune system. Others include chlorella, bromocriptine, aminoglutethimide, and lastly, urea, which is written up, for instance, in Moss (1992).

Martin continued his discussion about colorectal cancer and its prevention and cure in a letter published posthumously in the August/September 2006 issue of the *Townsend Letter*. He continued to push cimetidine, but noted that it is no longer available, the pharmaceutical company having dropped its production when the patent ran out.

(Cimetidine is listed in the Sigma-Aldrich catalog *Biochemicals, Reagents & Kits*, with the stoichiometric formula $C_{10}H_{16}N_6S$ , and is described as an $H_2$ histamine receptor antagonist, $1_1$ imidazoline receptor agonist, and an antiulcer agent. A search of the Internet yields the finding that there are side effects.)

Martin also returns to Coley's Toxins in a letter in the same issue, but notes that it is illegal in the United States and Canada. However, its use is legal in the Bahamas, and as of June 2006 MB Vax Science (or Bioscience) will supply free Coley's Toxins to the ITL Clinic in the Bahamas.

The amount of valuable information supplied by biochemist Martin in his cumulative letters to the *Townsend Letter for Doctors & Patients* is enough to fill a book.

A previous letter by Martin on pages 96–99 of the October 2000 issue of the *Townsend Letter for Doctors & Patients* had connected iron in high-meat diets to cancer and heart disease. The article in *The Lancet* was cited, and reference was made to Denmark during 1914–1918, when it was necessary to cut down on meat consumption and the cancer rate dropped. The Hopi Indians of the American

Southwest are also cited, who have a largely vegetarian diet and a cancer rate of only one per thousand.

Martin also describes treatment with cesium as producing remission in late-stage cancer patients. Another possibility described is a killed vaccine from the dead bacteria of the streptococcus of erysipelas. This vaccine is better known as Coley's Toxins. The genus is *Streptococcus* and the disease is known as erysipelas, an acute feverish condition with intense local inflammation of the skin and subcutaneous tissue. The treatment can be described as a form of immunotherapy.

In the February/March 2003 issue of the *Townsend Letter for Doctors & Patients*, beginning on page 140, chemical engineer/biochemist Wayne Martin has a long letter to the editor furnishing additional information about Coley's Toxins for sarcoma and intractable cancer. (Solid malignancies are customarily divided into sarcomas and carcinomas, the former occurring in nonepithelial cells or tissues, that is, in connective tissue, lymphoid tissue, cartilage, bone, etc., whereas carcinomas pertain to epithelial cells or tissue proper, that is, that lining the internal free surfaces or body cavities.) Much of the early history is provided, starting with the practice in New York City of a certain William Coley, M.D., who was then, in 1891, already a successful surgeon at the age of 29 (and was later to become chief bone surgeon at Memorial Hospital, which became the world-renowned Memorial Sloan-Kettering Cancer Center).

The initial discovery was made when a patient with a sarcoma on the neck in the form of a huge ulcerous malignancy — considered a hopeless case — also developed a severe infection of erysipelas. The patient survived the infection and at the same time, in just a few days, the malignancy healed, the patient leaving the hospital in good health. Coley subsequently tried this route on other patients, with mixed results; another trial worked with a spectacular healing, whereas with others the infection could not be induced, or else the patient died from the infection.

Accordingly, Coley prepared a killed vaccine of the streptococcus of erysipelas, but which had little anticancer activity until the newly discovered bacterium *Seratia marcescens* was added — which, moreover, in itself was known to be nonpathogenic against humans. The first trial of the killed vaccine, though slower acting, was a pronounced success, and other doctors were soon beginning to use the vaccine, despite an editorial in the *Journal of the American Medical Association* stating the Coley's Toxins were useless. On the other hand, the Mayo Brothers advised their patients who had had cancer surgery to go home and find a doctor who would administer Coley's Toxins.

In 1898 Coley joined the staff of New York's Memorial Hospital which, as mentioned, later became the Memorial Sloan-Kettering Cancer Center (MSKCC). But at about the same time, a Dr. James Ewing also joined the hospital as a pathologist, and became an ardent proponent of using x-rays and radium, meanwhile developing a hatred for the alternative use of Coley's Toxins. By interesting the Phelps Dodge Corporation, a large mining company in the American Southwest, in the potential for using its mined radium in the treatment of cancer, Ewing gained a powerful ally. Interestingly, however, the use of radium in treating the breast cancer of the Phelps Dodge CEO's daughter failed, although Coley's Toxins had been successful in other cases. Nevertheless, the CEO of the corporation, by now a major radium producer, made a large gift of radium to Memorial Hospital, with the proviso that Ewing be made medical director — who then cut off Coley and his toxins, notably for use against bone sarcoma, which heretofore had been successful. This in spite of the fact that, over the next 7 years, every patient who was treated with radium for bone sarcoma died.

Nevertheless, there were continued successes using Coley's Toxins at other hospitals, by other physicians, amply cited, with further refinements on dosage levels. Coley himself was not so fortunate, losing all his money in the stock market crash of 1929, and dying in 1936. This could have been the end of the story, except that Coley's daughter Helen Coley Nauts (now deceased) subsequently founded the Cancer Research Institute, which has since grown large and prestigious. (Address: 681 Fifth Avenue, New York, NY 10022, Jill O'Donnell-Tormey, Exec. Dir. at 212-688-7515.) Nauts reviewed and documented the many successful cases, and publishing 18 monographs on using Coley's Toxins. Along the way there have been attempts to suppress the use of these toxins, including blacklisting by the American Cancer Society as an unproven therapy — with the FDA making its use illegal, although it was used not only against cancer, but against such vascular diseases as thromboangiitis obliterans (Buerger's disease), and maybe against arteriosclerosis — and could be a potential alternative to angioplasty or heart bypass surgery.

As for the biochemistry involved, it has been proposed that the L-arginine to nitric oxide metabolic pathway is activated, whereby the greater amount of nitric oxide produced is cytotoxic to cancer cells. Not only this, but the nitric oxide produces a greater vascular blood flow, and the enzyme streptokinase naturally present in the toxins may lyse or destroy blood clots. Another beneficial effect was apparently against osteoarthritis.

It is noted that the Parke Davis Company produced and sold a weaker vaccine from 1898 to 1962, which proved ineffective at ordinary dosages, but was effective at much greater dosages. The therapy continues at present on a limited basis using laboratory-made vaccines, with dramatic remissions in evidence, and overdoses can be monitored and controlled by a rectal suppository of Tylenol. It is concluded that, with larger dosages under Tylenol control, the results should be far better than in Coley's time.

A further testimony is furnished in an article by Wayne Martin in the February/March 2006 issue of the *Townsend Letter for Doctors & Patients*. Titled "Coley's Toxins: A Cancer Treatment History," a number of almost unbelievable remissions or cures are described involving cancerous tumors of immense size. The toxins were injected directly into the tumor, producing an intense reaction, with chills and fever. Some of the remissions or cures were relatively rapid, others took longer treatment regimens. Martin also details several alternative methods for preparing the toxins, and notes that it can now be injected intravenously, whereas the original protocol was that the toxins should only be injected directly into the cancerous mass. Reemphasized is the fact that a Tylenol suppository can be used to offset the toxin in case things get out of hand. (There are a number of Internet entries on the subject, including "Wayne Martin on Coley's Toxins.")

There is an intriguing letter to the editor on page 118 of the November 2003 issue of the *Townsend Letter for Doctors & Patients*. The letter, titled "A Simple

Treatment for Flu," was written by Sherry A. Rogers, M.D. The subject is Dr. Miller's treatment for flu, as developed and used since 1968 by Joseph B. Miller, M.D. of Mobile, Alabama. It is described by Dr. Rogers as "one of the simplest, inexpensive, harmless, quick and effective treatments for the flu," providing relief for acute flu in less than 30 minutes, with complete eradication in a matter of a few days. (Along the way, Dr. Rogers mentions how Dr. Miller's food allergy injections not only cured a case of severe facial eczema, but could be used against such hidden food allergy symptoms as ulcerative colitis, arthritis, migraines, asthma, prostatitis, chronic sinusitis, relentless irritable bowel, fibromyalgia, and chronic fatigue, and much more.)

The treatment is said to be similar to an allergy testing technique, and first involves making a succession of one to five dilutions of current flu vaccine. A tiny amount (0.05 cc) is injected just under the first layer of skin, in similar fashion to a TB test, making about a 7-mm diameter wheal, that is, a pronounced eminence on the skin. If within 10 minutes the wheal does not disappear, or worsens, then the next order of dilution is employed, which would be a weaker 1 to 25. And so on, as necessary. It is further stated that, "The strongest negative weal is the treatment dose given as a very tiny 0.10 cc subcutaneously." This is to be the dosage that the patient himself or herself can administer four times a day. The flu will be gone in 24 to 48 hours. Although the author notes that serious reactions were never observed, the wrong dosage will expectedly worsen symptoms, indicating the necessity to go back and retest.

The subject leads to cancer because, as Dr. Rogers states, many types of viruses also cause many kinds of cancers — so, enter the topic of diluted flu vaccine. "It makes sense that the simple inexpensive flu vaccine should be considered as having a role in a variety of cancers, if we could only educate physicians about it." Thus, Dr. Rogers notes the many other cancers triggered by the herpes virus, such as Kaposi's sarcoma (in HIV patients), multiple myeloma, lymphomas, Hodgkin's disease, cancer of the nasal and throat passages, and others. He mentions a rampant liver cancer occurring in Taiwanese children during the 1980s. But 12 years later a marked decrease in hepatocellular carcinoma was seen because the children were inoculated against hepatitis B.

Concluding, Dr. Rogers states that "the majority of practice guidelines are created by physicians on pharmaceutical payrolls," as pronounced in the February 2002 issue of the *New England Journal of Medicine*.

## THE CONTINUING LEGACY OF WAYNE MARTIN AND COMPATRIOTS

Speaking further of inorganic metals or metallic compounds, in a letter on page 111 of the June 2002 issue of the *Townsend Letter for Doctors & Patients*, frequent contributor Wayne Martin first mentions how iron-deficient anemia develops in patients with a bacterial infection; hence, iron supplements can be viewed presumably as advisable. He then reports on work by Professor Harold Foster of the University of Victoria, Canada, about selenium being antiviral, which was earlier reported by Foster in the December 2000 issue. It was noted in particular that in regions of Africa with soils of high selenium content, the incidence of AIDS is much lower. Thus, Zimbabwe has 26% of its population infected, whereas Senegal with its high-selenium soils has only 1.77% infected. It may be added that selenium (or its compounds) is known to be an anticancer agent, as per Moss (1992). Another viral infection is caused by the Coxsackie B virus, resulting in a severe disease of the heart called *cardiomyopathy*. This infection has been correlated against patients who have had a myocardial infarction, as was reported in the April 23, 1977, issue of *The Lancet*. (More about the Coxsackie virus is reported by Martin in a letter in the July 2002 issue of the *Townsend Letter for Doctors & Patients*.)

In the same June 2002 issue, Wayne Martin writes about the potential of using thyophylline against cancer, as well as against asthma. His letter also discusses the use of evening primrose oil (from the seeds), which contains a high percentage of gamma linolenic acid, and which in its pure form has been used directly as an injection against cancer.

Still in the same issue, there is an advertisement in the initial pages for Vas-cuStatin as an inhibitor for angiogenesis. Said to be 100 times stronger than shark cartilage, it is produced by the Allergy Research Group of Hayward, California. There is an increasing progression of anticancer drugs poised to enter the market. For instance, there is Gleevec (called Glivec overseas), produced by Novartis. (This substance is a tyrosine kinase inhibitor as per Chapter 10.) Interestingly, it is but one of a number of oral chemotherapies — which caused an uproar upon its intro-duction, as Medicare at the time did not pay for pill prescriptions. (The main target is chronic myeloid leukemia, or CML, although it is under study against still other cancers. Full-page advertisements have appeared in publications such as the *New Yorker*, which announce testimonials of turnarounds or remissions for particular patients. It is given space in Guy B. Faguet's *The War on Cancer*.)

Another intriguing letter by Martin occurs on page 125 of the August/September 2001 issue of the *Townsend Letter for Doctors & Patients*. He questions the net benefits of fiber in preventing colon cancer, for the sharp silica fibers in the fiber is apparently conducive to esophageal cancer, as per an article in the May 29, 1982, issue of *The Lancet* titled "Silica Fragments from Millet Bran in the Mucosa Sur-rounding Oesophageal Tumors in Patients in North China." Thus, the Chinese and Iranian esophageal cancer rate was 50 times that in England.

The August/September 2001 issue was devoted to cancer, as was the June 2004 issue, the cover declaring "Alternative Therapies for Cancer," and similarly for the August/September 2006 issue, whose cover was headlined "Cancer Treatment: The Best of Conventional and Alternative Medicine," and subtitled "The Cancer Journey: Finding the Healing Path." The featured section, starting on page 71, was titled "Cancer Conquest," edited by Burton Goldberg, with a note by Jonathan Collin, M.D., publisher, titled "The Cutting Edge of Alternative Medicine and Cancer Treatment: The Video Every Alternative Practitioner Should See." (Details of the video are as follows: *Cancer Conquest: The Best of Conventional and Alternative Medicine*, edited by Burton Goldberg, www.curing-cancer.com, Do No Harm Pro-ductions LLC, DVD or VHS @$39.95 at: www.burtongoldberg.com.) The video is mainly concerned with therapies practiced in Germany, for example, the Scheller

Clinic Treatment Strategy, and does not include Mexican or U.S. clinics. (Goldberg, or the Goldberg Group, has published *Alternative Medicine: The Definitive Guide* and *An Alternative Medicine Definitive Guide to Cancer.*)

In further comment, in the August/September 2005 issue of the *Townsend Letter for Doctors & Patients*, Martin cites the work of Dr. David Horrobin of Magdalen College, Oxford University, that a diet low in red meat but high in vegetables and whole cereal grains acts against arthritis, as well as against colon cancer. A culprit was said to be arachidonic acid, a principal source being red meat.

In the August/September 2006 issue of the *Townsend Letter for Doctors & Patients*, on the very last page, Melvyn R. Werbach, M.D., writes about the Cancer Prevention Diet. "The results of animal studies suggest that the single most powerful and consistent dietary influence on carcinogenesis is simply energy restriction." In other words, eat less.

Subsequent issues of the *Townsend Letter for Doctors & Patients* in the former time frame were also informative, for example, in the February/March 2002 issue holistic cancer therapist W. Douglas Brodie, M.D., is profiled by Morton Walker in his regular column. Brodie has indicated that the most common cancer personality trait is "worrying for others."

The article also describes what is called insulin-potentiated hypoglycemic therapy, or IPHT, as used by Dr. Brodie. In this regard it can be mentioned that insulin-taking diabetics are at potential risk for cancer, in that an imbalance between insulin and its metabolic opposite, glucagon, may be conducive to a cancerous condition, as mentioned on pages 332 and 385 in Hoffman (1999). That is to say, the inhibition of insulin may inhibit cancer, whereas an excess may be carcinogenic.

More comes to light in the February/March 2003 issue of *TL* in an article titled "Diabetes, Cancer and Weight: A Metabolic Typing Survey," by Harold J. Kristal, DDS, with James M. Haig, NC. The article divided people into two metabolic groups, those of Group I who were slow oxidizers and sympathetics, and those of Group II who were fast oxidizers and parasympathetics. The categories sympathetic and parasympathetic pertain to the autonomic nervous system (ANS), with a different metabolic pathway than for the oxidative system. (The sympathetics were characterized by a blood pH that was acid, the parasympathetics by alkaline blood pH.) It was found that those of Group I were less prone to Type II (adult-onset) diabetes, but more prone to cancer, whereas those of Group II were more prone to Type II diabetes but less prone to cancer, especially those who were parasympathetic. (Moreover, Group II on the average tended to be more overweight, especially for the fast oxidizers). It is noted that fast oxidizers have an aggressive insulin response, which may lead to long-term insulin resistance for the typical high-carbohydrate diet. In any event, the conclusion may be inferred from the foregoing that there is an inhibition of the insulin balance, which translates to the inhibition of cancer. Or, in other words, there is less than normal insulin present or remaining in the bloodstream for the fast oxidizers. However, this is a condition also manifested as diabetes.

On pages 83 and 84 of the June 2000 issue of *Townsend Letter for Doctors & Patients*, Wayne Martin reports on a visit to the BioPulse Clinic in Tijuana, described as a large alternative medicine clinic. Here, the treatment called "insulin-induced hypoglycemic therapy" or IHT is overviewed as a treatment for cancer. Another method mentioned is the use of naltrexone, and still another, digitoxin. Naltrexone, for instance, is described as a harmless drug that can be used at home.

A further update by Wayne Martin appeared in the "More Letters" section of the January 2003 issue of *Townsend Letter for Doctors & Patients*. This particular letter was titled "When Being Anemic and Eating Blue Corn May Prevent Cancer." The letter starts off with input from Ralph Moss, who had mentioned that there were fewer deaths from cancer some 200 years ago, and who tells of the findings of the renowned Albert Schweitzer, M.D., at his hospital in Gabon, in West Africa. When Schweitzer established his hospital in 1913, he was astounded to find no cancer among the natives. Their diet was vegetarian, mainly cassava. Schweitzer, a German national, was interned during World War I and did not return until 1923, at which time many of the natives were dying of cancer. It was noted that these natives, employed in a newly formed timber industry, had since been eating a European-style diet. Three other doctors confirmed Schweitzer's original findings, and it was noted that the usual native diet had a very low iron content.

In turn, Martin brings up the subject of Dr. Maria de Sousa, who was for many years with the Memorial Sloan-Kettering Institute for Cancer Research. She found that excess body iron was immunosuppressive and hence cancer causing. It was found that white cells detect harmful bacteria by the latter's iron content. And that white cells, which usually detect and kill cancer cells, are instead attracted to normal cells by the fact of the latter's high iron content. So not only does the iron content in red meat act against us, but there is still more iron added to bread and other foods, plus the iron in vitamin pills. Returning to her native Portugal, de Sousa subsequently wrote that leukemic children survived longer when on low-iron diets.

As an aside, Martin mentions that the cyanide-bearing nitrilosides in the African natives' cassava diet might also have been responsible in part for a reduction in cancer occurrence (as similar to the nitrilosides in laetrile, for instance, which is still advanced in some quarters as a curative for cancer).

Martin next brings up the matter of cesium in the diet, citing studies by Keith Brewer among the Hopi and Pueblo Indians of Arizona. Their basic diet was blue Indian corn, supplemented by other foods and the ash derived from burning green chamisa leaves, and which were raised in volcanic soil high in cesium, rubidium, calcium, and potassium. It is stated that their diet had about 35 times as much of these 4 elements as the average U.S. diet. In fact, in 1940, the cancer incidence among the Hopi was only 1 in 1000, whereas the white U.S. population had an incidence of one in four. In turn, when the Pueblo Indians were introduced to the American diet, courtesy of the U.S. Public Health service, the incidence among them subsequently increased to one in four. The Hopi later followed, whereby the death rate increased to 6 per 1000 per year, but which was still less than the U.S. rate of 32 per 1000 per year. (As for the nearby Navajo, their cancer incidence — or lack thereof — has been reported upon elsewhere by John Heinerman.)

The term *incidence* is to be distinguished from the term *death rate*, but the distinction seems not clear in the cited reference, nor are the terms. If, say, there are 500,000 cancer deaths per year out of a population of 250 million, the death rate would be about 2 per 1000 population per year. If there was an incidence of

1,500,000 new cases per year, the incidence of new cases would be about 3 per 1000 population per year.

Of course, the total number of cases, new and old, which are in existence during each year is much higher. So, presumably, we could speak of a total of, say, about 15,000,000 cases of cancer in existence during the year, which in round numbers would yield a figure of about 30 existing cases per 1000 population per year. This incidence figure of 30 can be compared with the incidence figure for the Hopi cited in the reference, of 1 existing case per 1000 population (per year).

Furthermore, the total of 15,000,0000 existing cases among a population of 250 million would be at a ratio of about 1 in 17. However, the comparison ratio of 500,000 deaths to 1,500,000 new cases is 1 in 3. If there were 2,000,000 new cases, the comparison ratio would be 1 in 4, which is the ratio value cited in the reference for the United States as a whole.

On the other hand, if there were 500,000 deaths each year among the, say, 15 million existing cancer cases, the death rate would be about 33 per 1000 existing cases per year. This is close to the number cited in the reference, of 32 per 1000 per year.

In any event, the Hopi and Pueblo Indians were ever so much better off, cancerwise, before adopting the typical American diet, as were the Navajo.

Comparing the United States and Canada, the findings of Professor Harold Foster of the University of Victoria are reported as follows: there were 520,930 deaths in the United States during 1994 compared to 54,950 deaths in Canada. Foster maintains that calcium and selenium in the water are an important factor, citing an area in China where the death rate from esophageal cancer was reduced from 275 per 100,000 per year to 54 by adding calcium to the drinking water. Another example provided is that of Senegal, which as a very high selenium content in its soil. It has the lowest rate of esophageal cancer in the world, and virtually no cancer of the lung, breast, colon, and prostate.

These findings are also translatable to HIV/AIDS; Senegal has only 1.77% of its population infected with HIV-1, whereas Zimbabwe — with a very low selenium content in its soil — has an incidence over 25%.

Martin notes that many areas of beneficial high-calcium content have offset this advantage by installing water softeners. He adds that, "A water softener may be considered an instrument of death." (It may be noted that water softeners exchange calcium ions for sodium ions. An excess of the latter in drinking water is a no-no, leading to high blood pressure and other ailments. That is, an excess of sodium increases water accumulation in the body tissues, in turn producing higher blood pressures. Hence, the use of diuretics to counteract high blood pressure.)

Further studies cited include those reporting the beneficial effect of vitamin D (and calcium) against colon and other cancers. Some continuing investigations are currently under way.

Another report concerns the work of Helen Coley Nauts, Ph.D., who founded the Cancer Research Institute, initially to study the effect of her father's vaccine against cancer, better known as Coley's Mixed Toxins. Interestingly, early data on cancer incidence show that there was very little lung cancer among men who smoked. Thus, in 1930 some 80% of the men smoked, but the death rate from lung cancer was only one death per 100,000 per year. Yet by 1948, with only about 40% of the men smoking, the rate had increased to 60 — a 60-fold increase.

Significantly, Nauts attributes this astounding increase to the introduction, use, and overuse of antibiotics, which were, at least then, highly immunosuppressive. In confirmation, it turns out that bacterial infections are effective in the treatment of cancer; 449 cases are cited that were cured of cancer when the patients suffered from bacterial infections. In other words, it can be said that bacterial infections activate the immune system.

Further details are furnished based on the work of Dr. Eric Newsholme, who was head of the Biochemistry Department at Oxford University. Newsholme found that the polyunsaturated fats are highly immunosuppressive. Yet, these are the very kinds of fats and oils which are now pushed, as derived from, say, corn and sunflower seeds. Not so, however, with animal fats.

However, there are some diseases that require immunosuppression, and Newsholme tells how two children were cured of the disabling Guillain-Barré syndrome by taking 50 cc of sunflower seed oil each day, whereas the conventional drugs were ineffective.

Another paradox is that these polyunsaturated oils contain linoleic acid, which, in a series of steps, will convert cancer cells back to normal cells. A similar effect is observed for the theophylline contained in tea, whereas none was observed in coffee.

Mention is made that vitamin C seems to be effective against bladder cancer, with studies cited. An interesting example is furnished of petrochemical plant workers whose urine would give off light, the phenomenon of chemiluminescence, and which was indicative of bladder cancer. Vitamin C countered this, presumably by preventing the formation of cinnabarinic acid, which is associated with tumor formation.

Lastly, Martin returns to Dr. Schweitzer and the subject of gangrene and amputations. The African natives refused to allow amputation, so Dr. Schweitzer treated bacterial infections with the dyestuff methylviolet. The stuff worked, and may have been among the "first" of the antibiotics, a precursor to the discovery of the dyestuff called Prontosil, which is half sulfonamide (and resulted in a Nobel Prize for Germany's Gerhard Domagk, its discoverer). In confirmation, the case of Dr. Frederick Banting is cited, who later shared the Nobel Prize in 1923 for discovering insulin. Early on, as a battle surgeon with the Canadian Medical Corps in World War I, he was wounded on the front line, and developed gangrene in his right arm. Instead of going along with the recommended amputation, he cured himself with methylviolet.

Martin concludes that maybe some doctors will now consider methylviolet in treating infected wounds.

In the October 2005 issue of the *Townsend Letter for Doctors & Patients*, a letter from Wayne Martin addresses the use of intravenous dilute hydrochloric acid solutions as a defense against bacterial infections. He cites many letters from doctors that appeared in the journal *Medical World* between 1932 and 1935. The successes were such that Martin now thinks that the discovery of antibiotics would not have been necessary. He describes the dramatic recovery of a young patient as reported by William Howell, M.D., of Lexington, Kentucky. (The injections used were stated as 10 cc of 1 part in 1000 hydrochloric acid.)

Martin writes about appendix removal, stating that it increases the risk for colon cancer twofold. It is noted that the appendix constitutes an important part of the immune system — for instance, producing cancer-killing cells — thus, there is an argument for retaining an infected appendix, presumably by treatment.

In a letter appearing in the December 2003 issue of the *Townsend Letter for Doctors & Patients*, Wayne Martin returns to the subject of amputations — a consequence of diabetes. Martin first cites a study by a certain Isadore Snapper, M.D., of Brooklyn, New York, who spent 10 years at a hospital in North China and published a book about his experiences. None of the Chinese diabetic patients had the vascular disorders of the modern West, and lived on a vegetarian diet mainly of millet and soya food.

The experiences of a Dr. M. S. Mazel, then owner of the Edgewater Hospital in Chicago, are next described. He was successful in avoiding amputations by using the proteolytic enzyme urokinase.

In turn, the pioneering work on vitamin E of Canada's Evan Shute, M.D., Sc.D., is described. Shute was able to avoid amputations by the use of vitamin E as d-alpha tocopherol, administered at 800 units per day.

Martin also has a word about the harm from the use of homogenized milk, as per the work of cardiologist Kurt Oster, M.D., of Fairfield University. Thus, natural milk contains xanthine oxidase, an oxidizing enzyme, in large particles, which, consequently, do not get into the bloodstream. Homogenization reduces the particle size, allowing entry into the bloodstream, which Oster claims is harmful to the vascular system.

Martin continues by citing the work of Professor Stephen Seely of the University of Sheffield, who studied the effect of milk and cheese consumption on heart attacks. At the time of the study, milk homogenization was practiced worldwide. In Finland, which had the highest death rate from heart attacks in the entire world, the consumption of protein from liquid (homogenized) milk was 30.4 g per day, as compared to 2.5 g per day in Japan. Correspondingly, the death rate in Finland was ten times that in Japan. A further study by Seely on milk protein in cheese found no increase in heart attacks from eating cheese. Thus, in cheese making, homogenized milk is never used.

Martin adds the fact that Coley's Toxins were effective in treating patients having foot ulcers and a gangrenous condition, with symptoms of cold feet and lack of a pulse in the lower leg. Conducted by a Dr. Harry Gray at a Veterans Administration Hospital in the 1930s, amputation was avoided. This treatment is presumed to be effective for diabetic patients with foot ulcers. It is further noted that, at the present, physician Glen Wilcoxson, M.D., of Spanish Fort, Alabama, is treating patients with Coley's Toxins.

Returning to the subject of iron in the diet, Wayne Martin's letter in the October 2004 issue of the *Townsend Letter for Doctors & Patients* uses the Atkins Diet as the leadoff item. Martin questions the high-red-meat diet involved, for there is past evidence that a vast increase in deaths from cancer and heart attacks can be expected. Moreover, human teeth can be judged as much more suitable for a vegetarian diet than for a carnivorous diet. The incisors perform the cutting off of fibrous plant food, and the flat molars grind up such foods. This is as distinguished from the fangs of carnivores, for slashing, piercing, and tearing. (The point has been made that humans have an alimentary canal more like the shorter digestive system of carnivores, although a similar argument can be made for similarities with the longer canal of herbivores.)

In substantiation, the example of Denmark during World War I is given. Denmark had been getting about half its food from abroad, but the British blockade shut these foreign sources down, so a certain Mikkel Hendhede in the Danish Institute of Health recommended that Denmark go on a vegetarian diet. Instead of feeding grain to animals, and then eating the animals, the Danes could eat the grain themselves for a five-to-one benefit in grain consumption, at the same time selling most of the livestock to Germany. Outcries were made that the proteins in grain were incomplete (Martin asserts they are not). After much heated debate, including statistics on deaths from protein malnutrition countered by the longtime success of vegetarianism in Africa and India, the plan was adopted by the Danish government. Surprisingly, or not so surprisingly, there were no deaths at all from protein malnutrition, and the overall death rate had showed a decrease of 17% by the end of the war, mostly due to fewer cancer deaths.

The experiences of Albert Schweitzer are recounted, in that when he established his hospital in Gabon, in Africa in 1913, the natives there were noted to be free of cancer. Vegetarians, their two main items of diet were cassava and millet. In June and July of 1923, letters from three English doctors appeared in the *British Medical Journal* noting the absence of cancer among natives in various parts of Africa who had not had contact with Europeans. Again, the diet was cassava and millet with very little protein.

Consider next the United States and the Hopi Indians, who were free or nearly free of cancer, at lest until circa 1970. The background supplied introduces A. Keith Brewer, who in early World War II was working with the U.S. Navy on atomic energy, and became involved with the element cesium and its properties and effects. Although cesium did not fit into the atomic energy program, Brewer concluded that cesium was important in the defense against cancer, recommending 3 to 10 g a day as a treatment for cancer (which seems a lot to this observer). In fact, he later founded the A. Keith Brewer Library in Richland, Wisconsin, in support, but died in 1986.

However, in 1984 Brewer's report on the cancer benefits of cesium treatment was published in *Pharmacology, Biochemistry and Behavior*, Vol. 1, Supplement 1, pp. 1–5. Many cases of remission were supplied for late-stage cancer patients on treatment with cesium. Cesium treatment is not further addressed by Martin, but in Brewer's report mention is made of the Hopi Indians of northeastern Arizona, who were found to be nearly free of cancer as late as 1974.

At the time, the Hopi consumed their traditional vegetarian diet, mostly of calico corn (the multicolored Indian corn, or blue corn). In 1974 they were reported to have only 1 case of cancer per 1000 population, whereas in white Arizona it was 1 case in 4.

Brewer thought this very low cancer incidence among the Hopi was due to the high cesium content in their diet, attributable to the high cesium content of the volcanic soil. Moreover, the Hopi burned the leaves of the chamisa plant and added the ash to their corn meal, further adding to the cesium content.

(The chamisa or chamiso plant is a dense southwestern shrub of the rose family, with the scientific name *Adenostoma fasciculatum*. One may speculate that the plant itself may have anticancer properties, being of the family Rosaceae, which includes almonds and the like, and their amygdalin or laetrile content. As cited in Appendix U of Hoffman (1999), members of Rosaceae also contain diterpene alkaloids. However, reducing the leaves to ash would apparently destroy any bioactive organic constituents.)

Martin's article also mentions the Pueblo Indians (apparently not the Navajo) who lived close by to the Hopi (either in northern New Mexico or Arizona?) and who had a similar very low cancer incidence until the "do-gooders" in the government decided to issue food stamps so that these native Americans could enjoy a high meat diet like everyone else, after which the cancer incidence rose to one in four, the same level as the Arizona whites.

The Hopi for their part refused the offer of a high meat diet and thereby, as late as 1974, had the very low incidence of 1 case of cancer per 1000 population.

Martin cites again the editorial in the April 27, 1974, issue of *The Lancet* titled "Beware of the Ox." The article found that the incidence of colon cancer worldwide correlated with high beef consumption. Elsewhere, with low beef consumption, the incidence drops. An example given is a comparison between Scotland and England; red meat consumption is higher in Scotland, as is colon cancer incidence. Moreover, there was a small Asian population of about 15,000 living in Scotland, who were mostly from India and were lactovegetarians. In the January 13, 1990, issue of *The Lancet* it was reported that there were only 2 cases of colon cancer, whereas over the same time period the native Scots would have had an average of 14.2.

The native population in and around Kampala, Uganda, circa 1960 was found to be colon cancer free. This grain vegetarian population subsisted mainly on corn and millet, and was also found to be free from death by myocardial infarction. Earlier, the investigators Shaper and Jones had found the same population to be free or nearly so from myocardial infarction, as reported in 1959 in *The Lancet* ii, pp. 534–537. At about the same time, the January 1960 issue of the *American Journal of Cardiology* had a report on this population, whereby the hearts of the men who had died were examined for evidence of infarction. Of the 1427 hearts of middle-aged men, only one slight and well-healed infarction was found. On the other hand, as a reference point, a similar examination was carried out at St. Louis, Missouri, on both blacks and whites. Of the same number of hearts examined, about one fourth of the deaths were due to myocardial infarction. Furthermore, in both Kampala and St. Louis, the autopsies showed the same degree of atheroma (the condition of fat being deposited on the arterial walls). The big differences were in vascular thrombosis formation (the formation of arterial or venous blood clots), with much present in the U.S samples and none in the Kampala ones.

*The Lancet*, the November 27, 1978, issue had an article by Allen Cunningham titled "Lymphomas and Animal Protein Consumption." A comparison was made with Japan, where a vegetarian diet with much seafood was the rule. Whereas in 1963–1965, the industrial Western nations had an averaged death rate of 181 per

100,000 for all cancers, in Japan the figure was 107 per 100,000. The difference was greater for lymphomas and reticulo sarcomas.

Interestingly, in Japan about 80% of the men are said to smoke cigarettes, whereas in the United States the figure is only 30% — yet the U.S. death rate from lung cancer is about four times that of Japans.

With regard to leukemia, in 1976 *The Lancet* reported on the work of Stanislaw Garwicz of the University Hospital in Lund, Sweden. Garwicz had observed earlier that leukemia, especially childhood leukemia, correlated with the amount of protein in the diet and recommended that a low-protein diet be investigated as a treatment for leukemia- and lymphoma-type malignancies.

This report produced a parallel comment from the National Cancer Institute's W.A. Priester, who noted that squamous cell carcinoma of the eye developed much faster for cattle fed on a supplemental feed of animal protein.

Wayne Martin further takes up the matter of how high iron content affects the meat-eating population of the United States He notes that a high-iron diet is greatly immunosuppressive, which in turn elevates the risk of cancer. Also, he notes that the African diets previously mentioned contained very little iron, and the same holds true for the Hopi. The conventional medical wisdom would be that such diets would result in iron deficiency anemia.

Thus, Maria de Sousa of the prestigious Memorial Sloan-Kettering Institute for Cancer Research proclaimed the cancer-causing consequences of a diet too rich in iron. The effects are twofold, in that both cancer cells and bacteria have strong need for iron. This is evidenced by the fact that prolonged bacterial infections produce iron deficiency anemia. Ordinarily, the body's white cell immunocytes fight both cancer cells and bacteria by distinguishing the iron present in these cells. The immunosuppressive effect of the iron, however, is by virtue of the elevated iron content of the blood, which attracts these cancer-killing immunocytes, which become attached to the blood's iron content and are no longer available to act against cancer and bacterial cells.

Consider the further findings of Helen Coley Nauts, founder of the Cancer Research Institute and the daughter of William B. Coley, the developer of what are called Coley's Toxins. These findings resulted in Cancer Research Institute Monograph No. 8, dated 1980, which documented some 449 cases of cancer remission in patients with bacterial infections.

A biographical sketch of the career of William B. Coley is next presented. In 1981, Coley was a young surgeon in New York City, and had earlier developed a friendship with John D. Rockefeller, Jr., at Yale University. Rockefeller sent a dear friend to Coley for treatment, the lady suffering from bone sarcoma in one leg. Coley performed an amputation, but the cancer had metastasized to the lungs, liver, and brain, resulting in a terrible death. Rockefeller then asked Coley to investigate the medical literature for ways to better treat cancer, to be paid by Rockefeller. Going through the records of the many hundreds of cancer patients at New York Hospital, Coley found a clue in the 1884 case of one patient who miraculously recovered from cancer of the head and neck. The patient had had surgery thrice and was declared incurable, but somehow the patient became infected with erysipelas, a local infection caused by a streptococcus bacterium, and which resulted in a high fever. The patient recovered from the infection, and unexpectedly his cancer went into complete remission. Moreover, when Coley located the patient in 1891, 7 years later, the patient was still cancer free.

In treating subsequent hopeless cases, some went into complete remission but others died from the infection — and in still others the infection could not be induced. However, he made a killed vaccine of the streptococcus of erysipelas, and the successful result was called Coley's Toxins.

Upon reviewing the favorable results, Maria de Sousa of Sloan-Kettering found that the remission in Coley's patients was because the infection produced iron-deficient anemia, which then liberated the immunocytes to kill the cancer cells.

In another substantiation, Indiana University's E.D. Weinsberg reported in 1984 on how the withholding of iron from the diet — including meat — would act against cancer. This was reported on at length in *Physiology Review*, 64, pp. 65–102. The *New England Journal of Medicine*, October 20, 1988, carried a report by R.G. Stevens of the National Cancer Institute, according to which more cancer was found in men with higher body iron content.

Maria de Sousa left Sloan-Kettering at about this time to return to her native Portugal at the University of Oporto. Subsequently she responded to the Stevens report, stating that children with acute lymphocytic leukemia responded with longer survival times when continued on a low-iron diet.

(As an aside, Martin notes, as per the previously cited Hendhede report, that Denmark's vegetarian diet during the period 1914–1918 was very low in iron.)

It is further noted that, at the turn of the last century, the diet of the natives of Africa was low in iron, only about 20% of that occurring in today's high-meat diet.

As for freedom from myocardial infarction, as seen in the native population of Uganda, a lowering of dietary iron may be far more effective than reducing the serum cholesterol. In further substantiation, Martin cites Jerome L. Sullivan of the Department of Pathology at the South Florida College of Medicine in Tampa. In an article in the June 13, 1982, issue of *The Lancet* titled "Iron and the Sex Difference in Heart Disease," on page 1293 Sullivan reported the obvious, that the United States has a population of about 50 million who avoid death from myocardial infarction. These are premenopausal women (who are on the anemic side). Although these women are on a high-meat diet, the iron is lost by bleeding during menstruation. However, once past menopause, the women also become at risk, the same as men. Thus, Sullivan also notes that high body iron stores are cardiotoxic, particularly those in the heart.

As a counter, blood donations may be in order, and Sullivan recommends that iron in vitamin–mineral pills be avoided by taking those with no iron. Furthermore iron-added breads and cereals should be avoided, the exceptions being whole-grain breads and the cereal named Shredded Wheat®.

Jerome L. Sullivan mentions the disease named thalassemia major, in which body iron stores are much too high and death can occur owing to fibrosis of the myocardium caused by the iron stores therein.

In Africa, the conventional wisdom of the European doctors located there is that iron deficiency anemia is the rule, and pregnant women are given iron supplements. However, the August 10, 1974, issue of *The Lancet* contained a report that the resulting immunosuppression soon resulted in escalating bacterial infections and malaria.

Another line of work indicates that the low-grade (so-called) protein content of vegetarian diets may also act against cancer. Thus, Mark F. McCarty of the Pantox Laboratories reviewed the situation at length in *Medical Hypotheses*, 6, pp. 459–483 (1999). Titled "Vegen Proteins May Reduce the Risk of Cancer, Obesity, and Cardiovascular Disease by Promoting Increased Glucagon Activity," the indicators are that veggie proteins are high in the nonessential amino acids and low in the essential amino acids. (The inverse occurs in animal proteins.) The result is the increased production of glucagon, which has anticancer activity.

More specifically, glucagon is an inhibitor for pyruvate kinase, the enzyme involved in the pyruvate-producing Reaction 9 of the glycolyis sequence represented in Figure 3.1 of Chapter 3 (e.g., in Hoffman, 1999, p. 331). Thus, an excess of glucagon can be viewed as retarding glycolysis, whereby less pyruvate will be formed. Given that the pyruvate formed for the most part further converts to carbon dioxide and water via the carboxylic acid cycle, or Krebs cycle, or carboxylic cycle, there will be less pyruvate available for conversion to lactic acid or lactate. As the latter conversion supports cancer cell metabolism, this support is reduced, yielding an anticancer action.

Thus, the effect of enhanced glucagon activity can therefore be viewed as an anticancer condition, and is signaled by a person (usually) having hypoglycemia, or low blood sugar.

Conversely, the effect of reduced glucagon activity can therefore be viewed as a procancer condition, and is signaled by a person (usually) having hyperglycemia, or high blood sugar. Thus, as hyperglycemia, or high blood sugar, is the usual problem with diabetes, diabetics could be considered at risk for cancer. But this risk would be offset by an insulin-taking regimen. (So far, evidently, the definitive statistics are not there, one way or another.)

In further comment, as set forth in the section "Diet Extremes," there are the two opposing and offsetting pancreatic hormones known as glucagon and insulin. (The hormone glucagon is as distinguished from the polymeric form of glucose called glycogen.) An increase in the activity or concentration of the one decreases that of the other. It so turns out that glycolysis is inhibited by increased glucagon activity, or reduced insulin activity; that is, by the diabetic condition of hyperglycemia, or high blood sugar (James B. Blair, in *The Regulation of Carbohydrate Formation and Utilization in Mammals*). That is, the glucose or glycogen content of the blood is not sufficiently converted by glycolysis.

On the other hand, glycolysis is favored by reduced glucagon activity and increased insulin activity, resulting in the inverse diabetic condition of hypoglycemia, or low blood sugar. That is, the sugar in the blood is more readily converted to its end products.

(A mitigating factor is whether conversion is selective to yield lactic acid or lactate, as in cancer cells, or selective to yield carbon dioxide and water, as in normal cells. This depends on the absence or presence of, say, inhibitors for the enzyme lactic dehydrogenase, as set forth in Chapter 3. That is, absence of inhibitors for lactate dehydrogenase would favor cancer cell metabolism.)

Moreover, the nonessential amino acid alanine supports this discrepancy by enhancing glucagon activity at the expense of insulin activity, and has been denoted a biomarker for anaerobic glycolysis, or at least total glycolysis, whichever prevails. In particular, L-alanine inhibits the enzyme pyruvate kinase, as listed in Appendix Y of Hoffman (1999a). Hence, L-alanine can also be regarded as an anticancer agent, as explained for glucagon earlier, limiting anaerobic glycolysis to produce lactic acid or lactate.

We know that anaerobic glycolysis is the principal pathway for cancer cell metabolism (e.g., Guerra et al., 1993). There is the inference, therefore, that alanine and either insulin or glucagon levels may be indicators for cancer progression or regression, as has been suggested in cancer studies, and may also imply a pro- or anticancer action. The situation is more complicated, however, and there are other enzymes that affect glycogen (or glucose) storage in the liver and cause hypoglycemia, for instance (Voet and Voet, 1995, p. 509). Nothing is ever clear-cut.

McCarty, in the article cited earlier, first explains his finding in terms of cyclic AMP levels, which others have found to make cancer cells liable to contact inhibition, and thus more benign. A possible scenario is that glucagon inhibits a growth factor supporting cancer proliferation, and also induces cancer cell death by apoptosis. The cancers especially noted to be inhibited by a vegan diet are of the breast, prostate, and colon.

Lastly, Wayne Martin refers to a report in the May 18, 1991, issue of *The Lancet* that compares breast cancer incidences for young Chinese women in Singapore. Half were put on a typical high-meat Western diet, the other half on a vegan diet typical of northern China, with much soya food. The former were at three times the risk.

In sum, a low-meat or no-meat (or vegan) diet is seen as the way to go, reducing the odds for having both cancer and heart attacks.

Wayne Martin continues with his recommendations for a low-iron and vegetarian diet, but takes up the immolation of metastatic cancer in the July 2005 *Townsend Letter for Doctors & Patients*. It was found that blood-thinning agents such as coumarin would nullify angiogenesis by dissolving the fibrin jell that surrounds cancer cells. Ordinarily taken as a control against myocardial infarction (MI), a study in the October 17, 1964, issue of *The Lancet* reported that MI patients never died from cancer metastasis. Hence the recommendation of coumarin as an anticancer agent.

At this point, some further reconnoitering is in order about statistics. The Japanese and U.S. death rates mentioned earlier translate to 1.81 and 1.07 per 1000, respectively, which is of the order of the cancer incidence reported for the Hopi Indians. This requires a further distinction to be made between death rate and cancer incidence.

Thus, if the cancer death rate in the U.S. was about 500,000 per year out of a population of 250 million, then this translates to 2 deaths per year per 1000 population — the same number as the cancer incidence reported for the Hopi, which is very low as compared to the cancer incidences in the United States of 1 in 4, or 250 per 1000. The inference is that cancer incidence is greater or much greater than the death rate, or there may be a significant time lag between incidence and death, also called *holdup*. A resolution requires putting cancer incidence on a yearly basis, the same as for death rates.

If we take cancer incidence as given above to occur over an average life span, then the U.S. incidence of 1 in 4, or 250 per 1000, would be divided by the average age to obtain the yearly incidence. Given an average nominal life span of say 70 years for the U.S. population, then the preceding figure becomes about 270/70 or about 4 per 1000 population, becoming the average cancer incidence per year. This would in turn imply that, if the death rate were 2 deaths per year per 1000 population, then on the average half the cancer incidences result in death.

By contrast, the Hopi average cancer incidence per year is virtually nil, depending on the average nominal life span assigned.

A letter from A. Hoffer, M.D., Ph.D., FRCP(C), that has a bearing on the subject appeared in the October 2004 issue of the *Townsend Letter for Doctors & Patients*. Appropriately headed "Lies, Damn Lies and Statistics: The Statistics Game," the letter emphasizes that counting was the original criterion for success or the lack thereof. This was simply a matter of counting whether something worked or did not work — the "go" vs. "no-go" concept. This has been succeeded in today's world by what are called double-blind randomized clinical trials with a calculated 0.05 probability point as the holy of holies, of which Dr. Hoffer is no advocate. The history of clinical trials is briefly reviewed, starting with Daniel from the Book of Daniel who observed that his charges were healthier when they stuck to their accustomed diet. All Daniel did was count. Observing the effect of vitamin-C-containing fruit against scurvy was similarly simple. The same with eating rice bran against beri beri. The observations were convincing. The game of statistics emerged when English gentlemen wanted to win when they rolled the dice at Monte Carlo, thereby beating the odds.

Ralph W. Moss's article in the May 2006 issue of the *Townsend Letter for Doctors and Patients* is titled "Playing with Numbers." He questions the statistics whereby cancer mortality rates are reported to be diminishing slightly or at least staying essentially constant. For one thing, this apparent trend correlates with a decline in autopsies; in other words, the cause of death is not known definitively.

(In *Chances Are ...: Adventures in Probability*, by Michael Kaplan and Ellen Kaplan, an exercise is described in which doctors and hospital administrators graded four different cancer-screening programs. In Program A the death rate was reduced by 34%. In Program B there was an absolute reduction in deaths by 0.06%. In Program C, the survival rate increased from 99.82 to 99.88%. With Program D, some 1592 patients would have had to be screened to prevent 1 death. The doctors and administrators overwhelmingly advocated Program A, but the authors note that the four sets of numbers pertain to the same program. Thus, it all depends upon how the statistics are to be presented.)

Enter the use of probability theory in agriculture on plants and animals, and then in biosocial experiments. There are, however, two basic premises: (1) that the phenomenon studied never changes, and (2) that the sample drawn truly represents the population at large. As for the first, nature is never so accommodating. As for the second, its confirmation would require the expanse and trouble of sampling the entire population.

(Meeting the second premise, however, would merely be a reversion to counting. In sum, probability theory is an idealization, an invention of the mind. Any correlation to reality is *post factum*, that is, after the fact, which applies to pollings and elections.)

The situation was examined by Sir Lancelot Hogben in his book *Statistical Theory: The Relationship of Probability, Credibility and Error*, published in 1957. Hogben's conclusion was that probability theory cannot be used in evaluating human clinical studies, but nevertheless its use continues. For one important thing, there is the placebo effect, for humans respond to hope, faith, belief, and the like. The question then arises of whether this effect is real, and how to measure for it. And, "If the placebo is an essential element of all healing, removing it removes the healing and will injure the patients."

The presumed answer applies to the double-blind study, the gold standard of clinical research, but whose efficacy itself has never been tested. It is perhaps useful in cases where officials have to make decisions that do not involve life vs. death, as judgment can be readily made merely on a probability call (a number) rather than on a time-consuming, subjective evaluation of all the information.

In opposing double-blinds where presumably neither the doctors nor the patients know what is going on, Dr. Hoffer considers these experiments not only inefficient and expensive but unethical — based on lies to the patient and the doctors running the test. Furthermore, Dr. Hoffer doubts that very many of the trials are really double-blinded, as this is very difficult to accomplish.

Instead, Dr. Hoffer cites a rather novel way to proceed to achieve positive results — "if that is one of the objectives" — that involves determining the percentage change in the percentages. As an example, if, say, 5% of the treated group responds whereas 3% of the untreated group responds, this is ordinarily reported as a 66% improvement. A more precise and honest way to report these results is to state that "there was a 66% improvement in the percentage values, not in the improvement rate."

Moreover, there is the problem of emerging side effects. Thus, consider the double-blind study on using Femara (Letrozole®) on 2600 women who had already survived 5 years on the breast cancer drug Tamoxifen. It has been reported that the study was stopped early because it was concluded that, "women taking Letrozole were much less likely to have their cancer return than women taking the placebo, without serious side effects." However, in actual numbers, the differences were relatively minor between the treated group and the placebo, both in recurrences and in deaths. This was countered by the side effect of an increase in osteoporosis for the Letrozole group. Dr. Hoffer further asks, if the treated group had been taking, say, vitamin C instead of Letrozole, with the comparative results the same, would there have been the same upbeat reaction from the cancer specialists?

(An update of orthodoxy vs. alternative treatments for breast cancer is featured in the October 2004 issue of *Life Extension*, and relates to actress Suzanne Somers' bout with breast cancer, as further described in her best-selling book *The Sexy Years*. Without referring directly to the book, the gist of an interview with Ms. Somers is that she forsook the conventional route of treatment and essentially treated herself. However, the author does not proselytize, allowing people to choose for themselves.

Although the conventional wisdom is that natural estrogen or estrogen-like, or bioidentical, hormone drugs are conducive to breast cancer and should be a no-no, Ms. Somers chose to maintain a hormone balance instead — notably via estrodiol, progesterone, and testosterone (and also DHEA, or dehydroepiandrosterone, sometimes called a superhormone), as well as the European anti-breast cancer drug Iscador®. The monitoring of blood tumor biomarkers was only on a yearly basis, as the biomarkers can fluctuate so markedly. She compares her case with a close friend who went the conventional route, unfortunately with disastrous results. The use of conventional drugs such as Tamoxifen, Femara®, and bisphosphonates like Zometa® for maintaining bone integrity was scratched. What works, evidently works.)

An article by David F. Horrobin in *The Lancet*, Vol. 361, pp. 695–697 (2003) is titled "Are Large Clinical Trials in Rapidly Lethal Diseases Usually Unethical?" Horrobin answers the question in the affirmative, writing that the patients do not enter these trials because they are altruistic, but rather because they want to survive, and the trial gives them some hope. Furthermore, these large-scale trials use up skill, time, and money, thus preempting smaller-scale trials. Horrobin's policy is, "… we largely abandon large-scale trials looking for small effects and instead do large numbers of small trials, often in single centers, looking for large effects."

(We note that Dr. Horrobin's philosophy agrees with the concept of creating a countrywide network of cancer clinical research centers, or CCRCs, as previously noted. Dr. Horrobin was also cited in Part 2 of Marcus Cohen's articles on medical censorship.)

Dr. Hoffer agrees with Horrobin's view that drugs should be considered ineffective if very-large-scale trials must be conducted to reveal minor differences. The emphasis should be on real observable differences, so obvious that the results appear at a glance. "We need to continue to count. We need to use statistical analyses very rarely."

## MORE OF THE LATEST ON ALTERNATIVES

Turning to the June 2004 issue of the *Townsend Letter for Doctors & Patients*, as mentioned earlier, a number of alternative cancer therapies are further explored: for example, saunas, what are called vitaletheine modulators, photodynamic therapy, homeopathy, the oncotest, Coley's Toxins, and an overview of protocols.

With regard to the last mentioned, an article by Own R. Fonorow titled "The Cure for Cancer" includes the following therapeutic avenues. Thus, Scottish embryologist John Beard reported in 1902 that certain pancreatic enzymes would inhibit fast-growing cancers, these being the digestive enzymes trypsin and its precursor chymotrypsin. This resulted in what is called the Wolf/Benitez WoBenzym® systemic enzyme formula, which is reported to be the second largest selling over-the-counter product in Europe, second only to aspirin. The Kelley pancreatic enzyme therapy is mentioned, as carried on by Dr. Nick Gonzalez, who was awarded a $6 million grant from the NIH to continue this work.

Furthermore, recent information about pancreatic enzymes is furnished by Ralph W. Moss in the November 2004 issue of the *Townsend Letter for Doctors & Patients* in an article titled "Of Enzymes, Worms, and Cancer." (Moss has a section "Enzyme

Therapy" in his book *Cancer Therapy: The Independent Consumer's Guide to Non-Toxic Treatment and Prevention.*) Earthworms, for instance, can digest just about anything, as was noted by Charles Darwin. Along with insects, worms have been a staple of traditional Chinese medicine for thousands of years. The common earthworm, *Lumbricus rubellus*, is in fact the source of a number of proteolytic enzymes collectively known as lumbrokinase (LK), now available as a food supplement. Taking digestive enzymes is part of the enzymatic treatment of Nicholas J. Gonzales, M.D., and was originally proposed by embryologist John Beard of the University of Edinburgh, in his book *The Enzyme Treatment of Cancer and Its Scientific Basis*, published in 1911. Further positive benefits were reported in the 1950s and 1960s by Franklin H. Shively, M.D., in his self-published manuscript *Multiple Proteolytic Enzyme Therapy for Cancer Administered by Intravenous Infusions*. The work of Dr. Gonzalez has been languishing although supported by an NIH grant, as reported by Peter Chowka in an Internet document; this in spite of the about $200 billion spent so far in the War on Cancer, as stated by Clifton Leaf in his article in *Fortune*, mentioned in Chapter 9.

Moss reflects that the opponents of alternative medicine take the view that enzymes taken orally will be broken down by the digestive processes, and thereby will be ineffective. This was refuted by three physiologists at the University of California–San Francisco, however, who found that the enzymes in fact remained active via what is called enteropancreatic circulation. Hence, the intravenous infusions recommended by Shively are not necessary. (Compare with antibiotics, where oral administrations mostly superseded intravenous injections.)

Fonorow, in the article cited earlier, mentions that the enzymatic connection is supported by the "laetrile" clinics in Mexico, which claim a "100%" cure rate, but only if the patient has not undergone previous chemotherapy or radiation, and if the patient takes the pancreatic enzymes.

It is also mentioned by Fonorow that the University of Michigan Cancer Center has found that chemotherapy targets the wrong cancer cells, killing the harmless cancer cells but missing the small number that proliferate no matter what. Professor Michael F. Clarke, M.D, assumes these to be the cancerous stem cells, as described in Chapter 10.

Also cited is the less expensive cesium protocol, apparently using a total of 6 g of cesium chloride over a 30-day period. The Rath vitamin C protocol is next described; Matthias Rath, M.D., was a former associate of Linus Pauling. In addition to megadoses of vitamin C, there are megadoses of lysine, proline, and green tea extract. Lastly, there are arguments for adding Coenzyme 10 (CoQ10) to any protocol.

Dr. Emanuel Revici's approach is described in a letter from Harold J. Kristal, DDS, based on meeting Dr. Revici's niece Elena Avram, who is carrying on his work, and on William Kelly Eidem's book *The Doctor Who Cures Cancer*. Dr. Revici's analysis is aimed at striking an optimum balance between anabolic and catabolic cellular processes, the one building and the other tearing down. Called metabolic typing, the pH of the blood can be used as a marker, 7.46 being called the ideal, and which can be adjusted by nutrition.

Coley's Toxins received an update by Helen Coley Nauts, cited elsewhere, with an introductory letter from Wayne Martin. Martin furnishes some remarkable "for instances" of cures, and Nauts gives the history behind the development of the toxins. In the course of the article it is mentioned that the toxins produce a beneficial fever.

We now turn to saunas and cancer, in an article by Lawrence Wilson, M.D. An enumeration of beneficial effects is given, which starts off by comparing saunas to hyperthermia, a well-known but underused method for killing cancer cells.

In treating cancer with homeopathy, Dale D. Moss speaks of the Ramakrishnan approach, or plussing method, which uses certain agents in minute quantities — e.g., for lung cancer, the agents *Lycopodium*, Lachesis, and still others are used. There is a dosing schedule that requires several hours in a day to succeed. Some remarkable success percentages are quoted.

Photodynamic therapy (PDT) is said to light-activate a photosensitizer accumulated in a tumor, but not in healthy cells, and which creates a photochemical reaction that selectively destroys the tumor cells. Prominently mentioned as activating agents are tetrapyrrol compounds (e.g., chlorophyll derivatives).

In an article on vitalethine, Galen D. Knight, formerly at the University of New Mexico, describes the substance as a naturally occurring component in mammals that is regulated by modulators so as to influence the course of cancer (www.vital-therapeutics.org). Prominently mentioned are sulfur compounds such as cystamine ($H_2NCH_2CH_2SSCH_2CH_2NH_2$) that influence sugar metabolism. The substance itself is formed in the mammalian body from the amino acid L-cysteine and pantothenic acid (vitamin B5). The actions and interactions furnished are complicated, but it is concluded that niacin has a beneficial therapeutic effect against cancer — although it was surmised that vitamin C may have an adverse effect.

(This course of therapy has its detractors, as can be discerned from the Internet. There seems to be opposition to everything, rightly or wrongly. A criterion that can be used is whether anyone is making money off the therapy. However, this degree of rigor would disqualify the entire health care system.)

This brings us to an article by Savely Yurkovsky, M.D., titled "Guided Digital Medicine: The Law of Unintended Consequences and Non-Disease Treatment of Diseases." Speaking in terms of stress causing strain, a point made is that only the symptoms are treated, not the underlying disease. The side or adverse effects of drugs may be controlled, for instance, with antibiotics and beta-blockers, causing fatigue, insomnia, and depression, as well as with prednisone, producing diabetes and osteoporosis, etc. And vitamin supplements, for instance, may do more harm than good, especially in megadoses — and sometimes become a case of Russian roulette — with the best source of nutrients being old-fashioned foods. (An argument, perforce, for using natural food substances against cancer, such as in the Gerson diet, and such specifics as garlic, even vitamin C, although the beneficial results may be ever so slow in appearing, whereas we are used to immediate action when taking drugs.) A book referenced is Walter A. Heiby's *The Reverse Effect: How Vitamins and Minerals Promote Health and Cause Disease*, published in 1988. (Fat-soluble vitamin A and D overdoses are most usually cited, but even here there is a degree of controversy.)

In substantiation, Dr. Yurkovsky cites the well-known law of pharmacology, called the *Arndt–Schultz law*, that low doses excite physiological activity, moderate doses favor it, but high doses retard or arrest it. An analogy is to Le Chatelier's principle, that chemical systems at equilibrium tend to resist imposed external effects. Further, there are the observations of Dr. Denis Parsons Burkitt, discoverer of Burkitt's lymphoma, about chemotherapy dosage levels. His viewpoint was that smaller is better (possibly serving to stimulate the immune system). It is a protocol favored in Britain but not in the United States.

Thus, a quandary may exist, in light of what has already been said, and what more will be said about the treatment of cancer. But what else to do? It is presumably playing one thing against another, the usual catch-22 situation.

However, this argument may be countered, according to *Natural Strategies for Cancer Patients*, published in 2003. Written by Russell L. Blaylock, M.D., who also authored the book *Excitotoxins*, to be described subsequently, the beneficial role of nutritional supplements is emphasized. Thus, Dr. Blaylock states that in 30 years of practice treating cancer patients with nutritional supplements he has "never seen a single case of tumor-growth acceleration or interference with conventional treatments."

The well-publicized substance known as Coenzyme Q10, or CoQ10, receives favorable mention as an anticancer agent in an article by Christi Yerby appearing in the October 2005 issue of *Life Extension*. He states that low levels of CoQ10 were found in patients with myeloma, lymphoma, and cancers of the breast, lung, prostate, pancreas, colon, kidney, head, and neck. In one case study, a woman with breast cancer experienced a stabilized tumor from taking 90 mg/day of CoQ10. When the daily dose was increased to 390 mg, the tumor disappeared. It was mentioned that CoQ10 is synthesized from the amino acids tyrosine and phenylalanine in a cascade of reactions that involve vitamin C and the B vitamins B2, B3, B5, B6, B12, plus folic acid. Although the body produces CoQ10 naturally, this is sometimes not enough. An earlier reference is S.T. Sinatra's *The Coenzyme Q10 Phenomenon*, published in 1998.

## MAGNESIUM

Having earlier discussed calcium, we now turn to its twin, magnesium; the metals are neighbors in the periodic table and are major components of hard water. In this regard there is the Magnesium Web Site at http://www.mgwater.com, which is devoted to the benefits of magnesium and is maintained by Paul Mason (POB 1417, Patterson, CA 95363). Abstracts and articles are provided from significant scientific contributions in the medical research literature, worldwide.

Another cancer Web site is http://www.mgwater.com/cancer.shtml which has a contribution by Mildred S. Seelig, M.D., MPH, of the Department of Nutrition, School of Public Health, North Carolina University Medical Center. This contribution was published as Chapter 15 in *Adjuvant Nutrition in Cancer Treatment*, P. Quillan and R. M. Williams, Eds., Cancer Treatment Research Foundation, 1993. Titled "Magnesium in Oncogenesis and in Anti-Cancer Treatment: Interaction with Minerals and Vitamins," the material first addresses the epidemiological correlation of magnesium with cancer, stating that there is an increased longevity in hard-water areas. In the United States, these regions comprise the north and central plains, whereas the southeastern coastal area, which is a soft-water region, exhibits decreased longevity. A worldwide comparison is also made.

Other highlights presented are as follows. In studies on magnesium-deficient rats, spontaneous neoplasmas — that is, cancerous tissue — were observed to occur. On the other hand, large magnesium supplements may actually increase the growth rate of already established tumors. However, magnesium reduced the oncogenicity of the heavy metals lead, nickel, and cadmium. It was found also that cancerous tumors have higher magnesium levels than do normal cells, probably owing to the high magnesium requirements of growing cells. Other studies concerned the inter-relationships among magnesium, zinc, and vitamins B6 (pyridoxine) and E. Both magnesium and zinc are needed for many enzyme systems, and deficiencies in vitamin B6 and E will lower tissue magnesium levels. Treatments using irradiation and antineoplastic (anticancer) agents were found to be accompanied by reduced magnesium levels.

Accordingly, it was thought that inducing magnesium deficiency would be a way to treat cancer. This seemed at first to work. However, once magnesium levels were normalized, the tumor would again start to grow. Some 219 references were furnished.

A series of article abstracts about various magnesium-deficiency symptoms, syndromes, conditions, or diseases are supplied at http://www.mgwa-ter.com/abstract.shtml. These include the following: alcohol-related hypertension and strokes, alcohol-induced contraction of cerebral arteries, amyotrophic lateral sclerosis and aluminum deposition in the central nervous system, cardiac arrhyth-mias, asthma therapy, attention deficit disorder (ADD), cerebral artery disorders, constipation, diabetes, heart muscle disorders or myocardial infarction, hypertension, HIV, kidney stones, menopause, migraine, multiple sclerosis, osteoporosis, and premenstrual syndrome. In all cases, an increase in magnesium levels had beneficial effects.

(With regard to aluminum deposition in cerebral arteries, there is the recurring thought that this might be related to Alzheimer's disease and in turn, to a magnesium deficiency.)

Magnesium deficiency has been linked to sudden death in an article by Mark J. Eisenberg, M.D., MPH, of the Cardiology Division of the Department of Medicine, University of California, San Francisco. Published in 1992, the article is reproduced at http://www.mgwater.com/sudden.shtml. What is called *sudden death* continues to be significantly associated with cardiovascular mortality, and the consensus has emerged that a low magnesium content in drinking water correlates with high rates of sudden death. This has been confirmed by autopsy studies and by animal and clinical studies. Magnesium supplementation is advanced, and the addition of mag-nesium (salts) to municipal water supplies, the same as has been done for (or instead of) fluoridation. As the data on which this is all based is mostly from observational studies, further interventional studies are recommended. The article supplies 61 references.

Still another Web site is www.coldcure.com, with the name of George Eby mentioned. Of note is the idea that taking lithium against depression serves to increase the benefits of magnesium, although lithium in itself can be toxic.

## PERIPHERALS

Attention deficit disorder (ADD), mentioned earlier, and now much more often called attention deficit hyperactivity disorder (ADHD), is the subject of an illuminating update and overview by Tim Batchelder in the October 2003 issue of the *Townsend Letter for Doctors & Patients*. First emphasizing the cultural aspects, the article is appropriately titled "Attention Deficit Hyperactivity Disorder and Modern American Culture." A study by Ken Jacobson of the University of Massachusetts is cited whereby the diagnosis rates of British children having ADHD was found to be only about one fifth that of American children. Thus, children considered normal in England would probably be classified as having ADHD in the United States, for hyperactive behavior is to a degree regarded as normal by the English. In fact such labels as "learning disabled," "gifted," and "abnormal" are socially constructed and subjective descriptors that vary with the culture. Researcher Thomas Armstrong (http://www.thomasarmstrong.com/) notes that ADHD provides a neat catchall for explaining the complexities of modern life, and has racist overtones.

Accordingly, perhaps a better way of looking at things is to speak of multiple intelligences, rather than by IQ. Thus, there are linguistic, logical–mathematical, spatial, bodily–kinesthetic, musical, interpersonal, intrapersonal, and naturalist intelligences, although only the first two are measured by conventional IQ tests, and those inclined otherwise are too often lumped as having ADHD. The same criteria may be applied to adults where, so to say, square pegs do not fit into round holes, and vice versa.

Still another way of looking at things is furnished in the *Townsend Letter for Doctors & Patients* of October 2004. A letter submitted by a certain Bill Dueease is titled "Attention Deficit Disorder (ADD): Blessing? Or Disorder?" Dueease indicates that a better name should by "Attention Expansion Advantage," or AEA, for these people have very special advantages that offset the disadvantages, especially if the latter are understood and overcome. He lists a number of prominent persons believed to have had ADD/AEA. People with ADD/AEA do not filter the amount of information the brain receives from the five basic senses: smell, sight, touch, hearing, and taste. Accordingly, they become much more attuned to their surroundings. Not only this, but the brains of these people work much faster than normal, maybe two to three times faster. The result is manifested as a higher intelligence level, with their brains operating mostly on full throttle. Additionally, these people think differently; they operate outside the box. Also, they have an extra sixth sense, their hunches being remarkable and sometimes almost scary. Other attributes are boundless energy, the ability to focus on a problem, and the capacity to conduct multiple activities, or multitasking.

Among the drawbacks of ADD/AEA are a difficulty in sitting still, being disorganized, and being distracted. These people seemingly cannot focus on anything for a very long time, yet can concentrate on a single issue so as to reach important conclusions — which they may forget. Difficult to converse with, they interrupt and bounce from one subject to another. They are impulsive and challenge information, but also are often correct. They become bored easily and do not welcome repetitive tasks, preferring challenges and change.

Against drugs, Dueease recommends overcoming the drawbacks by an understanding of the behavioral differences, and working to adjust and accommodate on a practical and desirable level. (There is also a school of thought that hormonal imbalances may be partly involved.) Himself a person with ADD/AEA, Dueease has founded The Coach Connection. (Contact 800-887-7214, 239-415-1777, or coaches@findyourcoach.com, or see www.findyourcoach.com/00-add-coach.htm. A free copy of the article "The Ten Paths to Human Improvement" is available.)

Other researchers take an evolutionary approach, tracing the ADHD propensity back to the genes, as originally proposed by Thom Hartmann (http://www.thomhartmann.com), with ongoing research at the University of California, Irvine.

More than this, there is something called the "rewards deficiency syndrome," whereby some people are deficient in neurotransmitters, especially dopamine, and as a result seek dopamine augmentation via junk foods and drugs, even gambling.

Another aspect is that the ADHD personality fits in with our very survival, and has its modern counterpart in the movers and shakers of our time.

Such drugs as Ritalin and Dexedrine act to suppress spontaneous behavior, and also can have severe side effects, which are then modulated by antidepressants, in a vicious circle. Furthermore, herbal or nonorthodox wild foods may aggravate the situation, whereas domesticated foods are more benign.

Nevertheless, some herbal substances may prove beneficial in counteracting ADHD, such as curcumin (turmeric), ginger, ginseng, ginkgo, even algae. A listing is available from the Life Extension Foundation (http://www.lef.org).

Illustrative also of the important information to be found in the *Townsend Letter for Doctors & Patients* is an article in the July 2002 issue by David Perlmutter, M.D., and board-certified neurologist, as adapted from the publication *BrainRecovery.com*. Titled "Alzheimer's Disease — A Functional Approach," the article discounts the modern drugs used in the treatment of the disease. Causes are described, which include electromagnetic fields, aluminum, and homocysteine, and documentation is provided. A listing is furnished for antacids and analgesics with aluminum, as well as some of the latter category that do not contain aluminum or its compounds. Effective therapies against Alzheimer's disease encompass the following: reducing inflammation, limiting free radicals, and enhancing neuronal function. For the first mentioned, essential fatty acids are a requirement. For the second therapy, vitamin E, gingko biloba, alpha lipoic acid, $N$-acetyl cysteine, and vitamin D are advocated. For the latter, Coenzyme Q10 (CoQ10), nicotinamide adenine dinucleotide (NADH), acetyl-L-carnitine, phosphatidylserine, vitamin B12, and folic acid are listed.

Digressing in another direction, an editorial by Alan R. Gaby, M.D., appears on page 126 of the July 2002 issue of the *Townsend Letter for Doctors & Patients*. Titled "Thoughts on Adaptation and Evolution," the subject of protein-deficient diets is addressed relative to native peoples with low-protein diets who are nevertheless healthy. Thus, the inhabitants of Australian New Guinea, who subsisted mainly on a sweet potato diet chronically low in protein, were obviously strong and healthy.

It was subsequently found that a nitrogen-fixing bacterium, *Klebsiella aerogenes*, existed in the intestinal tract. It is presumed that the sweet potato diet promoted the growth of these bacteria, which are capable of synthesizing essential amino acids, and the human host thereby becomes a "walking legume."

In the same editorial, it is mentioned that some 80% of the diet for people in regions of tropical Africa comprises sorghum, millet, cassava, and yams. These foods contain nitrilosides that can react to form thiocyanate, which in turn may be oxidized to cyanate. And cyanate is a known inhibitor of sickle cell anemia. Whereas sickle cell anemia occurs in roughly 1 out of 50 genetically disposed persons in the United States, the rate in tropical Africa is less than 1 in a 1000. The inference is that the nitriloside-containing diet is counteractive. An aside is that people who have sickle cell anemia (the natives of Africa) do not contract malaria.

(Nitrilosides are labeled by Dr. Gaby as beta-cyanogetic glycosides. The topic of cyanogenetic glycosides, more familiarly known as laetrile and amygdalin, as anticancer agents is explored elsewhere in this book, and in Hoffman [1999, pp. 76ff, 228, 351ff]. It would be informative to determine whether the corresponding regions of tropical Africa have low, or extremely low, rates of cancer incidence. Cancer clinics in Mexico utilize laetrile, but the track record mostly seems to be missing, although there are a few authorities who have done some follow-up investigations, but they proclaim the treatment has proved ultimately ineffective. Laetrile is also known as vitamin B17, and there are some books concerning this treatment, even a "Little Cyanide Cookbook." Although these kinds of natural compounds occur in such common foods as beans, the cyanide or cyanic content is destroyed by the higher temperatures usually reached in cooking.)

Speaking further of the effectiveness of alternative medicine, and article appeared in the Denver & the West section of the Saturday, June 22, 2002, issue of the combined *Rocky Mountain News* and *Denver Post*. It was written by Amy Bernard Satterfield who, among other things, teaches journalism at Colorado State University, and the article was titled "TCM More than Just Silkworm Poop." The acronym pertains to traditional Chinese medicine, which employs an array of remedies, including acupuncture, herbs, and "silkworm poop." Satterfield was suffering from an undisclosed female complaint, which medical orthodoxy proposed to treat with surgery and massive amounts of hormones. Satterfield opted instead to go to a TCM doctor, who prescribed herbal potions and acupuncture treatments. She writes that she has undergone treatment for 6 months, and since starting the treatment has not had any problems with "my aforementioned unmentionable condition." Although she does not recommend TCM instead of antibiotics for deadly infections or "whiskey for a broken leg," she views it as an alternative to "sharp knives, harsh drugs and magazines about famous people."

While on the subject of Chinese medicine, there is an informative volume titled *Ancient Herbs, Modern Medicine: Improving Your Health by Combining Chinese Herbal Medicine and Western Medicine*, published in 2003, and written by Henry Han, OMD, Glenn E. Miller, M.D., and Nancy Deville.

(The acronym OMD stands for Doctor of Oriental Medicine. Dr. Han, internationally known, founded the Santa Barbara Herb and Wellness Center in 1998. His credentials are included at the end of the book, as well as those of the other authors.

It may also be added that there is a series publication called *Chinese Journal of Integrated Traditional and Western Medicine*.)

The chapter on cancer concerns for the most part the experiences of a 22-year-old American woman diagnosed in 1998 with a dermoid cyst, which is ordinarily nonmalignant, and is formed from the replication of an unfertilized egg. In this case, however, there were symptoms of malignancy, and major surgery ensued, although at the same time there was a search for Chinese medical alternatives, which is where Dr. Han, the first-named author of the book, came in. Dr. Han prescribed an unspecified regimen of some 23 different herbs that was designed to reduce bleeding, promote healing, and strengthen the immune system. In turn, the radical 3-hour operation removed fluid, the tumor and related cancerous tissue, parts of the ovaries, and the entire greater omentum, the connective tissue that covers the abdominal organs, which contained metastasized tumors.

Resisting follow-up chemotherapy, the patient again contacted Dr. Han, who knew of no Chinese alternatives to chemotherapy, save as an adjuvant. Nevertheless, Dr. Han consulted with his mother in China, Dr. Huiwen Luo, who was a Western-trained gynecologist and surgical oncologist. Having been sent by the Cultural Revolution to the remote Hui County of western China, she had found abnormally high rates of uterine, ovarian, and cervical cancer. In response she developed a combination treatment involving surgery, chemotherapy, immunotherapy, and Chinese herbal medicine. The success rate was impressive, with a 10-year survival rate of 42% for stage three cervical patients, and 37% for stage four, the latter the most serious and commonly fatal. (This is as compared to only a 5 to 7% usual survival rate for ovarian carcinoma for stage three and four victims in the United States.)

After a follow-up operation and further treatments, the patient in question was declared in remission, at least at the time of publication, in 2003. The chapter closed with discussions of the side effects of chemotherapy and ways to strengthen the immune system.

## SUBVIRAL AGENTS: PRIONS

As has been previously noted, there are subviral agents called prions that may be responsible for some baffling neurological diseases affecting the brain, such as Alzheimer's disease, and for others such as bovine spongiform encephalitis, or BSE, the so-called mad cow disease. In turn, there are the human counterparts of the latter, namely, Creutzfeldt-Jakob disease and what is called kuru, as once found in the hill tribes of New Guinea. (The last mentioned disease was apparently caused by eating the brains of infected persons, a cannibalistic practice since discontinued.) The increased incidences of BSE has been attributed to the use of rendered animal parts in domestic animal feed, particularly in Britain. (A form occurring in wild animals — either penned in game farms, notably, or even roaming free — is called chronic wasting disease.) And Creutzfeldt-Jakob disease may be the result of crossing the species barrier. There is the inference, therefore, that the ingestion of contaminated meat products could lead to the human Creutzfeldt-Jakob form — and similarly even for dairy products, considering that milk cows may also be fed contaminated feed.

Another neurological disorder has been traced to eating the bat called "the flying fox," and was described by medical anthropologist and columnist Tim Batchelder in the November 2003 issue of the *Townsend Letter for Doctors & Patients*, an issue devoted mainly to multiple sclerosis, or MS. These findings were courtesy of the work of ethnobotanist Dr. Paul Cox, who lives on the Hawaiian island of Kauai and is director of the National Tropical Botanical Garden. Thus, on the Pacific island of Guam the Chamorro people consume flying foxes, washed and boiled, at weddings, fiestas, and religious events. Unfortunately, the flying foxes consume cycad seeds, which contain the neurotoxin beta-methylamino L-alanine (BMAA), and which is retained in the bats at the high levels of 90%. A result is the neurological disease called ALS-PDC, for amytrophic lateral sclerosis–Parkinsonian dementia complex. This disease is related to Lou Gehrig's, Parkinson's, and Alzheimer's diseases.

Batchelder also notes that people in Guam and the West Indies consume the pawpaw fruit, as is, or as a tea — and have abnormally high rates of Parkinsonism (related to Parkinson's disease), due to certain alkaloids present in the fruit (and which also serve as insecticides). The reference is not specific about just which pawpaw is involved. The North American species is *Asimina triloba*, although there is also *A. parviflora*, both of the plant family Annonaceae. There are still other species that occur in tropical Central America, *A. squamosa* and *A. reticulata* — with the common name custard apple sometimes used. Also of the same family, there is the species *Annona muricata*, better known as graviola, about which much has been said of late as an anticancer agent. On the other hand, the common papaya is sometimes called a pawpaw, but is of the species *Carica papaya* of the family Caricaceae. It may be noted that the family Annonaceae contains aporphine and other alkaloids, and the species *Carica papaya* contains the alkaloid carpaine, which has also been used as an anticancer agent (Hoffman, 1999, pp. 504, 506, 518).

Batchelder in turn notes that the outlawed liqueur called absinthe is making a reappearance, although with much lower concentrations of wormwood. (There are now only about 10 parts per million of the active neurological ingredient alpha-thujone — presumably the inducer of artistic genius — rather than the 260 ppm in days of yore.) A few of the celebrated imbibers in times past include Van Gogh, Baudelaire, Rimbaud, Verlaine, Toulouse-Lautrec, and Picasso.

Lastly, Batchelder has a few remarks about multiple sclerosis, latitude, and evolution. Thus, it is well known that MS occurs more frequently at higher latitudes, which may be attributed to a lack of intense sunlight, the natural agent producing vitamin D synthesis in the body. In comparing the prairie provinces of Canada to the fish-eating eastern provinces, there is also a correlation of MS with a higher consumption of dairy products, glutinous grains (such as wheat), and saturated fats — the principal elements of the civilized diet. It is worth recalling here that vitamin D has been found to be an anticancer agent in other studies.

For a review of the situation, an article by Jonathan V. Wright, M.D., in the May 2004 issue of the *Townsend Letter for Doctors & Patients* spells out the role of vitamin D in preventing a number of illnesses. He argues that its insufficiency has resulted in a dramatic increase in these illnesses. It is titled "Vitamin D: Its Role in Autoimmune Diseases and Hypertension," and cites the work of Michael Holick, M.D., Ph.D., of Boston University. For our purposes, we note that the prevalence of prostate, breast, and eleven other cancers is affected by vitamin D deficiency. Discounting the benefits of milk, to which vitamin D is routinely added, Wright is in favor of sunshine as the primary source for producing vitamin D in the body, and is in favor of a little sunburn — that is, enough to produce only a shade of pink. He notes that the body naturally protects itself against an overdose of vitamin D, as we try to avoid severe sunburn, and, at the same time, the tanning or browning process reduces the amount of sunshine absorbed. There is again a correlation with the 35° latitude (Circa Louisiana and Charleston, South Caroline) — as with MS — above which latitude the incidence of these cancers markedly increases. Hence, enter the role of vitamin D supplements, which have the beneficial side effect of lowering blood pressure.

(Interestingly, according to the studies of Valhjalmur Stefansson on the Far North, the Eskimos did not suffer from cancer incidence on their native high-fat diet — a source of vitamin D — until they yielded to the typical modern, "civilized" diet.)

MS and its treatment and cure are further addressed in a letter from Wayne Martin in the January 2005 issue of the *Townsend Letter for Doctors & Patients*. He details the treatment protocol used by Dr. Frederich Klenner of Reidsville, North Carolina. Reference is made to the successful cure of a certain Dale Humpreys using the Klenner treatment as described in Humphrey's letter appearing in the November 2004 issue of the *Townsend Letter for Doctors & Patients*. The basis is that a virus (possibly the Coxsackie virus) produces small hemorrhages in the nerves, resulting in scars when healing takes place. These scars restrict the flow of blood to the nerves. To counter this effect, Dr. Klenner used vitamin E (3200 IU per day) and niacin (from 100 mg to 3000 mg per day), the latter to induce flushing, thus dilating the blood vessels compressed by the scars. Cell regeneration in the damaged myelin sheath of the nerves was countered by massive amounts of vitamin C (10 to 20 g per day). This was complemented by the respiratory enzymes thiamine and riboflavin. The former was taken orally in dosages of 300 to 500 mg four times a day, and 500 mg per day by hypodermic injection. The latter consisted of oral doses of 25 mg taken four times per day, and 40–80 mg per day by injection. In turn, 200 mg of calcium pantothenate was taken orally four times a day. Needed choline was supplied by 3600 mg of soya lecithin, and there were daily injections of 1 cc of crude liver extract. Included were 40 g of glycine, notably from gelatin, as well as 100 mg of magnesium per day taken orally. This comprises the Klenner treatment; it is complicated and involved, but then MS is a serious disease.

In this same letter Martin notes the immunosuppressive effect of polyunsaturated fats, as addressed in his letter appearing in the August 2002 issue of the *Townsend Letter for Doctors & Patients*. He cites Dr. Newsholme of the University of Oxford as to how polyunsaturated fats act against autoimmune diseases, of which MS is one. A treatment protocol is described using 1 g of fish oil per day (or maybe more, up to 12 g per day). Sunflower seed oil, which is an omega-6 fat, or fatty acid, is said to act similarly, whereas fish oil is an omega-3 fat.

(Technically speaking, for the record, the essential fatty acids, or EFAs — which are not synthesized in the human body — have been distinguished as having an unsaturated bond occurring within the last seven carbons of the methyl end of the fatty acid chain, designated the "omega" end. Thus, omega-3 fatty acids will have a first unsaturated bond between carbons numbered three and four from the omega end, whereas omega-6 fatty acids will have a first unsaturated bond between carbons numbered six and seven. The former are more prevalent in fish oils, and the latter in vegetable oils, although flaxseed oil favors the former. Each group will have different metabolic pathways, for better or worse, and it is a controversial subject that is not yet resolved. A reference is Boik, 1996.)

However, Martin raises the question that if the polyunsaturated fats are immunosuppressive, can they also be a cause of cancer?

## MORE ON DNA

The subject of prions leads to Barry Commoner's elegantly written report published in the February 2002 issue of *Harper's Magazine*. Titled "Unraveling the DNA Myth: The Spurious Foundation of Genetic Engineering," it has much broader implications. Barry Commoner is senior scientist at the Center for the Biology of Natural Systems at Queens College, City University of New York. Long known for his proenvironment stance, he now serves as director of the Critical Genetics Project. For starters, Commoner notes that biology has displaced physics as the "science of the century," with the promise of godlike powers of creating artificial forms of life. He cites the cloning of the sheep Dolly, a rhesus monkey that carries the genes of a luminescent jellyfish, and faster-growing pigs having a gene that begets bovine growth hormone, soybean plants engineered to resist herbicides, and corn plants with a bacterial gene causing them to be poisonous to earthworms.

On the downside, conveniently ignored or suppressed, are the developmental flaws and abortive failures in the cloned animals, the fact that the monkey does not glow like a jellyfish, and that the genetically engineered pigs have many side effects such as ulcers, arthritis, enlarged hearts, and kidney disease. As for the engineered plants, their own genetic system has been altered, with the potential consequences yet unknown.

These consequences aside, there is more to the story in that the total complement of DNA genes, called the genome, cannot fully account for the organisms' characteristics. This is contrary to the premise known as the "central dogma," which was disproved by the facts uncovered in the highly publicized Human Genome Project, conducted between 1991 and 2001. In short, despite the biotechnological industry's claims, genetic engineering cannot produce results that are "specific, precise, and predictable" — and therefore safe. Other factors are at work, which Barry Commoner proceeds to elucidate, although in increasingly technical language.

Thus, it had been theorized by Francis Crick — who with James Watson had discovered the DNA double helix — that the sequence of about 3 billion nucleotides in human DNA were necessary and sufficient, absolutely and exclusively, to identify and enumerate all the genes in the human body. In further explanation, if that is the word, DNA (or deoxyribonucleic acid) is the molecular agent of inheritance, and is an extremely long linear molecule composed of four kinds of nucleotides, which occur in a particular order within each gene. The molecule, however, is tightly coiled within each cell's nucleus. Segments of DNA form the genes, which in turn uniquely determine our individual inherited characteristics, or traits.

(The foregoing suggests a discrete structural unit of definite and invariable length for the hereditary unit that is called a gene. In the abstract, it may instead be thought of as an operational entity with properties dependent on the mode of measurement. See, for instance, the appropriate section in the *Encyclopedia Britannica*. Thus, there is the proposition that the functioning of a gene not only depends on its intrinsic properties but on those of neighboring genes. Moreover, the gene segments exist in some sort of position-dependent continuum, or in some most-probable arrangement. The notion of probability is thus introduced.)

The sequence of events may be diagrammed as DNA→ RNA→ protein. By providing instructions to RNA (or ribonucleic acid) as the intermediary or translator or transcriptor, DNA thereby initiates the generation of protein, although there is a reverse sequence, whereby RNA provides the genetic instructions to DNA, a feature of retroviruses, including HIV and the Ebola and Marburg viruses. Retroviruses have also been associated with the formation of cancerous cells, as have still other kinds of viruses.

(We now briefly recapitulate what has been discussed in Chapter 3: A nucleotide or nucleoside can be described as a monomeric unit of certain so-called "bases" containing nitrogen, which are combined with a deoxyribose, or ribose sugar, and a phosphate group, respectively. The word *ribose* signifies a pentose, a form of sugar containing five carbon atoms. What is called deoxyribose is ribose with a hydroxy, or OH, group absent. The polymer of nucleotides and nucleosides is a nucleic acid, either deoxyribose nucleic acid or ribose nucleic acid. The resulting nucleic acid, designated as DNA or RNA as the case may be, is found in chromosomes, mito-chondria, bacteria, and viruses, that is, in virtually all living cells. A chromosome is the structure in the cell nucleus containing the DNA. The mitochondria, for instance, are membranous subunits or organelles within a cell, and are involved in producing cellular energy and related functions.)

However, it was already known that cell proteins come into contact with numer-ous other proteins and with molecules of DNA and RNA (Commoner, 2002, p. 42). This fact was theorized away by assuming that the cellular proteins were "chaste" rather than "promiscuous." Nevertheless, the assumption was incorrect, for the genome research teams reported that the number of genes predicted from the esti-mated number of human proteins was awry. Instead of the predicted 100,000 or more genes, there were only about 30,000. The latter figure is compatible with a mustardlike weed having some 26,000 genes, and is only about twice as great as the gene count for a fruit fly or worm. It is hardly the criterion for distinguishing a human life from that of a fly or a carrot. A human would, in fact, be barely distinguishable from a mouse, "99 percent of whose genes have human counterparts."

Another significant objection to the theorizing of the central dogma occurs in terms of what is called alternative splicing. For in alternative splicing, the gene's original nucleotide sequence may be split into fragments, which then recombine in various (and unexpected) ways. In Commoner's words: "Alternative splicing thus has a devastating effect on Crick's theory" (Commoner, 2002, p. 43). Not only this, but other research has tended to contradict the double helix itself as central to the theorizing: "The precise duplication of DNA is accomplished by the living cell, not by the DNA molecule alone."

Moreover, in the living cell, replication of the gene's nucleotide sequence requires the assistance of specialized proteins called *chaperones*, which determine the way that the newly created protein molecule is folded in a three-dimensional sense. This affects the enzymatic action for such traits as creating eye color. However, some proteins may become misfolded, and remain inactive unless a special chaperone protein folds them.

These refolded proteins, however, lack nucleic acid, having neither DNA nor RNA, and the name given is *prions*, denoting nuclear-acid-free proteins (or, with a reshuffling of letters, for *pro*teinaceous *in*fectious particles). Their existence was confirmed by Stanley Pruisner, in the 1980s, to be the infectious agents found in scrapie, mad cow disease, and the corresponding almost always fatal human diseases (such as Creutzfeldt-Jakob disease and kuru).

The very fact that these subviral-sized prions exist without having either DNA or RNA also contradicts the central dogma that DNA, and DNA alone, is central to life.

Barry Commoner writes that the delay in dethroning the all-powerful theoretical role given to the gene in the 1990s permitted the invasion of genetic engineering into American agriculture, although the errors had already been noted a decade earlier (Commoner, 2002, p. 45). Thus, in a genetically engineered plant, the alien bacterial gene, say, will interact with and disrupt the plant's own genetic system in unknown ways (Commoner, 2002, p. 45). Furthermore, the biotechnology industry is not required to furnish any basic information about the composition of these transgenic plants.

In his concluding remarks, Barry Commoner states that "DNA did not create life; life created DNA. DNA is a mechanism created by the cell to store information." He further comments that the central dogma has been to a degree protected from criticism in ways more akin to religion than to science, for scientific dissent can be a punishable offense, leading to professional ostracism. An irony is that the biotechnology industry is based on 40-year-old science, and conveniently ignores more recent results. "What the public fears is not the experimental science but the fundamentally irrational decision to let it out of the laboratory into the real world before we truly understand it."

Lastly, we may add that cancerous cells can be perceived as another example of genetic modification, by one or another of the routes indicated in Barry Commoner's article. It may be asked, furthermore, can these kinds of genetic modifications in turn lead to a cure or cures?

## MORE ON DIET

In his exposé *Fast Food Nation: The Dark Side of the All-American Meal*, published in 2001, Eric Schlosser has some revealing findings about the meat industry, or the beef trust as he calls it. It has echoes of Upton Sinclair's blockbuster, *The Jungle*, published back in 1906. Or the more things change…. Among other things, Schlosser tells how the traditional ranchers and cattlemen are being superseded by the giants of agribusiness. He takes up the matter of commercial feedlots, slaughterhouses, meat processing, and inspections — and the lack thereof of the last mentioned. There is a reminder of other volumes challenging the meat industry, for example, Jeff and Jessica Pearson's *No Time but Place: A Prairie Pastoral*, published in 1980, about what happened in southeastern Colorado, as feedlots took over. Another polemic, casting a wider net, is Jeremy Rifkin's *Beyond Beef: The Rise and Fall of the Cattle Culture*, published in 1992.

Among other things, Schlosser notes the increasing occurrences of the deadly mutant bacterium species *E. coli* 157:H7 as well as other pathogens (Schlosser, 2001, p. 194ff). Concerning the outbreaks of "mad cow disease," or BSE (bovine spongiform encephalitis), he notes that about 75% of the cattle in the United States had been routinely fed rendered livestock wastes until August 1997 (Schlosser, 2001, p. 202ff). These wastes include the rendered remains of dead sheep and cattle, plus millions of dead cats and dogs every year, as acquired from animal shelters. It may be added that it may take 10 or more years after exposure for the human variant of BSE, Creutzfeldt-Jakob disease, to show up.

(The recycling of undigested feed is a standard operational procedure, or SOP, whereby the manure proper is separated from the residual grains, the latter to serve again as feed. The coined term is *anaphage*.)

The routine testing for *E. coli* 157:H7 and other pathogens has been obstructed by Republican-controlled presidencies and Congresses, for which some names are furnished (Schlosser, 2001, pp. 206–210). Thus, Schlosser maintains that the Reagan and earlier Bush administrations cut spending on public health measures, and staffed the U.S. Department of Agriculture with officials more interested in deregulation than in food safety, although the newly elected Clinton administration attempted to reverse this trend. Reversal was blocked, however, when the Republicans gained control of Congress in 1994, to wit: "Both the meatpacking industry and the fast food industry have been major financial supporters of the Republican Party's right wing." For instance, it is mentioned that Congressman Newt Gingrich, who became speaker of the House, received more money from the restaurant industry than any other congressman. The meatpacking industry also directed most of its campaign expenditures in similar directions, for example to Senators Mitch McConnell (KY), Jesse Helms (NC), and Orrin Hatch (UT). Senator Phil Gramm (TX) received more money from the meatpacking industry than any other senator.

Schlosser addresses the use of "natural flavors" to enhance the taste of such fast food products as fries (Schlosser, 2001, p. 120ff). These additives are required only to be GRAS (Generally Recognized As Safe), and do not require public disclosure. Schlosser names a few. Thus an artificial strawberry flavor may contain the following: amyl acetate, butyrate, and valerate; anethol; anisyl formate; benzyl acetate and isobutyrate; butyric acid; cinnamyl isobutyrate; cinnamyl valerate; cognac essential oil; diacetyl; dipropyl ketone; ethyl butyrate, cinnamate, heptanoate, heptylate, lactate, methylphenylglycidate, nitrate, propionate, and valerate; heliotropin; hydroxyphenyl-2-butanone (10% solution in alcohol); α-ionone; isobutyl anthranilate and butyrate; lemon essential oil; malltol; 4-methylacetophenone; methyl anthranilate, benzoate, cinnamate, heptine carbonate, napthyl ketone, and salicylate; mint essential oil; neroli essential oil; nerolin; neryl isobutyrate; orris butter; phenethyl alcohol; rose; rum ether; γ-undecalactone; vanillin; plus a solvent.

And although mixtures of many volatile chemicals are the rule, a single chemical may instead furnish the dominant aroma. Thus, ethyl-2-methyl butyrate smells unmistakably like apple. A popcorn smell is provided by methyl-2-peridylketone. A marshmallow taste is given by adding ethyl-3-hydroxybutanoate. There is a constituent called hexanal (an aldehyde) that smells like freshly cut grass. On the other hand, body odor is approximated by 3-methyl-butanoic acid. (It may be noted that butyric acid smells like rancid butter and is considered an anticancer agent.)

## THE NAVAJO AND CANCER

It has been mentioned several times in this book that the Navajo have a very low natural incidence of cancer, attributed mainly to avoiding the consumption of poultry and poultry products. Thus, the admissions records of the Monument Valley Hospital in southeastern Utah showed only 13 cases of cancer out of 13,000 admissions over a 5-year period. John Heinerman in his *The Spiritual Wisdom of the Native Americans* makes the connection with Navajo cooking and eating habits. Admittedly eating their fair share of junk food, two practices stand out: boiling their mutton for a long time, thereby killing any cancer-provoking viruses, and the tribal taboo against eating chickens and eggs — sources of some weird viruses, which may include cancer-causing retroviruses. One exception prominently cited, for a 30-year period, was the single case of prostate cancer among 5000 Navajos, and he had flouted the taboo by raising and eating chickens.

The subject of viruses in various meat products was investigated in Part 7, "Viruses and Cancer," in Hoffman (1999a). There has not been much published information, but what there is, is of definite concern, and is set forth in Section 7.8, "Viruses in Animal Products," of the cited reference. Although the emphasis has been mostly on bacterial microorganisms, the emergence of BSE, or mad cow disease, and its fatal human counterpart called Creutzfeldt-Jakob disease, has stirred an interest in viruses and subviruses, or prions. An array of different viruses are noted to appear in animals at the time of slaughter, notably in the feces, and for the most part cause disease only in the animals. The list includes foot-and-mouth disease, hog cholera and African swine disease, fowl and sheep cholera, and Newcastle disease in birds and domestic fowl. Ordinarily considered not transferable to humans, there is nevertheless the possibility of a crossing or mutation of these viruses with human viruses, as in the case of influenza strains. Milk is also a potential source, and may include viruses causing hepatitis. Viruses are found in seafoods, not to mention human animal and human waste. Inasmuch as a rigorous system of classification has not been developed for viruses, they are categorized by size and shape and include picornaviruses, reoviruses, adenoviruses, caliciviruses, astroviruses, etc. An unknown is whether or not they may transmute to retroviruses, considered a prime factor in cancer causation.

However, despite the fact that in the natural state the Navajo are mostly free from cancer, there are tragic uranium-derived consequences for the Navajos and other tribes, and for their land and water; and also for others who have lived and worked around the uranium mines and mine tailings, near test sites, and at the Los Alamos National Laboratory (LANL). These facts are amplified at a personal level in Alex Shoumatoff's *Legends of the American Desert: Sojourns in the Greater Southwest* (Shoumatoff, 1997, pp. 87–91, 457, 458, 463, 477–480). For starters, the largest radioactive spill in history, called the Churchrock incident, occurred on July 19, 1979, when a containment dam burst, spilling hundreds of millions of gallons of water and immense tonnages of uranium mine tailings into the Rio Puerco. Not only were the river and riverbed contaminated for miles downstream, but the contamination has spread into the water table, not only from this spill but from water-filled abandoned mines. Leukemia and cancer are high on the list of causes of death, but the government has been reluctant ever to admit that radiation was the source. While discussing the effects of radiation, Shoumatoff furnishes some observations and quotes about the personnel at LANL and their families. Thus, the laboratory society has been called a "self-selected incestuous culture," and Los Alamos itself has been called "an island of paranoia and privilege." In laboratory jargon there are three strata: the longhairs or cones — with several racial or religious subdivisions — then the plumbers or technicians, and lastly the creeps. The longhairs or cones, or "labbies," have developed the left side of the brain, the pragmatic and technical side, at the expense of the right side, the intuitive and compensatory side. "This has made them smart and brilliant, but lopsided, and has made for a lot of marital problems." In addition to being mostly workaholics, they are in a place where no brownie points accrue for having a good marriage. In a way of speaking, Los Alamos is dedicated to death, and is "our entire culture's collective shadow."

For other chilling details about the fallout from the bombs and nuclear energy, there is award-winning reporter Eileen Welsome's *The Plutonium Files: America's Secret Medical Experiments in the Cold War.* On the dust cover it is described as "A harrowing account of inhumanity … " whereby "Welsome uncovered a grotesque series of experiments in which American atomic scientists turned eighteen unsuspecting citizens into human guinea pigs, with tragic results." And more, much more, within the book itself, including further accounts of the goings-on at LANL.

Although there may be some temporary beneficial effects for being exposed to radiation —gaseous radon therapy consists of sitting around in a radon-containing atmosphere — the effects are not long-lived. Thus, as Eileen Welsome mentions in her book, radiation irritates  blood-forming organs, causing a temporary increase in red and white blood cell production, which is accompanied by a feeling of well-being (Welsome, 1999, p. 50). After this, even after a period of years, devastation sets in.

Returning to cancer's natural incidence, the aboriginal Eskimos, who lived essentially on a diet of meat and fat, evidently did not contract either cancer or scurvy, according to the previously mentioned Valhjalmur Stefansson, noted explorer of the Canadian Arctic. Nor apparently do the Hunzas of the Himalayas, who have a lactovegetarian diet. Stefansson believed the intestinal bacterial flora adjusted to the one or to the other, and that it is the mixed diet that causes the trouble. Among other things, Stefansson declared that occurrences of cancer correlated with appendicitis, constipation, and corpulence. As for the recipe for health, in the few months before birth, there should be a healthy mother on a healthy diet, followed by prolonged breast-feeding, and finally a diet of fresh and raw foods with a minimum of processing. Stefansson's books dealing with these subjects are *Cancer: Disease of Civilization?* and *The Fat of the Land.*

# 9 Cancer Esoterica

An understanding of cancer cell behavior and the effects of the body's defenses and other phenomena will influence treatment protocols. These extraneous phenomena may include viruses or microorganisms, assorted chemicals or biochemicals, and even electromagnetic interactions. The following constitutes a partial review and a deeper examination of some of the topics from the preceding chapters.

## THE MORPHISM OF CANCER CELLS

In the formation of oncogenes, depending on the action of still other viruses, or helper viruses, the end result will be either a solid tumor or a blood-related cancer such as leukemia. In turn, solid tumors may be classified as carcinomas or sarcomas, depending on what kind of body tissue is involved. Furthermore, cancerous cells mimic the normal cells from which they originated, resulting in the classification of more than 100 different kinds of cancer, with some figures above 300, or even as many as 600 different kinds.

Moreover, the fact that cancerous cells mimic normal cells prevents a triggering response from the immune system. The immune system simply cannot recognize a person's cancerous cells. Nevertheless, it can recognize another person's cells, including cancerous cells, as evidenced by the fact that organ transplants require suppression of the immune system. Research is proceeding, however, on ways to trigger an individual's own immune response against cancer cells. (This line of investigation was described by Stephen S. Hall in the April 1997 issue of the *Atlantic Monthly* and in his book, *A Commotion in the Blood* [1997], and it pertains principally to melanoma.)

There is also the consideration that the action of gut flora may produce carcinogenic biochemicals that enter the bloodstream and result in the formation of cancerous cells.

As for the skin cancer named melanoma, its formation involves the action of an enzyme called tyrosinase, which is required for the production of the skin pigment called melanin. The processes are said to be entirely different than for the formation of solid cancers and blood-related cancers.

Speaking further of viruses and cancer again brings up the subject of polymorphism or pleomorphism, whereby the same microbe, microorganism, virus, or virus-like organism may exist in two or more forms, as large as a bacterium, or maybe even as a subviral particle, such as a prion (e.g., as implicated in mad cow disease, or bovine spongiform encephalitis, and in the human form called Creutzfeldt-Jakob disease). The general subject has been reviewed, for instance, in Moss's *Cancer Therapy: The Independent Consumer's Guide to Non-Toxic Treatment and Prevention* (1992), Hoffman's *Cancer and the Search for Selective Biochemical*

*Inhibitors* (1999a), and in an article by Schaefer and Majnarich appearing in the August/September 2001 issue of the *Townsend Letter for Doctors & Patients*. A partial listing of prominent investigators who have been involved includes the names of Rife, Livingston, and Naessens — plus many others cited in the previous references, which also serve as a critique for the state of affairs.

Adding to the confusion is that there are as yet no systematic methods of cataloguing or classifying viruses that exist in terms of species of other microorganisms, and organisms. Most viruses are thought to remain unknown, and the relatively few that are known are merely classified by size and shape.

The subject is in flux, but the existence of polymorphism or pleomorphism is confirmed by such everyday examples as insect larva and their morphological transformation, for example, the caterpillar–pupa–butterfly sequence. The oceanic phenomena called red tide include a metamorphic organism that in one form exists as an animal-like flagellate, evidencing a trailing appendage, but in another form is more like a plant or alga (e.g., Hoffman, 1999a, pp. 187, 188). These are the concerns of Rodney Barker's *And the Waters Turned to Blood: The Ultimate Biological Threat* (1997). In any event, toxins are produced that can be life-threatening.

While on the subject of pleomorphism and the like, there is a video out titled *The Rise and Fall of a Scientific Genius*, about the career and findings of the much-cited Royal Rife, written and directed by Shawn Montgomery. A review was furnished in the January 2004 issue of the *Townsend Letter for Doctors & Patients*, and another in the November 2005 issue. Mentioned is the fact that in the early part of the twentieth century, Rife's work was respected by eminent medical researchers and physicists and was financially supported by Henry Timken, Jr., of the Timken Roller Bearing Company. (A device invented by Rife had saved the company millions of dollars.) A laboratory was provided by Timken in San Diego, and Rife received the cooperation of a Dr. Milbank Johnson, head of the local medical society, who was affiliated with the University of Southern California. Two prominent bacteriologists also worked with Rife: Dr. E. C. Rosenow of the Mayo Clinic and Dr. Arthur Kendall of Northwestern University.

Rife's work included the development of the Universal Microscope, which achieved magnifications of up to 31,000X on living organisms — rather than on dead organisms as with the electron microscope. A result was confirmation of Antoine Béchamp's conclusions that disease developed within the biochemical environment of the body by various ongoing and changing processes, rather than upholding the rigid view of Pasteur and Koch, that of "One bug — one disease." A prominent discovery was that of a fungus in people with cancer, a fungus that is said to have started out as a virus and is called the Bx cancer virus.

It is further added that Rife's Beam Ray Instrument (the radio frequency device) was clinically tested in a University of Southern California study on 16 terminally ill cancer patients in 1934, all supervised by a panel of medical experts. Fourteen were pronounced cured within 70 days; the other two required 20 more days before being clinically cured. Nevertheless, Rife's work was discounted by certain of the medical establishment, who succeeded in restrictedly defining a "virus" only as a particular microorganism that proliferates by modifying the genetic machinery of the host cells, rather than as encompassing the pleomorphism phenomenon discovered by Rife and others.

The video is subtitled *Part I: Rife's Rise* and is followed by *Part II: Rife's Fall*. The latter highlights the (successful) efforts at suppression with examples, courtesy of Morris Fishbein of the American Medical Association. A further application is furnished in Bryan Rosner's *When Antibiotics Fail: Lyme Disease and Rife Machines, with Critical Evaluation of Leading Alternative Therapies*; it was reviewed in the November 2005 *Townsend Letter for Doctors & Patients*.

Interestingly, in the December 2005 issue of the same periodical, Ralph Moss's column "The War on Cancer," asks the question, "Do Radio Frequency Energy Fields Cause Cancer?" The question pertains mostly to mobile phones. The American Cancer Society says no, but Moss offers some information to the contrary. In any event, there is the work of Rife and others using radio frequency electromagnetic fields (RFEMFs) against cancer.

In the same issue there is a remarkable article by Gitte S. Jensen, Ph.D., an immunologist and cancer researcher affiliated with McGill University. Descriptively titled "Microscopy and the Search for the Soul," it updates present research and laboratory instrumentation and also, interestingly, reinforces Béchamp's view that there is more to life than meets the eye via mere microscopy, contrary to Pasteur's restricted outlook. Among the findings is that the blood from patients with various chronic and acute illnesses can look drastically different than the blood from healthy people. A number of other researchers were pursuing work along the same lines, and their findings resulted in two world conferences on pleomorphism put together by Jensen.

A prominent discovery indicates that bacteria can exchange genetic information, resulting in evolutionary forms that thrive even under extreme circumstances. A further assessment is that there is no single cancer-causing bacterium, symbiont, or parasite, though bacterial presence and inflammation are linked to cancer (Personnet, 1999). There are still other considerations, with references supplied. Thus, biophysical forces and their interactions are mentioned (see L. McTaggart, *The Field: The Quest for the Secret Force of the Universe*.) Bioelectric potentials also enter (Becker and Selden, 1985). It is noted that the DNA decoding has been viewed as the near end of the search for the essence of life, whereas the subject is much more complex even than this, because DNA interacts with electromagnetic phenomena. Caution is advised in genetic manipulations, because our views are oversimplistic, there being so much not yet known in the interactions that could occur.

Jensen discusses several unusual concepts, that of the somatid (Naessen's symbiont, a particle associated with lifelike qualities), the protit (a living protein particle), and the bion (a transitional form between nonliving and living matter). Mention is made of Naessen's 714X, which can be described as a camphor compound used against cancer; however, it was conversely found to reduce the ability of natural killer cells to kill cancer cells *in vitro*.

Other references listed include Clark (1997) and Lockshin et al. (2004), as well as the earlier work of Germany's G. Enderlein, mentioned elsewhere.

In partial conclusion, the foregoing ties in with the more recent advances in medicine: chronic inflammation, or the inflammation response, is a common characteristic associated with all sorts of diseases, including heart disease, cancer, diabetes, arthritis, asthma, and maybe even Alzheimer's. In other words, over the long term, the body's immune system or immune response to a particular condition can eventually turn against itself, causing still other diseases or manifestations. (A term used is *autoimmune disease*.) The marker for the inflammatory condition is called the C-reactive protein, but the counter is yet in abeyance, and may be more a matter of diet and lifestyle rather than immunity per se.

The subject is explored, for instance, by Christine Gotman and Alice Park in the February 23, 2004, issue of *Time*, with the article reprinted in the July 2004 issue of *Life Extension*. Of special interest is a paragraph relating to the broader implications of inflammation and its treatment: "The concept is so intriguing because it suggests a new and much simpler way of warding off disease. Instead of different treatments for, say, heart disease, Alzheimer's and colon cancer, there might be a single inflammation-reducing remedy that would prevent all three." (Or, in comment, there might well be a single treatment for all kinds of cancer.)

The same issue of *Life Extension* contains an article by Dean S. Cunningham, M.D., Ph.D., where the possibility is brought up that the herb *Stephania tetranda* (stephania), long used in China against various ailments, might act against inflammation. (Aspirin is the most well-known anti-inflammatory chemical substance, with Celebrex® a newer drug on the scene.) The herb stephania, known in China as han-fang-chi or fen-fang-qi, contains a number of identified compounds: tetrandine, fangchinoline, cyclanoline, stephanathrine, oxofangchinoline, 2-*N*-methyltetrandine, and cyclanine. Some can be classed as alkaloids, and it is noted that in Chinese medical philosophy, the use of multiple ingredients is considered to be more effective than a single ingredient.

The subject is further examined in terms of chronic drug treatment by Sherry A. Rogers, M.D., in *The High Blood Pressure HOAX!*, published in 2005, and reviewed in the August/September 2006 issue of the *Townsend Letter for Doctors & Patients*. One readily becomes a "heart" patient if a first reading is above the current guidelines for risk (which sometimes change). Doctors who study sudden cardiac arrest have found that C-reactive protein was the most predictive risk factor rather than cholesterol. Because C-reactive protein is a marker for inflammation, for example, from infections and the environment, finding the source is a critical task. Furthermore, statin drugs counter cholesterol, which is necessary for many body functions, and attempts at resolution lead to still other problems, and the start of "the drug merry-go-round."

Some interesting facets of cancer cell behavior were furnished in biologist Lyall Watson's *The Romeo Error: A Matter of Life and Death*. Thus, there is something called the Hayflick limit, which occurs in all cell cultures, but presumably not for cells in their proper place in the body (Watson, 1975, pp. 24–26). In an isolated culture, say after about 50 generations, a limit is reached, which is different for different species, and the cells die out. Moreover, the cells change their identity during this period, "losing their memories" and "forgetting" what they are supposed to represent. Furthermore, all cells ultimately look the same, regardless of their origins. They retain all the cellular instructions but have forgotten how to "read."

These cells may be rejuvenated, however, by furnishing new instructions, even though these instructions may be different. For example, if exiled human cells are treated with horse serum, they become more horselike. Or if a mutation takes place in one or another of the cells, furnishing new instructions, the new proliferation will then grow beyond the Hayflick limit, no longer being constrained by the old cellular restraints. The new cellular line thus becomes cancerous.

If a flagging cell culture is placed back in its host, cancer may be produced if the cells had mutated; otherwise, the cells will function normally. Interestingly, it is noted that if cells from the orbital area of a frog embryo are placed somewhere in the stomach region, these cells will act to produce new gut lining, and not internal eyes. In other words, there is a coordinating system that ensures that all the cells in a given area act or function in the same way.

In Chapter 5 of Watson (1975), he first introduces the subject of vital energy, identified in Hindu writings as *prana*, which, by means scientifically unknowable, coordinates the living organism as a patterned and functional whole (Watson, 1975, p. 122ff). He next considers the body vital centers called *chakras*, which can be located by photographs without light. These chakras are related to the practices of acupuncture, which presuppose twelve main channels or meridians through which energy flows, and which correspond to the chakras. When these channels come close enough to the surface, manipulation can take place via acupuncture. More than 700 such points have been pinpointed empirically, and an electronic device called a *tobiscope* locates these points with an accuracy of less than one tenth of a millimeter (Watson, 1975, p. 125).

The jury is still out on acupuncture per se as a treatment against cancer, although there have been some positive results for electroacupuncture (Moss, 1975, pp. 373–375). The subject is further explored in the following section. Like so much in the arena of cancer therapies, there is no consensus, apparently with nothing absolutely definitive.

## ELECTROMAGNETIC PHENOMENA AND CANCER

There have been investigations into the use of electromagnetic treatments for cancer. Among the more interesting is the use of radio frequency waves in what is called Rife therapy, which seemingly has never been duplicated, although there are modern devices on the market. An exposé about the suppression of this therapy has been written by Barry Lynes, and will again be cited subsequently. There may be additional support in terms of the work of Harold Burr of Yale University on the effects of electrodynamic fields (Watson, 1975, pp. 138–142). Burr thought in terms of a life field that served as an organizer for cells of the body — how and why new cells arrange themselves in a pattern and function like the old cells (although we now think more in terms of DNA and RNA). Central to the consideration are enzymes, whose structure turns out to be extremely malleable, so as to lock into the substrate (or reactant) key, or vice versa. This is affected by electrical fields, and Burr and associates have determined, presumably beyond reasonable doubt, that every living thing, plant, or animal, possesses an electrical field. This field can be measured at some distance from the body, and mirrors or even controls changes in the body.

Experiments by Burr showed that chromosomal changes relate to life fields. For instance, in studying the seeds from pure and hybrid strains of maize, which differed by only one altered gene, there was a difference in the voltage patterns, permitting a distinction even before the seeds had sprouted.

(Versions of the Rife generator may be found for sale on the Internet. For instance, there is the Ultrasonic Rife Generator at about $1695 and the portable battery-operated unit at about $395, available from Transformation Technologies, POB 2698, North Hills, CA 91393, 877-287-0912, in care of Gary Wade. It is indicated that the generator can dissolve blood clots, so healing must first take place after surgery and phlebitis cases must be avoided. Also to be avoided are patients having strokes caused by artery rupture in the brain, and pregnancies, real or suspected. Another source is the International Center for Nutritional Research, 303 Corporate Drive East, Langhorne, PA 19047, 215-968-4324. There are in addition the names of the Royal Rife Research Society, Rife Technologies, Horizon Technology, and JW Labs. The qualifier is that the units must be used for investigational purposes. However, clinical treatments are routinely permitted in Canada and Mexico. Quackwatch notes that the attorney general of Minnesota filed a suit circa 1997–1998 for nonperformance. There is the observation that although ultrasonic waves can act against cancer cells, these units are not sufficiently energy intensive. An update is the Energy Wellness Frequency Instrument offered by Natural Energies Inc., 1825 Tamiami Trail A6-108T, Port Charlotte, FL 33948, 914-851-5383. These Rife-based generators developed for home use have the trademark Energy Wellness™ and are priced at about $3000. The included brochure mentions "exciting reports on experiments" involving many diseases and conditions other than cancer. There is a warning to consult a physician if the patient is epileptic, or has a pacemaker or other electronic heart implant.)

A letter from a certain Daniel Haley of Daingerfield, Texas, appeared in the April 2004 issue of the *Townsend Letter for Doctors & Patients*, with the heading "The Benefits of Medical Freedom." Successful treatments against cancer and other ailments using the Rife Blue Light device, and other devices, are described as having occurred under the auspices of a Dr. Hector Romero at Hermosillo, Sonora, Mexico. Without attempting here to pass judgment, an e-mail address for Dr. Romero's alternative clinic is: qaborq@yahoo.com.mx. (For confirmation of the treatment's effectiveness, at least for a particular patient's Stage IV liver cancer, one can call Haley's brother-in-law, Tex, at 512-556-3424.)

A lengthy article that appeared in the June 2000 issue of the *Townsend Letter for Doctors & Patients* may have some bearing on this. Titled "A Far-Infrared Ray Emitting Stone (SGES) to Treat Cancer and Degenerative Diseases," the article was written by Professor Serge Jurasunas of Natiris, LDA (Centro Indústrial de Abóboda, Estrada de Polima, Armasém D, 2785-543 Sao Domingos de Rana, Portugal, 21-448-04-10, FAX: 21-448-04-18 or 21-448-04-19, e-mail: natiris@mail.telepac.pt). The note is provided that Tenko-Seki stone (SGES, or "super growth ray-emitting stone) is extracted from hills on the island of Kyushi in Japan, where it has been used extensively in baths for therapeutic purposes, and some of the Japanese studies are cited. In the initial paragraphs of the article, as an aside, there is mention of the medical importance of organic germanium in treating many diseases, including cancer. The far-infrared ray wavelength is 4 to 14 microns and can be called a "growth ray" because it is apparently involved in the growth of plants, animals, and humans. Theories and case histories are furnished in the article.

Continuing in a somewhat similar vein, there is a long letter appearing in the October 2004 issue of the same periodical, titled "Effective Alternative Cancer Treatments Suppressed." Written by a certain Dr. Curt Maxwell of Winterhaven, California, a young patient had been receiving the insulin potentiation treatment (IPT), which involves dropping the blood sugar way down with insulin and then killing the cancer cells with low-dose methotrexate or some other recognized cyto-toxic chemotherapy drug. (The treatment was developed by Dr. Donato Perez Garcia at his Tijuana clinic, and is carried on by his grandson.) Dr. Maxwell was concerned that the patient was not receiving any protocols to build up health at the same time — such as IV vitamin C, a Myers cocktail, and the like. It was also mentioned that patients who attend the Mexican cancer clinics have a very high survival rate if no prior chemotherapy was involved. In speaking of double-blind scientific studies on alternative treatments, he wonders what these studies say about chemotherapy, a proven "scientific" treatment that poisons several hundred thousand people to death every year. In turn, he gives a plug for a number of alternative physicians, starting with Dr. Hariton Alivazatos of Greece, whose treatment or formula is available from the International Biologies Hospital in Tijuana, under the direction of Roberta Tapia, M.D. Other names listed, for the record, are Virginia Livingston Wheeler, Kurt Donsbach, Geronimo Rubio, Ernesto Contreras, Harold Manner, Johanna Budwig, Gerhard Ohlenschlager, Heinrich Kremer, Xavier Mayr, Abram Hoffer, Robert Brad-ford, Hulda Clark, Hans Nieper, Emanuel Revici, William B. Coley, Jese Stoff, Hariton Alivazatos, Lawrence Burton, Stanislaw Burzynski, Joseph Issels, Keith Brewer, and Jimmie Keller.

Dr. Maxwell cautions against the request to forward names to the National Cancer Institute of doctors actively treating cancer using alternatives, — at least without the doctors' permission, for in some states the practice of alternatives can lead to prosecution. Nevertheless, it may be added, merely belonging to ACAM (American College for the Advancement of Medicine) may be a giveaway. In fact, the editorial, or letter from the publisher, in the same issue of the periodical lists a number of prominent names of alternative practitioners: Jonathan Wright, Alan Gaby, Robert Atkins (deceased), Abram Ber, Emmanuel Cheraskin, Deepak Chopra, Elmer Cranton, Charles Farr, Garry Gordon, Abram Hoffer, Evarts Loomis, Theron Ran-dolph, Norman Shealy, Bernie Siegel, Lendon Smith (deceased), Melvyn Werbach, Julian Whitaker, James Carter, James Gordon, John Lee, Christiane Northrup, Wil-liam Philpott, Doris Rapp, Bernard Rimland, Hugh Riordan, and Andrew Weil.

The extrapolation may be to healing or faith healers Watson (1975, Chapter 9). In this regard, experiments once conducted at the University of California using a "high-frequency apparatus" showed that the photographic aura produced by a healer is significantly different from that for an ordinary person, and during healing is dramatically different (Watson, 1975, p. 221). Matters of uneducated medical diag-nosis are described, as performed by a Brazilian nicknamed Arigó, and of inexpli-cable surgical operations by the unwashed. (Exposés of these kinds of operations have been aired on TV from time to time.) The Israeli psychic Uri Gellor, who could presumably bend eating utensils and stop clocks from a distance, rates a paragraph. (There has subsequently been an exposé, however, by magician James Randi, better known as "The Amazing Randi.")

## SOME INEXPLICABLES

Nevertheless, these things said, there are examples here and there of cures, or at least remissions. Thus, there is Elaine Nussbaum's *Recovery from Cancer: A Personal Story of Sickness and Health*, published in 1997. And there is the organization called Institute for Noetic Sciences in Sausalito, California, that keeps track of such cases ("noetic," pertaining to the mind). It would be extremely informative to determine if there is any sort of a common thread that links these recoveries.

Another set of such circumstances is set forth in Michael Gearin-Tosh's *Living Proof: A Medical Mutiny*, published in 2002, which furnishes some more "for instances." (A favorable review of the book in the June 2002 issue of the *Townsend Letter for Doctors & Patients* cites a couple more.) Gearin-Tosh, a don or teacher of literature at St. Catherine's College, University of Oxford, was diagnosed with myeloma, a usually fatal cancer of the bone marrow. He consulted a number of orthodox cancer specialists or oncologists, whose advice uniformly was to commence chemotherapy immediately, and expect to live only two or three years. (Another option is a double marrow transplant, costing about $150,000 to $200,000 at the time — if there are no complications — as per p. 39 of the book.)

Nevertheless, Gearin-Tosh decided otherwise, and kept seeing yet other M.D.s, and found a few who thought differently. One in particular, who is cited several times in the book, was Ernst L. Wynder, M.D. and D.Sc., of Sloan-Kettering, considered preeminent in cancer research. Wynder's credentials within medical orthodoxy are simply outstanding (Gearin-Tosh, 2002, pp. 84, 85). Wynder's thoughts, relayed to Gearin-Tosh, were: "If your friend touches chemotherapy, he's a goner" (Gearin-Tosh, 2002, pp. 42, 43, 84, 85, 87, 88, 117, 130, 145, 165). Another citation worth noting is that of the eminent Professor Sir David Weatherall, Regius Professor of Medicine at the University of Oxford, who stated that "we know so little about how the body works" (Gearin-Tosh, 2002, pp. 165, 166). Gearin-Tosh also consulted with Dr. Gonzalez of New York City, an M.D. noted for utilizing alternative therapies (Gearin-Tosh, 2002, pp. 80–84, 92).

Accordingly, Gearin-Tosh went with alternatives, mainly the Gerson Therapy, which utilizes a vegetarian-type diet and coffee enemas (Gearin-Tosh, 2002, pp. 80ff, 113ff, 106), although Wynder said, "I would not put my dog on Gerson" (Gearin-Tosh, 2002, p. 117). Another therapy used was acupuncture, courtesy of a certain Dr. H. (Gearin-Tosh, 2002, pp. 112ff, 144, 145). A Chinese breathing exercise as described by a Dr. Jan de Vries was also utilized (Gearin-Tosh, 2002, pp. 55,56, 59, 66, 92). The work of Linus Pauling and A. Hoffer, M.D., Ph.D., is cited, particularly with regard to vitamin C (Gearin-Tosh, 2002, p. 111, 142–145, 260). Garlic is also mentioned (Gearin-Tosh, 2002, p. 249).

Gearin-Tosh followed these regimes for about a year, then wrote the book after about 7 years, and although not in perfect health was still alive in 2002. The first half of the book is a personal chronicle, with the last half consisting of a critique.

Among other things, it is recommended that one should not rush to treatment, and one should not be bullied and crushed into submission (Gearin-Tosh, 2002, p. 200, 201, 207). Philosopher Byron Magee is also quoted, who speaks of atheistic humanism among the "able and intelligent" and which "tends to identify itself with rationality as such, and to congratulate itself on its own sophistication" (Gearin-Tosh, 2002, p. 239).

The comment can be added that those of medical orthodoxy agree to certain protocols of treatment to protect their backsides. In other words, even if the treatment fails (or almost always fails), it will still be recognized (in court) by the attending physician's medical peers as the therapy of choice. Not necessarily so with alternatives, although a consent form is signed.

## METASTASIS, RESISTANCE, AND ABERRATIONS

There are other differences in behavior between normal cells and cancerous cells, as noted in Francis X. Hasselberger's *Uses of Enzymes and Mobilized Enzymes*. Thus, cancer cells tend to lose adhesion, breaking away from the normal cells of their origins (Hasselberger, 1978, pp. 143, 144). These mobile cancerous cells then travel elsewhere, displaying a low level of adhesion but a high degree of stickiness, which is diametrically different from the behavior of normal cells. In other words, cancer cells may metastasize, spreading to other parts of the body, and proliferating at these other locations. Perhaps most importantly, there are differences in metabolism, to be further discussed subsequently, especially in terms of enzymes and enzyme inhibitors.

In principle, chemotherapy of some kind is the way to go, if only it could be made selective against cancer cells. Conventional chemotherapy drugs are nonselective, however, and for this reason are referred to as "cytotoxic," or cell toxic, indicating that they act against all body cells to some degree. That is, it kills normal cells as well as cancerous cells, especially the faster-growing cells of the immune system and gastrointestinal tract, whereas cancer cells are generally slower-growing, although much longer-lived. The action ordinarily is to block key enzymes involved in the sequence for DNA→ RNA→ protein synthesis.

Another facet is that cancer cells themselves can build up an immunity or resistance to the chemotherapy agent, a fact well known but not publicized. Reasons for this behavior are set forth by Madeline Drexler in *Secret Agents: The Menace of Emerging Infections*. Though directed primarily at pathogens that exist as bacteria and viruses, there is a mention that cancer cells, fungi, and parasites all deploy what is known as the drug efflux mechanism (Drexler, 2002, p. 146). The drug is pumped out faster than it can accumulate inside, as in the case of tetracycline-resistant bacteria.

Furthermore, microorganisms that produce antibiotics contain resistance genes that act against these same antibiotics (Drexler, 2002, p. 147). These genes can in fact be deployed by still other bacteria to resist the drug. In comment, and extended to anticancer chemotherapy agents, the cancer cell itself can be suspected of harboring genes that will confer resistance. There is the further note that genes move around, so what, in absolute fact, is a species? (Drexler, 2002, p. 149).

Drexler's book carries a wealth of other information, making nearly all foods suspect of carrying disease-inducing pathogens. There are observations about the overuse of antibiotics causing the buildup of resistance, which is compounded by their routine use in the livestock industries (Drexler, 2002, p. 150ff).

As for influenza viruses, a subject in itself, it is stated that "the primordial source of all flu strains is migrating aquatic birds" (Drexler, 2002, p. 171ff). Moreover, not only can these viruses leap the species barrier per se, but the mixing of human and animal strains is even more worrisome. As for the latter, relating to novel flu strains, southeast China is today's presumptive source, what with its close proximity of humans, domestic animals (pigs), and domestic birds (ducks).

In jumping the species barrier between animals and humans, the AIDS virus is apparently the most prominent example. However, we can also wonder if a virus cannot jump (or mix) the species barrier between animals and insects, or animals and plants? And thence between humans and animals? Or, more directly, between humans and insects, or humans and plants? The as-yet-unknown sources for the Marburg and Ebola viruses give pause for thought.

In a chapter "Infection Unmasked," Drexler first underscores the point that some 70% of all deaths are due to lingering or chronic illnesses rather than to the abrupt severity of acute afflictions. Furthermore, there is the statement that "today, a growing number of researchers claim that these disabling conditions may be caused by infection." Thus, more than 90% of cervical cancer cases are caused by the human papillomavirus, and more than 60% of liver cancer cases result from the hepatitis B virus. The retrovirus HTLV-1 is the precursor for adult T cell lymphoma, with the cancerous condition occurring decades after the infection. The Epstein-Barr virus, a herpes-type virus causing mononucleosis, also has an effect on people with malaria, producing a cancer known as Burkitt's lymphoma, the leading cause of childhood cancer deaths worldwide. Kaposi's sarcoma, known as a complication of AIDS, is said to be caused by human herpesvirus 8.

(The foregoing is in line with the mechanism presented in the chapter "Cancer and Viruses" in Hoffman [1999] and stated early on herein, whereby viruses invade the cell chromosome to produce oncogenes.)

Peptic ulcers are induced by a spiral-shaped bacterium named *Helicobacter pylori* (and which may also be an agent for stomach cancer, as per the illustration on p. 206 of Drexler's book). Foodborne pathogens are guilty on many counts, triggering such chronic and autoimmune diseases as Guillain-Barré syndrome and reactive arthritis.

Drexler comments that the foregoing may very well be only the starting point. Whereas the germ theory of disease, as attributed to Robert Koch, paved the way for discoveries about acute infections, emerging ideas about the nature of chronic infections may prove similarly fruitful — although, expectedly, "some of these theories are based on wild hope and dubious information, and will yield nothing," but yet others "may change the practice of medicine." For instance, the Epstein-Barr virus has now been implicated in Hodgkin's disease and in aggressive breast cancers. Even multiple sclerosis (MS) behaves as if from an infection, and juvenile onset diabetes (Type I) may follow from a Coxsackie B enterovirus (intestinal virus) producing an immune response that adversely affects the pancreas. The chronic inflammation of the bowel called Crohn's disease acts like an infection suspiciously similar to intestinal tuberculosis, and *Mycobacterium paratuberculosis*, a relative of the TB bacterium, has been implicated. Not only this but nearly half the asthma cases in this country, and even juvenile rheumatoid arthritis, can be linked to *Mycoplasma pneumoniae*, described as a free-living organism smaller than most bacteria.

Meningitis, pneumonia, and deaths of newborns, as well as childhood asthma, can be traced to the sexually transmitted organism *Ureaplasma urealyticum*. Clostridia and eubacteria in the intestines are associated with a far higher incidence of gallstones, and kidney stones have been linked to what are called nanobacteria, being much smaller even than viruses. A woman infected with bacterial gum disease (or periodontal infection) has a dramatically greater chance of birthing a premature baby. It is thought that schizophrenia may be initiated just before or after birth by a viral infection that cross-circuits neural connections in the developing brain. Another theory attributes schizophrenia to a parasite transmitted from cats. Now, rather than a one-to-one, cause-and-effect relationship between the agent and the acute disease; the new thinking in chronic ailments is that "sly viruses and bacteria" act more subtly. The organisms always present in us, labeled "benign commensals," may in partial fact be hostile. This new attitude has been variously designated as the *Second Golden Age of Bacteriology, Koch's Postulates Part II*, and the *New Germ Theory.*

In a major development with widespread ramifications, the plaque formed in heart disease, or arteriosclerosis, has been traced in part to the action of the organism *Chlamydia pneumoniae*, although the picture in its entirety is more complex (Drexler, 2002, pp. 207–209). Interestingly, it was once thought that yeasts could transmute into bacteria, and that the bacterial hordes found in body tissue contributed to disease (Drexler, 2002, p. 210). In comment, transmutation may not have been too far off the mark, for now there is (controversial) evidence of pleomorphism or polymorphism, whereby microorganisms assume different embodiments and characteristics, say, between viral and bacterial forms. As for Koch's postulates regarding rigorously confirming the relationship between the organism and the disease by using an animal host, it has been found that many human diseases have no animal equivalent (Drexler, 2002, p. 211). The new attitude, as furnished by microbiologist Hal Nash, is that "the nature of acute disease allowed for the development of 'rules' and 'postulates.' The nature of chronic diseases is likely that there are no rules."

(Along these lines, a reading of Atul Gawande's very readable *Complications: A Surgeon's Notes on an Imperfect Science* indicates that in surgery, as well as in other branches of medicine, the protocols are not always clear-cut. Blind luck can play as big a part as expertise, and the interaction between physician and patient can be equally important. In other words, the rule is that there are sometimes no rules. Dr. Gawande's book, published in 2002, was followed up by an article in the December 6, 2004, issue of the *New Yorker* in the section "Annals of Medicine" titled "What Happens When Patients Find Out How Good Their Doctors Really Are?" Enter the bell curve, here with an emphasis on the treatment of cystic fibrosis.)

Some generalizations are in order, however, in that illnesses occurring in people with compromised immune systems are likely to be infectious (Drexler, 2002, p. 212). An example is Kaposi's sarcoma in AIDS victims and organ transplant patients. If a disease is negated by taking antibiotics, the indication is that it is (bacterial) infectious. When people living in poverty are disproportionately affected, the indication again is infection (as in the case of stomach cancer induced by *Heliobacter pylori*). The same may be said when occurrences vary with the time of year (a notable example being respiratory diseases). Or if the disease varies geographically (a notable example being MS, whose incidence increases with the distance away from the equator). And scientists are beginning to realize just how much they do not know about what is living on and in the human body. For instance, the estimate is that less than 1% of bacterial species have been identified. (Not to mention viruses, for which there is no systematic system of classification other than size and shape. There is, however, what is called "Virus databases on-line," courtesy of the BioInformation Group, Research School of Biological Sciences, Institute of Advanced Studies, Australian National University, PO Box 476, Canberra, ATC 2601, Australia.)

Speaking further of ubiquity, the human bowel itself contains hundreds of organisms, called the intestinal flora, or gut flora, which serve many purposes, such as breaking down foods, countering carcinogens, and synthesizing vitamins (Drexler, 2002, p. 213). About 1% of the human genome itself is said to contain endogenous retroviruses, an internal heritage from times past. (Intestinal flora constitute a subject taken up in Hoffman, 1999a, based in considerable part on Rowland, 1988.)

Nor are these endogenous microorganisms necessarily benevolent, for they may also initiate disease, simply by persistence (Drexler, 2002, p. 214ff). Whereas replicating viruses ordinarily destroy cells, those that produce persistent infections may merely replicate continuously in what are called differentiated or specialized cells, such as endocrine cells that make hormones, such as insulin. The cell is not destroyed per se, but its specialized function is. Possibilities include MS, juvenile diabetes, and assorted psychiatric illnesses as caused by viral infections and sustained by the immune system's response to still other infections.

The last-mentioned item brings up the subject of autoimmune diseases, which have chronic inflammation as the common denominator. (Examples range from rheumatoid arthritis and MS to lupus and Crohn's disease.) Thus, infectious agents can manage to make themselves look like human cells and avoid action by the immune system, or else make themselves slightly different so that the body responds against both the human cell and the infectious agent. Although the infectious agent may be ultimately destroyed, the immune system will still think that the corresponding human cells are foreign. The conclusion provided by David Relman, Stanford physician and microbiologist, is that an autoimmune disease becomes the "consequence of this imperfect balance between the immune system's need for vigilance and its need for tolerance of structures that should not be attacked."

Speaking of inflammation, it is now recognized that heart disease is strongly associated with inflammation via an agent having the designator C-reactive protein, whose increased level serves as a marker for all kinds of inflammation, as previously noted. There also may conceivably be an association with cancer, evidenced by a low-grade fever, or night sweats. In turn, the extrapolation may be to viruses as the causative agent.

In an article titled "The Prudent Heart Diet and Cholesterol Lowering Drugs: Why They Don't Prevent Heart Attacks" in the August/September 2002 issue of the *Townsend Letter for Doctors & Patients*, frequent contributor Wayne Martin takes a long look at the track record of polyunsaturated fats vs. saturated fats in preventing heart attacks. Referring frequently to articles in *The Lancet*, the unnerving conclusion after several rounds of comprehensive tests on various populations is that myocardial infarction (MI), as coronary thrombosis is now called, is not only not alleviated by a diet in polyunsaturated fats, but the cancer rate goes up. (The term "infarction" pertains to hemorrhaging and necrosis in an organ from obstruction of the local circulation by a thrombus, or embolus, i.e., blood clot.) And although MI was seemingly not known circa 1900, despite a diet of saturated fats such as butter and lard, there are now some 400,000 deaths per year.

(No explicit mention is made of the effect of trans-fatty acids or hydrogenated vegetable oils, nor of monounsaturated vegetable oils such as olive oil, as per the Mediterranean diet.)

In the same issue of the periodical just cited, an article by Owen Richard Fonorow of the Vitamin C Foundation reaffirms that vitamin C works against heart attacks, as suggested by Linus Pauling.

A year later, in the August/September 2003 issue, Wayne Martin again addresses the prudent diet vs. saturated fats in an article titled "The Role of Dietary Polyun-saturated Fats in Heart Disease and Atherosclerosis." (Atherosclerosis is a form of arteriosclerosis.) The data overwhelmingly indicate that saturated fats, whether butter or lard or whatever, are preferable to polyunsaturated fats, contrary to the present conventional wisdom. Moreover, aspirin was found to have no beneficial effect against heart attacks.

As if all the foregoing were not enough, Wayne Martin reported on hyperbaric oxygen for stroke in a letter in the June 2005 issue of the same periodical. Following surgery, his daughter had a seizure that showed the symptoms of paralytic stroke: she was completely blind and could not walk nor use her hands to feed herself. A doctor friend recommended hyperbaric oxygen therapy at once, but the resistance of medical orthodoxy was virtually unanimous, save for the counsel of another family friend who was an M.D. So after about a year, getting nowhere, Martin himself bought a hyperbaric oxygen chamber. The husband of the patient reported that after 3 weeks of daily treatments, she was showing definite improvement. After about 10 weeks, the patient was mobile, could feed and dress herself, and could watch TV. The husband, in his comments, thanked his father-in-law profusely. A follow-up letter from Martin in the January 2006 issue provides an update. His daughter continues to improve, and is using air under pressure with no added oxygen. Martin further discusses the problems of obtaining hyperbaric treatment for stroke, outside of buying one's own unit, which costs about $13,000. Also mentioned is that he — now 94 — has been an amputee since the age of 17, and that hyperbaric oxygen treatments might prevent diabetic amputations.

(As for oxygen therapy against cancer, the subject is discussed in Chapter 7 in the section titled "Still Other Options.")

## MORE ON IMMUNITY

Autoimmune diseases may involve "molecular mimicry," whereby organisms exhibit the surface substances called antigens that can at times mimic substances in human tissues (Drexler, 2002, p. 216). Ordinarily the antigens will initiate specific antibody and T cell (or T-lymphocyte) responses that act only against diseased cells. However, if the diseased cells or tissue cannot be distinguished from the normal condition, then the antibodies and T cells may attack both diseased and normal cells. An example provided is that of an antigen as per the Coxsackie B virus, whereby the T cells may sometimes also attack an enzyme occurring in the pancreatic cells that make insulin. The result is diabetes. Still other viruses may compound the damage. Another example of autoimmune misbehavior is that of obsessive-compulsive disorder (OCD), which may arise from childhood infections with *Streptococcus pyrogenes*, denoted as Group A strep.

Retroviruses inherent in the human genome may in fact produce certain psychiatric conditions, including schizophrenia (Drexler, 2002, p. 217). The retrovirus involved may possibly be activated by herpes simplex viral infections, and by hormones and immune cells. Some cases can possibly be attributed to a mother-transmitted infection of the fetal brain with the parasite *Taxoplasma gondii*, as occurs in cat feces. These theories are in line with some earlier medical literature, whereby many nineteenth century doctors thought schizophrenia an infectious condition.

Evolutionary biologist Paul Ewald of Amherst College, previously cited, advances the idea that many bacteria and viruses have evolved in ways that cause chronic diseases to be mysterious or "cryptic," so to say, rather than obvious (Drexler, 2002, pp. 218–220). Speaking further on the subject, he classifies diseases as being of genetic, environmental, and infectious origins, with the last-mentioned by far the most common and damaging, of which examples are atherosclerosis, strokes, many or most cancers, brain malfunctions, and autoimmune disorders. Even some diseases of genetic origins such as sickle cell anemia and cystic fibrosis may be initiated by infections. The major pestilences of malaria, smallpox, TB, typhoid, bubonic plague, cholera, yellow fever, etc., had to be infectious, by virtue of their having been commonplace. And the major cause of female infertility in the 1970s, the sexually transmitted *Chlamydia trachomatis*, became commonplace, due to freewheeling sexual mores — as are other pathogens transmitted by intimate contact. The list includes the Epstein-Barr virus, human papillomavirus, hepatitis B virus, that virus designated HHV8, and HIV. The catchall designator is STPs (sexually transmitted pathogens). Although there may be some argument as to whether a disease is infectious or not, Ewald's distinction is to the point: if the infectious agent were eliminated, so would be the disease, whether we are speaking of acute or chronic diseases.

Additional space is given to the work of Stanford physician and microbiologist David Relman regarding the curved rod-shaped bacteria causing bacillary angiomatosis, a skin condition associated with immunocompromised patients, for example, those having AIDS (Drexler, 2002, pp. 221, 222). Using what are called genetic angling techniques, Relman found that the bacterium was closely related to *Bartonella quintana*, the cause of trench fever in World War I, and was in fact *B.*

*benselae,* the source of cat-scratch disease, which produces mild, flu-like symptoms in humans. Similarly, the wasting syndrome called Whipple's disease was found to be infectious by Relman, and his experiments are now regarded as definitive.

In another turn of events, Kaposi's sarcoma (KS) was found to be infectious by other investigators, namely pathologist Yuan Change of Columbia University, and her husband epidemiologist Patrick Moore (Drexler, 2002, pp. 222, 223). A formerly benign form of cancer confined to elderly men of the Mediterranean and Middle East, and to equatorial Africa, and an occasional immunosuppressed organ transplant patient, KS became rampant with the emergence of AIDS. Eventually, Chang showed that KS was caused by a previously unknown herpesvirus, now called Kaposi's sarcoma herpesvirus (KSVH) or human herpesvirus 8 (HHV8).

Another work cited by Drexler is a 2001 report from University of Michigan researchers, whereby the herpesvirus known as the Epstein-Barr virus counters a block to cell migration and thereby permits (cancer) cells to metastasize or spread (Drexler, 2002, p. 223). In turn, Drexler mentions the work of Peyton Rous of the Rockefeller Institute, who in 1909 discovered a tumor virus occurring in chickens (the Rous virus), and who belatedly (in 1966) received the Nobel Prize in medicine and physiology. In fact, it is cited that there have been five recent Nobel Prizes awarded for the study of tumor viruses. These viruses are described as having the ability to trigger the genes that cause cells to become malignant. Newer technologies called DNA chips or DNA microarrays can register the tens of thousands of genetic sequences in bacteria and viruses, which can be compared with human tissue's binding properties. The prospect is that this technology could be used to compare normal and abnormal conditions.

The remaining pages of Drexler's chapter are devoted to critiquing these new discoveries about chronic diseases. However, medical oncologist Beatriz G. T. Poge of the Mt. Sinai School of Medicine in New York has studied more than 1000 samples of breast tumors from the operating room and found that more than a third have genetic swatches that are nearly identical to those of the mouse mammary tumor virus (Drexler, 2002, p. 229). This is a slow-growing retrovirus transmitted through the mouse mother's milk, resulting in cancer in the female offspring. Moreover, in humans, the virus is evidently exogenous, not being part of the woman's genome. The hypothesis that breast tumors could be caused by a virus produces much opposition in some quarters.

## BIOTERRORISM

In a concluding chapter, Drexler takes up the subject of bioterrorism, in which bioagents kill by suffocation via pneumonia, septic shock, massive bleeding, or paralysis (Drexler, 2002, p. 233ff). The spores and vegetative cells from the anthrax bacterium, *Bacillus anthracis,* are prominently discussed. Under stress, the bacteria change into deadly spores, and will revert to the rapidly multiplying vegetative form when conditions are ripe.

Past efforts at biowarfare are also presented, notably the Japanese program, which ran from 1932 to 1945 (Drexler, 2002, p. 244ff). The following are listed by Drexler as having been studied: plague, typhoid, paratyphoid A and B, typhus, smallpox, tularemia, infectious jaundice, gas gangrene, tetanus, cholera, dysentery, glanders, scarlet fever, brucellosis, tickborne encephalitis, hemorrhagic fever, whooping cough, diphtheria, pneumonia, venereal diseases, tuberculosis, and salmonella. Conducted near the small Manchurian village of Ping Fan under the direction of Japanese army doctor Shiro Ishii, the human testing was inhuman in the extreme, involving shrapnel bombs, tainted food, and vivisection. The victims were predominantly Chinese citizens, but also white Russians, Soviet prisoners, criminals, and mental patients. Estimates of those who died in these experiments range from 10,000 to at least 270,000. In 1947, the American military debriefed Shiro Ishii and others involved, and made a bizarre secret deal whereby immunity from prosecution was granted in exchange for the details of the experiments.

Bioweapons developed in the United States between 1950 and 1969 in the project designated "Operation Whitecoat" comprised seven biological disease-causing agents, as follows (Drexler, 2002, p. 248): *Bacillus anthracis* (bacterium causing anthrax), *Clostridium botulinum* (a soil bacterium causing botulism), *Francisella tularensis* (bacterial agent for tularemia or rabbit fever), various *Brucella* species (bacteria causing brucellos or undulant fever), the mosquito-borne virus for Venezuelan equine encephalitis, *Staphyloccus* enterotoxin B (bacterial food poisoning), and *Coxiella burnetii* (the rickettsial organism causing the highly contagious Q fever).

In 1973, after signing a treaty the previous year prohibiting the development of bioweapons, the USSR embarked on a massive buildup that peaked in 1980 with some 50-plus labs and 65,000 researchers and technicians (Drexler, 2002, p. 249). Dubbed Biopreparat as a cover-up, ostensibly to develop pharmaceuticals, some 52 agents were studied or in production, including those for smallpox, anthrax, plague, Ebola and Marburg fevers, yellow fever, tularemia, brucellosis, Q fever, botulism, Venezuelan equine encephalitis, and assorted genetic hybrid agents.

In the last chapter of Drexler (2002), the worldwide infectious disease situation is brought up to date, noting in particular the work of the Centers for Disease Control and Prevention (CDC) and director Bill Foege, M.D. The catchall term is "emerging infections." The latter include Legionnaire's disease, the Marburg and Ebola hemorrhagic fevers and, of course, AIDS, as well as some that have been around for awhile, such as smallpox and TB. The top three infectious killers worldwide are in fact AIDS, TB, and malaria, all being closely associated with poverty (Drexler, 2002, p. 383).

More on anthrax, the Ebola virus, and especially the smallpox virus, are presented in firsthand accounts in Richard Preston's *The Demon in the Freezer: A True Story*, published in 2002. Following the format of his previous book *The Hot Zone: A Terrifying True Story*, Preston interviewed many of the principals involved in the CDC and, in particular, in the U.S. Army Medical Research Institute of Infectious Diseases at Fort Dedrick, Maryland. He gives particulars about the highly successful program to eradicate smallpox, and about still-remaining sources of the stored virus. Included is the fact that genetic modification has produced a new strain that is not affected by conventional vaccinations.

There are also food concerns, as per Marion Nestle's *Safe Food: Bacteria, Biotechnology, and Terrorism* (2003). Nestle, chair of New York University's

Department of Food Studies and Nutrition, has also written *Food Politics: How the Food Industry Influences Nutrition and Health* (2002), and *What to Eat* (2006). She is coeditor with L. Beth Dixon of *Taking Sides: Clashing Viewes on Controversial Issues in Food and Nutrition* (2004). In this regard, there is also Russell L. Blaylock's *Excitotoxins: The Taste That Kills* (1997) and Carol Simontacchi's *The Crazy Makers: How the Food Industry is Destroying Our Minds and Harming Our Children* (2000). Christopher D. Cook's *Diet for a Dead Planet: How the Food Industry Is Killing Us* (2004), will be further cited subsequently.

## THE HALOGENS AND CAUSE AND CURE

The observation can be made that anything that kills the patient will also destroy cancer cells. In fact, in his *Cures Out of Chaos*, M. Lawrence Poldolsky, M.D., notes that mustard gas (dichloro-diethyl-sulfide) was found early on to be an anticancer agent. Presumably, this observation could be extended to phosgene (carbonyl dichloride) or to other deadly chemical warfare agents. The presence of the halogens fluorine, chlorine, bromine, and iodine is in fact indicative of toxicity — for example, polychlorinated or polybrominated biphenyls known as PCB and PBB, which rate a chapter in Podolsky's book — and continue on to the chlorinated solvents that are used routinely, and to such common plastics as vinyl chloride, which have become sources of environmental pollution. Along these lines, the routinely used chemotherapy drug 5-fluorouracil (5-FU) contains halogen, and its side effects are devastating.

As for halogens, the routine use of chlorine in municipal water supplies comes under occasional attack, for example, in an article by Joseph G. Hattersley titled "The Negative Health Effects of Chlorine." Originally published in the *Journal of Orthomolecular Medicine*, it was republished in the May 2003 issue of the *Townsend Letter for Doctors & Patients*. Early on, Hattersley comments on the highly reactive nature of chlorine, and characterizes it as another industrial waste product that is "profitably disposed of by using people as garbage cans." He notes that chlorine oxidizes certain contaminants in the water to create excessive free radicals, which damage arteries and initiate cancer, among other kinds of harm. For one thing, chlorine in water destroys the protective acidophilus that nourishes the immunity-strengthening "friendly" bacteria lining the colon, where most immune cells are located. Chlorine also combines with impurities in water to produce trihalomines (THMs), also called chloramines, which are carcinogenic. Free radicals generate dangerous toxins in the body, and contribute to arteriosclerosis, among other diseases: notably gastrointestinal, bladder, and rectal cancers. As for drinking water purity in general, an estimated 5000 different chemicals have shown up, and aquifers occurring below 8000 ft altitude are contaminated with heavy metals, not to mention that some drinking water may have been recycled from sewage wastes. Pesticides and other toxic wastes from farmlands and pastures add to the stream of industrial wastes, and this totality of chemical pollution is compounded by microbial pollutants. Nevertheless, there are alternatives to the chlorination of drinking water, including such means as ozone contacting and ultraviolet light absorption, and carbon-bed filtration.

The previous mention of fluorine toxicity brings up the subject of the fluoridation of municipal water supplies, an ongoing issue. We here defer to *Tooth Truth: A Patient's Guide to Metal-Free Dentistry* by Frank J. Jerome, D.D.S. Although the main emphasis is on the avoidance of utilizing metals such as mercury amalgams for fillings, Jerome also has a chapter on fluoridation. Thus, Jerome notes that most European countries, which formerly used fluoridation, have abandoned the practice, with the only major countries continuing the practice being the United States, Canada, and Britain (Jerome, 2000, p. 385ff). Moreover, the purported benefits have not been definitively substantiated: for instance, Toronto, which has fluoridated for 36 years, has a higher rate of decay than does Vancouver, which has never fluoridated. Moreover, the source of the fluoride used is from an industrial waste that also contains lead, arsenic, and radium, all of which are carcinogenic (Jerome, 1995, p. 387).

As for cancer, a multiyear study, authorized by Congress, finally concluded that fluoride does indeed cause cancer (Jerome, 1995, p. 392). In response, the FDA merely recommended that the safety limit for fluoride in water be doubled. The study was rebuked, not scientifically, but politically, accompanied by a call for "more studies," although nothing changed except an increasing death rate.

In a section "Protecting Reputations, Not the Public," Jerome indicts many public health officials and organizations, including the American Dental Association, which has staked its esteem on the advisability and safety of fluoridation: "Nothing is more tenacious than bureaucrats trying to protect their reputations."

More about the subject was presented in a series of three articles on "The Fluoride Controversy Continues: An Update," by Gary Null, Ph.D. and Martin Feldman, M.D., in the *Townsend Letter for Doctors & Patients,* starting December 2002. (Null is the author of numerous articles and some 50 books on health and nutrition. Feldman is assistant clinical professor of neurology at Mount Sinai Medical School in New York City.) In the first article, designated Part 1, the authors note that fluorides are indeed toxic. Most fluorides used are a major (toxic) waste from aluminum production, and rather than being simple sodium fluoride, these toxic-waste fluorides are more complex — for example, occurring as silicates — and are more rapidly absorbed in the gastrointestinal tract. The authors also cite mounting evidence that fluorides have in fact not reduced tooth decay, contrary to claims by the American Dental Association and others. Toothpastes come under fire, as do fluorides contained in fruit juices and other beverages, even in baby foods and infant formulas.

In the second article, appearing in the January 2003 issue and designated Part 2, it is added that ingested fluoride produces skeletal fluorosis, which may be a factor in arthritis and contribute to bone fracture, rather than enhancing bone strength. Fluoride also constitutes a thyroid-depressing substance, producing hypothyroidism, and is a known carcinogen. The authors quote Paul Connett of the Fluoride Action Network to the effect that "some of the earliest opponents of fluoride were biochemists and at least 14 Nobel Prize winners are among numerous scientists who have expressed their reservations about the practice of fluoridation." Other effects pinpointed by the authors are enzyme toxicity and genetic damage, adverse reproductive effects, reduced intelligence, interference with the functions of the pineal gland, which may contribute to early puberty and allied problems, and elevated lead levels in the blood. Of further note, a connection emerges between fluoride and aluminum in the form of aluminofluoride complexes, which may turn out to be the real culprit in Alzheimer's disease, rather than aluminum alone.

The third article, appearing in the February/March 2003 issue, is concerned with ways to avoid fluoride accidents, namely an overdose, and describes how a city can reject fluoridation, a course of action beset with difficulties, however. Among the adverse effects cited is that fluoride can affect the central nervous system and thus serves as a neurotoxicant. Moreover, there is a correlation between water fluoridation and increased hip fractures for persons 65 years and older, and a correlation for a decrease in fertility rates. Furthermore, fluoride is a potential carcinogen, and is a known inhibitor for many enzymes involved in cell metabolism. It is mentioned that fluoride disposal is costly, requiring a class-one landfill, and would be an added cost for the aluminum and fertilizer industries, which produce fluoride as a waste by-product. The ready alternative is to dispose of it via water fluoridation and toothpaste, although the risks have been found to outweigh the benefits, and fluoridation is outlawed in most of Western Europe, for instance.

In a follow-up article appearing in the April 2005 issue, Null and Feldman describe the neurotoxic and toxic effects of fluoride on the brain and thyroid gland. For instance, increased brain concentrations of aluminum compounds or complexes were observed in animal studies where aluminum or sodium fluoride was administered, the connection being that presence of aluminum is sometimes associated with Alzheimer's disease. The call is to "Stop Fluoridation Now."

## THE EFFECT OF TOXINS IN THE ENVIRONMENT

The analogy as per the foregoing is to Duff Wilson's *Fateful Harvest*, where toxic chemicals are disposed of by inclusion in fertilizer, to be spread across the land, as next discussed. Accordingly, any discussion of fluoride from industrial wastes further leads to the subject of industrial wastes that occur in commercial inorganic fertilizers, a subject exposed in Duff Wilson's book. Wilson was an investigative reporter for the *Seattle Times*, which had published a series of articles titled "Fear in the Fields — How Hazardous Wastes Become Fertilizer," beginning July 3, 1997, which were picked up by the wire services (but not the *New York Times*). Thus, there is the prospect, for instance, of toxic heavy metals being introduced into croplands and entering the food chain. Wilson's exposé traces the efforts of housewife and mayor Patty Martin of Quincy, Washington, to do something about the spread of toxic materials introduced with inorganic fertilizers as chemical wastes. Along the way she collided with the interests of corporate agribusiness and the chemical industry, and with political inertia, and in fact with the antagonism of the people, losing the next election for mayor of Quincy, a community that is part of the rich agricultural legacy of central Washington — and dependent on this same agriculture, fertilizer and all. In Duff Wilson's Epilogue, he summarizes the as yet vain efforts of Patty Martin, and notes that fundamental questions remain to be answered, both nationally and around the world. For instance, it is not known for sure how much toxic acid, ash, slag, dust, and other industrial wastes are being spread in the guise of fertilizer.

In fact, it is not necessary to list the entirety of the fertilizer contents on the bag or container, though supposedly this information can be found on the Internet for those who go to the trouble (Wilson, 2001, p. 242).

Some of the major contaminants are the heavy metals lead, cadmium, arsenic, mercury, etc., as well as, sometimes, radioactive wastes, even discarded wallboard. A difficulty of making a definitive assessment is that the dose makes the poison, or *Dosis sola facit venenum* (Wilson, 2001, p. 272), and the scenario has not yet been put together, including the long-term effects, if any. That is, there is a lengthy time gap between cause and effect. (One can wonder at what point the ancient Romans might have realized that they were being slowly poisoned by their lead cooking utensils?)

So far, neither the U.S Department of Agriculture nor the Environmental Protection Agency (EPA) wish to become embroiled in the issues. Vice president and presidential candidate Al Gore declined to become involved. Thus, the agricultural usage of these toxic wastes remains legal, though if declared a *hazardous waste*, it is illegal to use it, even if diluted (Wilson, 2002, p. 239). Thus, a "bustling toxic commerce" was found between factories and fertilizer makers (Wilson, 2002, p. 251). Between 1990 and 1995, there were 454 companies designated as farms and fertilizer manufacturers that received a nominal 271 million pounds of toxic wastes. Not only were heavy metals involved, but solvents and industrial chemicals, some 69 different types of toxics all told, with those designated carcinogens totaling some 13.9 million pounds.

Not only have toxic metals been implicated notably in cancer, but crops have been found to absorb these chemicals from the soil. Thus, lettuce absorbs cadmium "like a sponge" (Wilson, 2001, p. 251). During the controversy, a Colorado soil professor, John Mortvedt, called "Mr. Micronutrient," was consulted, who admitted that plants picked up various heavy metal compounds, notably cadmium, especially in acidic soils (Wilson, 2001, p. 172ff). His findings were watered down in subsequent hearings, when he waffled by stating that very little research had been done on heavy metals in micronutrient fertilizers (Wilson, 2001, p. 215); which, Wilson notes, is precisely the point.

Another volume of like genre is *Fatal Harvest: The Tragedy of Industrial Agriculture*, edited by Andrew Kimbrell and published in 2002. (The publisher is Island Press, Washington, D.C., and the sponsor is the Foundation for Deep Ecology, Sausalito, CA.) This extra-large, coffee-table-sized, important and colorful volume is divided into seven parts, with sections or chapters by various prominent authorities, and with other sections presumably by the editor. These seven parts are: "Farming as if Nature Mattered: Breaking the Industrial Paradigm;" "Corporate Lies: Busting the Myths of Industrial Agriculture;" "Diversity, Scale, and Beauty: Contrasting Agrarian and Industrial Agriculture;" "Industrial Agriculture: The Toxic Trail from Seed to Table;" "Biodiversity and Wildlife: The Overappropriation of Wildlife Habitat by Agriculture;" "A Crisis of Culture: Social and Economic Impacts of Industrial Agriculture;" "Organic and Beyond: Revisioning Agriculture for the 21st Century." The material is extensive and comprehensive, so only a few of the highlights of this extraordinary volume will be set forth here, as follows.

In Part One, Wendell Berry speaks of the preservation of the agrarian outlook, a local economy that rises from the fields, woods, and streams — being neither regional nor national, let alone global. He notes that the World Trade Organization itself contradicts the industrialist conservatives' professed anathema to big government, when in fact big business is the cause of big government. In turn, Helena Norberg-Hodge addresses the worldwide destruction of diversity in terms of economic globalization, once defined as "a world of homogeneous consumption." In the long term, a homogeneous planet is seen as disastrous to us all, "leading to a breakdown of both biological and cultural diversity, erosion of our food security, an increase in conflict and violence, and devastation of the global biosphere." Hugh H. Iltis, in a section dealing with the fallacies of agricultural hope, notes that there is a bioclimatic paradox, for instance, in the fact that tropical latitudes have low productivity for grains such as wheat, rye, barley, and rice. The plant respiration cycle that occurs during the long, warm, tropical nights burns up most of the carbohydrates formed during daytime photosynthesis. Wes Jackson, in a section on natural systems agriculture, compares the fossil-carbon equivalent of industrial fertilizers, noting that ten fossil-fuel calories are required to produce a single food calorie.

In Part Two, the editor addresses what are called the Seven Deadly Myths of Corporate Agriculture, being: (Myth One) Industrial Agriculture Will Feed the World; (Myth Two) Industrial Food is Safe, Healthy, and Nutritious; (Myth Three) Industrial Feed Is Cheap; (Myth Four) Industrial Agriculture is Efficient; (Myth Five) Industrial Food Offers More Choices; (Myth Six) Industrial Agriculture Benefits the Environment and Wildlife; (Myth Seven) Biotechnology Will Solve the Problems of Industrial Agriculture.

In Part Three, a section on monoculture vs. diversity sets forth the varieties of several staple crops lost from 1903 to 1983: tomatoes, 80.6% lost; lettuce, 92.8% lost; field corn, 90.8% lost, and sweet corn, 96.1% lost; apples, 86.2% lost; potatoes, out of over 5000 varieties worldwide, only 4 major commercial varieties are now grown. In discussing industrial grain production, only corn, rice, and wheat have emerged as staples. And in the case of wheat, for example, although there are over 30,000 natural varieties of wheat falling into 6 classifications, with some 1,500 developed for commercial production, this diversity amounts to only a miniscule part of the commercial wheat grown today. Most production is of hybrids and genetically modified varieties. The monoculture casualty is that of diversification, which protects the gene pool against unknown plant diseases. Sugar politics is also discussed, with the example given that during the Clinton administration, a call from a sugar producer (and campaign contributor) derailed a proposed tax on sugar that would offset environmental damage to the Everglades. As for cotton's devastating legacy, it is first noted that genetically modified cotton was found not to produce, a financial setback to scores of farmers. Not to mention that only one type of cotton, short-staple upland cotton, dominates 97% of the crop, another blow to diversity. This and devastation of the soil, as well as a dependence on cottonseed oil as a major food component, more usually known as vegetable oil or hydrogenated vegetable oil, never mind the presence of crop chemicals and genetic engineering. Apples, oranges, and grapes also get an evaluation, with the note that weeds can serve beneficially as ground cover among the orchard trees, instead of having only sterile soil.

In Part Four, while discussing the hazards of genetically engineered food, Joseph Mendelson III notes that pests eventually develop resistance to the gene-developed pesticides produced by the modified plant. Taking note of the "exotic" organisms that have invaded the United States in the past, causing the Dutch elm disease and chestnut blight, and other such exotics as killer bees and the kudzu vine, he mentions that crops altered by genetic engineering produce the same consequences, even mutating in unpredictable ways. As an example, the unpublicized case of a genetically engineered tomato is cited, which caused stomach lesions in laboratory rats, plus the case of genetically engineered fish, which fail to reproduce at a rate necessary for the long-term survival of the species. There is also the specter of "superweeds" as well as "superpests." The twin subjects of soil and water are also discussed, with the reminder that "death swamps" are being created from the runoff and seepage of chemically laden waters that have nowhere else to go. It is noted, in particular that, as the rate of pesticide use increases, so does the rate of breast cancer (Wilson, 2001, p. 256). Thus, the National Cancer Institute found 50 to 60% higher levels of organochlorine pesticides in the breast tissue of women with the cancer, compared to normal. The as yet unknown dangers of food irradiation are taken to task by Michael Colby, who observes that the consumer is the guinea pig.

In Part Five, Catherine Badgley asks whether (modern or industrial) agriculture and biodiversity can coexist. Thus, she notes that current estimates of extinction rates are three to four orders of magnitude greater than "background" extinction rates. (An order of magnitude nominally being a factor of 10, we are therefore speaking of rates 30 to 40 times normal.) With what is called habitat destruction, there is the extinction or endangerment of about 90% for threatened plant species. Soil degradation and erosion and pesticide contamination has been known to eliminate fish species (three extinct in Michigan, and another three reduced to relic populations). Large mammal species affected or endangered in North America include bison, bighorn sheep, elk, grizzlies, and wolves. Exotic plants introduced have taken over in a considerable part of the arid grazing lands in the western United States. Introduced bees are competing with native species. As for soil degradation and pesticides, some 80% of agricultural lands show moderate to severe soil erosion. Soil erosion of 1 in. per year compares with 1 in. of natural formation in 300 to 1000 years. The implementation of viable alternatives to present-day practices is recommended. Small farms are seen as a way to protect biodiversity.

In Part Six, the growing epidemic of hunger is addressed by Anuradha Mittal. The problem is seen as not that of not enough food, but of the faulty distribution of food not only worldwide but in the United States as well. The "Green Revolution" is perceived as a myth. However, it is noted that from 1970 to 1990, total food available per person worldwide increased by 11% and the estimated hungry people declined from 942 to 786 million. But if China is eliminated from the analysis, the number of hungry people in the rest of the world increased by over 11%. The discrepancies caused by China's inclusion or exclusion are attributed to a major redistribution of land, whereby the number of hungry people decreased from 406 to 189 million. And as for genetic engineering producing a "second Green Revolution," there are matters of high seed costs, royalties, and other inputs, plus the higher cost of cultivation, all accompanied by a higher market price.

In Part Seven, Texas author and populist Jim Hightower, publisher of the award-winning newsletter *The Hightower Lowdown*, describes the experiences of a certain Jim Crawford out in the Texas Panhandle, in the Muleshoe area, a region with more cattle than people. A graduate of Muleshoe High and Texas Tech University, for some 17 years Crawford farmed his corn crop the usual way using chemical fertilizers and pesticides. However, the price of fertilizer and pesticides kept going up, and the price of corn kept going down, so something had to change. Accordingly, Jim Crawford decided to try (feedlot) manure, of which there was aplenty thereabouts. The first year, his corn crop was about half of the usual, so the locals snickered. The second year, it was about even-steven, but the third year the crop was one-and-a half times the usual — and was of premium quality. The snickering stopped.

Whereas Wilson (2001) focuses on soil and crop contamination, epidemiologist Devra Davis emphasizes air quality, and the lack thereof, in *When Smoke Ran Like Water: Tales of Environmental Deception and the Battle Against Pollution* (2002). This, plus a large dose of the political machinations that abound. Thus, in the preface she notes that, though witnesses are under oath, the lawyers are not — and can say anything, whether outrageous or not. Her first chapter concerns the steel town of Donora, Pennsylvania, her home territory, which was enveloped by a killer fog starting on October 26, 1948. The massive fog that settled in was itself not toxic; it was the gaseous and particulate effluent it contained, variously from coke ovens, blast furnaces, and the zinc works, where part of the steel product received a coating of corrosion resistant zinc. Despite studies, there have been no final conclusions and many of the people involved did not want to talk about it — the same kind of situation uncovered in Wilson (2001), for jobs and economics are ubiquitous, and never mind that the initial fatalities were only the start, for there were the many who died later or much later, and those who were permanently debilitated. Moreover, there was the partial conclusion that the fluorspar (an ore of calcium fluoride) used in the operations was a major culprit, for the victims' lungs were not scarred as they would be from sulfur oxides, a sign that liberated fluorine gas was immediately absorbed into the lung tissue and bloodstream, causing death. The killer fog paralleled an earlier incident in Liege, Belgium, in 1930, which was also mostly swept under the rug.

In turn, the London killer fog of 1952 is discussed, with the note that here it was the sulfur oxides (i.e., sulfuric acid) from burning high-sulfur coal that was the major cause of death. The following chapter is about the Los Angeles Basin, variously highlighting ethyl lead in gasoline, carbon monoxide, and smog, and the efforts to eliminate or control these pollutants. Chapter 4 addresses the EPA, its teething troubles, and current problems. Chapter 6 takes on breast cancer, with the causes mostly yet inconclusive: for example, the National Cancer Institute's massive increase in funding has not resulted in any major developments about the environmental factors involved (Davis, 2002, p. 187). However, in the next chapter, notably about male sterility, distinct chemical causes are pinpointed. Along the way, DDT is discussed, and the last chapter is concerned with chlorinated fluorocarbons (CFCs) and global warming. Throughout there are many accounts, first-hand and otherwise, of the many-sided arguments and machinations that always occur whenever it is government vs. industry vs. the people.

Speaking more so about the effects of chemicals, one can tread further into the cancer-causing morass by mentioning that there are substances in minute or trace quantities which may act as anticancer agents, say, but in greater quantities may act as carcinogens. (Thus the old saying, that the dose is the poison.) Compounds of the heavy metal selenium are a purported example. Germanium compounds may be beneficial in minute quantities, but can be deadly in greater quantities or concentrations. Digitalis is another example.

A recent addition to the file of anticancer inorganic compounds is the chemical element indium, whose compounds constitute another instance of the trace minerals or metals. Its testing and beneficial effects have been described by Robert Lyons in *Indium: The Missing Trace Mineral* (2001). Most active as the water-soluble sulfate form, and although prolonging the lifetimes of patients, it was nevertheless found not to be a cancer cure in the complete sense of the word, in whatever form or concentrations used.

In sum, any good attorney can point all these things out, even as truisms, and forever muddy the waters. Reason enough for the saying that in many or most situations, we merely "muddle through," clear-cut decisions being a rarity.

## MORE ON CHEMOTHERAPY, ALKALOIDS, AND OTHER PLANT BIOCHEMICALS

For some of the reasons previously addressed, there is sometimes a preference for localized chemotherapy injections into the cancer growth itself rather than intravenous injections, which presumably confines the effects to the cancerous mass proper. There are problems here as well, however, including that of the cancer further spreading or metastasizing, one possibility being that the drug chemical may in itself be carcinogenic.

The body itself may try to fight off the chemotherapy via the immune system, manifested by fever and an increased white blood cell count, although the chemotherapy itself works against the immune system. Another quandary is that these symptoms may indicate that the immune system is reacting against the cancer, rather than against a conventional bacterial or viral infection. There are ways, in other words, that medical orthodoxy may misinterpret the body's resistance to cancer.

In a further and much-repeated comment regarding chemotherapy, Mathew Suffness and John M. Pezzuto, the former from the National Cancer Institute and the latter from the University of Illinois College of Medicine, declared that conventional chemotherapy is ineffective against solid tumors, and only works against blood-related tumors (Hostettmann, 1991, *Methods in Plant Biochemistry*, Vol. 6, *Assays for Bioactivity*, pp. 72ff, 116).

Such successes as there are against blood-related cancers can be judged intermittent, using such agents as *Catharantheus* and *Vinca* alkaloids, for example, vincristine and vinblastine, as derived from the Madagascar periwinkle *Catharantheus roseus* —

but which are cytotoxic, acting against normal cells as well as cancer cells, and producing the usual debilitating side effects. In fact, blood-related cancers are of different origins than solid tumors, and it may be added that the skin cancer called melanoma involves completely different biochemical processes. Thus, expectedly, in these instances the treatments need to be different. What may work for one type will not work for another. In fact, different words or wording may be used to distinguish between types; for example, with regard to solid tumors per se, there are sarcomas and carcinomas, depending on the body region of occurrence.

The *Vinca* alkaloids have the property of killing white blood cells, and thereby act against the proliferation of white blood cells that occurs with leukemia (Swerdlow, 2000, p. 220). At the same time, there are the harsh side effects from these toxic alkaloids in their use as chemotherapy agents.

It may be added that cancer specialist David Plotkin, M.D., in the June 1996 issue of the *Atlantic Monthly*, summarized the situation by noting that chemotherapy is most effective when needed least and least effective when needed most.

Alkaloids are among the most bioactive of plant constituents, ranging from the fairly innocuous to the deadly. The subject is reviewed in depth in Geoffrey A. Cordell's *Alkaloids: A Biogenetic Approach* (1981). In addition to the detailed chemistry of the subject, Cordell provides extensive information on what plants have which alkaloids, along with the history and other background knowledge. In fact, as has been noted, in screening the tropical rain forests for bioactive plants, the presence of alkaloids is the main indicator of bioactivity. Alkaloid compounds for the most part have a unique nitrogen-containing ring structure, which makes them basic or alkaline, and which may render them particularly active as enzyme inhibitors, with the total makeup of the compound determining which enzymes are deactivated or inhibited.

Alkaloids, however, are merely one category of bioactive compounds, which in general include classes or categories having such other names as glycosides (which may include cyanogenic compounds such as laetrile, or amygdalin), phenolics, saponins, flavonoids, certain vegetable proteins (some of which are deadly), and amino acids. The related subject is poisonous and medicinal plants, the two going together, and the title of the book by Will H. Blackwell, with a chapter on fungi by Martha J. Powell.

As for plants that may have anticancer properties, the baseline reference remains Jonathan L. Hartwell's extensive compendium *Plants Used Against Cancer*, published in 1982. As has been repeatedly indicated, Hartwell lists some 3000 different species as found in medical folklore, comprising 1430 genera from 214 plant families. Most are probably ineffective, and some may be exceedingly toxic, as Hartwell warns. There are still other and newer compilations of bioactive or medicinal plant species from around the world, for example, from North America, Central and South America (Neotropica), and the various divisions of Africa, as well as India, Southwest Asia, and China. Among these bioactive plants are those that native folklore prescribes against cancers. If mostly ineffective, these compilations are nevertheless a starting point for continued testing. Many are listed in Hoffman (1999a).

(The National Cancer Institute, or NCI, formerly had a program for testing tens of thousands of plant species, a fact previously mentioned. This was shut down about the time Hartwell's book was published, in favor of turning everything over to the pharmaceutical companies, as noted with dismay by botanist James A. Duke in the foreword. The testing has since been revived, but the search for new plant medicinals seems to have plateaued for a number of reasons, according to Swerdlow's book. For one thing it is easier and much faster to test synthetic compounds. Nevertheless, James A. Duke, prominent in phytochemicals, has gone on to write and compile a number of botanical books about bioactive plants and their uses, as cited elsewhere.)

China, in particular, is noted for its herbal medicines. To which can be added India, as embodied in the *yurveda Encyclopedia: Natural Secrets to Healing, Prevention, & Longevity* by Swami Sada Shiva Tirtha. (yurveda is the "science of life" or longevity, the holistic alternative science from India, said to be more than 5000 years old and the oldest healing science in existence.) The subject of cancer is taken up on pp. 499–501 among the many other diseases and illnesses discussed. Causes are first listed, then some therapies, with herbal therapies cited in terms of either English or Indian names. The chapters "Herbology" and "Herb Therapy" assist in the translation from one language to the other. No surefire therapy or cure emerges, however, and the Western reader is very likely to be turned off (at least this reader is, in spite of favorable reviews from other quarters).

## RECOURSES

It appears that everything is getting more and more complex, including the study of cancer and its treatment — which often translates into stasis. Thus, Jacques Barzun wrote in the prologue of his latest, about his 30th, *From Dawn to Decadence: 500 Years of Western Cultural Life: 1500 to the Present* (2001), that, in a stalled society, for any proposal or project, there are contrary arguments that seem equally sensible. And Isaac Newton declared that for every action there is an equal and opposite reaction.

Therefore, regarding cancer and other diseases, consider again Swerdlow (2000). On page 286, Swerdlow refers to Ernest Hemingway's warning never to confuse movement with action. "Screening provides considerable movement. Plants are gathered and checked, money is spent, jobs are created, numbers are added, scientific papers are published, and numerous plant chemicals demonstrate activity against disease. But how much action, in the form of actual treatment for disease, is there?" (Another observation is that screening is made on an *in vitro* and *in vivo* basis — but not on a clinical basis. In other words, the effect on humans may be different from what occurs in a culture dish or in mice — and likely is.) With the Internet and such sources as Medline, the proliferation of information is enormous, almost incomprehensible, but mostly inconsequential, making it impossible to see the forest for the trees, so to speak.

As for reporting on the status of alternative cancer therapies in general, there are, for instance, the frequently mentioned volumes Ralph W. Moss's *Cancer Therapy: The Independent Consumer's Guide to Non-Toxic Treatment & Prevention* and Richard Walters' *Options: The Alternative Cancer Therapy Book*. Moss also furnishes the Moss Report and is a regular contributor to the *Townsend Letter for Doctors & Patients*. It can be assumed that there will be much more information forthcoming. Suffice to say, no surefire, 100%, guaranteed cure is proffered. For each claim, it seems, there is a counter claim.

There are innumerable books concerned with orthodox treatments for cancer, the titles of which are readily found by a computer search, say under the subject of cancer (*Books in Print* lists those presently in print, and *First Search* or *WorldCat* lists all that have ever been published). And according to the computer-retrieval system Medline, there are on the average 15,000 to 20,000 papers, articles, and publications about cancer forthcoming every year, and likely increasing. Not to mention the millions of items accumulated on the Internet. Who knows, something useful may be buried in this mass of information. But in fact, as Swerdlow (2000) emphasizes, we seem to have a surfeit of information, almost too much.

As for the anticancer action of these plant-derived or herbal medicines, or still other chemicals, the most probable route is that of enzyme inhibitors. In fact, this is seen as the role of modern medicines such as antibiotics, which act against a critical enzyme in bacterial cells (prokaryotes), but in the dosages used, not against human cells (eukaryotes). Each and every body biochemical reaction in the body is in fact catalyzed and controlled by a particular enzyme. In turn, there are other substances that may inhibit, block, control, or modulate the action of these enzymes. These substances are known as enzyme inhibitors, and in rare instances may also promote a biochemical reaction. More than this, a particular substance will usually act against or inhibit more than one enzyme. This diversity produces side effects.

In brief review of previously presented findings, a distinction has been found in the metabolism of cancer cells vs. normal cells, dating back to the discovery of German biochemist Otto Warburg circa 1926, who later won a Nobel prize for other work (Voet and Voet, 1995, p. 595). And in the same reference there is the previously noted comment that understanding the metabolic differences between cancer cells and normal cells may be the key to successfully treating cancer.

As for human cells or eukaryotes, the metabolic path or sequence involves the conversion of glucose by what is labeled glycolysis. In a series of ten steps there is first produced a compound called pyruvic acid or pyruvate (the latter designating a so-called salt or compound of pyruvic acid). In the presence of oxygen, this is further converted to carbon dioxide and water in what is variously called the tricarboxylic acid cycle, or citric acid cycle, or Krebs cycle. The overall operation may be conveniently called aerobic glycolysis, with each step requiring a particular enzyme, and most usually requiring supportive reactions.

In cancer cells, however, the pyruvic acid or pyruvate is instead converted to lactic acid or lactate. This does not utilize oxygen, and the overall sequence can be referred to as anaerobic glycolysis. The conversion of pyruvic acid or pyruvate to lactic acid or lactate requires the action of a form, or forms, of an enzyme called lactate dehydrogenase.

In consequence, the inhibition of this particular enzyme has the potential of blocking cancer cell metabolism. The subject was further discussed by the author in the articles, "Enzyme Inhibitors for Cancer Cell Metabolism" and "Garlic and Allicin and Other Sulfur-Containing Compounds as Anticancer Agents," and in Hoffman (1999). There are still other metabolic pathways that can be considered, such as aminolysis, but in the main, cancer cells undergo anaerobic glycolysis.

Among the enzyme inhibitors noted is allicin, derived from freshly chewed garlic, whereby the enzyme allinase is contacted with certain sulfur compounds naturally present, notably alliin. There are still other inhibitors listed in the handbooks, some of which may be benign and some not. For the record, the handbook references include M.K. Jain's *Handbook of Enzyme Inhibitors* (1982), and H. Zollner's *Handbook of Enzyme Inhibitors*, in two editions (1989, 1993). Allicin as a chemical compound, unfortunately, has a half-life of only a few hours, negating its commercial preparation and use as such. This problem may have been solved however, as there are several brands of garlic tablets that are claimed to produce active allicin, and are so rated. (Examples being Garlicin®, Garlique®, and Garlinase®.) Further information appears in the previously cited references by the author.

More recently, an article appeared in the March 2003 issue of *Life Extension*, titled "Garlic May Reduce Risk of Prostate Cancer," by Elizabeth Heubeck. A study by the National Cancer Institute was cited whereby it was found that a diet rich in the allium food group — garlic, shallots, and onions — would cut the risk of prostate cancer in half. Eating as little as a tenth of an ounce of scallions each day reduced prostate cancer risk by 70% and the same amount of garlic reduced the risk by 53%. A clove of garlic a day was suggested. A China investigation was mentioned, where the diet is heavy on garlic, scallions, and onions, and where men have the lowest prostate cancer rate anywhere. A previous published study was also cited, where garlic was found to inhibit gastric cancer [Dorant et al., *British Journal of Cancer*, (1993)]. The principal component of crushed (and masticated) garlic, notably allicin, was found to inhibit the proliferation of human mammary, endometrial, and colon cancer cells [Hirsch, et al., *Nutrition and Cancer*, (2000)]. In the interim, until more comprehensive studies can be made, the outlook is that of cautious optimism at NCI. (The National Institutes of Health, of which the National Cancer Institute is part, is also studying the treatment of prostate cancer utilizing vitamin E and selenium, as reported by biochemist Wayne Martin via a letter to the editor in the January 2003 issue of the *Townsend Letter for Doctors & Patients*, but which mistakenly appeared as vitamin K because of a typo.)

It may be noted that other steps in the metabolic sequence are subject to the action of inhibitors, some of which appear in medical folklore as anticancer agents.

With regard to melanoma, which involves the enzyme tyrosinase, there are a number of inhibitors listed in the handbooks for this particular enzyme. Among them, interestingly, is ascorbic acid, or vitamin C, as well as some other commonly encountered substances such as lactic acid (from sour milk products) and butyric acid (from rancid butter). The aforecited alpine sunflower/yucca extract developed by Owen Asplund of the University of Wyonming may very well act as an enzyme inhibitor for tyrosinase.

It may be mentioned in passing that there are independent studies that found vitamin C or ascorbic acid to destroy cancer cells, as propagated by two-time Nobel laureate Linus Pauling, which was much resisted by the medical community. The update by Abram Hoffer, M.D., Ph.D., a former associate of Linus Pauling, titled *Vitamin C and Cancer*, merits another mention. Vitamin E has demonstrated some positive anticancer effects, according to the June 2001 issue of *Life Extension*. Milkweed is another candidate, and is a part of medical folklore. (Milkweed is of the genus *Asclepias*, named after Asclepius, the Greek god of the healing art.) The listings grow, as do the controversies.

Milkweed, for instance, contains an enzyme that digests or dissolves protein, and has been used as a folkloric remedy, notably for warts. Continuing along these lines, reference can be made to a book by Maud Oakes titled *Beyond the Windy Place: Life in the Guatemalan Highlands* (1995). Oakes was funded by a foundation to investigate ancient religious practices as may have been handed down from the Mayas. She chose an isolated village named Todos Santos, which was on the other side of a wind-swept pass from the larger village Huehuetenango, located in northwestern Guatemala, in fact near the Pan American or InterAmerican Highway. There, at Todos Santos, a cure for skin cancer came to light using poultices of the pulp from a small cactus that is rare and grows at great heights, but Oakes was not able to arouse any interest among her contacts in the United States (Oakes, 1951, pp. 70, 71, 81, 82).

There are a number of forms of human lactate dehydrogenase, that is, what are variously denoted as $LDH_1$, $LDH_2$, $LDH_3$, $LDH_4$, and $LDH_5$ (e.g., Voet and Voet, 1995, pp. 183, 164; Hoffman, 1999, pp. 386, 387). The fifth form of the enzyme, sometimes denoted as the M-type, for muscle (and liver), is presumably the most efficient for the conversion (or reduction) of pyruvate to lactate, or pyruvic acid to lactic acid.

The metabolism of the malaria parasite or protozoan (a one-celled organism) involves a form of the enzyme lactate dehydrogenase. (The malaria parasite can be any of several species of the genus *Plasmodium*, but is more commonly *P. falciparum*.) The inhibition of the form of lactate dehydrogenase occurring is the objective of studies under way at several institutions, notably by David L. VanderJagt and coworkers at the University of New Mexico School of Medicine, Leo Brady and coworkers in the Department of Biochemistry at the University of Bristol, and Karl Werbovetz and coworkers in the College of Pharmacy at the Ohio State University. The general subject is that of antiparasitic drug discovery, that is, the development of new and alternative (chemotherapy) agents for the treatment of such protozoal diseases as leishmaniasis and trypanosomiasis, as well as malaria. Another serious tropical parasitic disease is schistosomiasis (caused by a parasitic fluke of the genus *Schistosoma*), a disease better known as bilharziasis, or bilharzia. Further information and references about the foregoing antiparasitic work can be obtained from the Internet or Medline.

It would be interesting to know whether there is any (say, epidemiologic) connection between malarial immunity and cancer immunity. Thus, many native inhabitants of the tropical areas fortunately develop immunity to malaria, which may or may not be related to the inhibition of the malarial enzyme lactate dehydrogenase or other critical malarial enzymes.

Another drug under study against both malaria and cancer is artemisinin, derived from "sweet wormwood," *Artemisia annua*, which has a long history as an antimalarial agent, as well as for other purposes. (Of the sages or sagebrushes, *A. annua* is of the same genus as the more notorious *A. absinthium*, or "wormwood," the source of absinthe.) The foregoing subject is discussed in an article appearing in the December 2002 and July 2006 issues of *The Townsend Letter for Doctors and*

*Patients*, by Robert Jay Rowen, M.D., who is editor in chief of *Second Opinion*. Artemisinin is known to be cytotoxic in the presence of ferrous iron, and inasmuch as cancer cells are naturally high in iron influx, the connection can be made. The article presents a number of positive clinical results for various advanced cancer cases.

Artemisinin is classed as a lactone glycoside (e.g., in Hoffman, 1999, p. 111), one of a number of bioactive compounds in the genus *Artemisia* of the plant family Compositae or Asteraceae. The most notorious source of course is the species *A. absinthium*, which contains brain-damaging alkaloids (e.g., in Hoffman, 1999, p. 506). There is a revival of interest in artemisinin's potential as an anticancer agent, notably against colorectal cancer that has metastasized to the liver, as per the Web site Keep Michael Blair Alive! at www.blairalive.com, and which mentions other alternative therapies and causative agents — including parasites — as well as an extensive listing of supporting references.

Speaking further of parasites, there is the previously cited book by Hulda Regehr Clark titled *The Cure for All Cancers*, in which it is advanced that an intestinal fluke parasite, namely *Fasciolopsis buskii*, is the primary cause of all cancers. A deworming or anthelminthic procedure is recommended such as utilization of absinthe (that is, *Artemisia absinthium* of the family Compositae or Asteraceae). Absinthe, of course, has its own well-known toxic effects, or adverse side effects, but the plant is listed in Hartwell's compendium as an anticancer agent. Although there have been adverse comments regarding Clark's conclusions, it may at the same time again be remarked that British physician J. Jackson Clarke once wrote a series of books (the last published in 1922) in which, in a chapter "Cancer-Bodies," he mentioned that he had found protozoa in cancers, as well as elsewhere (Clarke, 1922, p. 92). These developments are presented notably in Section 7.7 of Hoffman (1999). (A layman's guide to the subject is provided in *The Parasite Menace* by Skye Weintraub, 1998.)

Increasingly, therefore, parasites (living things that live off other living things) are blamed for all sorts of ills. The classic example is the intestinal tapeworm, but there are myriad others, such as roundworms and hookworms, and trichonomads, the flagellate protozoa that cause trichomoniasis. The treatments can be as severe as the disease, ranging from using antimony compounds to using carbon tetrachloride (once used for hookworm). Accordingly, (herbal) intestinal purification has become a part of the medical subculture.

This discussion is not complete, however, as the methods of administration — oral, intravenous, or intramuscular — and the dosage levels and frequency, as well as other factors, must be established for successful clinical therapy. Thus, a drug or remedy may be effective if administered intravenously but not orally, because the digestive processes may affect the drug itself. An exception is penicillin and some other antibiotics, which can be successfully used orally. And it can be added that there are such peripheral matters that *in vitro*, *in vivo*, and clinical test results do not always agree. There is also biochemical individuality among patients, with the result that what works on one does not necessarily work on another.

(In an editorial on page 122 of the January 2002 issue of the *Townsend Letter for Doctors & Patients*, physician Alan R. Gaby, M.D., urges caution in extrapolating favorable test tube, or *in vitro*, results to the actual patient. For instance, "most natural substances that have shown antibacterial activity *in vitro* have not been found to be clinically useful as antibiotics." Thus, these substances may not achieve high enough concentrations in the infected tissues to be effective. These are variously involved: the absorption, transport through the bloodstream, and efficient penetration into the infected tissue, which in the case of bacterial infections may be barred by mucus, pus, and other debris. At the same time, the active substance must avoid sequestration by binding proteins, deactivation by body enzymes, and elimination by the normal body functions. In further comment, however, it may be noted that there are a few situations where a substance functions clinically, but not in *vitro* or *in vivo*. We must therefore distinguish clinical or human results from *in vivo* or animal tests. That is, what may work for mice, for instance, most likely will not work for humans, and vice versa, as cancer researchers have found out.)

In this regard it has been repeatedly suggested that cancer clinical research centers (CCRCs) or their equivalent be established to investigate and apply such alternative therapies as described, or still other therapies, initially to cases of advanced (or terminal) cancer, and presumably later to any case. Preferably on an outpatient basis, there would be close supervision by M.D.s and D.O.s, backed up by pharmacologists, biochemists, microbiologists, or molecular biologists, and botanists or ethnobotanists, as well as herbalists, homeopaths, naturopaths, and other support personnel. Different biochemical therapies could be tried, with the patients closely monitored for vital signs and side effects. (Even home test kits could be supplied for checking out different substances against, say, the enzyme lactate dehydrogenase.) Most helpful would be a near-instantaneous noninvasive test to determine whether the cancer is receding or not. And if something does not work, another route could be tried.

(It may be mentioned that almost any city of any substantial size now has some sort of cancer clinic, or several, but which utilize the orthodox cancer treatments. To be treated by alternative therapies, a patient has to leave the country, say, to Germany or Mexico, an avenue open only to the wealthy. The word is that our overseas neighbors are surpassing the United States in the arena of research, indicating that the ultimate breakthrough in cancer therapy may come from these directions.)

However, by establishing CCRCs or their equivalent in this country, the option should be open to everyone, rich and poor alike. (As Anatole France once wrote, the law in its majesty forbids the rich as well as the poor to steal a loaf of bread.) Moreover, by including the word "Research" in the descriptor, there is the inference that funding in total or in part would be borne by the federal government — part of the War on Cancer.

Beyond these considerations, there is another matter to be addressed. By using orthodox treatments, a physician is legally protected by his peers, that is, by the system or establishment, which is already in place. Therefore, legal means around this dilemma must be provided, which remains a touchy subject, even though the patient signs consent forms.

Plants or herbs are always considered a therapeutic possibility, although it should be mentioned that substitutions can occur, and that plant or herbal activity varies with geographic location, the season, even sometimes the time of day (storage time is another variable). Herbal identification and standardization are therefore problems, though Germany, for instance, has taken positive steps in this direction.

Substances that are mostly benign are preferred, especially those that do not adversely affect the liver and kidneys, nor respiration and the heart. For this reason, foods or foodstuffs are of primary consideration, having passed the test of time, and it may be noted that common garden vegetables and fruits contain an astounding array of bioactive compounds, including alkaloids, but usually in low or very low concentrations. It may be added that native peoples who live on vegetarian diets, such as the previously mentioned Hunzas, are found to be remarkably free from cancer.

Finally, there is both information and misinformation floating around about the curative powers of plants and herbs, and still other substances. No one can tell whether we are dealing with facts or with speculations. The National Institutes of Health is belatedly trying to sort it out, and is sponsoring a survey to accumulate information about unorthodox cancer cures or remissions that have been substantiated and documented by M.D.s or their equivalent. This is sound policy, given the fact that you do not know whom to believe, and people are liable to say anything. This brings up the point that an absolute cure that is both definitive and decisive is the objective.

(The NIH survey was being conducted by The Kushi Institute, a macrobiotics center at Beckett, Massachusetts, 413-623-5741, and by the University of Minnesota School of Public Health. The objective is to determine recoveries traceable to macrobiotics, that is, to a macrobiotic or vegetarian kind of diet. It may again be mentioned as well that the Institute for Noetic Sciences at Sausalito, California, has long kept records on the spontaneous remission of cancer. Mentioned earlier, there has been another investigation underway called the Cornell-Oxford-China Study or "The China Project," which is directed at linking diet and disease. In a preview, it is estimated that nearly 90% of all cancers, cardiovascular diseases, and other degenerative illnesses can be delayed until old age, and in fact the "normal" processes of aging are not normal at all. A resulting publication by T. Colin Campbell is titled *The China Study: The Most Comprehensive Study Ever Conducted and the Startling Implications for Diet, Weight Loss and Long Term Health*, published in 2005. Campbell is the project director. The statement is furnished that cancer can be turned on or off at will using only diet. Earlier, in 1987, T. Colin Campbell and L. Kinlen had published *Diet and Cancer*, courtesy of the Imperial Cancer Research Foundation. Another announced chronicler of cancer survival and survivors is *The Health Resource*, Conway, AR, 800-949-0090 or 501-329-5272.)

For the preceding reasons, an evaluation demands that theories or mechanisms be instituted that explain why a given substance works or does not work. In this connection, the most promising avenue appears to be the role of enzyme inhibitors, which, after all, have been declared the basis for modern medicine.

## CIRCLING THE WAGONS

Returning again to the War on Cancer, if there was a concerted, motivated, mission-oriented effort like the Manhattan Project, which developed the atomic bomb in 4 or 5 years, a cure would have been found long ago. The goal was clear-cut, the leadership outstanding, with the research directed by scientific and inspired genius Robert Oppenheimer, and sustained by down-to-earth Gen. Leslie Groves. As it is, and based on the dearth of life-saving results, one can wonder whether or not the medical establishment even wants a cancer cure. The cancer treatment business continues to do very well, economically at least; so why rock the boat? As for doctors per se, there is the remark circulated that during the two world wars, when the armed services had raided the medical profession, the country was in better overall health.

There is the unavoidable fact of business life that profit is the bottom line, and is necessary for continued existence and growth. And the drug companies cannot make a sufficient profit off a nonpatentable or nonproprietary substance such as from a plant. Some sort of chemical transformation of the plant substances will be required in order to obtain a proprietary position, which may not even be as effective. Hence, by definition, the drug companies cannot be overly concerned with plant cures, or plant-derived cures, and must turn to synthetics, as a matter of economic survival. An added complication is that many of the tropical countries expect to have a proprietary position on medicinal plants occurring in their particular countries, a piece of the action, so to speak. (The word is going out, however, that American drug companies are proceeding to patent, or at least to apply for patents on, plants whose medicinal usages date back to antiquity. If nothing else, this will hinder the use of a particular plant by others, most of whom do not have the financial and legal resources to challenge a large company in the courts.)

At the same time, one would think that the U.S. government should take up the slack and become more involved in plant remedies, say, via the National Institutes of Health and the National Cancer Institute. (An Office of Alternative Medicine, later called the National Center for Complementary and Alternative Medicine, was founded within the National Institutes of Health, but all seems quiet at the front lines.) Furthermore, as already indicated, musical chairs are being played by government and industry (and academia as well, which depends on research grants). Call it collusion if you will. It is the downside of capitalism in action. The human element always will out.

To further illustrate, the American Cancer Society, which generally seems to have its hand out, collecting about $400 million each year, has been accused of spending only about 30% of this cash hoard on cancer research, the rest going to salaries and nonresearch operations. No cures have been forthcoming, yet it maintains a blacklist called "Unproven Methods of Cancer Management" (Walters, 1993, p. 338, 6). The ACS manages to pay fat salaries, however, and has acquired an impressive investment folio, and in 1988 was said to have a fund balance of $426 million.

An article by Ellen Stark in the November 1996 issue of *Money* provides a more favorable appraisal. The spending program of the ACS is listed as 70.2% of its $382 million income. This, however, does not cite research as such. And it may be noted that the ACS is involved in information dissemination, for example, the publication of journals and reports. Otherwise, it may be asked just what is to be included in "programs"? Does this, for instance, include financial investments?

Much more about the ACS is furnished in Samuel S. Epstein's article, "American Cancer Society: The World's Wealthiest 'Nonprofit' Institution," published in 1999 in the *International Journal of Health Sciences*. Thus, an appraisal by James Bennett, a professor of economics at George Mason University and an authority on charitable organizations, found that in 1988 the ACS had a fund balance of $400 million plus another $69 million in land, buildings, and equipment. Of this total, only $90 million — about 26% — was spent on medical research and programs. Moreover, the board of the ACS Foundation comprises corporate executives from the pharmaceutical, investment, banking, and media industries, and *The Chronicle of Philanthropy* has mentioned that the ACS is "more interested in accumulating wealth than in saving lives." Epstein also lists the breakdown for several states as found by other investigators, including Thomas DiLorenzo, a professor of economics at Loyola College and veteran investigator of nonprofit organizations. At the time of writing (circa 1999), Epstein listed the current budget of the ACS at $380 million and cash reserves approaching $1 billion. As for lobbying, a March 30, 1998, Associated Press release addressed this issue, citing expenditures, the use of its own personal assets, and donations to political associations. And the national Charities Information Bureau is quoted as saying that it "does not know of any other charity that makes contributions to political parties."

(On a more positive note, there is the *American Cancer Society's Complete Guide to Prostate Cancer*, published in 2005.)

In the September 2005 issue of the *Townsend Letter for Doctors & Patients*, Ralph W. Moss asks, "Is There a Cancer Conspiracy?" A survey by the ACS finds that 27% of Americans believe that a cure actually exists, with another 14% suspicious. Moss goes on to say that maybe there is no conspiracy, precisely speaking, though there has been some foot dragging on alternative treatments for reasons outlined, with the term Big Pharma interjected. If the question were phrased without using the term "conspiracy," the negative survey results may be even more decisive, with the public saying that there is something terribly wrong in the search for new cancer treatments.

The contents of Epstein's paper, cited earlier, are featured in Winfield J. Abbe's report titled *An Unsuccessful Effort to Deny Use of State of Georgia Facilities for Fundraising by the American Cancer Society*, and is reprinted in full in the appendix of the report. Abbe, a professor of physics at the University of Georgia, objected to the ACS using University of Georgia facilities to promote its agenda and to raise funds, and so wrote university officials and the governor — to no avail. More than this, Abbe insisted that the university at least provide Samuel S. Epstein with a forum for rebuttal — also to no avail. Abbe's report damns the orthodox cancer establishment, with documentation furnished along with details of his wife's tragic fight against cancer. Not only is Abbe critical of the ACS, but also of the Race for the Cure. And he follows this up by citing correspondence with *The New England Journal of Medicine* (publication denied). Given the interlocking nature of medical orthodoxy, pharmaceuticals, finance, government, and the media, one may comment that public arousal — if any — will be slow. However, the fact that Michael Gearin-Tosh's *Living Proof: A Medical Mutiny* (2002) was published at all gives a degree of hope.

In a later communication sent to the *Townsend Letter for Doctors & Patients*, with references, the same Winfield J. Abbe reviewed and challenged a book by biologist Robert A. Weinberg titled *Racing to the Beginnings of the Road: The Search for the Origin of Cancer*, published in 1996. Weinberg was highly critical of Otto Warburg's work and conclusions about the metabolic origins of cancer cells as being anaerobic rather than aerobic. A similar criticism was leveled by Sidney Weinhouse in an article titled "Respiratory Impairment of Cancer Cells" appearing in *Science*, Vol. 124, in 1956. (Otto Heinrich Warburg, M.D., Ph.D., contributed an article titled "On the Origin of Cancer Cells" that was published *in Science*, Vol. 123, 1956, pp. 309–314, a translation from *Naturwissenschaften*, Vol. 42, 1955, p. 401ff. Warburg died in 1970, but his work on cancer cell metabolism dates back to 1923.) Abbe's further comments about the nature of cancer bear repeating. "The cancer industry believes cancer is hundreds of diseases, one for every type of cancer. It is as if they took hundreds of combinations for volume, temperature, and pressure but never discovered the single gas law linking all three together. Dr. Warburg, on the other hand, along with the thousands of others ... proved that cancer is one disease, not hundreds of diseases, and this proof is certainly not contradicted by anything from the pen of the biology professor in this book." Abbe in turn cites the long-recognized law of parsimony, that "only the simplest explanations, consistent with the experimental facts, are accepted in science."

A featured article by *Fortune* executive editor Clifton Leaf titled "Why We're Losing the War on Cancer" appeared in the March 2004 issue. This in turn caused some talk. Thus, in the June 2004 issue of the *Townsend Letter for Doctors & Patients*, Ralph W. Moss reviewed Leaf's article in his monthly column "The War on Cancer." Moss restates some of the facts uncovered by Leaf, namely that no improvements have occurred in the survival rate, with no dramatic breakthroughs (such as occurred for Hodgkin's disease). This, despite spending an estimated $14.4 billion per year on cancer research. In fact, cancer research has become irrelevant and compartmentalized, and is fundamentally flawed by utilizing animal rather than human models.

Moss emphasizes Leaf's findings about cancer regression or remission, whereby "regression is not likely to improve a person's chances for survival." Moreover, the phenomenon of metastasis remains largely understudied, because this is a difficult task and is not likely to produce quick, measurable results. Nor do new anticancer drugs come off unscathed, including Avastin® and Erbitux®, which maybe only extend lifetimes for a few months. A listing of "Miracle Cures That Weren't" includes radiation therapy, interferon, interleuken-2, endostatin, and Gleevec®.

(In his column in the April 2005 issue of the *Townsend Letter for Doctors & Patients*, Moss indicates that on a *monthly* basis Avastin costs $4,400, Erbitux costs $17,000, and the newer drug called Zevalin® costs $24,000 — for controlling, not curing, cancer. Assuming a median cost of $8,500 per month, the annual cost would be $100,000. Enough to bankrupt many or most patients, and to leave the less wealthy multitude out in the cold. Presumably, these treatments could go on until the victim succumbs. The prediction is that further new treatments will be accompanied by rising, even multiplying, costs. And, despite FDA approval, will the health insurance companies cooperate? In this regard, Moss mentions the much lower costs for alternative treatments.)

Moss concludes by faulting Leaf for not bringing up complementary and alternative medicine (CAM), from which scores of new ideas for cancer treatment have emerged. One noted in particular is called MTH-68, dating back to 1968, and as further developed by Eva and Laszlo Csatary, M.D. It is based on the nontoxic Newcastle disease virus vaccine, and has proved beneficial against some cancers, notably brain cancer. These and other alternative treatments are systematically ignored by mainstream medicine and the media.

Clifton Leaf appeared as a panelist on PBS's *The Charlie Rose Show* on the evening of April 29, 2004, along with the respective directors of the Memorial Sloan-Kettering Cancer Center (MSKCC) and the National Cancer Institute (NCI), together with Andrew Gove, CEO of Intel Corporation. By far the most gripping presentation was from Andrew Gove, who was a real-life suffering victim of cancer and its treatment. He dared ask the embarrassing questions and make the incisive comments, without the usual circumventing and backpedaling.

A prominent full-page advertisement appeared in the *New York Times* on Sunday, March 9, 2003 (National Edition, p. 5). The ad was placed by Matthias Rath, M.D., who had many provocative things to say about health maintenance and the inadequacies of our present health care system. Steps for turning things around are proffered, based on the need to take better care of ourselves, by ourselves. In other words, we need to take more control over our own destiny. Period. This would cut out much of the expense and wear and tear of eternally going to the doctor and of taking overly prescribed medications. There is the implication, both overt and covert, that we can avoid illnesses, notably by the means of better nutrition and, shall we say, by utilizing the unorthodox outlook and methods of CAM. Dr. Rath, educated in Germany, is an advocate of CAM for both heart disease and cancer, with books backing this up, and is founder of the Health Alliance (2901 Bayview Dr., Fremont, CA 94538).

The ACS, the AMA, and the NCI were all blasted by Barry Lynes, a proponent of the Rife radio frequency treatment, and author of *The Cancer Cure That Worked!: Fifty Years of Suppression* (1992) and *The Healing of Cancer* (1989). In Chapter 17 of his first-mentioned book, Lynes speaks to the suppression of alternative cancer cures, whereby the AMA guards its pocket book and the pharmaceutical companies push chemotherapy for profit. He calls the American Cancer Society a big-money public relations fraud, and characterizes the FDA as being owned by the cancer monopolies, with the media remaining "silent, silent, silent." (It is informative to note that the publisher put in a disclaimer at the end of the first edition of Lynes' book, published in 1987, to the effect that, though the American Medical Association may have misused its power several decades ago, this is not to imply that the AMA would act this way today.) In his book *The Healing of Cancer*, Barry Lynes made the following statement about the National Cancer Institute (1989, p. 61). "NCI created a bureaucratic haven for scientism, filled with committee procedures, payoffs, collusion with drug companies, and interminable roadblocks for the truly innovative cancer fighters."

(Along these lines, Ralph Moss described a somewhat similar electromagnetic treatment in his monthly column "The War on Cancer," which was published in the December 2002 issue of the *Townsend Letter for Doctors & Patients*. Referred to as

Cytoluminescent Therapy, or CLT, it is a form of what is called photodynamic therapy, or PDT. Electromagnetic radiation within the light spectrum is used against cancer cells that have been sensitized by a certain kind of drug. The therapy evidently works against different kinds of cancer. Moss provides successful examples variously involving colon, breast, and prostate cancer. Among the drugs employed is FDA-approved Photofrin®, but more effective photosensitizers are under development, such as from ox blood but especially from plants. The general subject of PDT was included in Moss 1992. A comment that can be made is that perhaps sensitizers could be involved, or should be involved, in the Rife radio frequency treatment.)

Continuing, Linus Pauling had considered the "War on Cancer" a fraud, calling both the ACS and the NCI derelict in their duties (Walters, 1993, pp. 4, 338). In his book, Walters adds that the ACS Blacklist of Unproven Methods has been used to smear promising new therapies. On the other hand, an official at the Memorial Sloan Kettering Cancer Center declared that the blacklist is the source for their best ideas (Walters, 1993, p. 339). And speaking of the MSKCC, it has been previously mentioned that Ralph Moss, author of *Cancer Therapy* and other cancer-related books, was fired for taking exception to the downgrading of a study which was favorable to laetrile.

In addition to Linus Pauling's statements, James Watson, another Nobel Prize-winner and codiscoverer of the DNA double helix, and who served on the National Cancer Advisory Board, once described the National Cancer Program as a bunch of crap, or worse (Walters, 1993, p. 4). This incompetence is in spite of the fact that the incidences of most common cancers — those of the lung, colon, breast, prostate, pancreas, and ovary — are either staying at the same level or increasing. Conventional treatments may ultimately fail because even a thumb-sized tumor has about 1 billion cancer cells, and if treatment kills or removes, say, 99.9% of the cells, a million cells remain.

As for scratching each other's back, 90% of the members of NCIs peer review committee get NCI funding for their own research, with 70% of the ACS budget allocated for research going to individuals or institutions represented by the ACS board members (Walters, 1993, p. 339).

And as for the interlocking relationships between government, finance, and the drug or chemical industry, we mention once more a sort of underground exposé in the form of Clarence E. Mullins' *Death by Injection: The Story of the Medical Conspiracy Against America* (1992). Though the title implies problems with inoculations, not to mention chemotherapy, the main thrust of the book is on the ties that bind. Institutional and business names are named, constituting a "who's who" of the business world. Further information is provided by James P. Carter, M.D., DrPh. (1993), in *Racketeering in Medicine*, as previously cited.

Another, wider look at the scene is Robert Bell's *Impure Science: Fraud, Compromise and Political Influence in Scientific Research* (1992). The major part of Bell's book is concerned with the falsification or distortion of data and results that had occurred within the academic biochemical and pharmaceutical community, and were investigated by Michigan's Congressman John Dingell and his Subcommittee on Oversights and Investigations. The most notorious was what became known as the "David Baltimore case." The remainder of the book is concerned with government agencies and their grants and contracts. Suffice to say, academics do not take kindly the challenging of one of their own by an outsider. This reflex action is most obvious in the realm of medical orthodoxy, where its practitioners do not want any interference or embarrassments from laypersons nor from alternative medicine proponents.

A more recent exposé, about certain ubiquitous food additives, is by Russell L. Blaylock, M.D., a neurosurgeon at the University of Mississippi Medical Center. Published in 1997 by the Health Press of Santa Fe, New Mexico, Blaylock's book is titled *Excitotoxins: The Taste that Kills*. A further subtitle is "How Monosodium Glutamate, Aspartame (Nutrasweet®) and Similar Substances Can Cause Harm to the Brain and Nervous System and Their Relationship to Nuerodegenerative Diseases Such as Alzheimer's, Lou Gehrig's Disease (ALS) and Others." For instance, it has been shown that increased instances of brain tumors are but one side effect. The degree of collusion between the FDA, the pharmaceutical companies, and the courts and the court of public opinion has to be read about to be believed. The thought again is of the Romans and lead cooking vessels.

A popularization of the same subject, the innocuous toxicity of certain food additives, by Carol Simontacchi, is titled *The Crazy Makers: How the Food Industry is Destroying Our Minds and Harming Our Children* (2000). Additionally, there is *Diet for a Dead Planet: How the Food Industry Is Killing Us* by Christopher D. Cook (2004). Cook takes on the corporate oligarchy that is increasingly controlling the food industry, from the farm to the consumer. Food-borne bacteria are a part of the subject, as are the large supermarket chains, the tail that can wag the dog to the disadvantage of the small and independent food producers.

Further addressing the subject of foods, and crops, there is Michael Pollan's *The Botany of Desire: A Plant's Eye View of the World* (2001). In this regard, Pollan contributed an article about corn to the *New York Times*, published as "When a Crop Becomes King" on page A21 of the July 19, 2002, issue. What with subsidies and other encouragements, the crop is almost a monoculture, and is ubiquitous in its conversion to the sweetener fructose for myriad uses, such as in soft drinks. Whether this is good or bad over the long term of course remains to be seen, as with another (artificial) sweetener used in diet drinks, namely the previously mentioned aspartame, which is said to be converted to methanol or methyl alcohol within the body, this being the scientific name for wood alcohol, long known as a serious poison. (Not to mention questions about genetically modified corn.) Whether the common usage of these and other such synthetics will eventually prove detrimental can be argued back and forth, interminably, and will never be fully resolved, even if most of the human race goes under, as long as someone shows a profit and can manipulate the system. That is, for every argument, there is a counterargument, just as Newton proclaimed about action and reaction.

## MORE ON GENETIC MODIFICATION OR ENGINEERING

A lengthy article appearing in the October 28, 2002, issue of the *Nation*, by Mark Shapiro, has the title "Sowing Disaster: How Genetically Engineered Corn has

Altered the Global Landscape." Shapiro introduces the article by focusing on Oaxaca, a state in extreme southern Mexico, in the Sierra Norte Mountains, where corn (i.e., maize), in all its genetic diversity, is a principal food crop. Presumably protected by its remoteness, the corn at the village of Capulalpan has nevertheless been found to be infiltrated with genetically altered genes — very likely from the planting of seeds from genetically engineered corn obtained from the local store. Here, the corn traditionally grows in some sixty different varieties, ranging from shades of blue, black, purple, and white to the ubiquitous yellow.

This is part of a region ranging from the Sierre Norte down through the south-ernmost state of Chiapas and on into Guatemala, where the genetic diversity of its corn is regarded as a hedge against unforeseen environmental changes, and which can be used to rejuvenate stressed-out domesticated varieties, whatever the cause, and is therefore a worldwide insurance policy. Thus, Shapiro quotes Mauricio Bellon of the International Maize and Wheat Improvement Center (CCMMYT), the world's foremost public research facility for corn: "The diversity of these land races, these genes, is the basis of our food supply.... We need this diversity to cope with the unpredictable.... The climate changes, new plant diseases and pests continue to evolve. Diseases we thought we had controlled come back. We don't know what's going to happen in the future, and so we need to keep our options open." The likely contaminate was probably Bt corn, as developed by Monsanto, which contains a bacterial gene causing the corn to produce its own insecticide against the corn borer. Another major Monsanto product is Roundup Ready soybean seed, which contains a bacterial gene making the plant resistant to Monsanto's herbicide Roundup. And so on, illustrating the emerging vastness of the agrichemical industry and its bio-technology (biotech), or biological engineering (BE). Shapiro supplies the estimates that, at this writing, some 34% of our corn, 75% of our soy, 70% of our cotton, and 15% of our canola are now genetically engineered, which is compromising the purity of organic farming. Moreover, many European countries refuse to import genetically altered crops, which therefore reduces demand, as a result of which there are calls for subsidies, which subsequently affects the U.S. taxpayer. Also, GE crops are resulting in resistant diseases and insects, and are not showing any greater yields. (In this latter connection, the word is that GE salmon interbreed with the native species, with the resulting hybrids showing a higher mortality rate. The inference is that GE could cause the extinction of a species.)

The subject merges with that of selective breeding, where the technical adjective for "breeding-true" is *homozygous*, with the converse described as *heterozygous*. And if selective breeding can produce "favorable" characteristics, it can also produce "unfavorable" characteristics. Extended to humans, famed biologist and Nobel lau-reate Peter Medawar declared that the objectives of "positive" eugenics can never be attained (Medawar, 1990, p. 108). "Human diversity is one of the facts of life, and the human genetic system does not lend itself to improvement by selective inbreeding." May we extend the analogy to crops and other animal life, where it is noted that the hybrids and the mongrels are the "fittest" ?

Apart from this, there was the previously cited article in the October 12, 2003, issue of the *New York Times* by Michael Pollan that traces current concerns about obesity to the overproduction of grains, notably corn. Corn is abundant and cheap, a staple for use directly as a food or in foods, and its conversion to sweetener adds myriad uses, carbonated drinks being the obvious example.

Another facet of the arguments about the ubiquity of corn usage has to do with corn-derived ethanol production and the latter's use as a supplemental motor fuel. Thus, syndicated columnist Michelle Malkin addressed ethanol as the other energy scandal (the oblique reference is to the Enron debacle), in her column on or about September 4, 2002. Malkin starts off by mentioning that agricultural conglomerate Archer Daniels Midland owns 41% of U.S. ethanol production capacity, and that 98% of the nation's ethanol plants are located in the farm belt, with the political ramifications seemingly obvious.

Features of the 2002 energy bill will require that gasoline refiners triple ethanol use in motor fuel by 2012 and thereafter, irregardless of the consequences. However, a little-publicized memo from the Office of Management and Budget noted that the president's Council of Economic Advisors and the Federal Trade Commission viewed the ethanol mandate as "costly to both consumers and the government and will provide little environmental benefit." The resulting increase in gasoline costs for ethanol blends would predictably be at least 3 to 5 cents per gallon, even 7 cents per gallon in New York, and in California nearly 10 cents per gallon. Not only this, but Cornell University agricultural researcher David Pimentel, who had chaired a Department of Energy panel commissioned to investigate energy production, performed a net energy analysis for ethanol production, with the following conclusion. About 70% more energy is required to produce ethanol than the energy that is actually in ethanol. Furthermore, "Abusing our precious croplands to grow corn for an energy-inefficient process that yields low-grade automobile fuel is unsustainable, subsidized food burning." As for environmental "benefits," the National Academy of Sciences also sees otherwise; namely, that there is little improvement in ozone air quality, and, although ethanol can reduce carbon monoxide emissions, this is offset by increased emissions of volatile organic compounds (VOCs) plus nitrous oxide, the usual precursors of smog.

Still another angle is provided by the western corn rootworm beetle, the species *Diabrotica virgifera virgifera* of the family Chrysomelidae. Originally attacking members of the plant family Cucurbitaceae, such as gourds and pumpkins, it has turned to corn and has become an ubiquitous pest in the Corn Belt of America's Midwest, destroying up to 80% of the crop in some places and costing up to an estimated 1 billion dollars per year in production losses. Moreover, it has been spreading to Western Europe, being first discovered in Serbia in 1992, with findings near airports in Italy and Switzerland, and may already be in France's great grain-raising area southwest of Paris, near Beauce. The subject has been given play in the *World Press Review*, December 2002, which reprinted an article by Hervé Morin that had appeared in *Le Monde*, published in Paris, September 26, 2002. Experiments using biological agents have so far proved ineffective, including the use of phero-mones and cheromones, with others such as natural predators in the offing. (This is always a gamble, for the unleashing of natural predators from foreign sources may have undesirable or fatal consequences for indigenous flora and fauna.) Which gets around again to GE, or genetic modification (GM), as it is also called. Whether this approach will be pursued remains to be seen, given the present European moratorium on genetically modified organisms.

The foregoing matters bring up the point that the corn crop in the United States for the most part comprises a monoculture, and increasingly (or pervasively) consists of genetically modified subspecies. This may conceivably make the corn crop more receptive to attack by the western corn rootworm beetle, or still other unexpected pests. In other words, there is the need, or make it a necessity, for diverse species or subspecies rather than having a uniform monoculture. It is the old saw about not putting all of one's eggs in one basket.

Although "science" seemingly assures us that all obstacles can be overcome, the emerging exceptions continue to confound the experts, one after another. It is as if Nature remains a contrarian, in the end able to thwart the best-laid plans of mice and men.

A notable instance is a situation exposed by the Union of Concerned Scientists. The case that has been cited concerns genetic engineering of a common soil bacterium named *Klebsiella planticola*. Developed by a German biotech company, the modified bacterium would successfully break down and rot wood chips, corn stalks, and other wastes from lumbering and agriculture, at the same time producing ethanol, which could be used as a fuel additive, as in gasohol. The rotted wastes in turn would serve to enrich soil. However, in tests conducted at Oregon State University, when the rotted wastes were added to soil, the seeds subsequently planted would sprout but then die. It turned out that the genetically modified bacterium countered the mycorrhizal fungi occurring naturally in the soil, which are vital to plant growth. The apocalyptic concerns were about the genetically modified bacteria persisting in the soil and eventually eradicating all plant growth. Thus we encounter another scenario with unexpected consequences. And if the genetically modified bacterium has this effect on one particular microorganism, what effect might it have on the millions of other microorganisms? Not to mention what unanticipated effects current and future genetically modified microorganisms might have on the global entirety of microorganisms ... and all other organisms.

## VACCINATION AND CANCER

Problems that occur with vaccinations constitute the principal thrust of books authored or edited by Robert S. Mendelsohn, M.D., as previously noted. The subject is also covered in Michael L. Culbert's comprehensive exposé titled *Medical Armageddon Update 2000: Behind the Healthcare Calamity of the Whole World and How to Fix It*. (Although Culbert doesn't get around to health maintenance organizations [HMOs] as such, he gets around to about everything else, including medical and health insurance, which he labels "a good idea gone wrong.") With regard to cancer cures and the lack thereof, apropos of medical orthodoxy, no punches are pulled in the pages of commentary furnished in *An Alternative Medicine Definitive Guide to Cancer*.

An update on the more conventional vaccinations requires mention of the vaccine preservative used — sodium ethyl mercury thiosalicylate, better known as thimerosal. The very presence of toxic mercury in routine childhood vaccinations raises a warning flag, and there are indications that this may be related to a marked increase of autism in children, especially in boys. The subject was explored in considerable depth, for instance, by Bette Hileman in the February 23, 2004 issue of *Chemical & Engineering News*, a weekly publication of the American Chemical Society. The pros and cons emerge occasionally as issues carried in the major media, although not very often, being for the most part carried in other sources.

Thus, according to a November 1998 newsletter from Johns Hopkins University Medical School, in addition to the neurotoxin thimerosal, flu vaccines are found to contain the preservative formaldehyde, a known cancer-causing agent, and also aluminum (or its compounds), and can be associated with an increase in Alzheimer's disease. In the serious influenza epidemic occurring circa January 2000, a large percentage of the elderly who had had the flu shots also contracted the disease. For instance, a nursing home in Toronto reported 32 cases of the flu, out of which 31 had been vaccinated the month before.

And from *Jane Russell's Health Facts* (www.jrussellshealth.com), information is cited as retrieved from Hugh Fudenberg, M.D., described as the world's leading immunologist (credited with some 850 papers or articles). Thus, if a person had five consecutive flu shots between 1970 and 1980 (being the interval studied), the chances of coming down with Alzheimer's disease were 10 times greater than for unvaccinated persons. This is attributed to a gradual buildup of mercury and aluminum in the brain.

Further information is furnished in *The Sanctity of Human Blood: Vaccination I$ not Immunization*, by Tim O'Shea (2004). It is noted that the flu virus constantly mutates, even over a single season. The vaccine, derived from a particular mutant form of the virus at a point in time, will be less effective, or no longer effective, by the time it is administered. Moreover, the sicker the person and the greater the number of persons affected, the faster the virus mutates, a phenomenon called *gene amplification*. What follows is a guessing game for the vaccine manufacturers, in trying to predict and match what mutant virus form will emerge for the next flu season, which is yet months away. In retrospect, there was the swine flu fiasco in 1976, a consequence being the paralysis of 565 infants with Guillain-Barre syndrome. A government scientist was fired for blowing the whistle and stating that there was really no persuasive evidence about a forthcoming swine flu epidemic and, moreover, that the vaccine had dangerous side effects.

An added note is that flu shots translate to a very big business — so, just follow the money.

The December 1999 issue of the *Townsend Letter for Doctors & Patients* contains articles bridging the connection between vaccinations and cancer. That is to say, vaccines carry viruses, some intended and some as contaminants. There is a poignant contribution by Raphaele Moreau-Horwin and Michael Horwin titled "Link between Increasing Rate of Pediatric Cancers and Childhood Vaccines" which connects cancer to viruses, and especially as pertains to childhood (mandatory) vaccinations. This is followed by an article titled "Vaccine Scene 1999: Overview and Update" by Harold E. Buttram, M.D. In particular, the work of W.J. Martin who is with the National Cancer Institute is cited, including the role of the African Green Monkey and the "stealth virus." Also, a voice from the past, an article containing some of

George Bernard Shaw's comments about vaccines, particularly the Pasteur treatment, which emphasizes that not everyone bitten by a rabid animal contracts rabies. (Nevertheless, who wants to play the odds? Further, the rabies virus may lie dormant, with the disease only showing up later, or many years later, as pointed out by Colin Kaplan et al., 1986, in *Rabies: The Facts.*)

Having mentioned routine vaccines, a letter by James A. Howenstine, M.D., in the February/March 2004 issue of the *Townsend Letter for Doctors & Patients* merits special note. He cites an astute observation made by Indiana physician Dr. W.B. Clarke back in the early 1900s: "Cancer was practically unknown until compulsory vaccination with cowpox vaccine began to be introduced. I have had to deal with two hundred cases of cancer, and I never saw a case of cancer in an unvaccinated person." Dr. Howenstine further mentions viral contamination from the very animals used to produce the vaccines. Thus, the Salk polio vaccine had some viruses that could not be eradicated, including the simian SV40 virus, a known cause of malignancies. (The vaccine had already been given to more than 10 million persons before the discovery of contamination.) Yellow fever vaccine, for instance, had been found to be contaminated with avian (bird) leukemia virus. More than this, mass immunization exhausts most of the immature immune cells from the thymus gland, thus compromising natural immunity.

(For more about viruses, and cancer and viruses, Part VII of Hoffman, 1999 discusses these aspects.)

Lastly, it may be mentioned that there is a treatise-size book published in 1999 by Little, Brown with the title *The River: A Journey to the Source of HIV and AIDS.* The author Edward Hooper makes a convincing case for the impact of simian viruses that have invaded such live-virus vaccines as the Sabin vaccine. Massive vaccination programs of this sort have the potential of infecting everyone with stray viruses, and may already have, with unknown consequences.

A comprehensive volume about the contamination of polio vaccine by the monkey virus SV40 and other viruses is by Debbie Bookchin and Jim Schumaker, titled *The Virus and the Vaccine: Contaminated Vaccine, Deadly Cancers, and Government Neglect*, published in 2004. Some of the highlights of this controversy are as follows.

Both the Salk and the Sabin vaccines have been, and are, derived from the ground-up kidneys of monkeys, usually rhesus monkeys but also from African green monkeys. Both have been found to carry the simian virus 40, SV40, as well as other viruses, the latter mostly as yet unknown. In the case of the Salk "killed" vaccine, the addition of formaldehyde or formalin was supposed to kill all viruses, including SV40, but the immolation proved not to be 100% effective (Bookchin and Schumacher, 2004, p. 86ff). In the case of the Sabin "live" oral vaccine, an antiserum agent had been developed that was supposed to kill any stray virus, including SV40 but also another called the vacuolating agent (Bookchin and Schumacher, 2004, pp. 76, 86, 87, 113). Sometimes called neutralization, the process was not totally effective (Bookchin and Schumacher, 2004, p. 271).

It may be noted that SV40 is a DNA virus, whereas most viruses contain only RNA (Bookchin and Schumacher, 2004, pp. 111, 116). Moreover, SV40 is also characterized as a polyoma virus, a classification found in other animals, even humans (Bookchin and Schumacher, 2004, p. 148).

More specifically, it may be commented in passing that an enzyme involved in the formation of cancerous cells via viruses is DNA-dependent RNA polymerase, also called DNA-directed RNA polymerase (Hoffman, 1999, p. 189). On the other hand, what are called retroviruses have notably been implicated in cancer and immunodeficiency diseases. The enzyme involved here is called reverse transcriptase, or RNA-dependent DNA polymerase (or RNA-directed DNA polymerase).

Further complicating the picture is the fact that viruses may have many different strains (Bookchin and Schumacher, 2004, p. 179). Thus, poliovirus has a few disease-causing strains but dozens more that are harmless, the implication being that SV40 may have different variants. It was found, moreover, that the skin of the SV40 virus contains three proteins, one of which regulates growth, the other two causing tumors (Bookchin and Schumacher, 2004, p. 205). The latter two proteins are labeled antigens, the one the larger T-antigen, the other the smaller t-antigen. However, the body has "brakes" for the activities of these proteins, notably the tumor suppressor genes called *p53* and the Rb genes. However, SV40 can block *p53* and Rb genes and can allow the telomeres to elongate, permitting cells to divide endlessly (Bookchin and Schumacher, 2004, p. 209). The comment has been made that "it is one of the most potent carcinogens that we know." Accordingly, there have been attempts to disable SV40 (Bookchin and Schumacher, 2004, p. 130).

Among the findings are the following: SV40 is a precursor or cause of the deadly cancers known as mesotheliomas, and still other cancers, even leukemia (Bookchin and Schumacher, 2004, pp. 140, 187, 192, 227, passim). Mesotheliomas occur in the lining that surrounds lungs, heart, and abdominal cavity, and are ordinarily associated with asbestos as the cause.

This cancer-causing action of SV40 was the center of much controversy between agencies of the U.S. government and the researchers involved, who had the viewpoint that SV40 occurred from laboratory contamination, and still other researchers who held the opposite view, that the SV40 was innate, or naturally occurring. The book goes into great detail about these controversies. Names are supplied, and among the names of the latter group are Bernice Eddy, Michele Carbone (originally from Italy), Harvey Pass, Robert Garcia, Janet Butel, and John Lednicky, as well as vocal opponents Hilary Koprowski and Leonard Haflick.

In Chapter 20, titled "Alexander's Tumor," a tragic case study is presented about a brain tumor in a young child that was linked to SV40, it being found in the tumor. The traditional chemotherapy treatments were unbearable, and the child died in his mother's arms.

In conclusion, the traditional viewpoint is that these polio vaccines were effective in stopping polio. The side effects are still moot, because epidemiological studies of only a few years are too short, for cancer can take many, many years to develop. The final chapter speaks of the conflicts among profits, safety, and best practices, with further mention of researcher Hilary Koprowski, who is experimenting with plants as a substrate to eliminate the risk of foreign animal viruses.

However, there is nevertheless some impressive work going on in the medical research establishment as per the series on cancer appearing in the aforecited November 7, 1997, issue of *Science*, as per Chapter 5.

One particular highlight, furnished in the series of news items and articles, involves the disabling of the tumor suppressor gene designated *p53*, which prevents viral DNA replication. Oddly enough, the inactivation is by means of a human respiratory virus called *adenovirus*, by removing the viral gene that disables *p53*. The reasoning was that the virus would selectively infect only cells in which the *p53* was nonfunctionals, that is, cancer cells. Clinical trials are encouraging, but the virus has to be injected directly into the tumor; if injected into the bloodstream, the immune system destroys the virus. The use will therefore be of limited value for cancers that have metastasization.

## TELOMERASE INHIBITORS

In further comment, the fact that the presence of the enzyme telomerase has been observed to be associated with tumors at least suggests a means for treating cancer, by utilizing inhibitors for telomerase. (The enzyme telomerase is not routinely available for experimentation, however, nor has it yet entered the handbooks that list known enzyme inhibitors.) Similar remarks apply to the enzyme tyrosinase, which is associated with melanoma, as indicated elsewhere. There is a likelihood, even, that the inhibition of reverse transcriptase (or RNA-directed DNA polymerase) could act against cancer, as well as retroviruses such as HIV (the AIDS virus), and the Ebola and Marburg viruses. (A number of inhibitors are listed in the handbooks of enzyme inhibitors for RNA-directed DNA polymerase, including such antibiotics as actinomycin, some of which are undoubtedly toxic.) These are, of course, speculative.

(In work under way at the Whitehead Institute for Biomedical Research in Boston by researcher Matthew Meyerson, a gene called human Ever Shorter Telomeres 2, or hEST2, has been found responsible for making a component of telomerase. Thus, it may very well be a key agent that switches on uncontrolled cellular growth.)

Very possibly, however, inhibitors for the previously mentioned enzymes may exist in the plant world, as distinguished from synthetic chemicals. And among these plant substances there will perhaps be some that do not have toxic or adverse side effects.

A significant development underway is by Nobel laureate Tom Cech and coworkers at the University of Colorado. A protein designated POT1 has been found to attach itself to the end of chromosomes and thereby keep telomerase away from the tips so that cancer cannot develop. Observed with mice, it is a long way to clinical confirmation in humans. (In comment, POT1 can be called an inhibitor for telomerase.)

## HISTONE DIACETYLASE INHIBITORS

Another recent development is the use of a histone diacetylase inhibitor (designated FK228), which is said to not add or delete DNA, but rather to normalize the existing DNA. The work has been carried out at the National Cancer Institute, and is described in the May 2004 issue of *Life Extension* in an article by Terri Mitchell. Still another treatment described in the article is the use of a methylation enzyme inhibitor. (The particular enzyme is also known as methyltransferase.)

With regard to using a histone dicetylase inhibitor for lymphoma treatment, a contact at the NCI is Robin Frye, RN, at (302) 402-5958, and is available at many cancer centers in the United States. A contact for treating thyroid cancer with histone diacetylase inhibitors has been reported to be Deborah Draper, RN, BSN, at (301) 435-8525.

## MARKERS FOR MONITORING CANCER GROWTH AND REMISSION

A section called "Cancer Markers" was furnished in Chapter 5, which emphasized the references by David Sidransky and others that appeared in the November 7, 1997, issue of *Science*. The references cited were more at the DNA level, however, but here the continuing and vital concern is the use of more prosaic markers to monitor the initiation, progress, and remission of cancer. Some are in routine use, such as prostate-specific antigen (PSA) for prostate cancer, and white blood cell count for leukemia.

Another more down-to-earth angle is that an insulin or glycogen imbalance may be a marker for cancer. Even such common measurements as blood pressure, pulse, and body temperature may influence cancer progression or regression, and their monitoring benefits from developments in modern technology. (Among the very latest may be skin- or palm-derived measurements for these and other body imbalances, as mentioned elsewhere. Beyond this possibility is work on spit, or saliva, tests as an indicator for cancer and other diseases, as per the work of Dr. David Wong, associate dean of the UCLA School of Dentistry.)

A newer angle is presented in an article by Mitch Jacoby in the March 29, 2004, issue of *Chemical and Engineering News*, a weekly publication of the American Chemical Society. Titled "Breath Analysis for Medical Diagnosis," many volatile organic chemicals carried in a person's breath are associated with a particular disease. These chemicals may be present only in extremely minute or picomolar-level concentrations. The challenge is to routinely and accurately analyze and correlate the breath chemistry to the disease.

It is certainly preferable that the means sought for monitoring the course of cancer be on a near-instantaneous basis, which translates to a near-continuous basis, if so needed.

## MORAL AND ETHICAL QUANDARIES

Finally, there are the ethical or moral ramifications, for it can be discerned that cancer is the disease of main concern in the arguments over euthanasia and assisted suicide. The situation is spelled out by Brian Eads in "A License to Kill," which appeared in the September, 1997, issue of the *Reader's Digest*. Eads' article pertains for the most part to the practice of euthanasia as it currently exists in the Netherlands (the naming of this country now seems prescient). Another reference is Wesley J. Smith's *Culture of Death: The Assault on Medical Ethics in America*, published in 2000.

Other information was furnished in *Seduced by Death: Doctors, Patients, and the Dutch Cure*, by Herbert Hendin, M.D., published in 1998. An update, a collection of essays edited by Kathleen Foley, M.D. and Herbert Hendin, is *The Case Against Assisted Suicide: For the Right to End-Of-Life Care*, published in 2002. The arguments do not address whether killing is wrong, but rather that legalization of assisted suicide would have an effect opposite to what its supporters claim. In other words, it would cause more suffering, give the patient less control, corrupt the practice of medicine, and decrease palliative care. Some of the contributors in particular speak of the prevalence of depression in the terminally ill, and note that it is eminently treatable. Treatment would counteract the terrible fear of abandonment, and it is noted that assisted suicide is "abandonment institutionalized." In this regard, it was noted in Hendin's book that Holland's legalization has been accompanied by the worst palliative care facilities in Europe. And in the United States., in Oregon, where assisted suicide has been legalized, there is now a "culture of silence."

This foregoing represents the collision between reason, that is, intellectualism, or ideology, and Biblical authority, that is, morality, or religion.

# 10 The Inhibition of Cancerous Stem Cells

## THE SUBJECT OF STEM CELLS AND CANCER

Consider an article that appeared under the heading of "Science Journal in the Marketplace" in the February 27, 2004, issue of the *Wall Street Journal*. It highlights an ongoing breakthrough in cancer research by Sharon Begley titled "'Stem Cells in Tumors May Help Explain Some Cancer Mysteries." The work described experiments from the 1950s concerning the injection of various cancer cell masses back into the patient (or into mice). It was found that another cancerous mass would result only if a sufficient number of cells were injected, may be a million or more.

The effect was ultimately thought to be due to the presence of a relatively small number of a particular kind of active cell, denoted as a *stem cell*. For the record, the *Academic Press Dictionary of Science and Technology* defines a stem cell as "a cell, capable of both indefinite proliferation and differentiation into specialized cells, that serves as a continuous source of new cells for such tissues as blood and testes." Cancer biologist Robert Weinberg of the Whitehead Institute, Cambridge, Massachusetts, and discoverer of the first human oncogene, is quoted in the article as follows. "Within a tumor mass, there is only a small population of cells that can spawn more tumor; other cells in the tumor cannot."

This selective behavior helps explain why anticancer drugs or treatments sometimes work and sometimes do not. Thus, with regard to specific drugs, the article notes that, "although Iressa® shrinks non-small-cell lung cancers, Erbitux® shrinks advanced colon cancers and the recently approved Avastin® shrinks metastatic colorectal cancer. In each case, in only some patients, the drugs prolong survival by mere months or sometimes not at all." As Dr. Weinberg has observed, "killing off the majority of cells in a tumor will still leave it with the ability to regenerate another tumor from these stem cells." A similar observation by University of Toronto molecular biologist John Dick is that non-stem cells "may result in a remission," but a relapse will occur "if the tumor-initiating cells are not eliminated."

Further information about Avastin and Erbitux was furnished by Ralph W. Moss in his monthly column "The War on Cancer" in the May 2004 issue of *The Townsend Letter for Doctors & Patients*. He mentions that the FDA approved Avastin (bevacizumab) in February 2004 for the treatment of advanced colorectal cancer. It will compete with Erbitux, which was also recently approved for advanced cases of this disease. Avastin, being an antiangiogenesis agent, works against the creation of blood vessels in the cancer mass, the treatment protocol consisting of intravenous drug administration along with IFL (also called the *Saltz regimen*). The acronym IFL stands for the combination of the already approved drugs irinotecan (Camptosar®

or CPT-11), 5-fluorouracil or 5-FU, and leucovorin. However, in random, double-blind clinical tests on 800 patients, the average survival time was 20.3 months for the treatment vs. 15.6 months for IFL alone, an increase of only 4.7 months. (And in either case, there is never a mention of a cure, and the baseline for no treatment whatsoever is not included. There is also no mention of alternative treatments.) Moss lists some of the side effects of the treatment, according to the Web site of the manufacturer (Genentech), which include gastrointestinal perforation and wound dehiscence (rupture of an organ or surgical wound), in some instances resulting in a fatality. In the treatment of small-cell lung cancer using chemotherapy and Avastin, hemoptysis has occurred (this being the expectoration of blood or blood-streaked sputum). High blood pressure as well as congestive heart failure may also occur. Still other side effects as listed by Moss include kidney damage, weakness, abdominal pain, headache, diarrhea, nausea, vomiting, anorexia, mouth sores, constipation, upper respiratory infection, nosebleeds, breathing difficulty, peeling skin, and protein loss in the urine.

(Moss also describes the financial and societal implications, for sales may reach perhaps $2 billion or more per year, with treatment costs set at about $4,400 per month or $44,000 for an expected survival time, which is more than the yearly income of the average American household. The effect of such rates on the insurance costs, particularly if treatment of the side effects is included, could be far-reaching. As a point of reference, Moss lists some of the alternative treatments against cancer angiogenesis as supplied by Boik [2001]: anthocyanidins and proanthocyanidins, the herb butcher's broom, horse chestnut, vitamins A and D3, anticopper compounds [e.g., alpha-lipoic acid], green tea catechins [e.g., EGCG or epigallocatechin-3-gallate], and resveratrol [as found in red wine]. But there are no substantiating clinical tests, as medical orthodoxy will quickly point out.)

Other landmarks in arriving at the previously mentioned conclusions about cancerous stem cells were furnished by Stanford biologist Irving Weissman and his colleagues, who in 1987 identified blood-forming stem cells in mice. Later, in 2003, a team of University of Michigan biologists led by Michael Clarke and Muhammad Al-Hajj discovered that breast cancer was composed of a relatively few cancer-initiating cells that presumably functioned interminably and were, in turn, surrounded by a multitude of non-cancer-initiating cells. Moreover, injection of the cancerous stem cells will always produce a tumor, whereas injection of the other cancer cells will not. In addition to breast cancer stem cells, brain cancer stem cells have been found, with the probability that such cancerous stem cells occur in other kinds of tumors.

A conclusion to be formed is that non-stem cancerous cells do not pose a very great danger, as they die off after a few divisions. Of more significance is the fact that standard chemotherapy practices do not interfere with the metabolism and proliferation of the cancerous stem cells, although they kill off non-stem cancerous cells.

Another conclusion reached is that metabolic or molecular pathways as uncovered for non-stem cancerous cells may prove inconsequential. The problem is that of discovering or distinguishing the metabolic pathways of the cancerous stem cells. We will attempt to take a closer look at these.

Regarding the phenomenon of bacterial infections building up a resistance to antibiotics, there is the consideration that certain bacteria are more resistant than others and they tend to survive and somehow build up immunity, proliferating in the meantime. There is the idea that this represents a kind of probability manifestation. That is, given a population of bacterial specimens, some will be more vigorous and resistant than the others, a sort of *survival of the fittest*, the fittest being those that survive. The next question is a method to selectively kill all of these strains. For bacteria, maybe another antibiotic may be advisable, at the necessary and sufficient dosage levels and frequency.

With cancer cells, we are talking of cells, or at least some cancer cells, that build up a resistance to conventional chemotherapy. These cells can be viewed as cancerous stem cells as described previously.

It should again be emphasized that thousands of National Cancer Institute (NCI)-sponsored tests utilizing plant substances or extracts against cancer suffer from the disadvantage that what works on cancer lines in the test tube or in an animal does not necessarily apply to clinical trials on humans. (Also, most of these substances do not work *in vitro* or *in vivo*, anyway.) As mentioned before, there may be thousands of ways to cure cancer in mice, but they need not work on humans. Moreover, medical folklore is sufficiently unreliable to be discounted, for the most part.

Furthermore, as mentioned earlier, most cancer cells are not of great consequence. It is the select populations, the cancerous stem cells, which proliferate uncontrollably. Accordingly, we are interested in distinguishing the metabolism of the cancerous stem cells from that of the ordinary cancerous cells (both of which differ from normal cells). In normal cells, the overall metabolism or conversion, or glycolysis of glucose or blood sugar is to carbon dioxide and water. In cancerous cells, mostly the ordinary cancerous cells, the overall conversion is to lactic acid or lactate, notably involving the enzyme called *lactate dehydrogenase*. Substances that inhibit this enzyme can be viewed as acting against cancer, at least against "normal" cancer cells. A number of these anticancer plants or plant substances occur in medical folklore, as indicated in previous chapters, such as certain sulfur compounds found in garlic or derived from garlic, etc.

On the other hand, if the metabolic pathway is different for the controlling cancerous stem cells, then different enzymes will be involved, calling for different enzyme inhibitors. An examination of the literature via the Internet (Google.com), Medline, and WorldCat so far reveals but few discernible patterns of findings in this area of metabolic pathways, of the critical enzymes involved, and of enzyme inhibitors selective for cancerous stem cells. The literature is highly technical and diffuse, with much ado about many things, but the specific information required is mostly not available.

A word or two is in order about the controversy over utilizing embryonic stem cells for research, including finding a cure for cancer. Thus, a qualification is that the adult stem cells are a known, potential alternative to embryonic stem cells. (And adult stem cells can be taken from the patient, whereas embryonic stem cells are not. For the latter, enter the complication and necessity of immunosuppression.) With regard to cancer per se, there is the idea that cancerous stem cells could be used for the exploratory research, assuming that they can be suitably isolated and proliferated. At the same time, there is a hope that a cure for cancer would emerge, based on blocking the metabolism of these cancerous stem cells. This will lead again to the subject of the critical enzyme or enzymes involved, as well as the enzyme inhibitors.

The article "Improved *Ex Vivo* Expansion of Functional CD⁺ Cells Using Stem-line™ II Hematopoietic Stem Cell Expansion Medium" by Allison et al. appeared in the Summer 2004 issue of the *Life Science Quarterly*, a publication of Sigma-Aldrich, St. Louis, MO. The term *hematopoietic* pertains to the formation of blood cells, and the article leads off by observing that hematopoietic stem cells (HSC) have the unique ability to differentiate variously into erythroid (pertaining to red blood), lymphoid (pertaining to blood plasma), and myeloid (pertaining to bone marrow) cell lineages. Consequently, it is noted that HSCs can be used as therapeutic agents against both malignant and benign diseases of the blood-forming and immune systems. Furthermore, HSCs can be isolated from three sources: umbilical cord blood (CB), bone marrow, and mobilized peripheral blood. At present, CB is regarded as the preferred source, being more disease resistant.

The problem is, the volume or number of CB cells is limited, as each umbilical cord has only enough cells to transplant into a small child. The thrust of the article, therefore, is the development of a method to proliferate or expand the number of CB cells by providing an appropriate medium. (The stem cells are designated *CD34⁺ cells*, as they are available not only from CB but also from bone marrow and peripheral blood.) The animals involved in the testing were denoted as *immunodeficient NOS/SCID mice* (where NOS/SCID pertains to nonobese diabetic/severe combined immunodeficient), and further denoted as the recipients of transplanted human CB cells, expanded (or proliferated) by the procedures described in the article.

The procedures were judged successful. The application of these procedures will be to greatly increase the number of stem cells available for clinical research and treatment.

## CANCEROUS STEM CELLS AND IMMUNITY

We take a brief look at the second edition of Voet and Voet's *Biochemistry*, published in 1990, 1995, in regard to immunity. Certain types of white blood cells (WBCs) called *lymphocytes* arise from common precursor cells (or stem cells) in the bone marrow (Voet and Voet, 1995, p. 1207). Obviously, the use of the term *stem cells* has been generalized to include other kinds and sources of cells. From there, things can get very complicated indeed, as per a discussion of antibodies and an immune system cancer called *myeloma*, as cited elsewhere (Voet and Voet, 1995, p. 74). It is stated in this reference that although antibody-producing cells usually die off after a few divisions, they can nevertheless be cloned to yield a single species of antibody in large amounts, henceforth designated as *monoclonal antibodies*. The cloning process involves the fusion of a cell that produces the desired antibodies with a cell of the immune system or one from the myelomatous tumor mass. "The resulting hybridoma cell has an unlimited capacity to divide, and when raised in cell culture, produces a large quantity of the monoclonal antibody."

The foregoing circumstance may or may not prove analogous to the initiation and proliferation of cancerous stem cells. Nevertheless, we choose to examine the technical complexities as furnished and described, for the record, in Figure 34.22 and on pages 1214 and 1215 of the aforecited reference. Developed by Cesar Milstein and Georges Kohler, monoclonal antibodies can be used to isolate and assay for small amounts of almost any biological substance, even in routine blood testing for HIV (AIDS virus). The caption for the cited figure pertains to producing monoclonal antibodies against an antigen designated X in a so-called *HAT medium*. (The acronym HAT stands for hypoxanthine, amethopterin, and thymidine, where amethopterin is also called *methotrexate*, which is an antifolate used against cancer but with devastating side effects.)

This HAT medium acts to block the growth of mutant cell lines lacking the enzyme hypoxanthine-guanine phosphoribosyl transferase. Labeled HGPRT, this is called a *purine salvage enzyme* that ordinarily catalyzes the formation of the AMP (adenosine monophosphate), GMP (guanosine monophosphate), and the precursor IMP (inosine monophosphate), all involved variously in metabolic processes. In short, the HAT medium serves as an inhibitor for the enzyme HGPRT. Further information supplied in the figure caption about the very complicated sequence involved is as follows:

> The amethopterin blocks the *de novo* synthesis of purines, which *HGPRT⁻* cells cannot replace through salvage pathways. Thymine, whose synthesis is also inhibited by the amethopterin, is available from the HAT medium. *HGPRT⁻* myeloma cells are fused with spleen-derived lymphocytes from a mouse immunized against X, and the resultant preparation is transferred to a HAT medium. This treatment is selective for fused cells (hybridomas): The *HGPRT⁻* myeloma cells cannot grow in HAT medium; lymphocytes that make HGPRT do not grow in culture; but the hybridoma cells that have the lymphocytes' HGPRT and the hybridoma cells' immortality, proliferate. Individual hybridoma cells are then cloned and screened for the production of anti-X antibody. A satisfactory clone can be grown in virtually unlimited quantities, either in culture or as a mouse tumor, so as to synthesize the desired amounts of monoclonal antibody.

If there is indeed some sort of a connection between the uninhibited growth of cancerous stem cells, then the application against the proliferation should be the inverse of the foregoing process. Thus, for a start, the HAT medium might be expected to act against stem cell proliferation. And, of course, amethopterin or methotrexate itself is considered an anticancer agent, although a highly toxic one (Hoffman, 1999a, p. 32). Nevertheless, the door is left open that other anticancer agents might serve by inhibiting the metabolism of the cancerous stem cells, as well as the anaerobic glycolysis of ordinary non-stem cancerous cells.

However, given that cancerous stem cells might have the same metabolism or metabolic pathways as other cancerous cells, and assuming that metastasis of cancer cell colonies to other locations is not a consideration here, there is the possibility of developing an immunity or immune response by the more active cancerous stem cells.

In further comment, apropos of bacterial infections building up a resistance to antibiotics, as mentioned previously, there is the parallel consideration for cancer cells in avoiding resistance to treatment. Thus, with cancer cells, we are talking of anticancer agents, mainly chemotherapeutic agents, that can be viewed as antigens and that may trigger a kind of immune response by the so-called cancerous stem cells.

Continuing along these lines, and citing the references in Voet and Voet (1995, Section 34.2), on immunity, it is noted that the myeloma proteins "are produced by cancer cells that originally proliferated in response to unknown, if any, antigens" (p. 1216). The reference further speaks of haptens that bind to particular myeloma proteins, creating hapten–myeloma complexes. A hapten is a small molecule having certain antigenic properties and can combine with an antibody, but by itself is not immunogenic. In turn, these antibody–hapten complexes resemble enzyme–substrate complexes.

As a further note, Stanford University has created an Institute for Cancer/Stem Cell Biology and Medicine. To ensure that the institute will be multidisciplinary in nature, it will be directed by Irving Weissman, M.D., whose work is prominently mentioned elsewhere, and who is the Karel H. and Avarice N. Beekhuis Professor in Cancer Biology. More about this line of investigation was described back in the November 1, 2001, issue of *Nature* in an article by Reya, Morrison, Clarke, and Weissman titled "Stem Cells, Cancer, and Cancer Stem Cells." The property of self-renewal is emphasized, signaling pathways involving a transformation of normal stem cells producing tumors and may also include cancer stem cells with an indefinite potential for driving tumorigenesis. An institute for stem cell research has been set up in New Jersey that is state-initiated and state-supported.

## INHIBITION OF CANCEROUS STEM CELLS

Depending on the category or search item, a survey of the Internet and the database Medline over the past year or so on stem cell research can yield hits ranging into the thousands, even tens of thousands. This may, of course, be markedly reduced by restricting the search to using appropriate keywords. For the record, a few items found of more than ordinary interest are described in the following text.

An article by Kendall Powell, appearing as a nature science update at news@nature.com, December 30, 2002, notes that stem cells and cancer cells have something in common, namely, a shared protein that serves to patrol cell proliferation. The shared protein is called *nucleostemin*, and several researchers such as Robert Tsai and Ronald McKay of the National Institute of Neurological Disorders and Stroke in Bethesda, Maryland, and Julia Polak, director of Tissue Engineering and Regenerative Medicine Centre, Imperial College, London, are cited in the context. It was found that the protein nucleostemin occurs prominently in self-renewing cells, for example, in embryonic and neural stem cells of mouse and in several human cancer cell lines. On the other hand, the protein hardly occurs in mature cells that no longer divide. It was also found in laboratory tests that decreasing nucleostemin levels in neural stem cells and cancerlike cells would reduce their proliferation. Another finding was that nucleostemin binds with the protein p53, a regulator of cell proliferation that is impacted in many cancers.

## TYROSINE KINASE

There is the implication that the enzyme tyrosine kinase is prominently involved in the initiation and growth of cancerous stem cells. Accordingly, we shall take a closer look at this enzyme.

In brief, enzymes are proteinaceous substances that catalyze biochemical reactions, and kinases constitute a subclass of the enzymes classified as *transferases*, which transfer functional groups. In turn, a kinase can be described as a phosphoryl-transfer enzyme utilizing ATP (adenosine triphosphate) or described as transferring a phosphate group from a nucleoside triphosphate to another molecule, according to the *Academic Press Dictionary of Science and Technology*. (Examples of some kinases and their actions occur in Figure 3.1 therein.)

In general, there are protein kinases and, in particular, there are tyrosine kinases; tyrosine is a nonessential amino acid present in most proteins and is synthesized metabolically from the essential amino acid phenylalanine. It is also said to be a precursor of thyroid hormones, melanin, and catecholamines. Not only is there more than one tyrosine kinase, but mutations can also occur.

A kinase is also defined as a substance that causes a zymogen to change into an enzyme, where a zymogen is further defined circuitously as a substance that will change into an enzyme, according to the *Random House Dictionary of the English Language*. They are also called *proenzymes* (or proteolytic enzymes), and include proteases, and are generally referred to as *proproteins* (Murray et al., 1996, p. 101). Zymogens are also called *relatively inactive precursors* to enzymes (Voet and Voet, 1995, p. 398). Therefore, we can consider that the tyrosine itself is transformed into an enzyme by the action of tyrosine kinase. Questions arise as to the type of enzyme and its purpose.

(Thus, we again mention proteases, the protein-digesting enzymes, as they have been cited contrarily both as cancer-inhibiting agents [recall enzyme therapy], as in Hasselberger, 1978, on page 146, and in other references as cancer-inducing agents, with protease inhibitors being of prime concern.)

Tyrosine is a (crystalline) amino acid with the formula $HOC_6H_4CH_2CH(NH_2)$ COOH. It results from the hydrolysis of proteins, that is, the reaction of proteins with water. The $-C_6H_4-$ group within the compound denotes a ring-type structure. Another definition provided is that tyrosine is found in most proteins and can be synthesized metabolically from phenylalanine. Furthermore, tyrosine is a precursor for thyroid hormones, melanin (the dark pigment of body parts, notably, the skin), and catecholamines (that affect the sympathetic nervous system).

(Phenylalanine is one of the 10 essential amino acids that must be obtained from outside the body, as distinguished from the 11 nonessential amino acids that occur naturally within the body, including tyrosine. Exclusive of the nonessential amino acid hydroxyproline, both sets comprise 20 common amino acids that are found in all proteins, and they conform with, or are derived from, the common genetic code. It may be further noted that a large array of alkaloids are derived from phenylalanine and tyrosine, according to Cordell's *Introduction to Alkaloids*, as presented by Hoffman (1999, p. 145).

Tyrosine kinase is the enzyme that catalyzes the transfer of a phosphoro group (or phosphate group) from ATP to tyrosine, according to the *Academic Press Dictionary of Science and Technology*. Apart from this short definition, the biochemical action of this enzyme is further described (Voet and Voet, 1995, p. 1280ff). The *receptor tyrosine kinases* (RTKs) are substances that mediate cell growth and differentiation. This involves binding with protein growth factors, which are proteins that cause their specific target cells to grow and/or differentiate (Voet and Voet, 1995, p. 268). Cell differentiation is the process by which two identical cells (with the same genome or gene complement) will somehow proceed along two different development pathways (Voet and Voet, 1995, p. 1168ff). Therein lies "the genetic basis of cancer, a group of diseases that have lost some of their developmental constraints."

Malignant cells are said to produce growth factors by a process called *autocrine secretion*, and several peptides have been found to be involved (Hoffman, 1999, p. 64). It is noted that tyrosine kinase favors autocrine activity, but it is also noted that (unspecified) inhibitors do exist.

As per the foregoing, the action of tyrosine kinase can be said to be that of transforming tyrosine into an enzyme that contains the phosphate group, presumably for the following purposes.

Insights are furnished about RTK inhibition of cancer in an article by Tsu-Tsair Chi in the August/September issue of the *Townsend Letter for Doctors & Patients*. This is mainly by angiogenesis, which was addressed in Chapter 6. To briefly recapitulate, the article noted that when tumors reach a certain size (approximately 2 mm in diameter), growth factors or proteins are released in overwhelming amounts into nearby tissues, thus initiating angiogenesis. "The growth factors subsequently bind to their RTKs within endothelial cells in the blood cells." The dormant endothelial cells ("endothelial" pertains to the internal cavities of the body) are activated, divide, and migrate towards the diseased tumorous or cancerous cells. The result is a network of new blood vessels.

The distinction between RTKs and tyrosine kinases per se, and their respective actions, and those between "normal" cancer cells and cancerous stem cells, would seem to be a "gray" area. Both involve malignancies, but the question remains: why does one kind of cell appear to be more refractory or resistant to treatment than the other?

An acronym that repeatedly occurs in searching Medline for the biochemistry of stem cells, for instance, is "KIT" or "kit," or "c-kit." According to the *On-Line Medical Dictionary*, this is "An oncogene, identified in feline sarcoma, encoding a tyrosine protein kinase that acts on the stem cell factor." Thus, there reemerges the subject of the enzyme tyrosine kinase, in this case being more than merely an enzyme, but classified as an oncogene. It may be added that the standard sources for enzyme inhibitors, now dated (e.g., Jain, 1982, Zollner, 1993), do not include the enzyme tyrosine kinase as such. (However, it may be mentioned that the extended series *The Enzymes*, published by Academic Press, is now up to 23 volumes at the time of this writing.)

Thus, the title of a highly technical journal article by Hochhaus et al., appearing in the September 2001 issue of *Onkologie*, published in Switzerland, is translated as "Selective Inhibition of Tyrosine Kinases — A New Therapeutic Principle in Oncology". The abstract of the article states the tyrosine kinases are enzymes that regulate mitosis, differentiation, migration, neovascularization, and apoptosis, or cell death. In the technical shorthand employed, for the record, it is further mentioned that chronic myelogenous leukemia (CML) would be an ideal target that utilizes a selective inhibitor for what is called BCR-AML tyrosine kinase (AML standing for acute myelocytic leukemia). The 2-phenylpyrimidine derivative designated *ST1571* was designed to function as inhibitors via competitive ATP-binding pocket interactions. (The acronym ATP stands for adenosine triphosphate.) It is further noted that there are protein tyrosine kinases with ATP-binding pockets structurally similar to ABL (defined as a proto-oncogene that is translocated in CML). Examples of such protein tyrosine kinases are designated *c-kit* and *PDGF-R* (where PDGF stands for platelet-derived growth factor). It is also mentioned that the gastric gastrointestinal stromal tumor (GIST) cells will overexpress the stem cell factor receptor designated as *CD-117*, which is the product of the proto-oncogene c-kit.

Significantly, it was found that the *in vivo* inhibition of c-kit produced an immediate metabolic change in the tumor cells. Further studies are under way against lung cancer cell lines, and clinical studies are being conducted against malignancies such as high-grade gliomas, prostate cancers, and leukemias.

A conclusion offered in the reference states: "The development of selective tyrosine kinase inhibitors is considered a promising approach for the design of new drugs."

An article of special note by Majid Ali, M.D., appeared in the November 2004 issue of the *Townsend Letter for Doctors & Patients*, titled "Cancer, Oxygen, and Pantotropha — Part 1." In further explanation, regarding the title, *Thiosphaera pantotropha* is called a metabolic two-timer, an aerobic/anaerobic bacterium that converts sulfur compounds such as sulfides and thiosulfates (hence the moniker "thio" for sulfur-containing) that occur in sewage. When oxygen is available, this is the oxidative source; when not available, an inorganic compound serves as the oxygen source, for example, nitric acid.

A cancer cell is also described by Dr. Ali as a metabolic two-timer, but with the difference that it (merely) survives in the presence of oxygen, but proliferates in its absence. The presence of oxygen denotes an aerobic condition, and its absence denotes an anaerobic or fermentative condition. Whereas Dr. Ali is in full agreement with the Warburg theory of cancer metabolism, he diverges with Warburg's viewpoint that cancer is irreversible.

(Warburg's Nobel Prize in Medicine, awarded in 1931, for his discovery of oxygen-transferring enzymes is again duly acknowledged. Furthermore, a second Nobel Prize was awarded 13 years later for Warburg's delineation of hydrogen-transferring enzymes, but he was prevented from receiving the award by the Hitler regime because he was Jewish.)

The question posed by Dr. Ali is whether an oxidative condition can be incurred such that the cancer cell will relinquish its anaerobic propensities. The aerobic condition is designated as *respiratory*, the anaerobic condition as *fermentative*, so that the object is to negate the cell's respiratory-to-fermentative (RTF) shift or propensity and to promote the fermentative-to-respiratory (FTR) shift. It is further noted that Warburg's theory about anaerobic cancer cell metabolism initiated much interest in offsetting oxygen therapeutics, both direct oxygenative treatments (e.g., nasal oxygen and oxygen baths) and indirect bio-oxidative treatments (intravenous infusions of ozone and hydrogen peroxide).

Accordingly, Dr. Ali speaks in terms of oxygen homeostasis (or metabolic constancy) and of an oxidative-dysoxygenative (OD) model for cancer (dysoxygenative pertains to an abnormal oxidative condition). This model can be used to explain such phenomena as the long-term quiescence in tumors, spontaneous regressions, and explosive growth, as induced by environmental, viral, and genetic factors.

All things said, Dr. Ali sees a limited future for conventional chemotherapeutic drugs, but much potential for "antibodies directed against signaling molecules that sustain and perpetuate malignant cell replication." For the record, a listing of chemo drugs is reproduced as follows: (1) imatinib (Gleevec®, a protein-tyrosine kinase inhibitor) for BCR-AML tyrosine kinase, (2) gefitinib (Iressa®, an inhibitor of intracellular phosphorylation of several tyrosine kinases), which binds the epidermal growth factor, (3) trastuzumab (Herceptin®, a DNA-derived humanized monoclonal antibody), which binds with the extracellular domain of the epidermal growth factor receptor 2 protein (HER2), (4) rituximab (Rituxin®, a chimeric murine(mouse)/human monoclonal antibody), which binds to CD20 antigens, (5) Avastin®, which targets angiogenesis, and others not mentioned.

In less technical terms, the following statement was made with regard to achieving and maintaining oxygen homeostasis. "The benefits of soy and other phytofactors, with or without therapies that modify specific molecular and genetic pathways, are often substantial in the sense that such therapies can alter the behavior of cancer cells for variable periods of time until oxystatic therapies begin to take hold."

Dr. Guy B. Faguet is particularly keen on imatinib mesylate, or Gleevec, against CML and is an advocate of the more fundamental gene therapy rather than the cell-toxic chemotherapy (e.g., Faguet, 2005, p. 46). He also notes it to be an inhibitor for tyrosine kinase. Interestingly, he skips the Warburg theory about cancer metabolism vs. normal cell metabolism and of enzymes and enzyme inhibitors.

Having mentioned soy again, a referral is made to a lengthy article appearing in the same November 2004 issue of the *Townsend Letter for Doctors & Patients*. By Vijaya Nair, M.D., and titled "Soy and Cancer Survivors: Dietary Supplementation with Fermented Soy Nutraceutical, Haelan 951 in Patients Who Survived Terminal Cancers," tyrosine kinase inhibition is not specifically cited, but components elsewhere identified with this particular inhibiting action are prominently included.

First, a distinction is made between the two categories of soy foods consumed, the nonfermented and the fermented. Traditional nonfermented soy foods include the following: fresh green soybeans, whole-dry soybeans, soy nuts, soy sprouts, whole-fat soy flour, soymilk and soymilk products, tofu, okara, and yuba. Traditional fermented soy foods include the following: tempe, miso, soy sauces, natto, and fermented tofu and soymilk products. In Asia, the fermented products are considered to have greater health benefits, presumably owing to the increased availability of isoflavones.

A study of miso found a particular rich mix of *isoflavone aglycones*, notably genestein and daidzein, both known to be anticancer agents derived from their isoflavone precursors, genestin and daidzin.

(We recall the biochemical, or phytochemical, or plant chemical called genestein, which is cited as an inhibitor for tyrosine kinase, as will be emphasized in the following section. Although we will not dwell on the chemical makeup of assorted compounds and classes of compounds, a few explanatory words are in order. Thus, the complex chemical intricacies and subtleties are that isoflavones are plant estrogens or phytoestrogens, which are heterocyclic phenols containing the –OH group and resemble estrogenic steroids. A steroid, in turn, has a "cyclopentanoperhydrophenanthrene" nucleus, whereas the nonsugar part of a glycoside is an aglycone. An aglycone is a glycoside, in full circle, being a sugar bonded to something that is not a sugar.)

The article states that health-conscious Americans, especially women concerned about breast cancer, are urged by media and consumer reports to consume (nonfermented) soy or soy proteins. However, this is not the form or forms traditionally consumed in Asian countries like Japan, China, Korea, and Indonesia. These countries use the cultured or probiotic form, that is, the fermented form, obtained from living things, like yeast, which is enhanced with genestein and daidzein. Furthermore, it has been found that cultures of *Saccharomyces cerevisiae*, or brewer's yeast, have a pronounced bio-antimutagenic and anticlastogenic activity ("clastogenic" refers to a breakup or disruption, e.g., of chromosomes). Thus, when this particular yeast source is used for the fermentation process, the cultured soy medium or product is reinforced in its anticancer activity.

(It is mentioned that in 1989, the NCI funded a $20 million 5-year program to investigate the role of common foods, including soybeans, in cancer prevention. This was supplemented in 1990 by $2.9 million for soy alone. The NCI published its report in the April 1991 issue of the *National Journal of Cancer* as "Commentary: The Role of Soy Products in Reducing Cancer Risks.")

The anticancer activity of soy is attributed to nutrients and micronutrients, broadly classified as isoflavones, protease inhibitors, saponins, phytosterols, and phytic (plant) acid compounds, as commonly reported in other references. Dr. Nair is more specific in describing the components of *Haelan 951*, a fermented soy product that has been available on the U.S. market for the past 12 years (and is a sequel to Haelan 851). The patented fermentation process involves the hydrolysis of soybean proteins into amino acids and other compounds rich in nitrogen and polysaccharides. It also includes the fermentation metabolites of isoflavones, protease inhibitors, saponins, phytosterols, and inositol hexaphosphate compounds that occur naturally in soybeans. The inoculum is described as an autogenic antiammonia azotobacter strain induced from *Azotobacter vinelandii* ("autogenic" signifies self-generating, and the prefix "azo-" pertains to the –N=N– group). The resulting product is said to contain soybean proteins, selenium, zinc, beta-carotene (vitamin A), riboflavin (vitamin B1), thiamine (vitamin B2), cyanocobalamin (vitamin B12), ascorbate (vitamin C), cholecalciferol (vitamin D3), alpha-tocopherol (vitamin E), and phylloquinone (vitamin K). Additionally, there are the micronutrients daidzein, genestein, protease inhibitors, saponins, phytosterols, inositol hexaphosphate, and essential fatty acids such as linolenic and linoleic acids, polysaccharide peptides, and 20 of the 22 amino acids, including ornithine. (It takes 25 lb of soybeans to make 8 oz of the Haelan 951 beverage.) Overall, the product is said to have antiviral, antibacterial, anti-inflammatory, antimutagenic, and anticarcinogenic activities.

(The so-called 20 common amino acids involved in synthesized proteins, as per the genetic code, do not include the dietary proteins ornithine and hydroxyproline, or such others as may occur.)

There are three fermented soy beverages available in the United States: EcoNugenics, Soy Unique, and Haelan. Haelan is marketed by Haelan 951 Products Inc., based in Seattle, but is manufactured in China. Based on the analyses, previously mentioned, it was decided to use this product in clinical trials, and the results were submitted to the NCI's Best Case Series Program. The results of seven cases are reported in the article, all with favorable, indeed, most favorable results. The tumor types treated were listed as follows, with the case scenarios detailed in the reference: (1) Infiltrating ductal carcinoma of the breast; (2) infiltrating ductal carcinoma with history of lymphatic spread, metastases to skin, lungs, bronchi, pericardium, and bones; (3) poorly differentiated adenocarcinoma of the gallbladder; (4) myeloproliferative disorder; (5) follicular lymphoma, grade 2; (6) prostate cancer, and (7) infiltrating adenocarcinoma of the prostate.

It is added by Dr. Nair that eight out of ten cancer patients now use some form of complementary and alternative medicine (CAM), mostly in conjunction with conventional medical treatments. (This, in comment, should supposedly lead to a significant decrease in cancer-related deaths.) Moreover, the use of Haelan 951 can apparently serve as an adjuvant in conjunction with conventional chemotherapy. Whereas thousands of patients in the United States, Europe, and Asia have been taking Haelan 951 as an adjunct or stand-alone treatment for cancer, most of the clinical trials have been conducted at medical and research institutions in China. More such clinical research is called for in the United States. (This is most likely, given the prevailing mind-set of the medical establishment. However, the creation of cancer clinical research centers [CCRCs] would fulfill this need, as described elsewhere.)

## PLANT SOURCES FOR TYROSINE KINASE INHIBITORS

A journal article of special interest by F. Hollósy and G. Kéri of the Hungarian Academy of Sciences is titled "Plant-Derived Protein *Tyrosine Kinase Inhibitors* as Anticancer Agents." Appearing in the March 2004 issue of *Current Medicinal Chemistry,* and published in the Netherlands, the article states that the protein tyrosine kinase is prominent in the regulation of cell growth, cell differentiation, and cell death. Thus, the interest lies in discovering sources for tyrosine kinase inhibitors, notably from the plant world. Specific screening techniques have uncovered structurally distinct inhibitors, for example, phenylpropanes, chalcones, flavonoids, coumarins, styrenes, quinines, and terpenes. There is the possibility that analogs that enhance the anticancer activity can be synthesized. (It may be added that several of these foregoing classes of chemical compounds have previously been found to have anticancer activity, and are so listed in the literature, and herein.)

Plant sources for several classes of compounds are presented in *Infraspecific Chemical Taxa of Medicinal Plants* by Péter Tétény and in Hoffman (1999, Chapter 3 and p. 116ff). The subject is Chemical Taxonomy, as per the title of Hoffman's Chapter 3, and information is tabulated in part in Appendix T of Hoffman (1999), as derived from Tétény. With further regard to Hoffman (1999), the aforementioned categories appear as follows: phenylpropanes (p. 495), flavonoids, (p. 496), coumarins, (p. 495ff), and terpenes, (p. 483ff). Chalcones (and flavones) are lipophilic (fat-soluble) compounds sometimes used as insecticides and fish poisons (Hoffman, 1999, p. 121). Flavones may be considered as a subclass of flavonoids; the flavonoids are described as aromatic oxygen-bearing heterocyclic compounds (aromaticity signifying the benzene ring structure).

Styrene is itself a (synthetic) cyclic hydrocarbon composed of a benzene ring with an unsaturated appendage, but may be projected to phenyl-type compounds. (Styrene is sometimes called *cinnamene*, there being an interesting parallel with cinnamon, e.g., the genus *Cinnamomum* of the family Lauraceae, which is classified under both terpenes and phenylpropanes [Hoffman, 1999, pp. 487, 495]. Quinines are alkaloids of the genus *Chinchona* of the family Rubiaceae [Hoffman, 1999, p. 502]. These categories present a wider enumeration of bioactive plant species as presented variously in Hoffman (1999).

As for flavones, or isoflavones, mentioned previously, the prefix "iso-" signifies a similarity or, more exactly, the same chemical composition but a different structure, with different physical and chemical properties. According to a letter and literature search presented by Sally Fallon and Mary G. Enig in the July 2004 *Townsend Letter for Doctors & Patients*, cited elsewhere, the soy isoflavone genistein has been found to act as an inhibitor for tyrosine kinase. However, it has also been found to damage the DNA and to have adverse estrogen-like effects. Apparently, there is a trade-off.

The subject of chemical taxonomy is briefly addressed in *Key Environments: Amazonia*, edited by Ghillean T. Prance and Thomas E. Lovejoy. In a chapter on "The Chemical Uses and Chemical Geography of Amazon Plants," written by Otto R. Gottlieb, such matters as arrow poisons, hallucinogens, and fish poisons are taken up. In a section on drugs, it is mentioned that *Rauwolfia* species (of the family Apocynaceae), with useful hypotensive alkaloids, seems never to have been used by the indigenous population. On the other hand, discoveries by modern scientific investigations, some patented, include *Pilocarpus jaborandi* (Rutaceae) containing the now widely used pilocarpine and *Ocotea glaziovii* (Lauraceae) containing glaziovine, an ansiolytic ("-lytic" pertains to lysis, the breaking open of a cell membrane).

*Tabebuia* species (of the family Bignoniaceae) contain lapachol, an anticancer agent.

Drugs used by traditional native healers include *Cephaelis ipecacuanha* (Rubiceae), containing the emetic emitine; *Chenopodium ambrosioides* (Chenopodiaceae), containing the vermifuge called *ascaridole*; *Dialyanthera otoba* (Myristicaceae), containing the fungicide otobain; *Quassia amara* (Simaroubaceae), containing quassin, used against stomach complaints; *Carpotroche brasiliensis* (Flacourtiaceae), with esters of glycerol and hydnocarpic acid once used against leprosy; *Stachytarpheta australis* (Verbenaceae), containing ipolamide, used as an antithermic and sudorific (sweat-inducing) agent; and *Calea pinnatifida* (Asteraceae), containing polyacetylene and a germacranolide, used as an amoebicide.

Also, *Maytenus illicifolia* (family Celastraceae) contains the antitumor agent pristimerin.

It may be added that the chemistry of plant biochemicals is every bit as interesting as that of synthetic biochemicals. The biochemicals that occur in each plant or plant extract are myriad in number, with some having more pronounced bioactivity than others. For an indication of the possibilities, one may consult James Duke's *Handbook of Phytochemical Constituents of GRAS Herbs and Other Economic Plants* (the acronym GRAS means "generally recommended as safe").

In general, stem cell inhibitors should ideally be specific to cancerous stem cells and should not affect vital stem cell proliferation by the blood cells.

# 11 A Summing Up

Generally speaking, the investigations regarding cancer occur at two levels. One may be categorized as more of nonclinical research per se, that is, laboratory studies about cancer in all its aspects, particularly at the molecular and genetic levels. The other may be classified as clinical research, that is, the effect of various treatment protocols on the actual patient. From all this, hopefully, a best, or most successful, treatment protocol or protocols will emerge, to be put into routine practice.

With regard to these levels, we attempt a further assessment of the cancer situation, as it now exists. However, a survey of Internet entries, the array of articles and books concerning the many interrelated subject categories (cancer and cancer therapy), health, medicine, alternative and complementary medicine (CAM), etc., produces an overwhelming flow of information that is almost self-defeating. The sources that we have cited (relatively a few) are viewed as the more prominent and reliable assessments. (And the information supplied by these sources is ample.) The inference is that, from all these sources, there should be some sort of consensus that at least a few, and maybe more, treatments or therapies constitute surefire cures for cancer. The fact that clinical substantiation has not been forthcoming is reason enough for medical orthodoxy to remain skeptical, if not hostile, to CAM. On the other hand, CAM remains skeptical about the underlying reasons for opposition by medical orthodoxy.

For starters, the indications are that we have inherited a valuable legacy of potential anticancer agents within the plant world. A vast array of medicinal plants has already been compiled, many of which contain substances that can potentially be of use. More substances are being uncovered. Both folklore and science have provided leads in these efforts. Alkaloids are a notable possibility (for example, the work once undertaken in Japan using hyoscyamine), but there are other possibilities, both inorganic and organic. The biochemical therapy theories are, for the most part, already in place, being in part the beneficial effects of foreign substances or antigens on the immune system and the action of enzymes, enzyme inhibitors, or promoters.

A particular difficulty is that apparently no one has ever bothered to figure out the optimum dosage levels and frequencies for plant-derived anticancer substances, in addition to, and in conjunction with, the purity and activity of the agent, which perforce includes composition. As it is, a plant or plant-derived substance or other substances are too often classified as toxic or nontoxic, poisonous or nonpoisonous, mostly with no in-betweens. This in-between, or gray, area may prove to be the window of opportunity.

A ready means of monitoring dosage, frequency, and activity of the cancer indicators is sorely needed, for example, in cancer cell presence and cancer cell proliferation. This is in conjunction with monitoring the patient's vital signs. In other words, a simple, effective, and a mostly noninvasive way is required for monitoring all the human process variables while a course of treatment is pursued. In this manner, the treatment can be tailored to the individual patient; not too much or too little and not too frequently or infrequently. It is the age-old ritual of trial-and-error approaches, the empirical means for closing in on the answer or the solution. Admittedly, some degree of this kind of testing is already in use with regard to conventional cancer therapies. But more, better, and quicker modalities of testing are demanded, preferably near-instantaneous. There is the necessity that this sort of monitoring be routinely applied to conventional as well as unconventional cancer therapies. In fact, it may be the only way to decide whether the treatment is working, and whether the patient is on the road to recovery.

The presence of cancer cells in blood serum may be indicated by the Ames test, which may or may not correlate closely enough to the growth or remission of solid tumors. X-rays and other electromagnetic devices (such as CAT [computerized axial tomography] scans and NMRs [nuclear magnetic resonance]) can, of course, provide a periodic indication of the progress of solid tumors, though a succession of tests can be debilitating. Vital signs such as pulse, blood pressure, and body temperature can be determined on the spot, whereas other analyses like the SMAC-17 blood test take longer. What is now needed is a quick, noninvasive, and exact method to tell whether the cancer mass is growing or receding at any given moment, and on a daily basis if not by the hour, minute, or second. This leads to the question: what further wonders might electronics come up with, combined with ultrasound or radio frequency waves and correlated to tumor behavior or size? It would then be possible to clinically chart the course of anticancer agents on a particular patient at any given time.

Continuing this line of thought, a skin test might be devised to indicate the presence or absence of cancer, in ways similar to an allergy test. That is, in an allergy test, the suspected allergens may cause a reddening of the skin, a so-called allergic reaction or response. There is the possibility that cancer cells might cause a similar allergic response, including a reddening of the skin. (In fact, there is progress in using the palm of the hand, as an indicator for various internal phenomena, as well as using spit or saliva as an indicator.)

Moreover, in this way, it might prove possible to test the effectiveness of a spectrum of anticancer agents on the individual patient merely by a skin test. That is, in this instance, the more effective anticancer agents might alleviate the reddening of the skin, if any, caused by the cancer cells.

By analogy, an allergic patient, for instance, can be given successive injections of the particular allergen or allergens causing the allergic response, which serve to counteract the allergy. The allergens so administered evidently act as antigens that stimulate the immune system, which in turn produces antibodies, as in immunotherapy. In other words, immunity is built up. This method is similar to immunization by vaccination.

The analogy can potentially be extended to cancer treatment, whereby successive injections or medicinal dosages of the anticancer agent or agents might either stimulate the immune system or act as enzyme inhibitors, or both. Increasingly, these procedures merge with the branch called *homeopathy*, though the word is an unmentionable in some circles of medical orthodoxy.

(There is the notion that cancer cells may, in fact, be generated all the time, only that they are kept in check by the action of the immune system. The counterargument is that cancer cells imitate normal cells such that the immune system cannot distinguish one from the other. The resolution awaits, and presumably will be tied in with the role of the major histocompatibility complex [MHC], as previously discussed.)

It is to be kept in mind, however, that at this point the foregoing is merely speculation, but may be worthy of further investigation. Considering all the effort that has gone into counteracting allergies, it is a wonder the analogy has not been given equal time in the case of cancer. Although there have been limited efforts toward developing cancer vaccines, they are mostly autovaccines derived from the biochemical makeup of the individual patient. Examples are Burton's Immuno-Augmentive Therapy (IAT) and the Livingston Therapy, as previously indicated. In the mainstream, this work has been discounted, in spite of some reported successes.

It is instructive to note that homeopathy is, in the broader sense, the administration of minute or trace amounts of any substance that will presumably stimulate the immune system or serve as an enzyme inhibitor or promoter. In the more restricted (and discounted) sense, it is presumably the administration of an agent that, in some way or another, bears a resemblance to the disease, the questionable doctrine of "signatures." This restrictive definition is as distinguished from traditional Western medicine, the practice of allopathy, and the administration of drugs or medicines that are different from the disease.

There are some renowned exceptions in the practice of allopathy, however, in conquering such viral diseases as polio and rabies. Here, immunity or cure is effected directly or indirectly, that is, by introducing minute amounts of the (killed or even live) virus into the patient; the patient's immune system then proceeds to develop antibodies against the disease. Alternately, the virus may be injected into an animal whose system develops antibodies, with the consequent serum injected into the patient. So, in full circle, there is evidence that allopathy merges with homeopathy sometimes, or vice versa, for the benefit of humankind.

A key, therefore, can most certainly be perceived as the use of minute or trace amounts of the bioactive agent. In other words, the objective is to destroy the disease without destroying the patient. The use of myriad bioactive plants and plant extracts can be perceived in the same manner. There is no doubt that some plant-derived substances can selectively act against cancer, yet are nontoxic to the patient, if administered in trace or minute (or required) amounts and with the necessary frequency. In fact, the same substances that, in larger amounts, cause cancer may be most effective. The reason or theory behind this apparent contradiction merits further investigation. It may turn out to have a striking similarity to the development and use of viral vaccines for immunization. As the causes of cancer are seen as virus-related or operating at the DNA level, the cancer itself is sometimes called an *immunodeficiency disease.*

(Inasmuch as cancer may be referred to as an immunodeficiency disease, so are many or most other diseases. This means that if the immune system were working at the optimum, a person would not get the disease in the first place, by definition. And there is the viewpoint that if antibiotics will not cure it, you are in for some major trouble.)

This line of investigation can be extrapolated to AIDS and to the retroviruses such as the Ebola and Warburg viruses, viruses yet unknown, or yet to be formed (or undergo mutations). In this context, we are not only talking about cancer but of all other kinds of virus-related diseases.

These kinds of plant-derived bioactive substances should therefore be tested for both general and specific antiviral activity and anticancer activity, a direction of medical research still in its infancy. Alkaloids may perhaps be the most prominent bioactive plant substances, as has been indicated, but there are no doubt others.

The same remarks can be extended to fungi and the substances derived from them, including alkaloids.

In terms of biologically active or bioactive substances, we return to the matter of degree, for most everything consumed or administered internally is bioactive, not to mention body substances such as hormones. There are, of course, the different foods and their myriad component compounds, including the vitamins and minerals, both natural and supplemental. Also included are medicinal-type substances taken in small or minute dosages in order not to be toxic, which is a back-handed way of saying that most medicinal substances are poisonous in larger doses.

Thus, we must confront the reluctance of medical orthodoxy to consider substances or drugs that are not synthesized in some kind of commercial operation, utilizing the technical expertise of the pharmaceutical industry. For everything, natural or synthetic, will ultimately have to be explained in the terms of high science. Everything, sooner or later, takes on the cast of modern scientific theory. Consider, for instance, Cordell's *Introduction to Alkaloids* (1981), which proceeds to discuss the chemistry of alkaloids that mostly occur naturally in plants and herbs. It is a technical work of the highest order, which not only describes plant sources, but provides routes for synthesis and production of many of the natural alkaloids.

The inference emerges, therefore, that much or most of this plant-based information lies in the public domain and cannot be patented or held proprietary by a drug or a pharmaceutical company. This is where the financial world intersects the natural world. This has been explained, for instance, by Ralph Moss and Clarence Mullins, as has been mentioned elsewhere. Hence, we may conclude that there is a large body of work that has not been further utilized because it is unprofitable. In other words, we may suspect that there are already broad-spectrum cures for cancer "out there," but no further studies or trials have been made because there is no profit at the end of the tunnel. It is suggested, therefore, that this nonproprietary domain should be a concern of the U.S. government through the support and activities of the National Institutes of Health (NIH), the National Cancer Institute (NCI), the Food and Drug Administration (FDA), or yet other agencies of the government.

The collusions that have been going on behind the scene are a suitable topic for investigation by Congress, assuming that the members of Congress are not beholden to the drug industry, which is a pretty broad assumption. The subject may be better addressed through the courts, for example, through class action lawsuits. The media can, of course, be an ally, but then the media also have their own marching orders.

Add to the complications the fact that the sequence of drug research, development, demonstration, and commercialization is partially paralyzed in the United States by the high costs incurred and the inordinate time period required to prove drug efficacy. All of this, as repeatedly acknowledged, demands that the drug be patentable in order to show a reasonable return on investment. It is this vicious cycle that must somehow be broken. It may be that new government agencies will have to be created or old ones recast, with the government playing either a greater or a lesser role.

We repeat that cancer clinical research centers (CCRCs) should be established in major cities and in not-so-major cities. These would be clinics that depart from the orthodox treatments of surgery, radiation, and conventional chemotherapy. These centers should be staffed not only by M.D. and D.O. physicians, but supported by biochemists, microbiologists, molecular biologists, pharmacists, pharmacologists, or ethnopharmacologists. The expertise of botanists and ethnobotanists should be drawn upon, as well as of herbalists and homeopaths, and other sorts of nontraditional specialists. Moreover, the operation should be made independent of the American Medical Association (AMA) and its dominions and membership, who are irrevocably tied to medical orthodoxy and its mind-set and limitations. It can be further advanced that the terms *oncologist* and *oncology* should be avoided like the plague, as these evil-sounding words have the ring of failure or of death.

Also consider excluding from the circle, such bastions of medical orthodoxy as the Memorial Sloan-Kettering Cancer Center (MSKCC), the M.D. Anderson Hospital in Houston, and maybe even the Mayo Clinic. Let them go their own way, as they have done and continue to do, with surgery, radiation, conventional chemotherapy, and such other avenues of their choosing. The last thing needed is negativism and obstructionism toward anything outside the domain of established medical orthodoxy.

There is the reminder of the energy crisis around the 1970s, which paralleled the War on Cancer. The government-sponsored and government-funded synthetic fuels program was to produce gaseous and liquid fuels from coal. After spending billions of dollars, and creating and funding the U.S. Department of Energy along the way, no new commercially viable industry has emerged as yet. Lots of studies, lots of people employed, lots of big names, but no commercial industry, as the required economics are not there. This, it seems, has been the progress of the War on Cancer. (An exception, of course, was the Manhattan Project during World War II, which took a period of about 4 years and an expenditure of about $4 billion to come up with the atomic bomb.)

The raising of funds for cancer research has in itself been a subject of controversy, with the role of a number of organizations being suspect. The ACS seems to be held in particular public esteem, its actions above reproach. But about these acclamations, Richard Walters' remarks in his book *Options: The Alternative Cancer Therapy Book* (1993), bear repeating, " ... the ACS collects around $400 million a year from the unenlightened American public, then spends less than 30% of this huge cash hoard on research. No major breakthrough in treating cancer has ever resulted from an ACS grant. ... Most of its money goes into fat salaries and other nonresearch expenses like land, buildings, and bank accounts (its 'fund balance' in 1988 was $426 million)." Walters also quotes from Dr. James Bennett, an economist from George Mason University, who did an exposé on health charities and made the statement that the ACS's lack of emphasis on research "... borders on dishonesty."

Moreover, Bennett stated that "it also fits perfectly with the highly politicized agendas of today's health charities."

Ralph Moss is an alumnus of the MSKCC. He had some pungent things to say about the cancer research business in his books (e.g., in *The Cancer Industry, Cancer Therapy, Questioning Chemotherapy*). Moss, being at one time on the Sloan-Kettering staff, has first-hand knowledge of its inner workings, but was fired when he disagreed with the official line that the anticancer drug laetrile was ineffective, whereas some research sponsored by MSKCC showed otherwise.

For more on such specific agencies and organizations as the NCI, ACS, and still other well-known institutions, the reader can consult *The Politics of Cancer Revisited*, published in 1998, by Samuel S. Epstein, M.D., of the University of Illinois Medical Center at Chicago. An encapsulation of some of Dr. Epstein's findings is therefore repeated in the following text.

The NCI was created in 1937 under the National Cancer Act, and became part of the National Institutes of Health (NIH) in 1944, but was provided semiautonomous status in the 1971 National Cancer Act (Epstein, 1998a, p. 200ff). The NCI Directors are appointed by the president as well as a three-member National Council Advisory Panel. Epstein supplies information about conflicts of interest and industrial ties that have existed with some of the board members, particularly on environmental carcinogens.

In Chapter 16, Epstein takes on the ACS, which he describes as the "world's wealthiest nonprofit institution." Epstein further states that, in 1988, with a fund balance of over $400 million, plus $69 million more in real estate and equipment holdings, the ACS spent $90 million, or only 26% of its budget, on medical research and programs. The rest of the budget covered "operating expenses," with about 60% for salaries, pensions, benefits, and overhead. The very next year, the cash reserves had increased to over $700 million. In 1992, *The Chronicle of Philosophy* stated that the ACS was "more interested in accumulating wealth than saving lives." By 1998, the ACS budget had increased to $380 million with cash reserves approaching 1 billion dollars. The American Cancer Society Foundation was created in order to allow larger contributions, and the composition of the foundation's board is further proof of influences of the pharmaceutical, investment, banking, and media industries.

The MSKCC, considered the nation's most prestigious cancer research and treatment center, is said to have close ties with the pharmaceutical industry, and Epstein provides some names and affiliations for MSKCC board members (Epstein, 1998a, pp. 494, 495).

Another prestigious institution, the University of Texas M.D. Anderson Cancer Center has been taken to task for claiming that "well over 50% of people with cancer who are cared for at the Center return home cured" (Epstein, 1998a, p. 475). This is as compared to other findings, for instance, about chemotherapy, which is described as merely a placebo for most patients, although the use of the so-called *Vinca* alkaloids (derived from the Madagascar periwinkle, *Catharanthus roseus*) have been successful in stopping blood-related cancers.)

A further word emerging from the medical underground is that some hospitals will not take on terminal cancer patients, as their deaths would impinge upon success statistics.

A step in the right direction, heretofore cited, comprises a grant by the NIH to find people who attribute their recovery from cancer to a macrobiotic diet. Their recovery must be documented by medical records, pathology reports, or other sources of substantiation. The survey is being conducted by The Kushi Institute, a macro-biotics center at Beckett, Massachusetts, and by the University of Minnesota School of Public Health. Michio Kushi, incidentally, is regarded as the leading proponent of macrobiotics and founded the Kushi Institute. The person to contact is Mercedes Gallagher at the Kushi Institute, 1-413-623-5741. However, the results have not yet been publicized.

Another step in the right direction, which has also been discussed earlier, is the *Cornell-Oxford-China Study*, or *The China Project*, which is directed at finding connections between diet and disease, with the inference that a plant-based diet is preventive. An estimate noted is that between 80 to 90% of all cancers, cardiovascular diseases, and other degenerative illnesses can be offset until old age, with the qualifier that the "normal" processes of aging are not so normal after all.

It may be added that there is a similarity between the latter investigative efforts and the "chemoprevention" program within the NCI. Maybe, at long last, there is a meeting of minds.

In fact, the entire cancer scene should be entered (objectively) into a computer data bank for analysis. This includes the type of cancer, the treatment or therapy, the successes, the failures, the life extensions, and all other variables or parameters of interest, not only for conventional treatments as obtained from the NCI and ACS, but especially for alternatives. (In this regard, the M.D. Anderson Cancer Center in Houston has made a stab at compiling such information.)

Finally, consider that it may be necessary (and sufficient) to settle only for a stalemate or standoff against the invading cancer. This would involve holding the cancer in check or remission without seeking an absolute cure, with the prospect of gradually conquering the adversary. This, in a way, is in line with the idea that some cancerous cells are always present in the body, in one way or another, including cancerous stem cells. But a healthy immune system keeps these cells under control and does not allow them to proliferate. It is also in line with the long-term proposition that the treatment may be slow-acting and long-term, as has been evidenced using megadoses of (intravenous) vitamin C, as per the Riordan clinic at Wichita, Kansas (Center for the Improvement of Human Functioning International [CIHFI], 3100 North Hillside Avenue, Wichita, KS 67219, 316-682-3100), or the practice of A. Hoffer, M.D., Ph.D., in Vancouver, BC (2717 Quadra Street, Suite 3, Victoria BC, Canada V8T 4E5, 250-386-8755). Another alternative for consideration is the poten-tial use of Coley's Toxins, as per the Cancer Research Institute (681 Fifth Avenue, NY 10022, 212-688-7515), and also the antineoplaston therapy of Stanislaw Burzyn-ski, M.D. (Burzynski Clinic, 9432 Old Katy Road, Ste 200, Houston, TX 77055, 713-335-5697, or Julian Whitaker, M.D., 4321 Birch St., Ste 100, Newport Beach, CA 92660, 714- 851-1550.)

As for overseas and Mexican alternative clinics and their treatment successes against cancer, this kind of information remains mostly in limbo, although fueled in one way or another by rumor and hearsay. (A possibility also is People Against Cancer, Otho, Iowa, for setting up treatments in Germany.) It may be presumed that their successes against terminal or advanced cancer are not any worse than with conventional medicine, the successes of the latter assumed nil, by definition. (Terminal cases are usually those where the cancer has metastasized or spread.) The situation is complicated by the fact that advanced or terminal patients may have already been treated by medical orthodoxy (such as by chemotherapy), which may compromise the success of alternative treatments. Otherwise, if the success rates for alternative treatments are markedly positive, this assessment should be trumpeted. Hence the need for impartial investigative journalism.

Lastly, the administration of cancer therapies is not cheap, whether alternative or orthodox. For those who wish to go it alone, as inexpensively as possible, perhaps the self-administered treatment of preference is that of megadoses of vitamin C. Although oral uptake is a possibility, the very large dosages that may be necessary indicate IV injection. And there are a few clinics around that perform this service for a relatively modest fee, including the administration of a *Myers cocktail*, which includes other nutrients as well as vitamin C.

# Bibliography

*A Cancer Survivor's Almanac: Charting Your Journey*, edited by Barbara Hoffman, with an introduction by Fitzhugh Mullin. 1996. Minneapolis, MN: National Coalition for Cancer Survivorship, Chronomed Pub.

*A Dictionary of Natural Products: Terms in the Field of Pharmacognosy Relating to Natural Medicinal and Pharmaceutical Materials and the Plants, Animals, and Materials from Which They Are Derived*, 2nd ed. 1997. Medford, NJ: Plexus.

Abramson, J.2004. *Overdosed America: The Broken Promise of American Medicine.* New York: HarperCollins.

Aikman, L. 1977. *Nature's Healing Arts: From Folk Medicine to Modern Drugs.* Washington, DC: National Geographic Society. (Photographs by Nathan Benn and Ira Block. Paintings by Tony Chen.)

Aisenberg, A.C. 1961. *The Glycolysis and Respiration of Tumors.* Publication no. 1023 of the Cancer Commission of Harvard University. New York: Academic Press.

Ali, M. 2004. "Oxygen Homeostasis." *Townsend Letter for Doctors and Patients*, no. 256 (November): 98–102.

Allison, D.W., Leugers, S.L., Pronold, B.J., Van Zant, G., and Donahue, L.M. 2004. "Improved *Ex Vivo* Expansion of Functional CD+ Cells Using Stemline™ II Hematopoietic Stem Cell Expansion Medium." *Life Science Quarterly* 5, no. 2 (Summer).

*Alternative Medicine® Review.* 2002. Monographs. Czap, K., Managing Editor. Dover, ID: Thorne Research.

*Alternative Medicine: The Definitive Guide.* 1993. Compiled by the Burton Goldberg Group. Puyallup, WA: Future Medicine Publishing.

Amdur, M.O., Doull, J., and Klaasen, C.D. Eds. 1991. *Casarett and Doull's Toxicology: The Basic Science of Poisons*, 4th ed. New York: Pergamon Press.

*An Alternative Medicine Definitive Guide to Cancer.* 1997. Puyallup, WA: Future Medicine Publishing.

Andrews, J. 1993. *Good and Hot: Capsicum Cookery.* New York: Macmillan.

Andrews, J. 1984. *Peppers: The Domesticated Capsicums.* Austin: University of Texas Press. (Foreword by W. Hardy Eshbaugh.)

Angell, M. 2004. *The Truth About the Drug Companies: How They Deceive Us and What to Do About it.* New York: Random House.

Antonio, M. 1993. *Atomic Harvest: Hanford and the Lethal Toll of America's Nuclear Arsenal.* New York: Crown.

Anzano, M.A., Byers, S.W., Smith, J.W., Peer, C.W., Mullen, L.T., Brown, C.C., Roberts, A.B., and Sporn, M.B. 1994a. "Prevention of Breast Cancer in the Rat with 9-*cis*-Retinoic Acid as a Single Agent and in Combination with Tamoxifen." *Cancer Research* 54: 4614–4617.

Anzano, M.A., Smith, J.M., Uskokovi, M.R., Peer, C.W., Mullen, L.T., Letterio, J.J., Welsh, M.C., Shrader, M.W., Logsdon, D.L., Driver, C.L., Brown, C.C., Roberts, A.B., and Sporn, M.B. 1994b. "1α,25-dihydroxy-16-ene-23-yne-26,27-hexafluorocholecalciferol (Ro24-5531), a New Deltanoid (Vitamin D Analogue) for Prevention of Breast Cancer in the Rat." *Cancer Research* 54: 1653–1656.

Apsley, J., Holtorf, K., Gordon, E., Anderson, W., and Buttar, R. 2006. "Nanotechnology's Latest Oncolytic Agent: Silver, Cancer, and Infection Associations." *Townsend Letter for Doctors and Patients*, no. 274 (May): 95–98.

Arpante, B.A. 1992. *The Recovery of a Cancer Patient: A Personal Diary*, edited by A. Melenski and P. Melenski. Missoula, MT: Mountain Press.

Atkins, R.C. 1982. *Dr. Atkins' Nutritional Breakthrough: How to Treat Your Medical Condition without Drugs*. New York: Bantam.

Atkins, R.C. 1990. *Dr. Atkins' Health Revolution: How Complementary Medicine Can Extend Your Life*. New York: Bantam.

Atkins, R.C. 1995 [1992]. *Dr. Atkins' New Diet Revolution*. New York: M. Evans,

Attenborough, D. 1957. *Zoo Quest to Guiana*. New York: Crowell.

Ausubel, K. 2000. *When Healing Becomes a Crime: The Amazing Story f the Hoxsey Cancer Clinics and the Return of Alternative Therapies, with a foreword by Bernie Siegel*. Rochester, VT: Healing Arts Press.

Avorn, J. 2004. *Powerful Medicines: The Benefits, Risks, and Costs of Prescription Drugs*. New York: Knopf.

Bagchi, D., and Preuss, H.G., Eds. 2005. *Phytopharmaceuticals in Cancer Chemoprevention*. Boca Raton, FL: CRC Press.

Bailey, L.B., Ed. 1994. *Folate in Health and Disease*. New York: Marcel Dekker.

Bailey, R. 1993. *Ecoscam: The False Prophets of Ecological Apocalypse*. New York: St. Martin's.

Ballentine, R. 1999. *Radical Healing: Integrating the World's Great Therapeutic Traditions to Create a New Transformative Medicine*. New York: Three Rivers Press.

Banik, A.E., and Taylor, R. 1960. *Hunza Land: The Fabulous Health and Youth Wonderland of the World*, with an introduction by Art Linkletter. Long Beach, CA: Whitehorn Publishing.

Barker, R. 1997. *And the Waters Turned to Blood: The Ultimate Biological Threat*. New York: Simon and Schuster.

Barzun, J. 2000. *From Dawn to Decadence: 500 Years of Western Cultural Life: 1500 to the Present*. New York: HarperCollins.

Bastien, J.W. 1987. *Healers of the Andes: Kallawaya Herbalists and Their Medicinal Plants*. Salt Lake City: University of Utah Press. (Illustrated by Eleanor Forfang Stauffer.)

Batchelder, T. 2003. "Attention Deficit Hyperactive Disorder and Modern American Culture." *Townsend Letter for Doctors and Patients*, no. 243 (October): 181–183.

Beard, J. 1911. *The Enzyme Treatment of Cancer and Its Scientific Basis*. London: Chatto and Windus.

Becker, R.O., and Selden, G. 1985. *The Body Electric: Electromagnetism and the Foundations of Life*. New York: Quill [Morrow, 1985].

Begley, S. 2004. "Stem Cells in Tumors May Help Explain Some Cancer Mysteries," *Wall Street Journal*, February 27.

Bell, R. 1992. *Impure Science: Fraud, Compromise and Political Influence in Scientific Research*. New York: John Wiley & Sons.

Bendich, A., and Butterworth, C.E., Eds. 1991. *Micronutrients in Health and Disease Prevention*. New York: Marcel Dekker.

Bennett, J.T. and DiLorenzo, T.J. 1994. *Unhealthy Charities*. New York: Basic Books.

Bennett, M. 2005. "Hospital-Spread Infection." *Townsend Letter for Doctors and Patients*, no. 268 (November): 61–65.

Benninga, H. 1990: *A History of Lactic Acid Making: A Chapter in the History of Biotechnology*. Dordrecht, the Netherlands: Kluwer.

Berlandier, J.L. 1980. *Journey to Mexico: During the Years 1826 to 1834.* 2 vols. Translated by Sheila M. Ohlendorf, Josette M. Bigelow and Mary M. Standifer, with an introduction by C.H. Muller. Botanical notes by C.H. Muller and Katherine K. Muller. Austin: The Texas State Historical Association in cooperation with the Center for Studies in Texas History, University of Texas.

Bilger, J.B. 2006. "Department of Food Science: The Search for Sweet: Building a Better Sugar Substitute." *New Yorker*, May 22, 40–46.

Bird, C. *The Persecution and Trial of Gaston Naessens: The True Story of the Efforts to Suppress an Alternative Treatment for Cancer, AIDS, and Other Immunologically Based Diseases.* Edited by Nancy Carleton. Tiburon, CA: H.J. Kramer.

Blackwell, W.H. 1990. *Poisonous and Medicinal Plants.* Englewood Cliffs, NJ: Prentice Hall. (Chapter 5 on Fungi written by Martha J. Powell.)

Blaylock, R.L. 1997. *Excitotoxins: The Taste that Kills*, with a foreword by George R. Schwartz. Santa Fe, NM: Health Press.

Blaylock, R.L. 2003. *Natural Strategies for Cancer Patients.* New York: Kensington Publishing.

Block, E. 1985. "The Chemistry of Garlic and Onions." *Scientific American, March: 114–119.*

Bogdanovich, W. 1991. *The Great White Lie: How America's Hospitals Betray Our Trust and Endanger Our Lives.* New York: Simon and Schuster.

Boik, J. 1996 [1995]. *Cancer and Natural Medicine: A Textbook of Basic Science and Clinical Research.* Princeton, MN: Oregon Medical Press.

Boik, J. 2001. *Natural Compounds in Cancer Therapy: Promising Nontoxic Antitumor Agents from Plants and Other Natural Sources*, with a foreword by Israel Barken. Princeton, MN: Oregon Medical Press.

Bolton, R., and Singer, M., Eds. 1992. *Rethinking AIDS Prevention: Cultural Approaches.* New York: Gordon and Breach.

Bonk, M., Ed. 1994. *Alternative Medicine Yellow Pages: The Comprehensive Guide to the New World of Health.* Puyallup, WA: Future Medicine Publishing.

Bookchin, D., and Schumacher, J. 2004. *The Virus and the Vaccine: Contaminated Vaccine, Deadly Cancers, and Government Neglect.* New York: St. Martin's Griffin.

Bostwick, D.G., Crawford, E.D., Higano, C.S., and Roach, M., Eds. 2005. *American Cancer Society's Complete Guide to Prostate Cancer.* Atlanta, GA: Health Promotions.

Bourke, J. 1950. *On the Border with Crook.* Columbus, OH: Long's College Book Co. [New York: Scribner's, 1891].

Bovard, J. 1994. *Lost Rights: The Destruction of American Liberty.* New York: St. Martin's.

Bovard, J. 1995. "Double-Crossing to Safety." *American Spectator* 28(1): 24–29.

Bratman, S., and Kroll, D. 1999. *Natural Health Bible.* Rocklin, CA: Prima Publishing.

Breggin, P.R. 1991. *Toxic Psychiatry: Why Therapy, Empathy, and Love Must Replace the Drugs, Electroshock, and Biochemical Theories of the "New Psychiatry".* New York: St. Martin's.

Bricklin, M. 1976. *The Practical Encyclopedia of Natural Healing.* Emmaus, PA: Rodale Press.

Brown, E. 1998. *Forbidden Medicine.* Murrieta, CA: Third Millennium Press.

Brown, M.H. 1979. *Laying Waste: The Poisoning of America by Toxic Chemicals.* New York: 1979.

Brown, M.H. 1987. *The Toxic Cloud: The Poisoning of America's Air.* New York: Harper and Row.

Brown, O.P. 1875. *The Complete Herbalist: Or, the People Their Own Physicians, By the Use of Nature's Remedies; Describing the Great Curative Powers Found in the Herbal Kingdom.* Jersey City, NJ: published by the author.

Brown, R., and Brown, B. 1942. *Amazing Amazon.* New York: Modern Age Books.

Bryson, C. 2004. *The Fluoride Deception*, with a foreword by Dr. Theo Colborn. New York: Seven Stories Press.

Buckingham, J., Ed. 1994. *Dictionary of National Products.* New York: Chapman & Hall.

Burkholz, H. 1994. *The FDA Follies: An Alarming Look at Our Food and Drug Administration.* New York: Basic Books.

Buttram, H.E. 1999. "Vaccine Scene 1999: Overview and Update." *Townsend Letter for Doctors and Patients* (December).

Calvino, N. 2004. "Integrative Medicine in Colon Cancer." *Townsend Letter for Doctors and Patients*, nos. 247/248 (February/March): 99–108.

Cameron, E., and Pauling, L. 1993 [1979]. *Cancer and Vitamin C: A Discussion of the Nature, Causes, Prevention, and Treatment of Cancer with Special Reference to the Value of Vitamin C.* Philadelphia: Camino Books.

Cameron, P. 1992 [1988]. *Exposing the AIDS Scandal: What You Don't Know Can Kill You.* Lafayette, LA: Huntington House.

Campbell, D.G. 2005. *Land of Ghosts: The Braided Lives of People and the Forest in Far Western Amazonia.* Boston: Houghton Mifflin.

Campbell, T.C., and Campbell, T.M. 2005. *The China Study: The Most Comprehensive Study Ever Conducted and the Startling Implications for Diet, Weight Loss and Long-Term Health*, with a foreword by John Robbins. Dallas: Benbella.

Campbell, T.C., and Kinlen, L. 1987. *Diet and Cancer.* Oxfordshire: Oxford University Press. (Prepared for the Imperial Cancer Research Foundation.)

Carper, J. 1997. *Miracle Cures: Dramatic New Scientific Discoveries Revealing the Healing Power of Herbs and Vitamins.* New York: HarperCollins.

Carter, J.P. 1993 [1992]. *Racketeering in Medicine: The Suppression of Alternatives.* Norfolk, VA: Hampton Roads Publishing Co.

Casura, L.G. 1998. "Twenty Questions with Ralph Moss, Ph.D." *Townsend Letter for Doctors and Patients*, no. 174 (January).

Cattaboni, F., Cavallaro, A., and Galli, G., Eds. 1978. *Dioxin: Toxicological and Chemical Aspects.* New York: SP Medical and Scientific Books.

Chandra, R.K., Ed. 1985. *Trace Elements in Nutrition of Children.* Nestle Nutrition Workshop Series, vol. 6. New York: Raven Press.

Chatwin, B. 1989. *What Am I Doing Here?* New York: Penguin Books.

Chi, T.-T. "Benefits of a Special Sea Cucumber Extract in Anti-Angiogenic Therapy and RTK Inhibition for Cancer." *Townsend Letter for Doctors and Patients*, nos. 277/278 (August/September): 91–95.

Childers, J.M., Chu, J., Voigt, L.F., Feigl, P., Tamimi, H.K., Franklin, E.W., Alberts, D.S., and Meyskens, F.L., Jr. 1995. "Chemoprevention of Cervical Cancer with Folic Acid." *Cancer Epidemiology Biomarkers and Prevention.* 4, no. 2: 155–159.

Chopra, D. 1993. *Ageless Body, Timeless Mind: The Quantum Alternative to Growing Old.* New York: Crown.

Chowka, P. 2002 (February 15). *Nicholas Gonzalez, MD: Two Years into an Unprecedented Study of Nutrition and Cancer, the Truth Is Still Out There.* (Retrieved September 1, 2004 from http://members.aol.com/pbchowka/)

Clark, H.R. 1993. *The Cure for All Cancers.* San Diego, CA: ProMotion Publishing.

Clark, J. 1956. *Hunza: Lost Kingdom of the Himalaya.* New York: Funk and Wagnalls.

Clark, L. 1953. *The Rivers Ran East.* New York: Funk & Wagnalls.

Clark, L. 1954. *The Marching Wind.* New York: Funk and Wagnalls.

Clark, W.R. 1997. *At War Within: The Double-Edged Sword of Immunity*, New York: Oxford University Press.

Clarke, J.J. 1902–1912. *Protozoa and Disease.* 4 parts. London: Baillière, Tindall, and Cox. (Part I, no title; Part II, *Sections on the Causes of Smallpox, Syphilis, and Cancer*; Part III, *The Cause of Cancer*; Part IV, *Rhizoid Protozoa: The Cause of Cancer and Other Diseases.*

Clarke, J.J. 1922. *Protists and Disease: Vegetable Protists: Algae and Fungi, Including Chytridiineae; Various Plassomyxineae; the Causes of Molluscum Contagiosum, Smallpox, Cancer, and Hydrophobia; Together with the Mycetoza and Allied Groups.* London: Baillière, Tindall and Cox.

Cohen, J.S. 2001. *Over Dose: The Case Against the Drug Companies. Prescription Drugs, Side Effects, and Your Health.* New York: Tarcher/Putnam.

Cohen, M.A. 2004a. "*Townsend's* New York Observer: News from the Cancer War." *Townsend Letter for Doctors and Patients*, no. 252 (July): 26–27.

Cohen, M.A. 2004b. "Emanuel Revici, M.D.: Efforts to Publish the Clinical Findings of a Pioneer in Lipid-Based Cancer Therapy, Part 1." *Townsend Letter for Doctors and Patients*, nos. 253/254 (August/September): 70–72.

Cohen, M.A. 2004c. "*Townsend's* New York Observer: The Impact of Medical Censorphip on Patient Care, Part 1." *Townsend Letter for Doctors and Patients*, nos. 253/254 (August/September) 142–144.

Cohen, M.A. 2004d. "*Townsend's* New York Observer: The Impact of Medical Censorphip on Patient Care, Part 2." *Townsend Letter for Doctors and Patients*, no. 255 (October) 38–40.

Cohen, M.A. 2004e. "Emanuel Revici, MD: Efforts to Publish the Clinical Findings of a Pioneer in Lipid-Based Cancer Therapy, Part 2." *Townsend Letter for Doctors and Patients*, no. 255 (October): 95-98.

Cohen, M.A. 2004f. "*Townsend's* New York Observer: The Impact of Medical Censorship on Patient Care, Part 3." *Townsend Letter for Doctors and Patients*, no. 256 (November): 107–109.

Cohen, M.A. 2004g. "*Townsend's* New York Observer: The Impact of Medical Censorship on Patient Care, Part 4." *Townsend Letter for Doctors and Patients*, no. 257 (December): 36–39.

Cohen, M.A. 2005a. "*Townsend's* New York Observer: AIDS in the U.S., Early Period (1981–87): Interview with Michael Ellner, President HEAL." *Townsend Letter for Doctors and Patients*, no. 265 (August/September): 88–89.

Cohen, M.A. 2005b. "*Townsend's* New York Observer: The Emergence of AIDS in the U.S.: Interview with Roberto Giraldo, M.D." *Townsend Letter for Doctors and Patients*, no. 267 (October): 44–45.

Cohen, M.A. 2005c. "*Townsend's* New York Observer: AIDS in Africa: Puzzling, Harrowing Pictures." *Townsend Letter for Doctors and Patients*, no. 268 (November): 32–34.

Cohen, M.A. 2005d. "*Townsend's* New York Observer: AIDS in Africa: Interview with Celia Farber." *Townsend Letter for Doctors and Patients*, no. 269 (December): 33–36.

Cohen, M.A. 2006. "*Townsend's* New York Observer: The Double Ordeal of Christine Maggiore, AIDS 'Heretic' and Grieving Parent." *Townsend Letter for Doctors and Patients*, no. 275 (June): 44–46.

Cohen, R. 1998. *Milk: The Deadly Poison*, with a contribution by Jane Heimlich. Englewood Cliffs, NJ:

Colborn, T., Dumanoski, D., and Myers, J.P. 1997. *Our Stolen Future: Are We Threatening Our Fertility, Intelligence, and Survival? A Scientific Detective Story.* New York: Penguin Books [New York: Dutton, 1996, 1997, New York: Little Brown, 1996].

Colt, G.H. 1996. "See Me, Feel Me, Touch Me, Heal Me." *Life*, September: 34–50.

Commoner, B. 2002. "Unraveling the DNA Myth: The Spurious Foundation of Genetic Engineering." *Harper's*, February: 39–47.

Cone, M. 2005. "Dozens of Words for Snow, None for Pollution." *Mother Jones* 30, no. 1 (January/February): 60–67.

Considine, D.M., and Considine, G.D., Eds. 1984. *Encyclopedia of Chemistry,* 4th ed. New York: Van Nostrand Reinhold.

Cook, C.D. 2004. *Diet for a Dead Planet: How the Food Industry Is Killing Us.* New York: New Press.

Cooke, R. 2001. *Dr. Folkman's War: Angiogenesis and the Struggle to Defeat Cancer,* with a foreword by C. Everett Cooke. New York: Random House.

Cordell, G.A. 1981. *Introduction to Alkaloids: A Biogenetic Approach.* New York: John Wiley & Sons.

Cousins, N. 1979. *Anatomy of an Illness as Perceived by the Patient.* New York: Norton.

Cousins, N. 1982. *Healing and Belief.* Cincinnati, OH: Mosaic Press.

Cousins, N. 1983. *The Healing Heart: Antidotes to Panic and Helplessness.* New York: Norton.

Cousins, N. 1989. *Head First: The Biology of Hope.* New York: Dutton.

Cousins, N. 1990. "The Laughter Prescription." *Saturday Evening Post*, September, vol. 262, no. 6.

*CRC Handbook of Identified Carcinogens and Noncarcinogens: Carcinogenicity-Mutagenicity Database*, 2 vols. 1982. Boca Raton, FL: CRC Press.

Crellin, J.K., and Philpott, J. 1990. *Herbal Medicine Past and Present, vol. 2, A Reference Guide to Medicinal Plants.* Durham, NC: Duke University Press.

Critser, G. 2005. *Generation RX: How Prescription Drugs Are Altering American Lives, Minds and Bodies.* Boston: Houghton Mifflin.

Culbert, M.L. 1997. *Medical Armageddon Update 2000: Behind the Healthcare Calamity of the Whole World and How to Fix It.* San Diego, CA: C and C Communications.

Damasio, A.R. 1995. *Descartes' Error: Emotion, Reason, and the Human Brain,* New York: Avon Books [G.P. Putnam's Sons: 1994].

D'Antonio, M. 1993. *Atomic Harvest: Hanford and the Lethal Toll of America's Nuclear Arsenal.* New York: Crown.

Davis, A. 1965. *Let's Get Well.* New York: Harcourt, Brace and World.

Davis, C.E. 1993. *The Politics of Hazardous Waste.* Englewood Cliffs NJ: Prentice Hall.

Davis, D. 2002. *When Smoke Ran Like Water: Tales of Environmental Deception and the Battle Against Pollution,* with a foreword by Mitchell Gaynor. New York: Basic Books.

Davis, W. 1987. *The Serpent and the Rainbow: A Harvard Scientist Uncovers the Startling Truth about the Secret World of Haitian Voodoo and Zombis.* New York: Warner Books [Simon and Schuster, 1985].

Davis, W. 1988. *Passage of Darkness: The Ethnobiology of the Haitian Zombie.* Chapel Hill: University of North Carolina Press.

Davis, W. 1996. *One River: Explorations and Discoveries in the Amazon Rain Forest.* New York: Simon and Schuster.

Day, L. 1991. *AIDS: What the Government Isn't Telling You: Censored.* Palm Desert, CA: Rockford Press.

Dean, W., and Morgenthaler, J. 1990. *Smart Drugs and Nutrients.* Menlo Park, CA: Health Freedom Publications.

Dean, W., Morgenthaler, J., and Fowkes, S.W. 1993. *Smart Drugs II: The Next Generation: New Drugs and Nutrients to Improve Your Memory and Increase Your Intelligence.* Menlo Park, CA: Health Freedom Publications.

de Duve, C. 1996. "The Birth of Complex Cells." *Scientific American*, April, 50–57.

*Desk Reference to Nature's Medicine.* 2006. Washington, DC: National Geographic Society.

de Villiers, M., and Hirtle, S. 2002. *Sahara: A Natural History.* New York: Walker and Company.

DeVita, V.T., Hellman, S., and Rosenberg, S.A., Eds. 1989. *Cancer: Principles and Practice of Oncology,* 3rd ed. Philadelphia: Lippincott Williams & Wilkins.

Devlin, T.M., Ed. 1986 [1982]. *Textbook of Biochemistry with Clinical Correlations,* 2nd edition. New York: John Wiley & Sons.

Dey, P.M., and Harborne, J.B., Eds. 1990–1991. *Methods in Plant Biochemistry.* London: Academic Press.

Dodge, Col. R.I. 1959 [1882]. *Our Wild Indians: Thirty-Three Years' Personal Experience among the Red Men of the Great West. A Popular Account of Their Social Life, Religion, Habits, Traits, Customs, Exploits, etc., with Thrilling Adventures on the Great Plains and in the Mountains of Our Wide Frontier,* with an introduction by General Sherman. New York: Archer House.

Dorner, F. and Drews, J. 1986. *Pharmacology of Bacterial Toxins.* New York: Pergamon Press.

Dreosti, I.E., Ed. 1991. Trace Elements, Micronutrients, and Free Radicals. Totowa, NJ: Humana Press.

Drexler, M. 2002. Secret Agents: The Menace of Emerging Infections. Washington, DC: Joseph Henry Press.

Duesberg, P.H., and Ellison, B.J. 1990. "Is the AIDS Virus a Science Fiction?" Policy Review no. 53 (Summer): 40–51.

Dufty, W. 1975. Sugar Blues. New York: Warner Books.

Duke, J.A. 1992a. Handbook of Biologically Active Phytochemicals and Their Activities. Boca Raton, FL: CRC Press.

Duke, J.A. 1992b. Handbook of Phytochemical Constituents of GRAS Herbs and Other Economic Plants. Boca Raton, FL: CRC Press.

Duke, J.A. 2002 [1985, 2001]. CRC Handbook of Medicinal Herbs. Boca Raton, FL: CRC Press.

Duke, J.A., and Ayensu, E.S. 1985. Medicinal Plants of China. Algonac, MI: Reference Publications.

Duke, J.A., and Vasquez, R. 1994. Amazonia Ethnobotanical Dictionary. Boca Raton, FL: CRC Press.

Ebadi, M. 2002. Pharmacodynamic Basis of Herbal Medicine. Boca Raton, FL: CRC Press.

Ehrenreich, B. 2001. "Welcome to Cancerland: A Mammogram Leads to a Cult of Pink Kitsch." Harper's, November: 43–53.

Eidem, W.K. 1997. The Doctor Who Cures Cancer: The Story of Emanuel Revici, M.D.: His Medical Breakthroughs, Innovative Treatments, and Struggle for Recognition. New York: Sullivan and Foster.

Eigenbrodt, E., Fiste, P., and Reinacher, M. 1985. "New Perspectives on Carbohydrate Metabolism in Tumor Cells." Pp. 141–179 in Regulation of Carbohydrate Metabolism, vol. 2, ed. R. Beitner. Boca Raton, FL: CRC Press.

Ellison, B., and Duesberg, P. 1995. Why We Will Never Win the War on AIDS. Visalia, CA: Inside Story Communications.

Encyclopedia of Chemical Reactions. 8 vols. 1946-1959. Compiled by C.A. Jacobsen, edited by C.A. Hampel. New York:Reinhold.

Epstein, S.S. 1979. The Politics of Cancer. New York: Anchor/Doubleday [San Francisco: Sierra Club Books, 1978].

Epstein, S.S. 1998a. The Politics of Cancer Revisited. New York: East Ridge Press.

Epstein, S.S. 1998b. The Breast Cancer Prevention Program. New York: Macmillan.

Epstein, S.S., and Steinman, S. 1997. *The Breast Cancer Prevention Program: The First Complete Survey of the Causes of Breast Cancer and the Steps You Can Take to Reduce Your Risks.* New York: Macmillan.

Ewald, P.W. 2000. *Plague Time: How Stealth Infections Cause Cancers, Heart Disease, and Other Deadly Ailments* New York: Free Press.

Faguet, G.B. 2005. *The War on Cancer: An Anatomy of Failure, a Blueprint for the Future.* New York: Springer-Verlag.

Farber, C. 2006a. "Out of Control: AIDS and the Corruption of Medical Science." *Harper's*, March, 37–52.

Farber, C. 2006b. *Serious Adverse Events: An Uncensored History of AIDS.* Hoboken, NJ: Melville House.

Fawcett, Col. P.H. 1953. *Lost Trails, Lost Cities: From His Manuscripts, Letters, and Other Records, Selected and Arranged by Brian Fawcett.* New York: Funk and Wagnalls.

Fayhee, J.M. 1994. *Mexico's Copper Canyon Country: A Hiking and Backpacking Guide to Tarahumara-Land*, revised ed. Boulder, CO: Johnson Books.

Fieve, R.R. 1989. *Moodswings*, revised and expanded ed. New York: Bantam.

Fink, J. M. 1992. *Third Opinion: An International Directory to Alternative Therapy Centers for the Treatment and Prevention of Cancer and Other Degenerative Diseases*, 2nd ed. Garden City Park, NY: Avery Publishing Group.

Fisher, J.A. 1994. *The Plague Makers: How We Are Creating Catastrophic New Epidemics — and What We Must Do to Avert Them.* New York: Simon and Schuster.

*Flora Neotropica.* 1968. Published for the Organization for Flora Neotropica by the New York Botanical Garden, New York. (As of 1994 there are 65 monographs, mainly by plant families.)

Folate in Health and Disease, Bailey, L.B., Ed., Marcel Dekker, New York, 1994.

Foley, K., and Hendin, H., Eds. 2002. The Case Against Assisted Suicide: For the Right to End-of-Life Care. Baltimore, MD: The Johns Hopkins University Press.

Fonorow, O.R. 2002. "The Long Neglected Theory of Cardiovascular and Heart Disease." Townsend Letter for Doctors and Patients, nos. 229/230 (August/September): 96–98.

Fonorow, O.R. 2004. "The Cure for Cancer: Theory, History and Treatment." Townsend Letter for Doctors and Patients, no. 251 (June): 118–120.

Foster, M.B., and Foster, R.S. 1946 [1945]. Brazil: Orchid of the Tropics. Lancaster, PA: Jacques Cattell Press.

Foster, S. 1995. Forest Pharmacy: Medicinal Plants in American Forests. Durham, NC: Forest History Society.

Foster, S., and Johnson, R.L. 2006. Desk Reference to Nature's Medicine. Washington, DC: National Geographic Society.

Fugate, F.L., and Fugate, R.B. 1991. Roadside History of Oklahoma. Missoula, MT: Mountain Press.

Fulder, S. 1997. The Garlic Book: Nature's Powerful Healer. Garden City Park, NY: Avery Publishing Group.

Fumento, M. 1990. The Myth of Heterosexual AIDS. New York: Basic Books.

Gallagher, C. 1994. American Ground Zero: The Secret Nuclear War. New York: Random House [Cambridge, MA: MIT Press, 1993].

Gardner, E.S. 1954. Neighborhood Frontiers. New York: Morrow.

Garrett, L. 1995. The Coming Plague: Newly Emerging Diseases in a World Out of Balance. New York: Viking Penguin [Farrar, Straus and Giroux, 1994].

Gawande, A. 2002. Complications: A Surgeon's Notes on an Imperfect Science. New York: Henry Holt.

Gearin-Tosh, M. 2002. Living Proof: A Medical Mutiny. New York: Scribner.

General George Crook: His Autobiography, Edited by M.F. Schmitt. 1960 [1946].Norman: University of Oklahoma Press.

"George Bernard Shaw on Vaccine from the Past." 1999. Townsend Letter for Doctors and Patients (December).

Gerard, J. 1975. The Herbal, or General History of Plants, the complete 1633 ed., revised and enlarged by Thomas Johnson. New York: Dover.

Gerson, M. 1958. A Cancer Therapy: Results of Fifty Cases. New York: Whittier Books.

Gheerbrant, A. 1955. The Impossible Adventure: Journey to the Far Amazon. London: Readers Union/Victor Gollancz, translated by Edward Fitzgerald. [Published 1953, 1954 as Journey to the Far Amazon. New York: Simon and Schuster.]

Gill, A.A. 2005 [2002]. AA Gill is away. New York: Simon and Schuster.

Gilmore, M.R. 1991. Use of Plants by the Indians of the Missouri River Region. Lincoln: University of Nebraska Press.

Girard, R. 1977. Violence and the Sacred, translated by Patrick Gregory. Baltimore, MD: The Johns Hopkins University Press.

Gitelman, H.J., Ed. 1989. Aluminum and Health: A Critical Review. New York: Marcel Dekker.

Givler, A. 2003. Hope in the Face of Cancer: A Guide fpr the Journey You Did Not Choose. Eugene, OR: Harvest House Publishers.

Gladwell, M. 2004. "Annals of Technology: The Picture Problem: Mammography, Air Power, and the Limits of Looking." New Yorker, December 13: 74–81.

Glum, G.L. n.d. Calling of an Angel. Los Angeles, CA: Silent Walker Publishing.

Goodman and Gilman's The Pharmacological Basis of Therapeutics, 9th ed. 1996. Molinoff, P.B., and Ruddon, R.W., Eds. New York: McGraw-Hill.

Goodman and Gilman's The Pharmacological Basis of Therapeutics, 10th ed. 2001. Hardman, J.G., Limbird, L.E., and Gilman, A.G., Eds. New York: McGraw-Hill.

Goodson-Kjome, P. 1995. This Adventure Called Life. Longmont, CO: Sunshine Press Publications.

Gordon, J.S., and Curtin, S. 2001 [2000]. Comprehensive Cancer Care: Integrating Alternative, Complementary, and Conventional Therapies. Cambridge, MA: Perseus.

Gordon, R. 1993. The Alarming History of Medicine: Amusing Anecdotes from Hippocrates to Heart Transplants. New York: Saint Martin's.

Gough, M. 1986. Dioxin, Agent Orange: The Facts. New York: Plenum.

Gould, D. 1987 [1985]. The Medical Mafia: How Doctors Serve and Fail Their Customers. London: Sphere [Hamish Hamilton, 1985].

Grann, D. 2005. "The Lost City of Z: A Quest to Uncover the Secrets of the Amazon." New Yorker, September 19, 56–81.

Graves, G. 1990. Medicinal Plants: An Illustrated Guide to More than 180 Plants That Cure Disease and Relieve Pain, with a foreword by A. Hollman, M.D., FRCP, FLS. [Originally published in 1834 as Hortus Medicus. Illustrations are from Hortus Medicus and Woodville's Medical Botany, published in 1790]. New York: Crescent Books.

Green, B.K. 1971. The Village Horse Doctor: West of the Pecos. New York: Knopf.

Green, B.K. 1972. A Thousand Miles of Mustangin'. Flagstaff, AZ: Northland Press.

Green, B.K. 1999. Horse Tradin'. New York: Knopf [Lincoln: University of Nebraska Press, 1967].

Greenwald, P. 1996. "Chemoprevention of Cancer." Scientific American, September, 96–99.

Greenwald, P., Kelloff, G., Burch-Whitman, C., and Kramer, B.S., 1995. "Chemoprevention." CA — A Cancer Journal for Clinicians 45, no. 1: 31–49.

Griggs, B. 1991 [1981]. *Green Pharmacy: The History and Evolution of Western Herbal Medicine.* Rochester, VT: Healing Arts Press.

Guerra, R., Tureen, J.H., Fournier, M.A., Makrides, V., and Tuber, M.G. 1993. "Amino Acids in Cerebrospinal and Brain Interstitial Fluid in Experimental Pneumococcal Meningitis." Pediatric Research 33, no. 5: 510–513.

Guppy, N. 1958. Wai-Wai: Through the Forests North of the Amazon. New York: Dutton.

Halamandaris, W. 1992. *The Care Gaps.* Lanham, MD: University Press of America.

Hall, S.S. 1997a. *A Commotion in the Blood: Life, Death, and the Immune System.* New York: Henry Holt.

Hall, S.S. 1997b. "Vaccinating Against Cancer." *Atlantic Monthly,* April, 66–84.

Han, H., Miller, G.E., and Deville, N. 2003. *Ancient Herbs, Modern Medicine: Improving Your Health by Combining Chinese Herbal Medicine and Western Medicine.* New York: Bantam Books.

Hardin, J.W., and Arena, J.M. 1974. *Human Poisoning from Native and Cultivated Plants,* 2nd ed. Durham, NC: Duke University Press.

Harper, D.W., and Culbert, M.L. 1980. *How You Can Beat the Killer Diseases.* New Rochelle, NY: Arlington.

Harris, T. 1991. *Death in the Marsh.* Covelo, CA: Island Press.

Hartwell, J.L., "Plant Remedies for Cancer," *Cancer Chemotherapy Reports,* 7: 19–24, May 1960.

Hartwell, J.L. 1982a. *Bioactive Plants, vol. 2, Plants Used Against Cancer: A Survey,* with a foreword by Jim Duke. Lawrence, MA: Quarterman Publications.

Hartwell, J.L. 1982b. *Plants Used Against Cancer,* with a foreword by Jim Duke. Lawrence, MA: Quarterman Publications.

Hasselberger, F.X. 1978. *Uses of Enzymes and Immobilized Enzymes.* Chicago: Nelson-Hall.

Hattersley, J.G. 2003 "The Negative Health Effects of Chlorine." *Townsend Letter for Doctors and Patients,* no. 238 (May): 60–63. (Previously published in *Journal of Orthomolecular Medicine* 15, no. 2 (2000): 89–95..

Heiby, W.A. 1988. *The Reverse Effect: How Vitamins and Minerals Promote Health and Cause Disease.* Deerfield, IL: MediScience Publishers.

Heinerman, J. 1977. *Healing Animals with Herbs.* Provo, UT: BiWorld.

Heinerman, J. 1982. *Aloe Vera, Jojoba and Yucca.* New Canaan, CT: Keats.

Heinerman, J. 1984 [1980]. *The Treatment of Cancer with Herbs,* with a special foreword by Robert Mendelsohn. Orem, UT: BiWorld. (Out of print; reported to be available from the author, P.O. Box 11471, Salt Lake City, UT 84147, (801)521-8824.)

Heinerman, J. 1989a. *Healing Secrets of the Maya: Health Wisdom from an Ancient Empire.* Foster City, CA: Human Energy Press.

Heinerman, J. 1989b. *The Spiritual Wisdom of the Native Americans.* San Rafael, CA: Cassandra Press.

Heinerman, J. 1991a. *Double the Power of Your Immune System.* Nyack, NY: Parker [Englewood Cliffs, NJ: Prentice Hall, 1991].

Heinerman, J. 1991b. *Health Secrets from the Ancient World.* San Rafael, CA: Cassandra Press.

Heinerman, J. 1993. *The Healing Power of Garlic: From Pharoahs to Pharmacists.* New Canaan, CT: Keats.

Heinerman, J. 1997. *Healing Animals with Herbs.* Provo, UT: BiWorld.

Hendin, H. 1998. *Seduced by Death: Doctors, Patients, and the Dutch Cure.* New York: Norton.

Hendler, S.S. et al. 1990. *The Doctors' Vitamin and Mineral Encyclopedia.* New York: Simon and Schuster.

Hiatt, H.H., Watson, J.D., and Winsten, J.A., Eds. 1977. *Origins of Human Cancer.* 3 vols. Cold Spring Conferences on Cell Proliferation, vol. 4. Cold Spring Harbor, NY: Cold Spring Harbor Laboratory. (Book A, *Incidence of Cancer in Humans*; Book B, *Mechanisms of Carcinogenesis*; Book C, *Human Risk Assessment.*)

Hochhaus, A., Lahaye, T., Kreil, S., Berger, U., Metzgeroth., G., and Hehlmann, R. 2001. "Selektive Hemmung von Tyrosinkinasen als neues therapeutisches Prinzip in der Onkologie [Selective Inhibition of Tyrosine Kinases: A New Therapeutic Principle in Oncology]." *Onkologie* (suppl. 5, September 24): 65–71.

Hoffer, A. 2000. *Vitamin C and Cancer.* Kingston, Ontario: Quarry Health Books.

Hoffer, A. 2006. *Adventures in Psychiatry: The Scientific Memoirs of Dr. Abram Hoffer.* Alton, Ontario: Kos Publishing.

Hoffman, E.J. 1997. "Enzyme Inhibitors for Cancer Cell Metabolism." *Townsend Letter for Doctors and Patients,* no. 166 (May): 58–66.

Hoffman, E.J. 1999a. *Cancer and the Search for Selective Biochemical Inhibitors.* Boca Raton, FL: CRC Press.

Hoffman, E.J. 1999b. "Garlic and Allicin and Other Sulfur-Containing Compounds as Anti-cancer Agents. *Townsend Letter for Doctors and Patients,* (January):

Hogben, L. 1957. *Statistical Theory: The Relationship of Probability, Credibility and Error.* London: Allen and Unwin.

Hollósy, F., and Kéri, G. 2004. "Plant-Derived Protein *Tyrosine Kinase Inhibitors* as Anti-cancer Agents." *Current Medicinal Chemistry. Anti-Cancer Agents* 4, no. 2: 173–197.

Holzer, H. 1973. *Beyond Medicine: The Facts About Unorthodox and Psychic Healing.* Chicago: Henry Regnery.

Hong, W.K., Lippman, S.M., Hittelman, W.N., and Lotan, R. 1995. "Retinoid Chemoprevention of Aerodigestive Cancer: From Basic Research to the Clinic." *Clinical Cancer Research* 1: 677–686.

Hooper, E. 1999. *The River: A Journey to the Source of HIV and AIDS.* Boston: Little, Brown.

Hostettmann, K., Ed. 1991. *Methods in Plant Biochemistry, vol. 6, Assays for Bioactivity.* London: Academic Press.

Houston, R. 2005. "Vitamins, Cancer and Hope." *Townsend Letter for Doctors and Patients,* no. 264 (July): 78–80.

Houston, R.G. 1989. *Repression and Reform in the Evaluation of Alternative Cancer Therapies.* Washington, DC: Project Cure. (Available from People Against Cancer, P.O. Box 10, Otho, IA 50569-0010, (515)972-4444.)

Hutchens, A.R. 1992a [1987]. *A Handbook of Native American Herbs.* Boston: Shambhala.

Hutchens, A.R. 1992b. *Indian Herbalogy of North America.* Magnolia, MA: Peter Smith [Windsor, Ontario: MERCO, 1969, 1970, 1973; Boston: Shambala, 1969, 1991].

Hylton, W.H., Ed. 1974. *The Rodale Herb Book: How to Use, Grow, and Buy Nature's Miracle Plants.* Emmaus, PA: Rodale Press.

Jackman, A., and Judson, I. 1994. "Oncology Drug Discovery and Clinical Trial Testing: Who's Listening?" *Cancer Investigation* (New York) 12, no. 1: 105–108.

Jacobs, M.M., Ed. 1991. *Vitamins and Minerals in the Prevention and Treatment of Cancer.* Boca Raton, FL: CRC Press.

Jain, M.K. 1982. *Handbook of Enzyme Inhibitors (1965–1977).* New York: John Wiley & Sons.

Jennings, E. 1993. *Apricots and Oncogenes: On Vegetables and Cancer Prevention.* Cleveland, OH: McGuire and Beckley Books.

Jerome, F.J. 2000 [1995]. *Tooth Truth: A Patient's Guide to Metal- Free Dentistry.* Chula Vista, CA: New Century Press.

Johnson, J.H. 1990. *How to Buy Almost Any Drug Legally Without a Prescription.* New York: Avon Books.

Jonas, W.B., and Levin, J.S., Eds. 1999. *Essentials of Complementary and Alternative Medicine.* Baltimore, MD: Lippincott Williams & Wilkins.

Joseph, S. 1992. *Dragon within the Gates: The Once and Future AIDS Epidemic.* New York: Carroll and Graf Publishers.

Jurasunas, S. 2006. "Mitochondria and Cancer." *Townsend Letter for Doctors and Patients,* nos. 277/278 (August/September): 83–86, 146–148.

Kamrin, M.A. and Rodgers, P.W., Eds. 1985. *Dioxins in the Environment.* Washingon, DC: Hemisphere Publishing.

Kane, C.W. 2006. *Herbal Medicine of the American Southwest: A Guide to the Medical and Edible Plants of the Southwestern United States,* with a foreword by Michael Moore. Tucson, AZ: Lincoln Town Press. (Paintings by Frank S. Rose.)

Kantak, K.M. 1990. ":Nutritional Aspects of Drug Addiction on Behavior." Pp. 149–169 in *Advances in Behavioral Pharmacology,* Vol. 17, ed. J. Barrett, T. Thompson, and P.B. Dewes. Hillsdale, NJ: Lawrence Erlbaum.

Kaplan, C., Turner, G.S., and Warrell, D.A. 1986. *Rabies: The Facts,* 2nd ed. New York: Oxford University Press.

Kaplan, M., and Kaplan, E. 2006. *Chances Are ...: Adventures in Probability.* New York: Viking.

Kenner, D. 2006. "Avemar—a Functional Food with Proven Anti-Cancer Effects." *Townsend Letter for Doctors and Patients,* nos. 277/278 (August/September): 96–100.

Kimbrell, A. Ed. 2002. *Fatal Harvest: The Tragedy of Industrial Agriculture.* Washington, DC: Island Press.

Kindscher, K. 1987. *Edible Wild Plants of the Prairie: An Ethnobotanical Guide.* Lawrence: University Press of Kansas.

Kindscher, K. 1992. *Medicinal Wild Plants of the Prairie: An Ethnobotanical Guide.* Lawrence: University Press of Kansas.

Kingsbury, J.M. 1964. *Poisonous Plants of the United States and Canada.* Englewood Cliffs, NJ: Prentice Hall.

Kingsbury, J.M. 1965. *Deadly Harvest: A Guide to Common Poisonous Plants.* New York: Holt, Rinehart and Winston.

Kingston, D.G.I., Cragg, G.M., and Newman, D.J., Eds. 2005. *Anticancer Agents from Natural Products.* Boca Raton, FL: CRC Press.

Kintzios, S.E., and Barberaki, M.G., Eds. 2004. *Plants that Fight Cancer.* Boca Raton, FL: CRC Press.

Knutson, R.M. 1987. *Flattened Fauna: A Field Guide to Animals of Roads, Streets, and Highways.* Berkeley, CA: Ten Speed Press.

Knutson, R.M. 1992. *Furtive Fauna: A Field Guide to the Creatures Who Live on You.* New York: Viking Penguin.

Koch, H.P., and Lawson. L.D., Eds. 1996 [1988]. *Garlic: The Scientific and Therapeutic Application of* Allium Sativum *L. and Related Species,* 2nd ed. Baltimore, MD: Williams & Wilkins.

Koonin, E.V. and Galperin, M.Y. 2003. *Sequence – Evolution – Function: Computational Approaches in Comparative Genomics.* Norwell, MA: Kluwer Academic.

Krakoff, I.H. 1996. "Systemic Treatment of Cancer." *CA— A Cancer Journal for Clinicians* 46, no. 3: 134–141.

Kramer, P.D. 1993. *Listening to Prozac: A Psychiatrist Explores Anti-Depressant Drugs and the Remaking of the Self.* New York: Viking Penguin.

Krebs, H., in collaboration with Schmid, R. 1981. *Otto Warburg: Cell Physiologist, Biochemist and Eccentric*, translated by Hans Krebs and Anne Martin. Oxford: Clarendon Press, New York: Oxford University Press.

Kristal, H.J., and Haig, J.M. 2003. "Diabetes, Cancer and Weight: A Metabolic Typing Survey." *Townsend Letter for Doctors and Patients*, nos. 235/236 (February/March): 108–110.

Krizay, J. 1986. *The Fifty Billion Dollar Drain: Alcohol, Drugs, and the High Cost of Insurance*. Newport Beach, CA: Care Institute.

Krochmal, A., and Krochmal, C. 1973. *A Guide to the Medicinal Plants of the United States*. New York: Quadrangle/New York Times Book Co.

Kroeger, H. 1997. *Free Your Body of Tumors and Cysts*. Boulder, CO: Hanna Kroeger Publications.

Kuralt, C. 1985. *On the Road with Charles Kuralt*. New York: Putnam's.

Lanctôt, G. 1995. *The Medical Mafia: How to Get Out of it Alive and Take Back Our Health and Wealth*. Morgan, VT: Here's the Key.

Lane, I.W., and Comac, L. 1993 [1992]. *Sharks Don't Get Cancer: How Shark Cartilage Could Save Your Life*. Garden City Park, NY: Avery Publishing Group.

Langford, J.O., and Gipson, F. 1973. *Big Bend: A Homesteader's Story*. Austin: University of Texas Press.

Lax, E. 2004. *The Mold in Dr. Florey's Coat: The Story of the Penicillin Miracle*. New York: Henry Holt.

Leaf, C. 2004. "Why We're Losing the War on Cancer." *Fortune*, March: 76–96.

Lee, J.G. 1961. "Navajo Medicine Man." *Arizona Highways* 37, no. 8, 2–7.

Lerner, M. 1992. *Choices in Cancer Therapy: A Complete Guide to Conventional and Alternative Cancer Treatments, Including Nutrition — Mind-Body — Newest Drugs — Surgery— and Much More*. New York: HarperCollins.

Lerner, M. 1994. *Choices in Healing: The Best of Conventional and Complementary Approaches to Cancer*. Cambridge, MA: MIT Press.

Lévi-Strauss, C. 1966. *The Savage Mind*. Chicago: University of Chicago Press.

Levy, S.B. 1992. *The Antibiotic Paradox: How Miracle Drugs Are Destroying the Miracle*. New York: Plenum Press.

Life Extension Foundation. 2003. *Disease Prevention and Treatment: Scientific Protocols that Integrate Mainstream and Alternative Medicine*, 4th ed. Hollywood, FL: Life Extension Foundation.

Lindorff, D. 1992. *Marketplace Medicine: The Rise of the For-Profit Hospital Chains*. New York: Bantam.

Lockshin, R.A., Zakari, Z., and Tilley, J.L., Eds. 2004. *When Cells Die, vol. 2, A Comprehensive Evaluation of Apoptosis and Programmed Cell Death*. New York: Wiley-Liss.

Ludwig, E. 1939. *The Nile: The Life-Story of a River*, translated by Mary H. Lindsay. New York: Garden City Publishing.

Lumholtz, C, 1971 [1912]. *New Trails in Mexico: An Account of One Year's Exploration in North-Western Sonora, Mexico, and South-Western Arizona 1909-1910*. Glorieta, NM: Rio Grande Press.

Lumholtz, C. 1973 [1902]. *Unknown Mexico: A Record of Five Years' Exploration among the Tribes of the Western Sierra Madre; in the Tierra Caliente of Tepic and Jalisco; and among the Tarascos of Michoacan*, 2 vol. Glorieta, NM: Rio Grande Press.

Lynch, J.J. 1977. *The Broken Heart: The Medical Consequences of Loneliness*. New York: Basic Books.

Lynes, B. 1989. *The Healing of Cancer*. Queensville, Ontario: Marcus Books.

Lynes, B. 1992 [1987]. *The Cancer Cure That Worked!: Fifty Years of Suppression.* Queensville, Ontario: Marcus Books.

Lyons, R. 2001. *Indium: The Missing Trace Mineral, The Newly Discovered Trace Mineral for Vibrant Health.* Henderson, NV: New Health Press.

Mabry, T.J., Hunziker, J.H., and DiFeo, D.R., Eds. 1977. *Creosote Bush: Biology and Chemistry of* Larrea *in New World Deserts.* Stroudsburg, PA: Dowden, Hutchinson & Ross.

Macfarlane, G. 1985. *Alexander Fleming: The Man and the Myth.* Oxford, England: Oxford University Press[London: Chatto and Windus, the Hogarth Press, 1984].

Machlin, L.J., Ed. 1991. *Handbook of Vitamins,* 2nd ed. New York: Marcel Dekker.

Madison, V. 1955. *The Big Bend Country of Texas.* Albuquerque: University of New Mexico Press.

Maggiore, C. 1996. *What If Everything You Thought You Knew About HIV Was Wrong?* Studio City, CA: American Foundation for AIDS Alternatives.

Mallis, A., Ed. 1982. *Handbook of Pest Control: The Behavior, Life History, and Control of Household Pests,* 6th ed. Cleveland, OH: Franzak & Foster.

Mallory, R. 1992. "Jalapeños — a Burning Issue." *Texas Highways* 39, no. 11, 4–9.

Markle, G.E., and Petersen, J.C., Eds. 1980. *Politics, Science, and Cancer: The Laetrile Phenomenon.* Papers from a symposium, American Association for the Advancement of Science 1979 National Annual Meeting, Houston, TX, January 3–8. Boulder, CO: Westview Press.

Martin, L.C. 1993 [1984]. *Wildflower Folklore.* Old Saybrook, CT: Globe Pequot Press.

Martin, W. 2000a. "Report on Visit to BioPulse Clinic in Tijuana." *Townsend Letter for Doctors and Patients* (June) 83–85.

Martin, W. 2002b. "The Prudent Heart Diet and Cholesterol Lowering Drugs: Why They Don't Prevent Heart Disease." *Townsend Letter for Doctors and Patients,* nos. 229/230 (August/September): 100–107.

Martin, W. 2003. "The Role of Dietary Polyunsaturated Fats in Heart Disease and Arteriosclerosis." *Townsend Letter for Doctors and Patients,* nos. 241/242 (August/September): 80–84.

Martin, W. 2006. "Coley's Toxins: A Cancer Treatment History." *Townsend Letter for Doctors and Patients,* nos. 229/230 (February/March): 113–118.

Matthews, R.A.F. 1991 [1970, 1981]. *Plant Virology,* 3rd ed. San Diego, CA: Academic Press.

Mathiessen, P. 1996. *The Cloud Forest: A Chronicle of the South American Wilderness.* New York: Pyramid Books [Viking, 1961].

Maurois, A. 1959. *The Life of Alexander Fleming: Discoverer of Penicillin,* translated by Gerald Hopkins. New York: Dutton.

McPhee, J.A. 1986. *Rising from the Plains.* New York: Farrar, Straus, Giroux.

McTaggert, L. 2002. *The Field: The Quest for the Secret Force of the Universe.* New York: HarperCollins,

Mead, J.R. 1986. *Hunting and Trading on the Great Plains, 1859-1875.* Norman, OK: University of Oklahoma Press.

Medawar, P. 1990. *The Threat and the Glory: Reflections on Science and Scientists,* edited by David Pyke, with a foreword by Lewis Thomas. New York: HarperCollins.

Mellor, J.W. 1922–1937. *A Comprehensive Treatise on Inorganic and Theoretical Chemistry.*16 vols. New York: Longmans, Green.

Mendelsohn, R.S. 1979. *Confessions of a Medical Heretic.* Chicago: Contemporary Books.

Mendelsohn, R.S. et al. 1985. *Dissent in Medicine: Nine Doctors Speak Out.* Chicago: Contemporary Books.

Meskin, M.S., Bidlack, W.R., Lewis, D.S., Davies, A.J., and Randolph, R.K., Eds. 2004. *Phytochemicals: Mechanisms of Action.* Boca Raton, FL: CRC Press.

Meyskens, F.L. 1990. "Coming of Age: The Chemoprevention of Cancer." *New England Journal of Medicine* 323, no. 12:

Meyskens, F.L., and Prasad, K. 1983. *Modulation and Mediation of Cancer.* Farmington, CT: S. Karger.

Meyskens, F.L., and Prasad, K., Eds. 1986. *Vitamins and Cancer.* Totowa, NJ: Humana Press.

Millard, C. 2005. *The River of Doubt: Theodore Roosevelt's Darkest Journey.* New York: Random House.

Mitchell, J. 1993. *Up in the Old Hotel, and Other Stories.* New York: Vintage Books, Random House.

Moerman, D.E. n.d. *Medicinal Plants of Native America,* 2 vols. Technical Reports: no. 19. Ann Arbor: Museum of Anthropology, University of Michigan.

Mooney, J. 1932. *The Swimmer Manuscript of Cherokee Sacred Formulas and Medicinal Prescriptions.* Bureau of American Ethnology, Smithsonian Institution, Bulletin 99. Washington, DC: U.S. Government Printing Office.

Moore-Ede, M. 1993. *The Twenty-Four Hour Society: Understanding Human Limits in a World That Never Stops.* Reading, MA: Addison-Wesley.

More, M. 1979. *Medicinal Plants of the Mountain West.* Santa Fe: Museum of New Mexico.

Morra, M. and Potts, E. 1994 [1980, 1987]. *Choices,* 3rd ed. New York: Avon.

Morris, N. 1976. *The Cancer Blackout.* Baton Rouge: B of A Communications, Louisiana State University.

Mors, W.B., Rizzini, C.T, and Pereira, N.A. 2000. *Medicinal Plants of Brazil,* edited by Robert A. DeFilipps. Algonac, MI: Reference Publications.

Morse, S.S., Ed. 1993. *Emerging Viruses.* New York: Oxford University Press.

Moss, F.E., and Halamandaris, V.J. 1977. *Too Old, Too Sick, Too Bad: Nursing Homes in America.* Germantown, MD: Aspen Systems Corp.

Moss, R.W. 1980. *The Cancer Syndrome.* New York: Grove.

Moss, R.W. 1988. *Free Radical: Albert Szent-Gyorgyi and the Battle over Vitamin C,* with a foreword by Studs Terkel. New York: Paragon House.

Moss, R.W. 1989. *The Cancer Industry: Unraveling the Politics.* New York: Paragon House. [Revised edition of *The Cancer Syndrome.* New York: Grove, 1980. Retitled *The Cancer Industry: The Classic Exposé on the Cancer Establishment.* New York: Paragon House].

Moss, R.W. 1992. *Cancer Therapy: The Independent Consumer's Guide to Non-Toxic Treatment and Prevention.* New York: Equinox Press.

Moss, R.W. 1995. *Questioning Chemotherapy.* Brooklyn, NY: Equinox Press.

Moss, R.W. 1997. *Alternative Medicine Online: A Guide to Natural Remedies on the Internet.* Brooklyn, NY: Equinox Press.

Moss, R.W. 1998. *Herbs Against Cancer: History and Controversy.* Brooklyn, NY: Equinox Press.

Moss, R.W. 2000. *Antioxidants against Cancer.* Brooklyn, NY: Equinox Press.

Moss, R.W. 2003. "The War on Cancer." *Townsend Letter for Doctors and Patients,* no. 245 (December): 36–38.

Moss, R.W. 2004a. "The War on Cancer: FDA Approves Avastin." *Townsend Letter for Doctors and Patients,* no. 250 (May): 30–31.

Moss, R.W. 2004b. "The War on Cancer: Intravenous Vitamin C." *Townsend Letter for Doctors and Patients,* no. 255 (October): 24–25.

Moss, R.W. 2004c. "The War on Cancer: Of Enzymes, Worms and Cancer." *Townsend Letter for Doctors and Patients,* no. 256 (November): 20–21.

Moss, R.W. 2005a. "The War on Cancer: A New View of Cancer's Origins." *Townsend Letter for Doctors and Patients,* no. 262 (May): 24–25.

Moss, R.W. 2005b. "The War on Cancer: Is There a Cancer Conspiracy?" *Townsend Letter for Doctors and Patients*, no. 267 (October): 34–35.

Moss, R.W. 2005c. "The War on Cancer: Do Radiofrequency Energy Fields Cause Cancer?" *Townsend Letter for Doctors and Patients*, no. 269 (December): 58–60.

Moss, R.W. 2006a. "The War on Cancer: Unmasking a 'Cure'." *Townsend Letter for Doctors and Patients*, no. 273 (April): 32–33.

Moss, R.W. 2006b. "The War on Cancer: Playing with Numbers." *Townsend Letter for Doctors and Patients*, no. 274 (May): 38–39.

Mott, L. and Snyder, K. 1987. *Pesticide Alert: A Guide to Pesticides in Fruit and Vegetables.* San Francisco: Sierra Club Books (Natural Resources Defense Council, 40 W. 20th St., New York, NY 10011).

Moyers, B. 1993. *Healing and the Mind*, with a contribution by David Grubin. New York: Doubleday.

Muenscher, W.C. 1939. *Poisonous Plants of the United States.* New York: Macmillan.

Mullarkey, B.A. 1993 [1992]. *Bittersweet Aspartame, a Diet Delusion.* Oak Park, IL: Health Watch Books.

Mullins, C.E. 1989. *The Rape of Justice: America's Tribunals Exposed.* Staunton, VA: Legal Studies Group, Commission for Judicial Reform.

Mullins, C.E. 1992a [1988]. *Death by Injection: The Story of the Medical Conspiracy Against America.* Staunton, VA: National Council for Medical Research.

Mullins, C.E. 1992b [1985]. *The World Order: Our Secret Rulers.* Staunton, VA: Ezra Pound Institute of Civilization.

Mullins, C.E. 1993 [1983, 1984, 1991]. *Secrets of the Federal Reserve: The London Connection.* Staunton, VA: Bankers Research Institute.

Murray, R.K. et al. 1996. *Harper's Biochemistry*, 24th ed. Stanford, CT: Appleton and Lange.

Naiman, I. 1999. *Cancer Salves: A Botanical Approach to Treatment.* Santa Fe, NM: Seventh Ray Press.

Naj, A. 1992. *Peppers: A Story of Hot Pursuits.* New York: Knopf.

Naj, A. 1993. "Peppers: Hot, Hotter, Hottest." *Reader's Digest*, July, 115–117.

Nauts, H.C. 2004. "Coley's Toxins — The First Century." *Townsend Letter for Doctors and Patients*, no. 251 (June): 107–116.

Nelson, R.A. 1992. *Handbook of Rocky Mountain Plants*, revised by Roger L. Williams. Niwot, CO: Roberts Rinehart.

Nestle, M. 2002. *Food Politics: How the Food Industry Influences Nutrition and Health.* Berkeley: University of California Press.

Nestle, M. 2003. *Safe Food: Bacteria, Biotechnology, and Bioterrorism.* Berkeley: University of California Press.

Nestle, M. 2006. *What to Eat.* New York: North Point Press.

Nestle, M., and Dixon, L.B., Eds. 2004. *Taking Sides: Clashing Views on Controversial Issues in Food and Nutrition.* Guilford, CT: McGraw-Hill/Dushkin.

Norden, M.J. 1995. *Beyond Prozac: Brain-Toxic Lifestyles, Natural Antidotes and New Generation Antidepressants.* New York: HarperCollins.

Null, G. 1988. *Gary Null's Complete Guide to Healing Your Body Naturally.* New York: McGraw-Hill.

Null, G., and Feldman, M. 2002. "The Fluoridation Controversy Continues: An Update, Part 1." *Townsend Letter for Doctors and Patients*, no. 233 (December): 58–62.

Null, G., and Feldman, M. 2003a. "The Fluoridation Controversy Continues: An Update, Part 2." *Townsend Letter for Doctors and Patients*, no. 234 (January): 72–78.

Null, G., and Feldman, M. 2003b. "The Fluoridation Controversy Continues: An Update, Part 3." *Townsend Letter for Doctors and Patients*, nos. 235/236 (February/March): 117–121.

Null, G., and Feldman, M. 2005. "Stop Fluoridation Now: New Research on Fluoride's Brain and Thyroid Toxicity." *Townsend Letter for Doctors and Patients*, no. 261 (April): 56–61.

Null, G., Robbins, H., Tanenbaum, M., and Jennings, P. 1997. "Vitamin C and the Treatment of Cancer. Part II. Abstracts and Commentary from the Scientific Literature." *Townsend Letter for Doctors and Patients*, (June): 130–134.

Nussbaum, E. 1997. *Recovery from Cancer: A Personal Story of Sickness and Health.* Garden City Park, NY: Avery Publishing Group.

*Nutrition and Cancer: New Insights into the Preventive Role of Phytochemicals.* 2001. New York: Kluwer Academic/Plenum Press[Washington, DC: American Institute for Cancer Research, 1999].

Oakes, M. 1951. *Beyond the Windy Place: Life in the Guatemalan Highlands.* New York: Farrar, Straus and Young.

O'Shea, T. 2004. *The Sanctity of Human Blood: Vaccination I$ not Immunization,* 8th ed. San Jose, CA: Two Trees.

Padrus, E. and the editors of *Prevention Magazine.* 1988. *The Complete Guide to Your Emotions and Your Health.* Emmaus, PA: Rodale Press.

Patterson, J.T. 1987. *The Dread Disease: Cancer and Modern American Culture.* Cambridge, MA: Harvard University Press.

Pauling, L. 1973. *Vitamin C and the Common Cold.* New York: Bantam Books.

Pauling, L. 1976. *Vitamin C, the Common Cold, and the Flu.* San Francisco: Freeman.

Pauling, L. 1987. *How to Live Longer and Feel Better.* New York: Avon [San Francisco: Freeman, 1986].

Pearson, D., and Shaw, S. 1983 [1982]. *Life Extension: A Practical Scientific Approach.* New York: Warner Books.

Pearson, D., and Shaw, S. 1987. *Life Extension.* New York: Warner Books.

Pearson, J., and Pearson, J. 1980. *No Time but Place: A Prairie Pastoral.* New York: McGraw-Hill.

Pelton, R., and Overholser, L. 1994. *Alternatives in Cancer Therapy: The Complete Guide to Non-Traditional Treatments.* New York: Simon and Schuster.

Perry, M.C., and Yarborough, J.W., Eds. 1984. *Toxicity of Chemotherapy.* Orlando, FL: Grune and Stratton, Harcourt Brace Jovanovich.

Personnet, J., Ed. 1999. *Microbes and Malignancy: Infection as a Cause of Human Cancers.* New York: Oxford University Press.

Peskin, B.S. and Habib, A. 2006. The Hidden Story of Cancer: Find Out Why Cancer has Medical Science on the Run and How a Simple Plan Based on New Science Can Prevent It. Houston, TX: Pinnacle Press.

Pfeiffer, C.C. 1975. Mental and Elemental Nutrients: A Physician's Guide to Nutrition and Health Care. New Canaan, CT: Keats.

Pfeiffer, C.C. 1978. Dr. Carl C. Pfeiffer's Updated Fact Book on Zinc and Other Micro-Nutrients. New Canaan, CT: Keats.

Pfeiffer, C.C., and Braverman, E.R. 1987. The Healing Nutrients Within: Facts, Findings and New Research on Amino Acids. New Canaan, CT: Keats.

Pfeiffer, C.C., Maillous, R., and Forsythe, L. 1988a. The Schizophrenias: Ours to Conquer. Wichita, KS: Bio-Communications Press (Center for the Improvement of Human Functioning International).

Pfeiffer, C.C., and the Publications Committee of the Brain Bio Center. 1988b. Nutrition and Mental Illness: An Orthomolecular Approach to Balancing Body Chemistry. Rochester, VT: Inner Traditions International.

Philpott, W.H., and Kalita, D.K. 1980. Brain Allergies: The Psychonutrient Connection, with a foreword by Linus Pauling; afterword by Roger Williams. New Canaan, CT: Keats.

Philpott, W.H., and Taplin, S. n.d. Biomagnetic Handbook: A Guide to Medical Magnetics, the Energy Medicine of Tomorrow. Choctaw, OK: Philpott Medical Service.

Physicians' Desk Reference, 42nd ed. 1988. Oradell, NJ: Medical Economics Company.

Piller, C., and Yamamoto, K.R. 1988. Gene Wars: Military Control over the New Genetic Technologies. New York: Morrow.

Plechner, A.J. 2004. "An Innovative Cancer Therapy That Saves Animals: Can it Help Humans as Well?" Townsend Letter for Doctors and Patients, nos. 247/248 (February/March): 110–118.

Plotkin, D. 1996. "Good News and Bad News about Breast Cancer." *Atlantic Monthly,* June, 53–82.

Podolsky, M.L. 1997. *Cures Out of Chaos: How Unexpected Discoveries Led to Breakthroughs in Medicine and Health*, with a foreword by Daniel E. Koshland, Jr. Amsterdam: Harwood Academic Publishers.

*Poisonous Grassland Plants.* 1959 [1957]. Section 4 of a Series on Pasture and Range Plants. Bartlesville, OK: Phillips Petroleum Company. (Plant illustrations are from original water colors by Nina Lea Burden, Zona Wheeler, and Alvin Pearson.)

Pollan, M. 2001. *The Botany of Desire: A Plant's Eye View of the World.* New York: Random House.

Powell, K., "Stem and cancer cells have something in common," News@nature.com, December 30, 2002.

Powis, G., and Hacker, M.P., Eds. 1991. *The Toxicity of Anticancer Drugs.* New York: Pergamon Press.

Prance. G.T., and Lovejoy, T.E., Eds. 1985. *Key Environments: Amazonia, with a* foreword by HRH the Duke of Edinburgh. New York: Pergamon Press. (Published in collaboration with the International Union for Conservation of Nature and Natural Resources.)

Preston, R. 1992. "A Reporter at Large: Crisis in the Hot Zone." *New Yorker*, October 26, 58–82.

Preston, R. 1994. *The Hot Zone: A Terrifying True Story.* New York: Random House.

Preston, R. 2002. *The Demon in the Freezer: A True Story.* New York: Random House.

*Prevention Magazine* Staff. 1976. *The Encyclopedia of Common Diseases.* Emmaus, PA: Rodale Press.

*Prevention Magazine's Complete Book of Vitamins and Minerals.* 1994. Emmaus, PA: Rodale Press.

Proctor, R.N. 1994. *Cancer Wars: How Politics Shapes What We Know and Don't Know About Cancer.* New York: Basic Books.

Proctor, R.N. 1995. *Cancer Wars: What We Know and Don't Know About Cancer.* New York: Basic Books.

Proctor, R.N. 1999. *The Nazi War against Cancer.* Princeton, NJ: Princeton University Press.

Pyle, E., *Home Country,* William Sloane Associates, New York, 1935-1940.

Quillan, P. and Williams, R.M., Eds. 1993. *Adjuvant Nutrition in Cancer Treatment.* Cancer Treatment Research Foundation.

Randolph, T.G., and Moss, R.W. 1990 [1989]. *An Alternative Approach to Allergies: The New Field of Clinical Ecology Unravels the Environmental Causes of Mental and Physical Ills.* New York: HarperCollins.

*Reader's Guide to Alternative Health Methods*, edited by A.W. Hafner et al. 1992. Chicago: American Medical Association.

Regenstein, L. 1982. *America the Poisoned: How Deadly Chemicals Are Destroying Our Environment, Our Wildlife, Ourselves and How We Can Survive.* Washington, DC: Acropolis.

Regenstein, L. 1986. *How to Survive in America the Poisoned.* Washington, DC: Acropolis.

Rifkin, J., in collaboration with Perlas, N. 1983. *Algeny.* New York: Viking.

Rifkin, J. 1992. *Beyond Beef: The Rise and Fall of the Cattle Culture.* New York: Dutton.

Rissler, J., and Mellon, M. 1996. *The Ecological Risks of Engineered Crops.* Cambridge, MA: MIT Press.

Robbins, J. 1992. "Care for a little Hellish Relish? Or try a Hotsicle." *Smithsonian*, January, 42–51.

Roberts, H.J. 1989. *Aspartame (NutraSweet) Is it Safe: A Concerned Doctor's View.* Philadelphia: Charles Press.

Rodale, J.I., and Staff. 1966. *The Complete Book of Vitamins.* Emmaus, PA: Rodale Books.

Rodale, J.I., and Staff. 1972. *The Complete Book of Minerals for Health.* Emmaus, PA: Rodale Books.

Rogers, S.A. n.d. *The High Blood Pressure Hoax!* Sarasota, FL: Sand Key Company.

Root-Bernstein, R.S. 1993. *Rethinking AIDS: The Tragic Cost of Premature Consensus.* New York: Free Press.

Rosedale, R. and Colman, C. 2004. *The Rosedale Diet.* New York: HarperCollins.

Rosner, B. n.d. *When Antibiotics Fail: Lyme Disease and Rife Machines with Critical Evaluation of Alternative Therapies.* South Lake Tahoe, CA: Lyme Innovations Press.

Rowen, R.J. 2006. "Artemisinin: From Malaria to Cancer Treatment." *Townsend Letter for Doctors and Patients*, no. 276 (July): 68–70 (first appeared in no. 233 [December]: 86–88).

Rowland, I.R., Ed. 1988. *The Role of Gut Flora in Toxicity and Cancer.* London: Academic Press.

Royte, E. 2002 [2001]. *The Tapir's Morning Bath: Mysteries of the Tropical Rain Forest and the Scientists Who Are Trying to Solve Them.* Boston: Houghton Mifflin.

Sachs, J.S. 2005. "Are Antibiotics Killing Us? *Discover*, September, 36–41.

Salisbury, F.B. and Ross, C.W. 1985 [1969, 1978]. *Plant Physiology.* Belmont, CA: Wadsworth Publishing.

Sandberg, A.A. 1994. "Cancer Cytogenetics for Clinicians." *CA — A Cancer Journal for Clinicians* 44, no. 3: 136–158.

Sanderson, I.T. and Loth, D. 1965. *Ivan Sanderson's Book of Great Jungles.* New York: Julian Messner.

Saunders, C.F. 1933. *Western Wildflowers and Their Stories.* Garden City, NY: Doubleday, Doran.

Sax, N.I. 1981. *Cancer Causing Chemicals.* New York: Van Nostrand Reinhold.

Schaller, G.B. 1980 [1979]. *Stones of Silence: Journeys in the Himalaya.* New York: Viking.

Schlosser, E. 2001. *Fast Food Nation: The Dark Side of the All-American Meal.* Boston: Houghton-Mifflin.

Schom, A. 1997. *Napoleon Bonaparte.* New York: HarperCollins.

Schroeder, H.A. 1973. *Trace Elements and Man: Some Positive and Negative Aspects.* Old Greenwich, CT: Devin-Adair.

Schroeder, H.A. 1974. *The Poisons around Us: Toxic Metals in Food, Air, and Water.* Bloomington: University of Indiana Press.

Schutte, K.H. 1964. *The Biology of Trace Elements: Their Role in Nutrition.* Philadelphia: Lippincott.

Schwartz, G.R. 1988. *In Bad Taste — The MSG Syndrome: How Living Without MSG Can Reduce Headache, Arthritis, Depression and Asthma, and Help You Get Control of Your Life*. Santa Fe, NM: Health Press.

Schweid, R. 1980. *Hot Peppers: Cajuns and Capsicum in New Iberia, Louisiana*. Seattle: Madrona Publishers.

Scippa, R. 1994. "Inside Belize." *Profiles* 7, no. 5, 40–45.

Seager, S.B. 1992. *Psychward*. New York: Berkley Books [New York: Putnam's, 1991].

Seligman, M. 1991. *Learned Optimism: The Skill to Conquer Life's Obstacles, Large and Small*. New York: Knopf.

Shapiro, M. 2002. "Sowing Disaster?: How Genetically Engineered American Corn Has Altered the Global Landscape." *Nation*, October 28: 11–19.

Shilts, R. 1987. *And the Band Played On: Politics, People, and the AIDS Epidemic*. New York: St. Martin's.

Shnayerson, M., and Plotkin, M.J. 2003. *The Killers Within: The Deadly Rise of Drug-Resistant Bacteria*. Boston: Little, Brown.

Shoumatoff, A. 1978. *The Rivers Amazon*. San Francisco, CA: Sierra Club Books.

Shoumatoff, A. 1997. *Legends of the American Desert: Sojourns in the Greater Southwest*. New York: Knopf.

Sidransky, D. 1997. "Nucleic Acid-Based Methods for the Detection of Cancer." *Science*, November 7: 1054–1058.

Siegel, B.S. 1986. *Love, Medicine, and Miracles: Lessons Learned about Self-Healing from a Surgeon's Experience with Exceptional Patients*. New York: Harper and Row.

Siegel, B.S. 1990. *Peace, Love and Healing: Body Mind Communication and the Path to Self-Healing: An Explanation*. New York: Harper and Row.

Simontacchi, C. 2000. *The Crazy Makers: How the Food Industry Is Destroying Our Minds and Harming Our Children*. New York: Putnam.

Sinatra, S.T. 1998. *The Coenzyme Q10 Phenomenon*. Los Angeles, CA: Lowell House.

Sinnott, M. Ed. 1998. *Comprehensive Biological Catalysis: A Mechanistic Reference*. 4 vols. San Diego: Academic Press.

Slagle, P. 1987. *The Way Up from Down: A Safe New Program That Relieves Low Moods and Depression with Amino Acids and Vitamin Supplements*. New York: Random House.

Smith, L.H. 1979. *Feed Your Kids Right: Dr. Smith's Program for Your Child's Total Health*. New York: Dell Publishing.

Smith, L.H. 1994. *Feed Your Body Right: For Proper Nutrition without Guesswork*. New York: M. Evans and Co.

Smith, W.J. 2000. *Culture of Death: The Assault on Medical Ethics in America*. San Francisco: Encounter.

Snodgrass, S.R. 1992. "Vitamin Neurotoxicity." *Molecular Neurobiology*. 6, no. 1: 41–73.

Sofowora, A. 1982. *Medicinal Plants and Traditional Medicine in Africa*. New York: John Wiley & Sons.

Solzhenitsyn, A. 1969. *Cancer Ward*, translated by Nicholas Bethell and David Burg. New York: Farrar, Straus and Giroux.

Sporn, M.B. 1991. "Carcinogenesis and Cancer: Different Perspectives on the Same Disease." *Cancer Research* 51: 62115–6218.

Sporn, M.B. 1993. "Chemoprevention of Cancer." *The Lancet* 342: 1211–1213.

Sporn, M.B., and Roberts, A.B. 1991. "Interactions of Retionoids and Transforming Growth Factor- in Regulation of Cell Differentiation and Proliferation." *Molecular Endocrinology* 5, no. 1: 3–7.

St. George, G. and the Editors of Time-Life Books. 1974. *Soviet Deserts and Mountains.* Amsterdam: Time-Life Books. (Photographs by Lev Ustinov, Novosti Press Agency, Moscow.)

Stark, E. 1996. "Which Charities Merit Your Money." *Money,* November: 100–103.

Starr, P. 1982. *Social Transformation of American Medicine.* New York: Basic Books.

Stefansson, V. 1956. *The Fat of the Land,* with comment by Stare, F.J. and White, P.D. New York: Macmillan. (Originally published as *Not by Bread Alone,* Macmillan, New York, 1946.)

Stefansson, V. 1960. *Cancer: Disease of Civilization?: An Anthropological and Historical Study,* with an introduction by Rene Dubos. New York: Hill and Wang.

Stephens, I. 1955. *Horned Moon: An Account of a Journey through Pakistan, Kashmir, and Afghanistan.* Bloomington: University of Indiana Press.

Suffness, M., and Pezzuto, J. 1991. "Assays Related to Cancer Drug Discovery." Pp. xx-xx in *Methods in Plant Biochemistry,* vol. 6, *Assays for Bioactivity,* ed. K. Hostettmann. London: Academic Press.

Swain, T., Ed. 1972. *Plants in the Development of Modern Medicine.* Cambridge, MA: Harvard University Press.

Swerdlow, J.L. 2000. *Nature's Medicine: Plants That Heal.* Washington, DC: National Geographic Society. (Photographs by Lynn Johnson.)

Szasz, T. 1977 [1970]. *The Manufacture of Madness: A Comparative Study of the Inquisition and the Mental Health Movement.* New York: Harper and Row.

Szasz, T. 1985. *Ceremonial Chemistry: The Ritual Persecution of Drugs, Addicts, and Pushers.* Holmes Beach, FL: Learning Publications [Garden City, NY: Anchor Press, 1974].

Szasz, T. 1988a. *The Myth of Psychotherapy: Mental Healing as Religion, Rhetoric, and Repression.* Syracuse, NY: Syracuse University Press.

Szasz, T. 1988b. *Schizophrenia: The Sacred Symbol of Psychiatry.* Syracuse, NY: Syracuse University Press.

Szasz, T. 1988c. *The Theology of Medicine: The Political-Philosophical Foundations of Medical Ethics.* Syracuse, NY: Syracuse University Press [Baton Rouge: Louisiana State University Press, 1977].

Szasz, T. 1990 [1977]. *Anti-Freud: Karl Kraus's Criticism of Psychoanalysis and Psychiatry.* Syracuse, NY: Syracuse University Press.

Taylor, F.S. 1939. *Inorganic and Theoretical Chemistry,* 5th ed. London: Heinemann.

Taylor, L. 1998. *Herbal Secrets of the Rainforest: The Healing Power of Over 50 Medicinal Plants You Should Know About.* Rocklin, CA: Prima Publishing.

Teresi, D. 2002. *Lost Discoveries: The Ancient Roots of Modern Science — from the Babylonians to the Maya.* New York: Simon and Schuster.

Tétényi, P. 1970. *Infraspecific Chemical Taxa of Medicinal Plants,* translated by Isván Finály and Peter Tétényi. New York: Chemical Publishing Co.

*The Complete German Commission E Monograph.* 1998. Austin, TX: American Botanical Council.

*The Rise and Fall of a Scientific Genius* (video), written and directed by Shawn Montgomery, Zero Zero Two Productions, 3 Baldoon Rd., Toronto, Ontario, Canada M1B 1V6; www.zerozerotwo.org, 2003, 2004. *Part I: Rife's Rise. Part II: Rife's Fall.*

Theroux, P. 2000. *Fresh Air Fiend: Travel Writings 1985–2000.* Boston: Houghton Mifflin.

Thomas, R. 1993. *The Essiac Report: The True Story of a Canadian Herbal Cancer Remedy and of the Thousands of Lives it Continues to Save.* Los Angeles, CA: The Alternative Treatment Information Network.

Tirtha, Swami Sada Shiva. 1998. *yurveda Encyclopedia: Natural Secrets to Healing, Prevention, and Longevity.* Bayville, NY: Ayurveda Holistic Center Press.

Tobyn, G. 1997. *Culpeper's Medicine: A Practice of Western Holistic Medicine*. Rockport, ME: Element Books.

Train, P., Hendrichs, J.R., and Archer, W.A. 1982. *Bioactive Plants, vol. 1, Medicinal Uses of Plants by Indian Tribes of Nevada*. Lawrence, MA: Quarterman Publications.

Tunçel, G., Nout, M.J.R., Brimer, L., and Göktan, D., 1990. "Toxicological, Nutritional and Microbiological Evaluation of Tempe Fermentation with *Rhizopus oligosporus* of Bitter and Sweet Apricot Seeds." *International Journal of Food Microbiology* 11: 339–344.

Tyler, V.E. 1992. *The Honest Herbalist: A Sensible Guide to the Use of Herbs and Related Remedies*, 3rd ed. New York: Pharmaceutical Products Press [Binghamton, NY: Haworth Press, 1993].

*Undesirable Grasses and Forbes*. 1959 [1956]. Section 3 of a Series on Pasture and Range Plants. Bartlesville, OK: Phillips Petroleum Company. (Plant illustrations are from original water colors by Nina Lea Burden, Zona Wheeler, and Alvin Pearson.)

Up de Graff, F.W. 1923. *Head Hunters of the Amazon: Seven Years of Exploration and Adventure*, with a foreword by Kermit Roosevelt. Garden City, NY: Garden City Publishing.

Varoni, V. 2001. *Nature's Cancer-Fighting Foods: Prevent and Reverse the Most Common Forms of Cancer Using the Proven Power of Great Food and Easy Recipes*. Paramus, NJ: Reward Books.

Velikovsky, I. 1950. *Worlds in Collision*. New York: Macmillan.

Venziale, C.M., Ed. 1981. *The Regulation of Carbohydrate Formation and Utilization in Mammals*. Papers from a symposium, Mayo Medical School, Rochester, MN, July 9–11. Baltimore, MD: University Park Press.

*Veterans and Agent Orange: Health Effects of Herbicides Used in Vietnam*. 1994. Report of the Committee to Review the Health Effects in Vietnam Veterans of Exposure to Herbicides. Division of Health Promotion and Disease Prevention, Institute of Medicine. Washington, DC: National Academy Press.

Voet, D., and Voet, J.G. 1990. *Biochemistry*. New York: John Wiley & Sons.

Vogel. V.J. 1990 [1970]. *American Indian Medicine*. Norman: University of Oklahoma Press.

Walker, M. 2003. *German Cancer Therapies: Natural and Conventional Medicines That Offer Hope and Healing*. New York: Kensington Publishing.

Walters, R. 1993. *Options: The Alternative Cancer Therapy Book*. Garden City Park, NY: Avery Publishing.

Warburg, O.H. 1956. "On the Origin of Cancer Cells." *Science* 123: 309–314. (Originally published in *Naturwissenschaften* 42 (1955): 401.)

Watson, L. 1975 [1974]. *The Romeo Error: A Matter of Life and Death*. Garden City, NY: Anchor Press/Doubleday.

Watt, J.M., and Breyer-Brandwijk, M.G. 1962. *The Medicinal and Poisonous Plants of Southern and Eastern Africa: Being an Account of Their Medicinal and Other Uses, Chemical Composition, Pharmacological Effects and Toxicology in Man and Animal*. Edinburgh: E.&S. Livingstone.

Webb, J.L. 1966 [1963]. *Enzyme and Metabolic Inhibitors*. 3 vols. New York: Academic Press.

Weinberg, R.A. 1994. "Oncogens and Tumor Suppressor Genes." *CA — A Cancer Journal for Clinicians* 44, no. 3: 160–170.

Weinberg, R.A. 1996. *Racing to the Beginning of the Road: The Search for the Origin of Cancer*. New York: Harmony Books.

Weinhouse, S. 1956. "On Respiratory Impairment in Cancer Cells." *Science* 124: 267–269.

Weintraub, S. 1998. *The Parasite Menace*. Pleasant Grove, UT: Woodland Publishing.

Welsome, E. 1999. *The Plutonium Files: America's Secret Medical Experiments in the Cold War.* New York: Dial Press, Random House.

Whitaker, J., Ed. n.d. *Health and Healing: Tomorrow's Medicine Today.* Potomac, MD: Phillips Publishing.

Whitson, T.D., Ed. 1987. *Weeds and Poisonous Plants of Wyoming and Utah.* Laramie, WY: Cooperative Extension Service, College of Agriculture, University of Wyoming.

Whitson, T.D., Ed. 1991. *Weeds of the West.* Laramie, WY: Western Society of Weed Science in cooperation with the Western United States Land Grant Universities Cooperative Extension Services, College of Agriculture, University of Wyoming.

Willard, P. 2001. *Saffron: The Vagabond Life of the World's Most Seductive Spice.* Boston: Beacon Press.

Williams, R.J. 1953. *Free and Unequal: The Biological Basis of Individual Liberty.* Austin: University of Texas Press.

Willis, J. C. 1973. *A Dictionary of the Flowering Plants and Ferns*, 8th ed., revised by H.K.A. Shaw. Cambridge, England: Cambridge University Press.

Wilson, D. 2001. *Fateful Harvest: The True Story of a Small Town, a Global Industry, and a Toxic Secret.* New York: HarperCollins.

Winfield, J.A. n.d. *An Unsuccessful Effort to Deny Use of State of Georgia Facilities for Fund Raising by the American Cancer Society.* Published by the author, Athens, GA.

Wittman, J. 1993. *Breast Cancer Journal: A Century of Petals.* Golden, CO: Fulcrum.

Wolinsky, H., and Brune, T. 1994. *The Serpent on the Staff: The Unhealthy Politics of the American Medical Association.* New York: Putnam's.

Woodward, L. 1985. *Poisonous Plants: A Color Field Guide.* New York: Hippocrene Books.

Wright, J.V. 1979. *Dr. Wright's Book of Nutritional Therapy: Real-Life Lessons in Medicine without Drugs.* Emmaus, PA: Rodale Press.

Wright, J.V. 2004. "Vitamin D: Its Role in Autoimmune Disease and Hypertension." *Townsend Letter for Doctors and Patients*, no. 250 (May): 75–78.

Yerby, C. 2005. "Coenzyme Q10: New Applications for Cancer Therapy." *Life Extension*, October: 50–56.

Yurkovsky, S. 2004. "Guided Digital Medicine: The Law of Unintended Consequences and Non-Disease Treatment of Diseases, Part 2." *Townsend Letter for Doctors and Patients*, no. 251 (June): 93–98.

Zimmer, C. 1993. "Climate Watch: The Case of the Missing Carbon." *Discover*, December, 38–39.

Zollner, H. 1989. *Handbook of Enzyme Inhibitors*, New York: VCH Publishers.

Zollner, H. 1993. *Handbook of Enzyme Inhibitors*, 2nd ed. 2 vols. New York: VCH Publishers.

Zumwalt, E.R. et al. 1986. *My Father, My Son.* New York: Macmillan.

# Index

5-fluorouracil (5-FU), 120, 209–210, 404
   action, 122
   cost of treatment, 294
   side effects, 160, 371
6-mercaptopurine, 120
13-cis-retinoic acid, 147
714X, 66, 71, 72

## A

Abscisic, 71
Acetylsalicylic acid, 290, 296
Aconite, 236, 248
Acrylamide, 8
ACS, *see* American Cancer Society (ACS)
Actinex, 240
Actinic keratosis, 240
Actinomycin D, 127, 139
Acupuncture, 21, 184, 292, 359, 362
Acute lymphoblastic leukemia (ALL), 153–154
Adenoviruses, 73, 133, 351, 399
Adjuvant cancer therapies, 284, 285
Adriamycin, 139
Adult respiratory distress syndrome (ARDS),
   26–27
Aflatoxin (AF), 178
Agave, 212, 248, 284
Agriculture, 40, 45, 373–378, 393–395
AIDS, 23–26, 65, 136
Alanine, 103, 130, 168, 333
Alcohol, 9, 23, 42, 47–48
Alfalfa, 251, 256
Alkaloids, 13, 34, 159, 247, 379
   and bioactivity, 227–228
   in fruits and vegetables, 38, 215
Allicin, 106, 140, 158, 172–179
Almonds, 164, 205, 209, 234
Aloe, 259, 297
Alpha-tocopherol, *see* Vitamin E
Alternative medicine, *see* Complementary and
   Alternative Medicine (CAM)
Aluminum, 8, 276, 342, 373, 396
Alzheimer's Disease, 8, 12, 217, 342, 344
AMA (American Medical Association), 237, 301
AMAS, 54
Amazonia, 31–32, 214, 238, 239, 276–277
American Cancer Society (ACS), 1

fundraising, 295, 388
   publications, 146–147
   spending, 387
   unproven methods blacklist, 223, 243,
      294–295
American College for the Advancement of
   Medicine (ACAM), 361
American Society for the Control of Cancer
   (ASCC), 1, 295
Ames bacterial test, 72, 145, 176, 255
Amethopterin, 407
Amino acids, 128–129, 131, 135, 409; *see also*
   Proteins
Amygdalin, *see* Laetrile
Anemia, 36, 90, 121, 168
   iron-deficient, 160, 169, 171, 321, 330, 331
   sickle cell, 234, 343, 368
"Aneuploidy," 25
Angiogenesis, 179, 220, 286, 403, 404
Animal studies, 178, 182, 279, 312–313, 373
Anthocyanosides, 259
Antibacterial agents, 32, 60, 145, 177, 217, 249;
      *see also* Antibiotics
Antibiotics; *see also* Penicillin
   administration, 384
   bacterial selectivity, 139
   and immunosuppression, 266, 326
   as protein synthesis inhibitors, 139–143, 311
   resistance, 15, 22, 60, 363–364, 405
   side effects, 60, 140
Antibodies, 23, 67, 77, 81, 368, 419; *see also*
   Immunity
   monoclonal, 222–223, 406, 407
Antidepressants, 21, 51, 268
Antifolates, 118, 119, 122, 407
Antigens, 88, 226, 305, 368, 408, 417
Antimalarials, 259, 383
Antimetabolites, 118, 120, 122, 241, 311
Antineoplaston Therapy, 156, 223, 224, 297, 423
Antioxidants, 15, 86, 202, 223, 241, 272
Antitumor agents, conventional, 284, 286–290
Antiviral agents, 32, 77–78, 195, 242, 321, 414
Apoptosis, 87
Arachidonic acid, 323
Arginine, 224
Argyria, 14
Arndt-Schultz law, 339
Arsenic, 44, 87, 108, 205, 236, 372

Artemisinin, 133, 383–384
Artesunate (ART), 133
Ascorbate, *see* Vitamin C
Ascorbic acid, *see* Vitamin C
Ashwagandha, 259
Asparaganase, 153–154, 311
Asparagine, 8, 129, 131, 135, 253, 256
Aspirin, 106, 268, 358
Assisted suicide, 400–401
Astragalus, 259
Atkins Diet, 5, 179, 273, 298, 327
Attention deficit disorder (ADD), 18, 259,
        341–342
Attention deficit hyperactivity disorder (ADHD),
        18, 259, 341–342
Autoimmune diseases, 346, 358, 364, 366, 368
Autumn crocus, 247, 259, 311
Avastatin®, 294
Avastin®, 403, 404
Avemar, 2–3
Ayurveda, 141
Azelaic acid, 318

**B**

Bacillus Calmette-Guérin (BCG), 12, 74, 80, 222,
        315
Bacteria, 11, 366, 405; *see also* Antibacterial
        agents; Antibiotics; Coley's Toxins;
        Infections; Pleomorphism
    Ames test, 72, 145, 176, 255
    as bioweapons, 369–370
    disease-causing, 364–365
    exchange of genetic information, 357
    immune reaction to, 78
    intestinal, 10, 62, 161, 189, 202, 366
    and iron overload, 170
    and the SOS response, 144–145
    in vaccines, 78–79
Bacterial metabolism, 85, 90
Bacteriophages, 73, 75
B-cells, 77
BCG (Bacillus Calmette-Guérin), 12, 74, 80, 222,
        315
Beale Treatment (Insulin), 165, 191
Beechnut, Virginia, 251
Benign prostatic hyperplasia (BPH), 270
Beta-carotene, 16, 121, 146, 151, 223, 276, 413
    forms used in chemoprevention, 291
Bethroot, 259
B-glucosidase, 235
Bilberry, 259
Bilyea, 140
Bindweed, 297

Bioactivity, 61, 180
    and alkaloids, 227–228
    variations, 205
Biochemical catalysis, 90
Biochemistry, 11–17, 83–84
Biochemotherapy, *see* Chemotherapy
Bioflavonoids, 223, 242
Biological response modifiers (BRMs), 133
Biomass, 42, 46, 89, 92, 94
Biotechnology, 85, 313, 349, 370, 393; *see also*
        Pharmaceutical industry
Bioterrorism, 369–371
Birch, 251
Bitterleaf, 259
Black cherry, 255
Black cohosh, 251
Black locust, 254
Black walnut, 251, 254, 258
Bladder cancer, 74, 182, 222, 225, 226
Blood-related cancers, 62, 120, 127, 311, 378; *see
        also* Leukemia
Bloodroot, 29, 33, 200–201, 211, 250, 259
Blueberry, European, 259
Bovine cartilage, 137, 199
Bovine pancreatic trypsin inhibitor (BPT1), 137
Bowman-Birk protease inhibitor (BBI), 137
Breast cancer, 14, 54, 147, 148, 294
    conventional drugs for, 335–336
    and mammography, 188, 317
    and organochlorine pesticides, 376
    and viral causes, 317
Bromelain, 151
Burdock root, 198, 201, 230, 251
Burkitt's lymphoma, 73, 255
Burton's Immuno-Augmentative Therapy (IAT),
        153, 224, 278
Burzynski therapy, 156, 199, 224, 267, 423
Buttercup, 251
Butterfly milkweed, 239

**C**

Cadmium, 374
Caffeine, 98, 105, 215, 221, 238
Calaguala (fernroot), 140
Calcium, 80, 104, 117, 317, 325
    deficiency, 15–16
California buckthorn, 259
CAM, *see* Complementary and Alternative
        Medicine (CAM)
Camptothecin, 247, 261, 296
Canaigre dock, 251
Cancer; *see also* Carcinogenesis; Remission;
        Stem cells

cells *vs.* normal cells, 83–84, 88–92, 102–104, 139
cure for, 241, 275–276, 280
death rate, 316, 324–325, 333–334
detection, 72, 181–185
formation, 59, 62–63, 271
incidence, 322, 324–325, 333–334
literature, 1–4, 417
metastasis, 407
microbial origins, 67–73
monitoring, 400, 417–418
morphism, 355–359
precursors, 48, 183, 364, 398
proliferation, 123, 126, 129, 407, 408
recoveries, 362–363
research and politics, 387–392
and stress, 19
theories, 64, 69, 72, 84–88
types, 63–64, 73, 355
Cancer clinical research centers (CCRCs), 48, 52, 163, 220–221, 272, 385, 421
Cancer Control Society, 284, 293, 295, 303
Cancer markers, 72, 181–185, 400
Cancer of unknown primary (CUP), 64
Cancer Research Institute, 71, 320, 325, 330, 423
Cancer Treatment Centers of America (CTCA), 48
Capsaicin, 31
Carbitine®, 268
Carbohydrates, 135
Carbolic acid, 30, 106, 314
Carbon dioxide, 42–43, 46
Carboplatin (CBDCA), 14
Carcinogenesis, 59–62, 147, 316
    chemical, 91
    and electrophilic behavior, 14–15
    and mutagenesis, 144
Carcinogens, 14, 62; *see also* Alcohol; Toxins
    and the SOS response, 144–145
Carcinomas, 63, 169, 183, 184, 319, 355; *see also* Cancer
Carnitine, 223
Carnivora®, 180, 298
Carrot, 251
Cascara sagrada, 259
Castor bean, 259
Catalase, 78, 113, 170, 196
Catalysis, 90
Cat's claw, 29, 201–202, 260, 277
Cell biochemistry, 11–17, 83–84, 125–129
Cell differentiation, 410
Cell metabolism, 61, 62, 88–92; *see also* Glycolysis
    byproducts, 84, 89, 90

in normal *vs.* cancer cells, 83–84, 102–104, 283
Cell resistance, 283, 405; *see also* Antibiotics
Cellular immunity, *see* Immunity
Cervical cancer, 123, 146, 184, 276, 344, 364
Cesium, 267, 319, 324, 328–329, 337
CFK (Cocancerogenic K Factor), 223
Chaparral, 29, 30, 241–245, 258, 260
Chelation therapy, 21, 269–270
Chemoprevention, 146–148, 178, 423
    preventive agents, 91, 291–292
Chemotherapy, 378–379
    cost, 302
    cytotoxicity, 147, 412
    dosage levels, 339
    drugs used, 255, 412
    as enzyme inhibitors, 118–121
    minimizing side effects of, 151, 246, 247–248, 253
    oral, 322
    resistance, 283, 363, 405
    selectivity, 61, 160
    term usage, 79
    using naturally occurring substances, 149
Chinese rhubarb, 260
Chinese therapies, 4, 6–7, 47, 257, 274, 343–344
    herbal, 213
    native plants used, 238, 246–248, 261
Chiropractic medicine, 4
Chlorine, 41–43, 371
Chocolate, 260
Choriogonadotropin (CG), 70–71, 114
Chronic myelogenous leukemia (CML), 183, 322, 411, 412
Cisplatin (DDP), 14
Clinical trials
    statistics, 191, 334–335
    support for, 420, 421–422
    *vs.* animal studies, 182, 185–186
Clover, 262
Cockleburr, 251
Coenzyme Q10, 337, 339, 342
Colchicines, 221, 247, 259, 289
Coley's Toxins, 78–79, 85, 189, 223, 228
    availability, 318, 327
    history of use, 319–320
Colon cancer, 80, 133, 268
    and fiber intake, 322
    and meat consumption, 318
Colorectal cancer
    and diet, 48, 318
    metastatic, 384, 403
    treatments, 71, 188, 286, 288, 290, 316
Comfrey, 200, 219, 227, 250, 256
    formulations, 254, 257

liver toxicity, 258
    for radiation side effects, 253
Complementary and Alternative Medicine
        (CAM), 5, 46, 189–193, 296, 414
    alternative practitioners, 361
    anecdotal evidence, 22, 163, 230
    centers for, 292
    complementary therapies, 283, 284, 285,
        292–299, 336–339
    controversies, 299–304
    database information, 49, 191
    opposition to, 68–69, 292–296
    success vs. failures, 278–279
Complementary medicine, see Complementary
        and Alternative Medicine (CAM)
Complement C1, 137
Compund-X, 29, 199–200, 275, 305–311
Condurango, 201, 230, 231
Conjugated linoleic acid (CLA), 136, 291, 310,
        322, 326
CoQ10, 337, 339, 342
Cori cycle, 186
Cortisol, 117, 133–134
Coumadin, 318
Coumarins, 249, 333, 414, 415
Crabgrass, 255
Cranberries, 251
Creatine, 86, 268
Creosote bush, see Chaparral
Creutzfeldt-Jakob, 12, 217, 344, 349, 351, 355
Crotoxins, 274
Cryogenic therapy (or cryotherapy), 223
Cundurango, see Condurango
Curare, 60, 108
Curcumin, 288, 298–299
Curly top gumweed, 239
Cyanate, 256, 343
Cyanide, 160–162, 234, 237, 257; see also
        Laetrile
Cyanobacteria, 121
Cyanogenetic glycosides, 34, 215, 284, 343
Cyclophosamide, 255
Cystamine, 338
Cytochromes P450, 221
Cytosan, 255
Cytotoxicity, 147, 158, 412

**D**

Da-huang, 260
Dandelion, 251
Daunomycin, 139
David Remedy, 246
Deoxyribonucleic acid, see DNA

Depression, see Mental illnesses
Diabetes, 140, 167–168, 218, 323, 332
Diet, 4–7, 164–168, 280–281, 349–351; see also
        Drinking water; Food; Nutritional
        supplements; Proteins, dietary;
        Vegetarianism
    Atkins Diet, 5, 54, 179, 273, 298, 327
    caloric restriction, 166, 255, 323
    carbohydrates, 135
    carnivorous, 166, 167
    and depression, 18, 20
    fats, 135–136, 166–167, 346–347
    fiber, 322
    food substitutes, 9–11
    hydrogenated oils (trans fat), 11, 62, 367, 375
    iron, 168–172, 324
    Livingston, 71
    macrobiotic, 256, 270, 277, 303, 386, 423
    micronutrients, 16, 413
    minerals, 267
    of Native Indians, 324, 351–353
    nutritional therapies, 71, 165, 189
    red wine, 48, 296
    refined sugar, 9, 71, 179, 273, 274, 332
    selenium, 34–35
    yeast, 4, 20
Dietary Health and Education Act, 7
Differential therapy, 71
Digitalis, 33, 216, 233, 318
Digitoxin, 318
Diisopropylphosphofluoridate, 136
Dipyridamole, 318
DNA, 347–349
    functions of, 126
    intercalators/crosslinkers, 286
    methylation, 145–146
    and protein synthesis, 125–126
    recombination, 145
    repair, 144
    replication, 124, 139, 143–144, 181
    synthesis inhibitors, 120, 287
    transcription inhibitors, 127, 139, 287
Dogwood, 251
Dongguei, 257
Doxorubicin, 139
Drinking water, 44, 53, 59, 325, 340
    chlorination, 371
    fluoridation, 16–17, 59, 96, 372–373
Drosnes-Lazenby Treatment, 165, 191
Drugs; see also Antibiotics; Chemotherapy
    biological response to, 279–281
    costs, 49, 50, 241, 302, 389–390, 424
    dosages, 52, 233, 236
    patents, 2, 49, 213, 220, 318, 387
    resistance to, 237

safety, 50, 61
side effects, 50, 51, 53, 335
testing, 6, 60, 240, 245, 279
universal, 64

# E

E. coli (Escherichia coli), 80, 120, 121
    DNA damage in, 144
Echinacea, 239, 240, 260
Elderberry, 260
Elder tree, 251
Elecampane, 28, 203, 246, 260
Electromagnetic radiation, 21, 68, 69, 162,
    359–362
Electrophilic behavior, 14–15
Elm, 263
Enderlein remedies, 70
Endoxan, 255
Energy medicine, 187, 311–312
Enterotoxins, 80
Enteroviruses, 62
Environmental toxins, 40–45
Enzyme inhibitors, 104–107, 158–163, 288,
    381–386
    chemotherpay drugs as, 118–121
    for melanoma, 164
    reluctance to investigate, 186–188
Enzymes, 151–157; see also Glycolysis
    breaking, 86
    digestive, 153, 337
    involved in anaerobic glycolysis, 107
    and metabolic pathways, 92–95
    pancreatic, 133, 152, 336
    study of, 85
    transformations, 123–124
    as treatments for cancer, 83–84
Epithelial cancers, 147, 148
Epstein-Barr virus, 73, 74, 317, 364, 368, 369
Erbitux®, 403
Erysipelas, 319
Escozul, 138
Esophageal cancer, 322, 325
Essaic tea, 197–198, 230
Essential fatty acids (EFAs), 135, 136, 272, 414
Estrogen, 105, 147, 336
Ethics, 400–401
European elder, 260
European mistletoe, 260
Euthanasia, 400–401

# F

Fats, 135–136, 166–167
    polyunsaturated, 326, 346–347, 367
Fatty acids, 135, 136, 272, 346, 414
FDA (Food and Drug Administration), 3, 50–51,
    191–192
Femara®, 335, 336
Fermentation, 84, 85
    of soy, 412, 413
Fernroot, 140
Fever induction, 80–81, 117–118
FK228 (histone diacetylase inhibitor), 399–400
Flavonoids, 169, 213, 228, 309, 379, 414; see also
    Alkaloids
Flax, 260
Fluoride, 16–17, 59, 96, 372–373
Folate, see Folic acid
Folic acid, 77, 112, 121–123
    as chemopreventive agent, 291
    deficiency, 119, 276
Folklore, 32, 204, 240, 276, 296; see also
    Complementary and Alternative
    Medicine (CAM)
Food; see also Agriculture; Alkaloids; Diet;
    Garlic; Onions
    additives, 8, 16, 350–351, 392
    anticancer agents in, 137
    apricot kernels, 206–208, 209, 234
    containing carcinogens, 145, 222, 280
    dairy, 3–4, 75, 165, 179
    legumes, 121, 164, 256
    meats, 165, 222, 318, 323, 350
    nuts, 178–179, 205–206, 209, 234
    poisonous, 36–37, 237
    safety, 65, 350, 370–371
    soy, 412, 413, 414
    tomatoes, 71, 252, 291, 296, 310
    vegetables, 40, 45, 71, 255, 309–310
Food and Drug Administration (FDA), 3, 50–51,
    191–192
Four Corners virus, 26–27
Free radicals, 16, 152, 185, 270, 342, 371
Fungi, 12, 38, 127, 202, 204
    anticancer action, 238, 247
    cancer causing, 189, 356
    drug resistance, 363
    immunity against, 77
    and pleomorphism, 70, 189
    source for enzymes, 85

# G

Garlic, 140, 172–179, 237, 251, 260

Gelotology, 6
Gemzar®, 294
Gene amplification, 396
Genes; *see also* DNA; Oncogenes
    regulation of, 288–289
    tumor-suppressors, 169
Genestein, 413, 415
Gene therapy, *see* Genetic engineering (GE)
Genetic engineering (GE), 121, 129, 131, 133, 349
    of crops, 376–377, 392–395
Genetic modification (GM), 133, 349, 392–395; *see also* Genetic engineering (GE)
Genetics, 130–134; *see also* DNA; RNA
Genome, 132, 347
Geranium, 86, 176, 251, 261, 360
German protocols, 297–298
Germ theory, 364–365
Gerson treatment, 151, 165, 189, 191, 257
Gestalt, 5
Giant foxtail, 254
Ginger, 250, 251, 285, 310, 342
Ginseng, 38, 240, 246, 248
    American, 259
Gleevec, 322
Glivec, 322
Gluconeogenesis, 97, 273
Glucose, 84; *see also* Glycolysis
Glucosides, 34, 213, 247
Glucosinolates, 309
Glutamine, 83, 84, 89, 92–93, 98
Glutaminolysis, 83, 89, 90, 93, 98
    inhibitors, 106–107, 186
Glutathione (GSH), 315
Glycogenesis, 84
Glycogenolysis, 84
Glycolysis, 84, 95–97, 154–157, 273–274
    aerobic, 100–101
    anaerobic, 100, 101–102
    inhibitors, 104–105
Goat's rue, 239
Goldenrod, 255
Goldenseal, 260, 306
Gold therapy, 186
Gonzalez cancer therapy, 297
Gotu kola, 261
Grape juice, 242
Graviola, 307
Greasewood, *see* Chaparral
Green tea, 175, 240
Growth factors, 147, 169, 410
Gut flora, 10, 62, 161, 189, 202, 366
    antibiotics effect on, 60

# H

Hackberry, 254
Haelan 951, 413
Hallucinogens, 238–239
Halogens, 371–373
Happy tree, 261
Harringtonine, 216, 238, 247
Hayflick limits, 215, 358
Health care, 48, 49
    outside U.S., 235, 237
Heat therapy, 79, 223
Hematopoetic stem cells (HSCs), 406
Hemp, 261
Hendricks Natural Immunity Therapy, 223
Herbalogy, 204–205; *see also* Herbs
Herbicides, 40
Herb of Cancer (yerba del Cancer), 237
Herbs, 245; *see also* Chinese therapies; Plants
    allelopathic, 254–255
    of the American Southwest, 239
    bioactivity, 205
    combinations of, 306
    preparation, 240
    reference guides, 32, 33, 308–309
    terminology, 205
    used for noncancer diseases, 217–221
    used in India, 380
Herceptin®, 294
HGPRT (hypoxanthine-uanine phosphoribosyl transferase), 407
Histone diacetylase
    inhibitors, 399–400
Histoplasmosis, 204
Hodgkin's disease, 252
Holistic medicine, 5; *see also* Complementary and Alternative Medicine (CAM)
Homeopathy, 50, 51, 236, 312, 418
Homoharringtonine, 216, 238
Hormesis, 312
Hormones, 110, 117–118, 268
    affecting rate of protein degradation, 138
    as enzyme inhibitors, 113–116
    protein-type, 128
Ho-Shou-Wu, 247
Hoxsey therapy, 200–201, 230, 243, 298, 302, 303
Huckleberry, 259
Human chorionic gonadotrophin (HCG), 70
Humoral immunity, *see* Immunity
Hunter's syndrome, 132
Hunzas, 166, 167, 206, 207, 208
Hydrazine sulfate, 71, 86, 186, 223, 273
Hydrogen cyanide, 36, 160, 162, 209, 234, 256
Hydrogen peroxide, 54, 152
Hydrogen sulfide, 162, 209

Hydroxyurea, 122
Hyperthermia, 81, 117, 223, 229, 236, 338
Hypothermia, 13, 223
Hypothyroidism, 167–168, 372

## I

IAT ( Immuno-Augmentative Therapy), 224, 274, 278
IFL, 403–404
Immune system; *see also* Immunity; Immunodeficiency; Immunotherapy
    antibodies, 81, 406, 407
    antigens, 88, 226, 305, 368, 408, 417
    biological enhancement agents, 222, 223, 224, 235, 236, 298
    cancer of, 406
    compromising, 87–88
    immune reactions, 78–82
    triggering, 180, 224, 235, 236
Immunity, 180–181, 368–369
    and cancerous stem cells, 406–408
    and diet, 71
    and microorganisms, 228–229
    types of, 77
Immunodeficiency, 70, 136, 181, 224, 419; *see also* AIDS
Immunosuppressants, 294, 326, 330, 346, 347
Immunotherapy, 78, 80, 267, 319
    nitrogen, 222–227
    orthodox therapies, 222–223
Indian tribes, *see* Native Indians
Indium, 378
Infections, 85, 170, 368, 370; *see also* Antibiotics
    and cancer recovery, 326, 330
    chronic, 365–366
    emerging, 316–317, 363, 370
    viral, 63, 77
Infectious diseases, 76, 368–369, 370
Inflammation, 217, 319, 357–358, 366
    and cancer, 64, 357
    treatments, 32, 310
Influenza, 22, 74, 76, 351, 364, 396
Inoculations, *see* Vaccines
Insulin, 115, 168, 191, 323
Insulin-induced hypoglycemic therapy (IHT), 323, 361
Insulin potentiation treatment (IPT), 361
Interferons, 121, 128, 222, 228, 249, 389
Interleukins, 117, 192, 222, 228, 389
Intestinal flora, 10, 62, 161, 189, 202, 366
Introns, 76
Iproplatin (CHIP), 14
Iressa®, 403

Iris, Blue flag, 251
Iron
    dietary, 168–172
    excessive, 324
    in high-meat diets, 318, 330–331
    supplements, 244
Iscador®, 336
Isoenzymes, 124, 151
Isoflavones, 137, 412, 413
Isotretinoin, 146
Issels' Whole Body Therapy, 80, 151, 229

## J

Juglone, 254
Juniper, 261
Juniper berry extract, 253

## K

Kaposi's sarcoma (KS), 256, 262, 321, 364, 369
Kelley's Nutritional Metabolic Therapy, 151, 153, 224, 256, 257, 336
Kelp, 261
Koch's postulates, 365
Koch Treatment, 165, 191
Krebiozen theory, 11, 165, 191

## L

Lactate, *see* Lactate dehydrogenase; Lactic acid
Lactate dehydrogenase, 62, 97, 176, 405
    forms of, 383
    inhibitors of, 103, 106, 107, 158, 196
Lactic acid, 62, 69, 89
    inhibitors of, 105–106
    production of, 97–98
    and the Warburg theory, 84–87
Laetrile, 1, 160–161, 205, 210, 234–237, 257
Lapachol, 308
Larrea, *see* Chaparral
L-asparaganase, 153–154, 311
Legionnaires' disease, 26
Letrazole®, 335
Leukemia, 62, 63
    treatments, 120, 140, 153, 220
Lignans, 137
Lincoln Therapy, 223
Linoleic acid, 136, 291, 310, 322, 326
Lipids, 135–136
Liver cancer, 46, 71, 241, 246–247, 277, 321
Livingston cancer diet, 71
Llantén, 140

Lobelia, 249–250, 251, 253, 258
Lumbrokinase (LK), 337
Lycopene, 240, 291
Lymphatic cancer, 77
Lymphocytes, 77, 180, 406; *see also* Immunity
Lysogeny, 63, 73–75

# M

Madagascar periwinkle, 139, 140, 141, 261
Madonna lily, 251
Magnesium, 16, 276, 339–341
Malignancies, 63, 410
Malpractice, 237
Mammography, 54
Mandrake, American, 219, 250, 258, 262
Marine life, 219, 220, 239
Markers, 72, 181–185, 400
Maté, 262
Matico, 140
Mayapple, 219, 250, 258, 262
Maytens, 140, 220, 246, 307, 416
Maytensine, 220, 246
Medical ethics, 20, 47, 400–401
Medical insurance, 22, 53, 269, 301, 395, 404
Medical orthodoxy, 1–3, 14, 22, 56–57, 188, 417
    opposition by, 24, 26, 71, 149, 367
MEDWATCH, 51
Melanoma, 62, 63–64, 73, 355
    -associated antigens (MAAs), 88
    enzyme inhibitors for, 164, 382
    Mexican treatments, 248
Melatonin, 21, 268, 289, 296, 298
Mental illnesses, 17–21
Mercury, 395, 396
Mesotheliomas, 398
Metabolism, *see* Cell metabolism
Metabolites, 89–90
Metals, 16, 80, 108, 340; *see also* Iron;
        Magnesium
    catalysis, 13, 87
    entering food chain, 373–374
    removal from body, 177, 270
    in water, 371
Metastasis, 153, 154, 183, 318, 363, 389
Methotrexate (MTX), 118, 119–120, 122, 255,
        361
Methylation, 145–146
Methyltransferase, 400
Micronutrients, 16, 413
Microorganisms, *see* Bacteria; Fungi; Viruses
Microsatellite analysis, 182
Microsatellites, 182, 183
Microtube inhibitors, 289–290

Milkweed, 239, 249, 251, 314, 382–383
Mind-body connection, 6, 13, 268, 269, 274, 303
    mental illness, 17–21
Minerals, 16, 71, 104, 267, 276, 378; *see also*
        Magnesium; Selenium
Mistletoe, 253, 260
Monkshood, 236
Monoclonal antibodies, 406, 407
MTH-68, 228, 390
MTH-68 vaccine, 228
MTX (methotrexate), 118, 119–120, 122, 255,
        361
Multiple sclerosis (MS), 44, 74, 264, 345–346,
        364
Mustard,wild, 252
Mutagenicity, 14, 63, 144, 145
Mutagens, 14, 310
"Mutant gene" theory, 25
Mutations, 89, 221–222
Mycoplasma, 12, 76
Mycota, 12, 39; *see also* Fungi
Myeloma, 321, 339, 362, 406–408
Myers cocktail, 424
Myrrh, 249, 262
Myrtle, 254

# N

Naessens theory, 66, 71–72, 186, 223
Naltrexone, 324
National Cancer Institute (NCI), 146, 190, 198,
        233, 241, 292
National Center for Complementary and
        Alternative Medicine (NCCAM), 5,
        284
Native Indians
    cancer incidence, 165
    medicine men, 142–143, 218, 242–243
    treatments with plants, 238, 239
Navajos
    diet, 65, 280, 351
    smallpox vaccine, 28–29
    uranium exposure, 75, 351–352
NCI, *see* National Cancer Institute (NCI)
NDGA, 86, 241–242, 244, 253, 273
Neo Tropica, 264–265, 276–277
Neuropeptides, 13
Neurotoxins, 13, 162, 239, 274, 345, 396
Neurotransmitters, 13
N-factor, 249
N-gene, 249
Niacin, 109, 110, 112, 268, 338
Nicotinamide, 95, 109, 112, 124, 342
Nicotine, 143, 215, 221, 249

Nicotinic acid, *see* Niacin
Nieper's therapy, 151, 199, 315
Nitric oxide, 320
Nitrilosides, 205, 234, 324, 343; *see also* Laetrile
Nitrogen, 34, 71, 86; *see also* Urea
    and immunotherapy, 222–227
Nitrosamines, 14, 222
Noni, 262
Nucleic acids, *see* DNA; RNA
Nucleostemin, 408
Nutrition, *see* Diet; Food
Nutritional supplements, 51, 52, 55, 339; *see also*
      Minerals; Vitamins
   regulation of, 241
   testing, 240
   *vs.* natural food sources, 178, 338

## O

Office of Cancer Complimentary and Alternative
      Medicine (OCCAM), 292
Omega-3 fatty acids, 54, 133, 272, 346–347
Oncogenes, 62–63, 67, 91, 129, 403
Oncogenicity, 61
Onions, 237, 252
Osteopathic medicine, 4
Osteosarcoma, 17
Oxalates, 29, 34, 158, 244
Oxygen therapies, 270–271, 367, 412

## P

P53 gene, 169, 181, 399
   as cancer marker, 183
   disabling, 399
   mutation, 182–183
   and nucleostemin, 408
   and SV40, 398
Pacific yew, 212, 262
Paclitaxels, 262, 290, 311; *see also* Taxol
Pancreatic cancer, 14
Papilloma viruses, 73
Parasites, 77, 187, 202, 384
Parthenin, 310
Patient information, 56, 190–193
   ethomedical references, 32–33
   internet sites, 52, 312
   misinformation, 55
   on poisonous plants, 33
   relevant books, 311–312
Pau d'arco, 29, 201, 231, 262, 277, 308
PDR Cancer Formula, 258, 263–264
Penicillin, 50, 60–61, 139, 299–300, 301

Peony root, 248
People Against Cancer, 293, 298, 316, 423
Peptidases, 136; *see also* Proteases
Peptide hormones, 128
Peptides, 80, 128, 156, 269
Periwinkle, 249, 252
   classification, 141
   Madagascar, 139, 140, 261
   rosy, 141, 215
Perwinkle, 261
Pesticides, 40, 376
Pharmaceutical industry, 47, 49–51, 387
Pharmocognosy, 219
Phenylalanine, 9, 409
Photodynamic therapy (PDT), 338, 391
Photofrin®, 391
Phytochemicals, 15, 61, 78
Pipsissewa, 252
Placebo effect, 6, 54, 191, 335
Plantain, 140
Plants, 140, 210–213; *see also* Alkaloids;
      Bioactivity; Chaparral; Herbicides;
      Herbs; Pesticides
   adjuvant cancer therapies, 284, 285
   adverse side effects, 240
   of the American Southwest, 237–241
   with anticancer properties, 137, 233, 259–263,
      306–307
   antitumor agents, 140
   of Australia, 249
   cataloging, 214
   of China, 246–248
   of Egypt and Israel, 249–250
   escharotic, 305–306
   garden and ornamental, 38
   of Great Britain, 255–258
   hallucinogens, 238
   of Mexico, 248
   oxalates, 29
   poisonous and medicinal, 33–38, 61,
      213–217, 236, 258
   in the rain forests, 31–32, 214, 238, 239, 265,
      276–277
   remedies in nature, 28–33, 39
   of the Rocky Mountains, 210
   screening, 254, 308
   of South Africa, 246
   of the Soviet Union, 248
   species extinction, 238, 376
   standardized remedies, 230
   substitutions, 180, 205
   taxonomy, 211, 216, 306, 307, 415
   terminology, 205
   of the United States, 250–255
   used for noncancer diseases, 217–221

weeds, 35–36
Platinum, 13, 14
Pleomorphism, 12, 26, 65–66, 69–70, 76,
        355–357
Plussing method, 338
Podophyllin, 219, 250, 258, 262
Poisons, *see* Plants; Toxins
Pokeroot, 252
Polyerga®, 297, 298
Polymorphism, *see* Pleomorphism
Polypeptides, *see* Peptides
Polyporus umbellata, 238
Potato, 252
Prenylflavonoids, 221
Preventive medicine, 1, 121, 146–147, 176–177,
        423; *see also* Chemoprevention
Prions, 12, 66, 76, 217, 344–347
Pristimerin, 416
Probability theory, 334–335
Probiotics, 189
Proenzymes, 409
Progenitor cryptocides (PC), 65, 70, 85
Prophage, 63
Prophylactic regimens, 88
Proproteins, 409
Prostate cancer, 74, 183–184, 270, 382, 411
Proteases, 136–138, 152, 413
Proteins, cellular; *see also* Proteases
    control of cell proliferation, 408
    degradation, 138–139
    digestion of, 134–135, 136–138
    influence of antibiotics, 139–143
    roles of, 128–129
    stress (or heat shock), 62
    synthesis, 125–126
Proteins, dietary, 134, 330, 342, 414
Proteolytic, 151, 152, 409; *see also* Proteases
Protoglycan molecules (PGMs), 133
Protovirus, 63
Provirus, 63
Prussic acid, *see* Hydrogen cyanide
PSA (prostate specific antigen), 54, 184
Psychosomatics, *see* Mind-body connection
PTK/ZK®, 294
Purple coneflower, 239
Pyrifer, 81
Pyruvate, 84, 89, 92, 93–98; *see also* Glycolysis
Pyruvic acid, 84, 89, 92, 93–98

## Q

Queen's root, 252
Quercetin, 105, 169, 212, 230, 237, 242, 310; *see
        also* Chaparral

for colon cancer, 133
    sources, 237, 242
Quinones, 3, 151, 197, 242, 308, 413

## R

Rabies, 22, 28, 164, 202–204, 236, 250, 258
Radiation, 67, 68
Radioactivity, 67, 68
Radio frequency ablation (RFA), 297
Radio frequency electromagnetic fields
        (RFEMFs), 357
Radiotherapy, 67–68, 162, 278, 359–360
Ramakrishnan approach, 338
Receptor tyrosine kinases (RTKs), 220, 410; *see
        also* Tyrosine kinase
Red cinchona, 262
Red clover, 252, 262
Religion, 53
Remission, 189, 389
    markers for monitoring, 400
    spontaneous, 151, 279, 280, 306
Resources, *see* Patient information
Respiration, 107–108, 161
Resveratrol, 285, 291, 296, 404
Retinoids, 146, 148
Retinoids differential therapy, 71
Retinol, *see* Vitamin A
Retroviruses, 23, 25, 28, 73
    and breast cancer, 317
    defective, 63
    distinguishing feature, 204
    in the human genome, 368
Reverse transcriptase, 27, 73, 143, 204, 212, 398,
        399
    as a cancer marker, 182
    inhibition of, 184
Revici therapy, 81–82, 229, 267
Rheumatism, 236
Rhodanase, 235
Rhubarb, Chinese, 260
Ribonucleic acid, *see* RNA
Rife generator, 68, 278, 360
RNA
    functions of, 127–128
    and protein synthesis, 125–126
    transcription regulators, 127, 287
RNA-directed DNA polymerase, *see* Reverse
        transcriptase
Rosemary, 257, 263
RTKs, *see* Receptor tyrosine kinases (RTKs)
Rue, 28, 202–203, 236

# S

Saffron, 247, 259, 311
Saltz regimen, 403
Salves, 201, 305–306
Saponins, 34, 213, 215, 247, 248, 413
Sarcomas, 63, 64, 111, 319, 355, 379; *see also*
        Cancer
Sassafras, 252
Saunas, 338
Savin, 253
Scorpion venom, 138
Scourges, 22–28, 47
Selectivity, 221–222
Selenium, 34–35, 87, 173, 256, 267, 276
    as an antiviral, 321
    concentrator, 29
    in garlic, 176
    testing, 240
Self-healing, 6
Senescence, 215
Serine proteases, 136, 137
Serum therapies, 37, 72, 153, 266, 274; *see also*
        Vaccines
Shaman, *see* Native Indians
Shark cartilage, 137, 198–199, 220
Sheep sorrel, 252
Silver, colloidal, 14
Skin cancer, *see* Melanoma
Sleeping cancer cells, 271
Slippery elm, 263
Slow viruses, *see* Subviruses
Snake venoms, 137–138, 274
Sodium, 8, 13, 21, 71, 134, 191, 199
Sodium selenite, 292
SOS response, 144–145
Soy, 412, 413, 414
Soybeans, 137, 253
Sphingomyelinase, 315–316
Sprouting vetch, 253
Spurge, 249, 258
St. John's wort, 19, 203, 248, 250, 268
Standard genetic code, 130
Statins, 304
Statistics, 333–335
Stem cells, 235, 403–406
    hematopoetic, 406
    and immunity, 406–408
    inhibition of cancerous stem cells, 408
    and role of tyrosine kinase, 409–414
    and stomach cancer, 64
    and tyrosine kinase inhibitors, 411, 414–416
Stomach cancer, 64, 177, 241, 305, 310, 364
Streptococcus, 78, 85, 319; *see also* Coley's
        Toxins

Styrene, 415
Subviruses, 12, 75–77, 344–347
    causing infectious disease, 76
    somatids, 66
Sugar,refined, 9, 71, 179, 273, 274, 332
Sugar substitutes, 9–11, 392
Sulfanilamide, 119
Sulfonamides, 60, 300, 326
Sulfur compounds, 87, 106, 172–179, 338, 411
Sunflower, Alpine, 253
Superoxide dismutase (SOD), 152, 185
Suppressor genes, 67
SV40 virus, 397–398
Sweeteners, *see* Sugar substitutes
Sycamore, 252
Synthetic drugs, *see* Drugs

# T

Tamoxifen, 54, 147, 148, 335
Tangkuei, 246, 247, 257
Tarceva®, 294
Taxol, 34, 139, 212, 216, 237–238, 311
T-cells, 77
Tecoma, 277
Telomerase, 62, 180–181, 182, 183, 184, 215
Telomerase inhibitors, 399
Tenko-Seki stone (SGES), 360–361
Thapsigargin, 290
The China Study, 178, 386, 423
Thiosulfinates (THS), 173, 174; *see also* Allicin
Thistle, Blessed, 251
Thuja, 263
Thyophylline, 322
Thyroid, 117, 118
TNF (tumor necrosis factor), 222–223, 228, 286
Toxins; *see also* Alkaloids; Metals
    bacterial, 78, 79–80
    chlorinated compounds, 41–43
    in drinking water, 44, 371
    environmental, 40–46, 221, 373–378
    flesh-eating, 37, 314
    in food, 8, 36–37, 178, 221, 239, 376
    hormesis, 312
    industrial chemicals, 67, 221, 373
    in plants, 33–38
Trace elements, 16–17, 35
Triacylglycerols, *see* Fats
Tricarboxylic cycle, 99–100, 107–108
Triglycerides, *see* Fats
Tris, 145
Trypsin, 83, 136, 137, 152, 336
Tumor necrosis factor (TNF), 222–223, 228, 286
Tumors, *see* Antitumor agents; Cancer

Turmeric, 298–299
Tyrosinase, 62, 382, 399
Tyrosine kinase, 220, 236, 288
    biochemical action, 410
    classification, 409
    inhibitors of, 411
    plant-derived inhibitors, 414–416

## U

Urea, 71, 86, 122, 224, 267–268

## V

Vaccinations, 3, 67, 87
    and cancer, 395–399
Vaccines, 22–23, 28–29, 228; see also Coley's
        Toxins
    and antigens, 305
    autogenous, 70, 73
    bacterial, 78–79
    contaminated, 396–397
    flu, 320–321, 396
    for metastatic malignant melanoma, 88
    Newcastle disease virus, 390
    preservatives in, 395–396
    universality, 82
VascuStatin, 322
Vegetarianism, 159, 255, 279, 303, 332
    benefits of, 256, 270
    and cancer incidence, 75, 164, 166, 319, 328,
        386
Venoms, 80, 137, 138, 274, 314
Venus flytrap, 180, 298
Vinblastine, 127, 139, 252, 290
Vinca alkaloids, 141, 219, 226, 311, 379
Vincristine, 255, 290
Vincrystine, 252
Violet, 252
Viral oncology, 67
Virion, 75, 76
Viroid, 76
Viruses, 26–28, 75–77, 364–367; see also
        Antiviral agents; Bacteriophages;
        Pleomorphism; Retroviruses;
        Subviruses
    cancer-causing, 67–73
    classification, 12, 356
    and gene repair, 133
    genetic crossovers, 74, 76
    genome, 75
    insect-carried, 315
    interference between, 204

    intestinal, 62
    lysogeny, 63, 73–75
Vitamin A, 60, 71, 111, 223
    deficiency, 300
    research with, 146, 147
    toxicity, 147
Vitamin C, 170, 173, 185–186, 193–197, 326, 338
    biochemcial role, 77–78, 113
    as chelating agent, 21
    in chemoprevention, 146
    discovery, 2, 299, 303
    intravenous, 269–270
    megadoses, 5, 189, 296, 337, 423
    and nitrosamine formation, 222
Vitamin D, 148, 223, 345–346
Vitamin E, 55–56, 72, 110, 113, 223, 247
Vitamins, 109–110, 185, 189, 223; see also
        Nutritional supplements
    as enzyme inhibitors, 111–113
    megadoses, 338
    review of, 240

## W

Warburg, Otto, 83, 84–88, 162, 271–272, 389
Warburg Cancer Theory, 84–88
Warfarin, 318
War on Cancer, 2, 64, 133, 196, 275, 386
Watercress, 253
Western medicine, 47, 218, 239, 309, 343–344,
        419
Wheatgrass therapy, 151, 255
White birch, 255
White lupine, 253
Wholistic medicine, see Holistic medicine
Whortleberry, 259
Wine, 48, 296
Wintergreen, 252
Wobe-Mugos, 83–84, 151, 152–153
Wolf/Benitez WoBenzym® systemic enzyme
        formula, 336
Woodland angelica, 251
Wormwood, 202, 254

## X

Xanthohumol, 221

## Y

Yarrow, 28, 203, 253
Yellow dock, 252, 255, 263
Yellow jasmine, 263

Yew, 33–34, 38, 139–140, 216, 238, 311
    for leukemia, 247
Yucca, 164, 210, 237, 253

**Z**

Zometa®, 336
Zymogen, 409